KU-508-390

Pharmaceutical Calculations

14th Edition

Pharmaceutical Calculations

14th Edition

Howard C. Ansel, PhD, ScD
Professor and Dean Emeritus
College of Pharmacy
University of Georgia
Athens, Georgia

Wolters Kluwer | Lippincott Williams & Wilkins
Health
Philadelphia · Baltimore · New York · London
Buenos Aires · Hong Kong · Sydney · Tokyo

Acquisitions Editor: David Troy, Sirkka Howes
Product Manager: Kristin Royer
Marketing Manager: Joy Fisher-Williams
Designer: Holly McLaughlin
Manufacturing Coordinator: Margie Orzech
Compositor: SPi Global

14th Edition
Copyright © 2013 Wolters Kluwer Health | Lippincott Williams & Wilkins.
Copyright © 2010, 2006, 2001, 1996, 1991, 1986 by Lippincott Williams & Wilkins.

This textbook is intended to provide the *underpinnings of the methods* used in pharmaceutical calculations. The drugs, drug products, formulas, equations, uses, and doses are included in this textbook for the sole purpose of providing examples in the types of calculations described. The information *is not intended* for use in any practice or clinical application, nor should it be considered or construed as specific for any individual patient nor as a substitute for current drug package inserts. The author, editors, and publisher make no warranty, express or implied, with regard to the contents and use of this publication and are not responsible, as a matter of product liability, negligence, or otherwise, for any injury resulting from any material contained herein.

9 8 7 6 5 4 3 2 1
Printed in China
First Edition, 1945

Not authorised for sale in United States, Canada, Australia, and New Zealand.

Library of Congress Cataloging-in-Publication Data
Ansel, Howard C., 1933-
    Pharmaceutical calculations / Howard C. Ansel. — 14th ed.
        p. ; cm.
    Includes bibliographical references and index.
    ISBN 978-1-4511-8680-2
    I. Title.
    [DNLM: 1. Drug Dosage Calculations. 2. Dosage Forms. 3. Drug Compounding—methods. 4. Drug Prescriptions. 5. Weights and Measures. QV 748]
        615.1'401513—dc23

                                                                                                        2012021655

Care has been taken to confirm the accuracy of the information presented and to describe generally accepted practices. However, the authors, editors, and publisher are not responsible for errors or omissions or for any consequences from application of the information in this book and make no warranty, expressed or implied, with respect to the currency, completeness, or accuracy of the contents of the publication. Application of this information in a particular situation remains the professional responsibility of the practitioner; the clinical treatments described and recommended may not be considered absolute and universal recommendations.

The authors, editors, and publisher have exerted every effort to ensure that drug selection and dosage set forth in this text are in accordance with the current recommendations and practice at the time of publication. However, in view of ongoing research, changes in government regulations, and the constant flow of information relating to drug therapy and drug reactions, the reader is urged to check the package insert for each drug for any change in indications and dosage and for added warnings and precautions. This is particularly important when the recommended agent is a new or frequently employed drug.

Some drugs and medical devices presented in this publication have Food and Drug Administration (FDA) clearance for limited use in restricted research settings. It is the responsibility of the health care provider to ascertain the FDA status of each drug or device planned for use in his or her clinical practice.

CCS0912

Preface

The 14th edition of *Pharmaceutical Calculations* includes many of the progressive changes recommended by a review team of pharmacy educators. These changes, together with the substantial input by a number of contributors, have rendered this edition especially relevant to today's basic practice requirements.

Among the most evident changes is a "CalcQuiz" section at the conclusion of each chapter. This section provides a limited number of *un*solved problems, which may serve as homework, quiz, or assessment exercises. Another new feature, the "Comprehensive Review Problems," at the end of the book provides a set of multipart solved problems for student use as a final self-assessment.

Other changes in this revision include a greater number of solved example problems within each chapter; an increased focus on institutional and patient-specific problems; an introduction of cholesterol ratio problems; greater attention to determinations of pediatric doses; additional examples of the use of dosing tables; newly added monoclonal antibody dosing problems; calculations on the preparation of isotonic solutions by volume adjustment; problems integrating compounding instructions with pharmaceutical formulas; an example of the prescription format in e-prescribing; and pharmacoeconomic problems of medication therapy management services. Popular features such as "Case-in-Point," "Calculations Capsules," and "Special Considerations" have been maintained and, in some cases, expanded.

Throughout its history, a distinguishing characteristic of this textbook has been the inclusion of relevant background information to explain the pharmaceutical or clinical purpose underpinning each type of calculation. This time-honored aspect has been continued in the new edition.

New Companion Website

Pharmaceutical Calculations, 14th edition, includes additional resources for both instructors and students, available on the book's companion website at http://thePoint.lww.com/Ansel14e.

Resources for Students and Instructors

- Interactive math calculations Quiz Bank, with more than 400 review problems and detailed solutions.
- Searchable Full Text Online

See the inside front cover for more details, including the passcode you will need to gain access to the website.

Acknowledgments

The author gratefully acknowledges the contributions to this revision by the following pharmacy practitioners and educators: Ted Chaffin and Tom Schoenbachler, for insights into contemporary community pharmacy practice; Deborah Elder, for contributions in the area of pharmacy compounding; Ken Duke, for problems in the area of nuclear pharmacy; Warren Beach, for Case-in-Point calculations; Flynn Warren, for a host of new problems including many relating to institutional pharmacy practice; and Shelly J. Stockton and Loyd V. Allen Jr, for their continued courtesy in enabling liberal use of their work published in the *International Journal of Pharmaceutical Compounding*.

Gratitude is expressed to the following reviewers, whose experience was drawn upon during the planning process and whose thoughtful analysis and constructive comments led to many of the changes in this revision: Payal Agarwal, Scott Asbill, Shelley Chambers-Fox, Nancy Culberson-Taylor, Andrew Draper, Jeff Fortner, Karla Foster, Daniel Parsons, James Pschirer, Melanie Reinhardt, and Hardeep Saluja.

Particular thanks are offered to David Troy, Senior Acquisitions Editor, and Kristin Royer, Product Manager, for their support and guidance during the revision process and to the other exceptional people at Lippincott Williams & Wilkins for masterful work in the design, preparation, and production of this revision.

Howard C. Ansel
Athens, Georgia

Contents

Introduction

Scope of Pharmaceutical Calculations

The use of calculations in pharmacy is varied and broad-based. It encompasses calculations performed by pharmacists in traditional as well as in specialized practice settings and within operational and research areas in industry, academia, and government. In the broad context, the scope of pharmaceutical calculations includes computations related to:

- chemical and physical properties of drug substances and pharmaceutical ingredients;
- biological activity and rates of drug absorption, bodily distribution, metabolism and excretion (pharmacokinetics);
- statistical data from basic research and clinical drug studies;
- pharmaceutical product development and formulation;
- prescriptions and medication orders including drug dosage, dosage regimens, and patient adherence to medication treatment plans;
- pharmacoeconomics; and other areas.

For each of these areas, there is a unique body of knowledge. Some areas are foundational whereas others are more specialized, constituting a distinct field of study. This textbook is foundational, providing the basic underpinnings of calculations applicable to pharmacy practice in community, institutional, and industrial settings.

In community pharmacies, pharmacists receive, fill, and dispense *prescriptions*, and provide relevant drug information to ensure their safe and effective use. Prescriptions may call for *prefabricated* pharmaceutical products manufactured in industry, or, they may call for individual components to be weighed or measured by the pharmacist and *compounded* into a finished product. In hospitals and other institutional settings, *medication orders* are entered on patients' charts. Prescriptions and medication orders may be handwritten by authorized health professionals or transmitted electronically.

In the preparation of pharmaceuticals, both medicinal and nonmedicinal materials are used. The medicinal components (*active therapeutic ingredients or ATIs*) provide the benefit desired. The nonmedicinal (*pharmaceutical ingredients*) are included in a formulation to produce the desired pharmaceutical qualities, as physical form, chemical and physical stability, rate of drug release, appearance, and taste.

Whether a pharmaceutical product is produced in the industrial setting or prepared in a community or institutional pharmacy, pharmacists engage in calculations to achieve standards of quality. The difference is one of scale. In pharmacies, relatively small quantities of medications are prepared and dispensed for specific patients. In industry, *large-scale* production is designed to meet the requirements of pharmacies and their patients on a national and even international basis. The latter may involve the production of hundreds of thousands or even millions of dosage units of a specific drug product during a single production cycle. The preparation of the various dosage forms and drug delivery systems (defined in Appendix B), containing carefully calculated, measured, verified, and labeled quantities of ingredients enables accurate dosage administration.

A Step-Wise Approach Toward Pharmaceutical Calculations

Success in performing pharmaceutical calculations is based on:

- an understanding of the purpose or goal of the problem;
- an assessment of the arithmetic process required to reach the goal; and,
- implementation of the correct arithmetic manipulations.

For many pharmacy students, particularly those without pharmacy experience, difficulty arises when the purpose or goal of a problem is not completely understood. The background information provided in each chapter is intended to assist the student in understanding the purpose of each area of calculations. Additionally, the following steps are suggested in addressing the calculations problems in this textbook as well as those encountered in pharmacy practice.

Step 1. Take the time necessary to carefully read and thoughtfully consider the problem *prior to* engaging in computations. An understanding of the purpose or goal of the problem and the types of calculations that are required will provide the needed direction and confidence.

Step 2. Estimate the dimension of the answer in both quantity and units of measure (e.g., milligrams) to satisfy the requirements of the problem. A section in Chapter 1 provides techniques for *estimation*.

Step 3. Perform the necessary calculations using the appropriate method both for efficiency and understanding. For some, this might require a step-wise approach whereas others may be capable of combining several arithmetic steps into one. Mathematical equations should be used only after the underlying principles of the equation are understood.

Step 4. Before assuming that an answer is correct, the problem should be read again and all calculations checked. In pharmacy practice, pharmacists are encouraged to have a professional colleague check all calculations prior to completing and dispensing a prescription or medication order. Further, if the process involves components to be weighed or measured, these procedures should be double-checked as well.

Step 5. Finally, consider the *reasonableness* of the answer in terms of the numerical value, including the proper position of a decimal point, and the units of measure.

Fundamentals of Pharmaceutical Calculations

1

Objectives

Upon successful completion of this chapter, the student will be able to:

- Convert common fractions, decimal fractions, and percentages to their corresponding equivalent expressions and apply each in calculations.
- Utilize exponential notations in calculations.
- Apply the method of ratio and proportion in problem-solving.
- Apply the method of dimensional analysis in problem-solving.
- Demonstrate an understanding of significant figures.

Pharmaceutical calculations is the area of study that applies the basic principles of mathematics to the preparation and safe and effective use of pharmaceuticals. Mathematically, pharmacy students beginning use of this textbook are well prepared. It is the *application* of the mathematics that requires study.

This initial chapter is intended to remind students of some previously learned mathematics. Most students likely will progress rapidly through this chapter. A student's performance on the practice problems following each section can serve as the guide to the degree of refreshment required.

Common and Decimal Fractions

Common fractions are portions of a whole, expressed at $\frac{1}{3}$, $\frac{1}{8}$ and so forth. They are used only rarely in pharmacy calculations nowadays. It is recalled, that when adding or subtracting fractions, the use of a *common denominator* is required. The process of multiplying and dividing with fractions is recalled by the following example problems.

If the adult dose of a medication is 2 teaspoonsful (tsp.), calculate the dose for a child if it is ¼ of the adult dose.

$$\frac{1}{4} \times \frac{2 \text{ tsp.}}{1} = \frac{2}{4} = \frac{1}{2} \text{ tsp., } \textit{answer}$$

If a child's dose of a cough syrup is ¾ teaspoonful and represents ¼ of the adult dose, calculate the corresponding adult dose.

$$\frac{3}{4}\text{tsp.} \div \frac{1}{4} = \frac{3}{4}\text{tsp.} \times \frac{4}{1} = \frac{3 \times 4}{4 \times 1}\text{tsp.} = \frac{12}{4}\text{tsp.} = 3 \text{ tsp., } \textit{answer}$$

NOTE: When common fractions appear in a calculations problem, it is often best to convert them to decimal fractions before solving.

A *decimal fraction* is a fraction with a denominator of 10 or any power of 10 and is expressed decimally rather than as a common fraction. Thus, $\dfrac{1}{10}$ is expressed as 0.10 and $\dfrac{45}{100}$ as 0.45. It is important to include the zero before the decimal point. This draws attention to the decimal point and helps eliminate potential errors. Decimal fractions often are used in pharmaceutical calculations.

To convert a common fraction to a decimal fraction, divide the denominator into the numerator.

Thus, $\dfrac{1}{8} = 1 \div 8 = 0.125$.

To convert a decimal fraction to a common fraction, express the decimal fraction as a ratio and reduce.

Thus, $0.25 = \dfrac{25}{100} = \dfrac{1}{4}$ or ¼.

Percent

The term **percent** and its corresponding sign, %, mean "in a hundred." So, *50 percent (50%)* means 50 parts in each one hundred of the same item.

Common fractions may be converted to percent by dividing the numerator by the denominator and multiplying by 100.

Convert ⅜ to percent.

$$\tfrac{3}{8} \times 100 = 37.5\%, \ answer.$$

Decimal fractions may be converted to percent by multiplying by 100.

Convert 0.125 to percent.

$$0.125 \times 100 = 12.5\%, \ answer.$$

Examples of equivalent expressions of common fractions, decimal fractions, and percent are shown in Table 1.1. A useful exercise is to add to the content of this table by working with common fractions that are not listed (e.g., $\frac{1}{400}$, $\frac{1}{60}$, etc.).

Table 1.1 ▼ EQUIVALENCIES OF COMMON FRACTIONS, DECIMAL FRACTIONS, AND PERCENT

COMMON FRACTION	DECIMAL FRACTION	PERCENT (%)	COMMON FRACTION	DECIMAL FRACTION	PERCENT (%)
$\frac{1}{1000}$	0.001	0.1	$\frac{1}{5}$	0.2	20
$\frac{1}{500}$	0.002	0.2	$\frac{1}{4}$	0.25	25
$\frac{1}{100}$	0.01	1	$\frac{1}{3}$	0.333	33.3
$\frac{1}{50}$	0.02	2	$\frac{3}{8}$	0.375	37.5
$\frac{1}{40}$	0.025	2.5	$\frac{2}{5}$	0.4	40
$\frac{1}{30}$	0.033	3.3	$\frac{1}{2}$	0.5	50
$\frac{1}{25}$	0.04	4	$\frac{3}{5}$	0.6	60
$\frac{1}{15}$	0.067	6.7	$\frac{5}{8}$	0.625	62.5
$\frac{1}{10}$	0.1	10	$\frac{2}{3}$	0.667	66.7
$\frac{1}{9}$	0.111	11.1	$\frac{3}{4}$	0.75	75
$\frac{1}{8}$	0.125	12.5	$\frac{4}{5}$	0.8	80
$\frac{1}{7}$	0.143	14.3	$\frac{7}{8}$	0.875	87.5
$\frac{1}{6}$	0.167	16.7	$\frac{8}{9}$	0.889	88.9

PRACTICE PROBLEMS

1. How many 0.000065-gram doses can be made from 0.13 gram of a drug?

2. Give the decimal fraction and percent equivalents for each of the following common fractions:
   (a) $\frac{1}{35}$
   (b) $\frac{3}{7}$
   (c) $\frac{1}{250}$
   (d) $\frac{1}{400}$

3. If a clinical study of a new drug demonstrated that the drug met the effectiveness criteria in 646 patients of the 942 patients enrolled in the study, express these results as a decimal fraction and as a percent.

4. A pharmacist had 3 ounces of hydromorphone hydrochloride. He used the following:
   $\frac{1}{8}$ ounce
   ¼ ounce
   1½ ounces

   How many ounces of hydromorphone hydrochloride were left?

5. A pharmacist had 5 grams of codeine sulfate. He used it in preparing the following:

   8 capsules each containing 0.0325 gram
   12 capsules each containing 0.015 gram
   18 capsules each containing 0.008 gram

   How many grams of codeine sulfate were left after he had prepared the capsules?

6. The literature for a pharmaceutical product states that 26 patients of the 2,103 enrolled in a clinical study reported headache after taking the product. Calculate (a) the decimal fraction and (b) the percentage of patients reporting this adverse response.

Exponential Notation

Many physical and chemical measurements deal with either very large or very small numbers. Because it often is difficult to handle numbers of such magnitude in performing even the simplest arithmetic operations, it is best to use exponential notation or *powers of 10* to express them. Thus, we may express *121* as *1.21 × 10²*, *1210* as *1.21 × 10³*, and *1,210,000* as *1.21 × 10⁶*. Likewise, we may express *0.0121* as *1.21 × 10⁻²*, *0.00121* as *1.21 × 10⁻³*, and *0.00000121* as *1.21 × 10⁻⁶*.

When numbers are written in this manner, the first part is called the ***coefficient***, customarily written with one figure to the left of the decimal point. The second part is the ***exponential factor*** or *power of 10*.

The exponent represents the number of places that the decimal point has been moved—positive to the left and negative to the right—to form the exponential. Thus, when we convert *19,000* to *1.9 × 10⁴*, we move the decimal point 4 places to the left; hence the exponent 4. And when we convert *0.0000019* to *1.9 × 10⁻⁶*, we move the decimal point 6 places to the right; hence the *negative* exponent⁻⁶.

In the *multiplication* of exponentials, the exponents are *added*. For example, *10² × 10⁴ = 10⁶*. In the multiplication of numbers that are expressed in exponential form, the *coefficients* are multiplied in the usual manner, and then this product is multiplied by the power of *10* found by algebraically *adding* the exponents.

Examples:

$$(2.5 \times 10^2) \times (2.5 \times 10^4) = 6.25 \times 10^6, \text{ or } 6.3 \times 10^6$$
$$(2.5 \times 10^2) \times (2.5 \times 10^{-4}) = 6.25 \times 10^{-2}, \text{ or } 6.3 \times 10^{-2}$$
$$(5.4 \times 10^2) \times (4.5 \times 10^3) = 24.3 \times 10^5 = 2.4 \times 10^6$$

In the *division* of exponentials, the exponents are *subtracted*. For example, $10^2 \div 10^5 = 10^{-3}$. In the division of numbers that are expressed in exponential form, the *coefficients* are divided in the usual way, and the result is multiplied by the power of *10* found by algebraically *subtracting* the exponents.

Examples:

$$(7.5 \times 10^5) \div (2.5 \times 10^3) = 3.0 \times 10^2$$
$$(7.5 \times 10^{-4}) \div (2.5 \times 10^6) = 3.0 \times 10^{-10}$$
$$(2.8 \times 10^{-2}) \div (8.0 \times 10^{-6}) = 0.35 \times 10^4 = 3.5 \times 10^3$$

Note that in each of these examples, the result is rounded off to the number of *significant figures* contained in the *least* accurate factor, and it is expressed with only one figure to the left of the decimal point.

In the *addition* and *subtraction* of exponentials, the expressions must be changed (by moving the decimal points) to forms having any common power of 10, and then the coefficients only are added or subtracted. The result should be rounded off to the number of *decimal places* contained in the *least* precise component, and it should be expressed with only one figure to the left of the decimal point.

Problem: $(1.4 \times 10^4) + (5.1 \times 10^3)$

Solution: first change 5.1×10^3 to have a common exponent, 0.51×10^4, then

$$\begin{array}{r} 1.4 \times 10^4 \\ + \, 0.51 \times 10^4 \\ \hline 1.91 \times 10^4 \end{array}$$ or, rounded off, 1.9×10^4, *answer.*

Problem: $(1.4 \times 10^4) - (5.1 \times 10^3)$

Solution: first change 1.4×10^4 to have a common exponent, 14×10^3, then

$$\begin{array}{r} 14.0 \times 10^3 \\ - \, 5.1 \times 10^3 \\ \hline 8.9 \times 10^3 \end{array}$$, *answer.*

CALCULATIONS CAPSULE

Exponential Notation

The factorized summary of some commonly used notations is as follows:

$10^9 = 1,000,000,000 = (10 \times 10 \times 10 \times 10 \times 10 \times 10 \times 10 \times 10 \times 10) = 1$ billion
$10^6 = 1,000,000 = (10 \times 10 \times 10 \times 10 \times 10 \times 10) = 1$ million
$10^3 = 1000 = (10 \times 10 \times 10) = 1$ thousand
$10^2 = 100 = (10 \times 10) = 1$ hundred
$10^{-2} = 1/(10 \times 10) = 1$ hundredth
$10^{-3} = 1/(10 \times 10 \times 10) = 1$ thousandth
$10^{-6} = 1/(10 \times 10 \times 10 \times 10 \times 10 \times 10) = 1$ millionth
$10^{-9} = 1/(10 \times 10 \times 10 \times 10 \times 10 \times 10 \times 10 \times 10 \times 10) = 1$ billionth

PRACTICE PROBLEMS

1. Write each of the following in exponential form:
   (a) 12,650
   (b) 0.0000000055
   (c) 451
   (d) 0.065
   (e) 625,000,000

2. Write each of the following in the usual numeric form:
   (a) 4.1×10^6
   (b) 3.65×10^{-2}
   (c) 5.13×10^{-6}
   (d) 2.5×10^5
   (e) 8.6956×10^3

3. Find the product:
   (a) $(3.5 \times 10^3) \times (5.0 \times 10^4)$
   (b) $(8.2 \times 10^2) \times (2.0 \times 10^{-6})$

   (c) $(1.5 \times 10^{-6}) \times (4.0 \times 10^6)$
   (d) $(1.5 \times 10^3) \times (8.0 \times 10^4)$
   (e) $(7.2 \times 10^5) \times (5.0 \times 10^{-3})$

4. Find the quotient:
   (a) $(9.3 \times 10^5) \div (3.1 \times 10^2)$
   (b) $(3.6 \times 10^{-4}) \div (1.2 \times 10^6)$
   (c) $(3.3 \times 10^7) \div (1.1 \times 10^{-2})$

5. Find the sum:
   (a) $(9.2 \times 10^3) + (7.6 \times 10^4)$
   (b) $(1.8 \times 10^{-6}) + (3.4 \times 10^{-5})$
   (c) $(4.9 \times 10^2) + (2.5 \times 10^3)$

6. Find the difference:
   (a) $(6.5 \times 10^6) - (5.9 \times 10^4)$
   (b) $(8.2 \times 10^{-3}) - (1.6 \times 10^{-3})$
   (c) $(7.4 \times 10^3) - (4.6 \times 10^2)$

Ratio and Proportion

Ratio

The relative magnitude of two quantities is called their ***ratio***. Since a ratio relates the relative value of two numbers, it resembles a common fraction except in the way in which it is presented. Whereas a fraction is presented as, for example, ½, a ratio is presented as 1:2 and is not read as "one half," but rather as "one is to two."

All the rules governing common fractions equally apply to a ratio. Of particular importance is the principle that *if the two terms of a ratio are multiplied or are divided by the same number, the value is unchanged*, the *value* being the quotient of the first term divided by the second. For example, the ratio *20:4* or $^{20}\!/_4$ has a value of 5; if both terms are divided by *2*, the ratio becomes *10:2* or $^{10}\!/_2$, again the value of 5.

The terms of a ratio must be of the same kind, for the *value* of a ratio is an abstract number expressing how many *times* greater or smaller the first term (or numerator) is than the second term (or denominator).[a] The terms may themselves be abstract numbers, or they may be concrete numbers of the same denomination. Thus, we can have a ratio of *20 to 4* ($^{20}\!/_4$) or *20 grams* to *4 grams* (20 grams/4 grams).

When two ratios have the same value, they are *equivalent*. An important fact about equivalent ratios is that the *product of the numerator of the one and the denominator of the other always equals the product of the denominator of the one and the numerator of the other; that is, the cross products are equal:*

$$\text{Because } \tfrac{2}{4} = \tfrac{4}{8},$$
$$2 \times 8 \ (\text{or } 16) = 4 \times 4 \ (\text{or } 16).$$

---

[a] The ratio of *1* gallon to *3* pints is not *1:3*, for the gallon contains *8* pints, and the ratio therefore is *8:3*.

It is also true that *if two ratios are equal, their reciprocals are equal:*

Because $\frac{2}{4} = \frac{4}{8}$, then $\frac{4}{2} = \frac{8}{4}$.

Proportion

A ***proportion*** is the expression of the equality of two ratios. It may be written in any one of three standard forms:

(1) $a:b = c:d$

(2) $a:b :: c:d$

(3) $\dfrac{a}{b} = \dfrac{c}{d}$

Each of these expressions is read: *a is to b as c is to d*, and *a* and *d* are called the *extremes* (meaning "outer members") and *b* and *c* the *means* ("middle members").

In any proportion, *the product of the extremes is equal to the product of the means.* This principle allows us to find the missing term of any proportion when the other three terms are known. If the missing term is a *mean*, it will be *the product of the extremes divided by the given mean*, and if it is an *extreme*, it will be *the product of the means divided by the given extreme*. Using this information, we may derive the following fractional equations:

If $\dfrac{a}{b} = \dfrac{c}{d}$, then

$a = \dfrac{bc}{d}$, $b = \dfrac{ad}{c}$, $c = \dfrac{ad}{b}$, and $d = \dfrac{bc}{a}$.

In a proportion that is properly set up, the position of the unknown term does not matter. However, some persons prefer to place the unknown term in the fourth position—that is, in the denominator of the second ratio. *It important to label the units in each position (e.g., mL, mg) to ensure the proper relationship between the ratios of a proportion.*

The application of ratio and proportion enables the solution to many of the pharmaceutical calculation problems in this text and in pharmacy practice.

If 3 tablets contain 975 milligrams of aspirin, how many milligrams should be contained in 12 tablets?

$$\frac{3 \text{ (tablets)}}{12 \text{ (tablets)}} = \frac{975 \text{ (milligrams)}}{x \text{ (milligrams)}}$$

$$x \text{ (milligrams)} = \frac{12 \text{ (tablets)} \times 975 \text{ (milligrams)}}{3 \text{ (tablets)}} = 3900 \text{ milligrams, } answer.$$

If 3 tablets contain 975 milligrams of aspirin, how many tablets should contain 3900 milligrams?

$$\frac{3 \text{ (tablets)}}{x \text{ (tablets)}} = \frac{975 \text{ (milligrams)}}{3900 \text{ (milligrams)}}$$

$$x \text{ (tablets)} = \frac{3 \text{ (tablets)} \times 3900 \text{ (milligrams)}}{975 \text{ (milligrams)}} = 12 \text{ tablets, } answer.$$

If 12 tablets contain 3900 milligrams of aspirin, how many milligrams should 3 tablets contain?

$$\frac{12 \text{ (tablets)}}{3 \text{ (tablets)}} = \frac{3900 \text{ (milligrams)}}{x \text{ (milligrams)}}$$

$$x \text{ (milligrams)} = \frac{3 \text{ (tablets)} \times 3900 \text{ (milligrams)}}{12 \text{ (tablets)}} = 975 \text{ milligrams, } answer.$$

If 12 tablets contain 3900 milligrams of aspirin, how many tablets should contain 975 milligrams?

$$\frac{12 \text{ (tablets)}}{x \text{ (tablets)}} = \frac{3900 \text{ (milligrams)}}{975 \text{ (milligrams)}}$$

$$x \text{ (tablets)} = \frac{12 \text{ (tablets)} \times 975 \text{ (milligrams)}}{3900 \text{ (milligrams)}} = 3 \text{ tablets, } answer.$$

Proportions need not contain whole numbers. If common or decimal fractions are supplied in the data, they may be included in the proportion without changing the method. For ease of calculation, it is recommended that common fractions be converted to decimal fractions prior to setting up the proportion.

If 30 milliliters (mL) represent ⅙ of the volume of a prescription, how many milliliters will represent ¼ of the volume?

$$\frac{1}{6} = 0.167 \text{ and } \frac{1}{4} = 0.25$$

$$\frac{0.167 \text{ (volume)}}{0.25 \text{ (volume)}} = \frac{30 \text{ (mL)}}{x \text{ (mL)}}$$

$$x = 44.91 \text{ or } \approx 45 \text{ mL, } answer.$$

Dimensional Analysis

When performing pharmaceutical calculations, some students prefer to use a method termed ***dimensional analysis*** (also known as ***factor analysis***, ***factor-label method***, or ***unit-factor method***). This method involves the logical sequencing and placement of a series of ratios (termed *factors*) into an equation. The ratios are prepared from the given data as well as from selected *conversion factors* and contain both arithmetic quantities and their units of measurement. Some terms are inverted (to their reciprocals) to permit the cancellation of like units in the numerator(s) and denominator(s) and leave only the desired terms of the answer. One advantage of using dimensional analysis is the consolidation of several arithmetic steps into a single equation.

In solving problems by dimensional analysis, the student unfamiliar with the process should consider the following steps:[1,2]

Step 1. Identify the wanted unit of the answer (e.g., mL, mg, etc.) and place it at the beginning of the equation. Some persons prefer to place a question mark next to it.

Step 2. Identify the given quantity(ies) and its (their) unit(s) of measurement.

Step 3. Identify the conversion factor(s) that are needed for the "unit path" to arrive at the arithmetic answer in the unit wanted.

Step 4. Set up the ratios such that the cancellation of the units of measurement in the numerators and denominators will retain only the wanted unit as identified in *Step 1*.

Step 5. Perform the arithmetic computation by multiplying the numerators, multiplying the denominators, and dividing the product of the numerators by the product of the denominators.

Ratio and Proportion

- A *ratio* expresses the relative magnitude of two like quantities (e.g., 1:2, expressed as "1 to 2.")

- A *proportion* expresses the equality of two ratios (e.g., 1:2 = 2:4).

- The four terms of a proportion are stated as:

$$a:b = c:d, \text{ or, } a:b::c:d, \text{ or } \frac{a}{b} = \frac{c}{d}$$

and expressed as "*a* is to *b* as *c* is to *d*."

- Given three of the four terms of a proportion, the value of the fourth, or missing, term may be calculated by cross multiplication and solution.

- The ratio-and-proportion method is a useful tool in solving many pharmaceutical calculation problems.

The general scheme shown here and in the "Calculations Capsule: Dimensional Analysis" may be helpful in using the method.

Unit Path

Given Quantity	Conversion Factor as Needed	Conversion Factor as Needed	Conversion Computation	Wanted Quantity and Unit
___ (Wanted Unit) =				=

Example Calculations Using Dimensional Analysis

How many fluidounces (fl. oz.) are there in 2.5 liters (L)?

Step 1. The wanted unit for the answer is *fluidounces.*

Step 2. The given quantity is *2.5 L.*

Step 3. The conversion factors needed are those that will take us from liters to fluidounces. As the student will later learn, these conversion factors are:
  1 liter = 1000 mL (to convert the given 2.5 L to milliliters), and
  1 fluidounce = 29.57 mL (to convert milliliters to fluidounces)

Step 4. Set up the ratios in the unit path

Unit Path

Given Quantity	Conversion Factor as Needed	Conversion Factor as Needed	Conversion Computation	Wanted Quantity and Unit
fl.oz. (Wanted Unit) =	2.5 L	1000 mL / 1 L	1 fl. oz. / 29.57 mL	=

Note: The unit path is set up such that all units of measurement will cancel out except for the unit wanted in the answer, *fluidounces*, which is placed in the numerator.

Step 5. Perform the computation:

Unit Path

	Conversion Factor as Needed	Conversion Factor as Needed	Conversion Computation	Wanted Quantity and Unit
Given Quantity				

$$\underline{\text{fl.oz.}}\ (\text{Wanted Unit}) = \frac{2.5\ \cancel{L}}{} \left| \frac{1000\ \cancel{mL}}{1\ \cancel{L}} \right| \frac{1\ \text{fl. oz.}}{29.57\ \cancel{mL}} \left| \frac{2.5 \times 1000 \times 1}{1 \times 29.57} = \frac{2500}{29.57} \right| = 84.55\ \text{fl. oz.}$$

or

$$2.5\ \cancel{L} \times \frac{1000\ \cancel{mL}}{1\ L} \times \frac{1\ \text{fl. oz.}}{29.57\ \cancel{mL}} = \frac{2.5 \times 1000 \times 1}{1 \times 29.57} = \frac{2500}{29.57} = 84.55\ \text{fl. oz.}$$

Note: The student may wish to see the problem solved by ratio and proportion:

Step 1.

$$\frac{1\ (\text{L})}{2.5\ (\text{L})} = \frac{1000\ (\text{mL})}{\text{x}\ (\text{mL})};\ \text{x} = 2500\ \text{mL}$$

Step 2.

$$\frac{29.57\ (\text{mL})}{2500\ (\text{mL})} = \frac{1\ (\text{fl. oz.})}{\text{x}\ (\text{fl. oz.})}$$

$$\text{x} = 84.55\ \text{fl. oz.,}\ \textit{answer.}$$

CALCULATIONS CAPSULE

Dimensional Analysis

- An alternative method to ratio and proportion in solving pharmaceutical calculation problems.

- The method involves the logical sequencing and placement of a series of ratios to consolidate multiple arithmetic steps into a single equation.

- By applying select conversion factors in the equation—some as reciprocals—unwanted units of measure cancel out, leaving the arithmetic result and desired unit.

- Dimensional analysis scheme:

Unit Path

	Conversion Factor as Needed	Conversion Factor as Needed	Conversion Computation	Wanted Quantity and Unit
Given Quantity				
___ (Wanted Unit) =				=

A medication order calls for 1000 milliliters of a dextrose intravenous infusion to be administered over an 8-hour period. Using an intravenous administration set that delivers 10 drops/milliliter, how many drops per minute should be delivered to the patient?

Solving by dimensional analysis:

$$8 \text{ hours } = 480 \text{ minutes (min.)}$$

$$? \text{ drops} = 1000 \text{ mL} \times \frac{10 \text{ drops}}{1 \text{ mL}} \times \frac{1}{480 \text{ min.}} = 20.8 \text{ or } 21 \text{ drops per minute, } answer.$$

Note: "drops" was placed in the numerator and "minutes" in the denominator to arrive at the answer in the desired term, *drops per minute.*

The student may wish to see this problem solved by ratio and proportion:

Step 1.

$$\frac{480 \text{ (min.)}}{1 \text{ (min.)}} = \frac{1000 \text{ (mL)}}{x \text{ (mL)}}; x = 2.08 \text{ mL}$$

Step 2.

$$\frac{1 \text{ (mL)}}{2.08 \text{ (mL)}} = \frac{10 \text{ (drops)}}{x \text{ (drops)}}; x = 2.08 \text{ mL } or \text{ 21 drops per minute, } answer.$$

The following problem is often used to demonstrate the process of dimensional analysis.

Calculate the number of seconds in a day.

$$? \text{ s} = 1 \text{ day} \times \frac{24 \text{ hr}}{1 \text{ day}} \times \frac{60 \text{ min}}{1 \text{ hr}} \times \frac{60 \text{ sec}}{1 \text{ min}} = 1 \times \frac{24 \times 60 \times 60}{1 \times 1 \times 1} = 86,400 \text{ seconds, } answer.$$

CASE IN POINT 1.1: A pharmacist consults with a parent on the use of a cough syrup for her 5-year-old child. The nonprescription cough syrup contains, in each 5-mL (milliliters), 10 mg (milligrams) of dextromethorphan HBr, a cough suppressant, and 100 mg of guaifenesin, an expectorant. The package label indicates the dose for a child 2 to 6 years of age is 1/4 of the adult dose of two teaspoonfuls. The pharmacist suggests using an oral syringe calibrated in 0.25-mL units for dosing. If a standard teaspoonful is equivalent to 5 mL, (a) how many milliliters should be administered to the child, and (b) how many milligrams of each of the two therapeutic ingredients would be administered per child's dose?

PRACTICE PROBLEMS

1. If an insulin injection contains 100 units of insulin in each milliliter, how many milliliters should be injected to receive 40 units of insulin?

2. An injection contains 3 mg of medication in each milliliter (mL). If a physician prescribes a dose of 0.5 mg to be administered to a hospital patient three times daily, how many milliliters of injection will be required over a 5-day period?

3. In a clinical study, a drug produced drowsiness in 30 of the 1500 patients studied. How many patients of a certain pharmacy could expect similar effects, based on a patient count of 100?

4. A formula for 1250 tablets contains 6.25 grams of diazepam. How many grams of diazepam should be used in preparing 350 tablets?

5. If 100 capsules contain 500 mg of an active ingredient, how many milligrams of the ingredient will 48 capsules contain?

6. Each tablet of TYLENOL WITH CODEINE contains 30 mg of codeine phosphate and 300 mg of acetaminophen. By taking two tablets daily for a week, how many milligrams of each drug would the patient take?

7. A cough syrup contains 10 mg of dextromethorphan hydrobromide per 5 mL. How many milligrams of the drug are contained in a 120-mL container of the syrup?

8. If an intravenous fluid is adjusted to deliver 15 mg of medication to a patient per hour, how many milligrams of medication are delivered per half minute?

9. The biotechnology drug filgrastim (NEUPOGEN) is available in syringes containing 480 micrograms (mcg) of filgrastim per 0.8 mL. How many micrograms of the drug would be administered by each 0.5 mL injection?

10. A prescription drug cost the pharmacist $42.00 for a bottle of 100 tablets. What would be the cost for 24 tablets?

11. How many 0.1-mg tablets will contain the same amount of drug as 50 tablets, each of which contains 0.025 mg of the identical drug?

12. Acyclovir (ZOVIRAX) suspension contains 200 mg of acyclovir in each 5 mL. How many milligrams of acyclovir are contained in a pint (473 mL) of suspension?

13. A metered dose inhaler contains 225 mg of metaproterenol sulfate, which is sufficient for 100 inhalations. How many micrograms (mcg) of metaproterenol sulfate would be administered with each inhalation if there are 1000 micrograms in each milligram?

14. A pediatric vitamin drug product contains the equivalent of 0.5 mg of fluoride ion in each milliliter. How many milligrams of fluoride ion would be provided by a dropper that delivers 0.6 mL?

15. If a pediatric vitamin contains 1500 units of vitamin A per milliliter of solution, how many units of vitamin A would be administered to a child given 2 drops of the solution from a dropper calibrated to deliver 20 drops per milliliter of solution?

16. An elixir contains 40 mg of drug in each 5 mL. How many milligrams of the drug would be used in preparing 4000 mL of the elixir?

17. An elixir of ferrous sulfate contains 220 mg of ferrous sulfate in each 5 mL. If each milligram of ferrous sulfate contains the equivalent of 0.2 mg of elemental iron, how many milligrams of elemental iron would be represented in each 5 mL of the elixir?

18. An estradiol transdermal patch is available in various patch sizes. The patch size is closely proportional to the amount of drug contained in the patch. If the patch containing 0.025 mg of estradiol is 6.5 cm^2 in size, calculate the approximate size of the patch containing 0.1 mg of estradiol.

19. If an ophthalmic solution contains 1 mg of dexamethasone phosphate in each milliliter of solution, how many milligrams of dexamethasone phosphate would be contained in 2 drops if the eyedropper used delivered 20 drops per milliliter?

20. A 15-mL package of nasal spray delivers 20 sprays per milliliter of solution, with each spray containing 1.5 mg of drug. (*a*) How many total sprays will the package deliver? (*b*) How many milligrams of drug are contained in the 15-mL package of the spray?

21. A penicillin V potassium preparation provides 400,000 units of activity in each 250-mg tablet. How many total units of activity would a patient receive from taking four tablets a day for 10 days?

22. If a 5-g packet of a potassium supplement provides 20 milliequivalents of potassium ion and 3.34 milliequivalents of chloride ion, (*a*) how many grams of the powder would provide 6 milliequivalents of potassium ion, and (*b*) how many milliequivalents of

chloride ion would be provided by this amount of powder?

23. If a potassium chloride elixir contains 20 milliequivalents of potassium ion in each 15 mL of elixir, how many milliliters will provide 25 milliequivalents of potassium ion to the patient?

24. The blood serum concentration of the antibacterial drug ciprofloxacin increases proportionately with the dose of drug administered. If a 250-mg dose of the drug results in a serum concentration of 1.2 micrograms of drug per milliliter of serum, how many micrograms of drug would be expected per milliliter of serum following a dose of 500 mg of drug?

25. The dosage of the drug thiabendazole (MINTEZOL) is determined in direct proportion to a patient's weight. If the dose of the drug for a patient weighing 150 pounds is 1.5 grams, what would be the dose for a patient weighing 110 pounds?

26. If 0.5 mL of a mumps virus vaccine contains 5000 units of antigen, how many units would be present in each milliliter if the 0.5 mL of vaccine was diluted to 2 mL with water for injection?

27. A sample of Oriental ginseng contains 0.4 mg of active constituents in each 100 mg of powdered plant. How many milligrams of active constituents would be present in 15 mg of powdered plant?

Alligation

Alligation is an arithmetic method of solving problems relating mixtures of components of different strengths. There are two types of alligation: *alligation medial* and *alligation alternate*.

Alligation medial may be used to determine the strength of a common ingredient in a mixture of two or more preparations. For example, if a pharmacist mixed together known volumes of two or more solutions containing known amounts of a common ingredient, the strength of that ingredient in the resulting mixture can be determined by alligation medial.

Alligation alternate may be used to determine the proportion or quantities of two or more components to combine in order to prepare a mixture of a desired strength. For example, if a pharmacist wished to prepare a solution of a specified strength by combining two or more other solutions of differing concentrations of the same ingredient, the proportion or volumes of each solution to use may be determined by alligation alternate.

Alligation medial and alligation alternate may be used as options in solving a number of pharmaceutical calculations problems. The methods and problem examples are presented in Chapter 15.

Significant Figures

When we *count* objects accurately, *every* figure in the numeral expressing the total number of objects must be taken at its face value. Such figures may be said to be *absolute*. When we record a *measurement*, the last figure to the right must be taken to be an *approximation*, an admission that the limit of possible precision or of necessary accuracy has been reached and that any further figures to the right would not be significant—that is, either meaningless or, for a given purpose, needless.

A denominate number, like 325 *grams*, is interpreted as follows: The 3 means *300 grams*, neither more nor less, and the 2 means *exactly 20 grams more*; but the final 5 means *approximately 5 grams more*, i.e., *5 grams plus or minus some fraction of a gram*. Whether this fraction is, for a given purpose, negligible depends on how precisely the quantity was (or is to be) weighed.

Significant figures, then, are consecutive figures that express the value of a denominate number accurately enough for a given purpose. The accuracy varies with the number of significant figures, which are all absolute in value except the last, and this is properly called *uncertain*.

Whether *zero* is significant, however, depends on its position or on known facts about a given number. The interpretation of *zero* may be summed up as follows:

1. Any zero between digits is significant.
2. Initial zeros to the left of the first digit are never significant; they are included merely to show the location of the decimal point and thus give place value to the digits that follow.
3. One or more final zeros to the right of the decimal point may be taken to be significant.

Examples.
Assuming that the following numbers are all denominate:

1. In *12.5*, there are *three* significant figures; in *1.256*, *four* significant figures; and in *102.56*, *five* significant figures.
2. In *0.5*, there is *one* significant figure. The digit 5 tells us how many *tenths* we have. The nonsignificant *0* simply calls attention to the decimal point.
3. In *0.05*, there is still only *one* significant figure, as there is in *0.005*.
4. In *0.65*, there are *two* significant figures, and likewise *two* in *0.065* and *0.0065*.

CALCULATIONS CAPSULE

Significant Figures

- Digits other than zero are significant.

- A zero between digits is significant.

- Zeros used only to show the location of the decimal point are not significant.

- The United States Pharmacopeia states that in performing pharmaceutical calculations, all figures are to be utilized until the calculations are completed and then only the significant figures retained in the final result.[3]

5. In *0.0605*, there are *three* significant figures. The first *0* calls attention to the decimal point, the second *0* shows the number of places to the right of the decimal point occupied by the remaining figures, and the third *0* significantly contributes to the value of the number. In *0.06050*, there are *four* significant figures, because the final *0* also contributes to the value of the number. [*It should be noted, however, that in pharmacy practice "trailing zeros" are not retained as a result of a calculation as they may lead to misinterpretation and error.*]

One of the factors determining the degree of approximation to perfect measurement is the precision of the instrument used. It would be incorrect to claim that *7.76 milliliters* had been measured in a graduate calibrated in units of *1 milliliter*, or that *25.562 grams* had been weighed on a balance sensitive to 0.01 gram.

We must clearly distinguish *significant figures* from *decimal places*. When recording a measurement, the number of decimal places we include indicates *the degree of precision with which the measurement has been made*, whereas the number of significant figures retained indicates *the degree of accuracy* that is sufficient for a given purpose.

Sometimes we are asked to record a value "correct to (so many) decimal places." We should never confuse this familiar expression with the expression "correct to (so many) significant figures." For example, if the value *27.625918* is rounded to *five decimal places*, it is written *27.62592*; but when this value is rounded to *five significant figures*, it is written *27.626*.

Rules for Rounding

1. When rounding a measurement, retain as many figures as will give only one *uncertain* figure. For example, in using a ruler calibrated only in full centimeter units, it would be correct to record a measurement of 11.3 centimeters but not 11.32 centimeters, because the 3 (tenths) is uncertain and no figure should follow it.
2. When eliminating superfluous figures following a calculation, add 1 to the last figure retained in a calculation if it is 5 or more. For example, 2.43 may be rounded off to 2.4, but 2.46 should be rounded off to 2.5.
3. When adding or subtracting *approximate* numbers, include only as many decimal places as are in the number with the *fewest* decimal places. For example, when adding 162.4 grams + 0.489 grams + 0.1875 grams + 120.78 grams, the sum is 283.8565 grams, but the rounded sum is 283.9 grams. However, when an instrument has the capability to weigh precisely all the quantities in such a calculation, rounding may be deemed inappropriate.

   In this regard, *there is an assumption made in pharmaceutical calculations that all measurements in the filling of a prescription or in compounding a formula are performed with equal precision by the pharmacist.* Thus, for example, if the quantities 5.5 grams, 0.01 gram, and 0.005 gram are specified in a formula, they may be added as if they are precise weights, with a sum of 5.515 grams.
4. When multiplying or dividing two approximate numbers, retain no more significant figures than the number having the fewest significant figures. For example, if multiplying 1.6437 grams by 0.26, the answer may be rounded from the calculated 0.427362 grams to 0.43 grams.
5. When multiplying or dividing an approximate number by an absolute number, the result should be rounded to the same number of significant figures as in the approximate number. Thus, if 1.54 milligrams is multiplied by 96, the product, 243.84 milligrams, may be rounded to 244 milligrams, or to three significant figures.
6. Oftentimes, logic plays a role. For example, when a calculation is performed to determine the *number of doses* available from a medication or the *number of drops* to be administered to a patient, it is both logical and practical to express the answer in whole units.

PRACTICE PROBLEMS

1. State the number of significant figures in each of the *italicized* quantities:
   (a) One fluidounce equals *29.57* milliliters.
   (b) One liter equals *1000* milliliters.
   (c) One inch equals *2.54* centimeters.
   (d) The chemical costs *$1.05* per pound.
   (e) One gram equals *1,000,000* micrograms.
   (f) One microgram equals *0.001* milligram.

2. Round each of the following to three significant figures:
   (a) 32.75
   (b) 200.39
   (c) 0.03629
   (d) 21.635
   (e) 0.00944

3. Round each of the following to three decimal places:
   (a) 0.00083
   (b) 34.79502
   (c) 0.00494
   (d) 6.12963

4. If a mixture of seven ingredients contains the following approximate weights, what can you validly record as the approximate total combined weight of the ingredients?
   26.83 grams, 275.3 grams, 2.752 grams, 4.04 grams, 5.197 grams, 16.64 grams, and 0.085 gram.

5. Perform the following computations, and retain only significant figures in the results:
   (a) $6.39 - 0.008$
   (b) $7.01 - 6.0$
   (c) 5.0×48.3 grams
   (d) 24×0.25 gram
   (e) $56.824 \div 0.0905$
   (f) $250 \div 1.109$

Estimation

It is important for pharmacy students and pharmacists to recognize the *reasonableness* of the result of a calculation. By performing an *estimation* of the answer *prior* to calculation, the approximate result may be predetermined. This helps assure the correct dimension of the answer including the critical placement of a decimal point.

The technique of estimation is demonstrated by the examples that follow. Rounding of numbers is a component of this process.

Add the following numbers: 7428, 3652, 1327, 4605, 2791, and 4490.
Estimation:
The figures in the thousands column add up to 21,000, and with each number on the average contributing 500 more, or every pair 1000 more, we get $21,000 + 3000 = 24,000$, *estimated answer* (actual answer, 24,293).

In *multiplication*, the product of the two leftmost digits plus a sufficient number of *zeros* to give the right place value serves as a fair estimate. The number of *zeros* supplied must equal the total number of all discarded figures to the left of the decimal point. Approximation to the correct answer is closer if the discarded figures are used to round the value of those retained.

Multiply 612 by 413.
Estimation:
$4 \times 6 = 24$, and because we discarded four figures, we must supply four zeros, giving 240,000, *estimated answer* (actual answer, 252,756).

In division, the given numbers may be rounded off to convenient approximations, but again, care is needed to preserve the correct place values.

Divide 2456 by 5.91.

Estimation:

The numbers may be rounded off to 2400 and 6. We may divide 24 by 6 mentally, but we must remember the two zeros substituted for the given 56 in 2456. The estimated answer is 400 (actual answer, 416).

PRACTICE PROBLEMS

1. Estimate the sums:

(a) 5641
2177
294
8266
3503

(b) 3298
368
5192
627
4835

(c) $75.82
37.92
14.69
45.98
28.91
49.87

2. Estimate the products:

(a) $42 \times 39 =$

(b) $596 \times 204 =$

(c) $8431 \times 9760 =$

(d) $0.0726 \times 6951 =$

(e) $6.1 \times 67.39 =$

3. Estimate the quotients:

(a) $171 \div 19 =$

(b) $184 \div 2300 =$

(c) $98,000 \div 49 =$

(d) $1.0745 \div 500 =$

(e) $458.4 \div 8 =$

CALCQUIZ

1.A. Digoxin (LANOXIN) pediatric elixir contains 0.05 mg (milligram) of digoxin in each milliliter (mL) of elixir. If there are 1000 µg (micrograms) in each milligram, how many micrograms of digoxin would be delivered in each dose of 0.6 mL?

1.B. A probiotic colon health product contains, in each capsule, 3 billion viable cells of *Lactobacillus acidophilus* and *Bifidobacterium longum*. Express, by exponential notation, the number of viable cells in a container of 30 capsules.

1.C. A liquid dietary supplement is packaged in 10-mL dropper containers to deliver 2000 international units of vitamin D_3 in each drop (0.027 mL). Calculate the number of drops delivered per milliliter.

1.D. The drug pramlintide (SYMLIN) is an antihyperglycemic agent for use in patients with diabetes treated with insulin. A 5-mL vial contains 600 µg of pramlintide per milliliter. A 0.05-mL dose measures 5 insulin units on the syringe used for injection and provides 30 µg of pramlintide. Calculate the number of micrograms of pramlintide and the corresponding measurement of insulin units on the syringe with the administration of 0.075 mL of injection.

1.E. A physician prescribed mometasone furoate monohydrate (NASONEX) nasal spray for a patient, with directions to administer two sprays into each nostril once daily. If each spray contains 50 µg of drug and the container can deliver a total of 120 sprays, how many micrograms of drug would the patient receive daily, and how many days of use will the prescription last the patient?

ANSWERS TO "CASE IN POINT" AND PRACTICE PROBLEMS

Case in Point 1.1

1. teaspoonful = 5 mL
   Adult dose = 2 teaspoonfuls = 10 mL

(a) Child's dose = 1/4 × 10 mL (2 teaspoonfuls) = 2.5 mL, *answer*.

(b) ? mg dextromethorphan HBr

$$= \frac{10 \text{ mg} \times 2.5 \text{ mL}}{5 \text{ mL}} = 5 \text{ mg}$$

dextromethorphan HBr, and

$$? \text{ mg guaifenesin} = \frac{100 \text{ mg} \times 2.5 \text{ mL}}{5 \text{ mL}}$$
$$= 50 \text{ mg guaifenesin,}$$
answers.

Proof of calculations: child's dose is ¼ of adult dose:

Child's calculated dose of cough syrup/ adult dose = 2.5 mL/10 mL = ¼ √

Child's calculated dose of dextromethorphan HBr/adult dose = 5 mg/20 mg = ¼ √

Child's calculated dose of guaifenesin/ adult dose = 50 mg/200 mg = ¼ √

Common Fractions, Decimal Fractions, and Percent

1. 2000 doses
2. (a) 0.029 or 2.9%
   (b) 0.43 or 43%
   (c) 0.004 or 0.4%
   (d) 0.0025 or 0.25%
3. 0.69 or 69%
4. 1⅛ or 1.25 ounces hydromorphone hydrochloride
5. 4.416 grams codeine sulfate
6. 0.012 or 1.2%

Exponential Notations

1. (a) 1.265×10^4
   (b) 5.5×10^{-9}
   (c) 4.51×10^2
   (d) 6.5×10^{-2}
   (e) 6.25×10^8

2. (a) 4,100,000
   (b) 0.0365
   (c) 0.00000513
   (d) 250,000
   (e) 8,695.6

3. (a) $17.5 \times 10^7 = 1.75 \times 10^8$
   (b) $16.4 \times 10^{-4} = 1.64 \times 10^{-3}$
   (c) $6.0 \times 10^0 = 6.0$
   (d) $12 \times 10^7 = 1.2 \times 10^8$
   (e) $36 \times 10^2 = 3.6 \times 10^3$

4. (a) 3.0×10^3
   (b) 3.0×10^{-10}
   (c) 3.0×10^9

5. (a) 8.52×10^4, or 8.5×10^4
   (b) 3.58×10^{-5}, or 3.6×10^{-5}
   (c) 2.99×10^3, or 3.0×10^3

6. (a) 6.441×10^6, or 6.4×10^6
   (b) 6.6×10^{-3}
   (c) 6.94×10^3, or 6.9×10^3

Ratio, Proportion, and Dimensional Analysis

1. 0.4 mL insulin injection
2. 2.5 mL
3. 2 patients
4. 1.75 g diazepam
5. 240 mg
6. 420 mg codeine phosphate
   4200 mg acetaminophen
7. 240 mg dextromethorphan hydrobromide
8. 0.125 mg
9. 300 mcg filgrastim
10. $10.08
11. 12½ tablets
12. 18,920 mg acyclovir
13. 2250 mcg metaproterenol sulfate
14. 0.3 mg fluoride ion
15. 150 units vitamin A
16. 32,000 mg
17. 44 mg elemental iron

18. 26 cm^2

19. 0.1 mg dexamethasone phosphate

20. (a) 300 sprays
    (b) 450 mg

21. 16,000,000 units

22. (a) 1.5 g
    (b) 1 milliequivalent chloride ion

23. 18.75 mL

24. 2.4 mcg ciprofloxacin

25. 1.1 g thiabendazole

26. 2500 units antigen

27. 0.06 mg

Significant Figures

1. (a) four
   (b) four
   (c) three
   (d) three
   (e) seven
   (f) one

2. (a) 32.8
   (b) 200
   (c) 0.0363
   (d) 21.6
   (e) 0.00944

3. (a) 0.001
   (b) 34.795
   (c) 0.005
   (d) 6.130

4. 330.8 g

5. (a) 6.38
   (b) 1.0
   (c) 240 g
   (d) 6.0 g
   (e) 628
   (f) 225

Estimation

1. (a) 20,500 *(19,881)*
   (b) 14,500 *(14,320)*
   (c) $240.00 *($253.19)*

2. (a) 40 × 40 = 1600 *(1638)*
   (b) 600 × 200 = 120,000 *(121,584)*
   (c) 8000 × 10,000 = 80,000,000
       (82,286,560)
   (d) (7 × 70) = 490 *(504.6426)*
   (e) 6 × 70 = 420 *(411.079)*

3. (a) 170 ÷ 20 = 8.5 *(9.0)*
   (b) 180 ÷ 2000 = 0.09 *(0.08)*
   (c) 9800 ÷ 5 = 1960 *(2000)*
   (d) 0.01 ÷ 5 = 0.002 *(0.002149)*
   (e) 460 ÷ 8 = 57.5 *(57.3)*

References

1. Available at: http://susanp3.tripod.com/snurse/id28.htm. Accessed June 5, 2012.
2. Craig GP. *Clinical Calculations Made Easy.* 4th Ed. Baltimore, MD: Lippincott Williams & Wilkins, 2008.
3. The United States Pharmacopeial Convention. *The United States Pharmacopeia 32 National Formulary* 27. Rockville, MD: The United States Pharmacopeial Convention, 2009;1:675.

International System of Units 2

Objectives

Upon successful completion of this chapter, the student will be able to:

- Demonstrate an understanding of the International System of Units.
- Convert measures within the International System of Units.
- Convert measures between the International System of Units and other systems of measure used in pharmacy.
- Apply the International System of Units correctly in pharmaceutical calculations.

The *International System of Units (SI)*, formerly called the *metric system,* is the internationally recognized decimal system of weights and measures. The system was formulated in France in the late 18th century. Over the years, effort has been made in the United States to transition from use of the common systems of weights and measures (e.g., pounds, feet, gallons) to the international system. Today, the pharmaceutical research and manufacturing industry, *The United States Pharmacopeia—The National Formulary,*[a] and all the health professions reflect conversion to the SI system. The advantages include the simplicity of the decimal system, the clarity provided by the base units and prefixes, and the ease of scientific and professional communications provided through the use of a universally accepted system.

The base units of the SI are the *meter* (for length), the *kilogram* (for weight), and the *liter* (for volume).[b] Subdivisions and multiples of these base units, their relative values, and their corresponding prefixes are shown in Table 2.1.

Guidelines for the Correct Use of the SI

The following are select guidelines for the correct use of the SI from the U.S. Metric Association, with additional considerations relevant to the practice of pharmacy:[1,2]

- Unit names and symbols generally are not capitalized except when used at the beginning of a sentence or in headings. However, the symbol for liter (L) may be capitalized or not. *Examples:* 4 L or 4 l, 4 mm and 4 g; *not* 4 Mm and 4 G.
- In the United States, the decimal marker (or decimal point) is placed on the line with the number; however, in some countries, a comma or a raised dot is used. *Examples:* 4.5 mL (U.S.); 4,5 mL or 4·5 mL (non-U.S.).
- Periods are not used following SI symbols except at the end of a sentence. *Examples:* 4 mL and 4 g, *not* 4 mL. and 4 g.

---

[a] *The United States Pharmacopeia—The National Formulary* (USP-NF) establishes standards for the quality, purity, and strength of prescription and nonprescription medicines. The standards, which are recognized and used by over 130 countries, are provided as printed volumes and electronically.

[b] Although not included in this text, the SI includes measures of force, viscosity, electricity, luminance, and many others in a variety of disciplines.

Table 2.1 ▼ **PREFIXES AND RELATIVE VALUES OF THE INTERNATIONAL SYSTEM (SI)**

PREFIX	MEANING
Subdivisions	
atto-	one quintillionth (10^{-18}) of the basic unit
femto-	one quadrillionth (10^{-15}) of the basic unit
pico-	one trillionth (10^{-12}) of the basic unit
nano-	one billionth (10^{-9}) of the basic unit
micro-	one millionth (10^{-6}) of the basic unit
milli-	one thousandth (10^{-3}) of the basic unit
centi-	one hundredth (10^{-2}) of the basic unit
deci-	one tenth (10^{-1}) of the basic unit
Multiples	
deka-	10 times the basic unit
hecto-	100 times (10^2) the basic unit
kilo-	1000 times (10^3) the basic unit
myria-	10,000 times (10^4) the basic unit
mega-	1 million times (10^6) the basic unit
giga-	1 billion times (10^9) the basic unit
tera-	1 trillion times (10^{12}) the basic unit
peta-	1 quadrillion times (10^{15}) the basic unit
exa-	1 quintillion times (10^{18}) the basic unit

- A compound unit that is a ratio or quotient of two units is indicated by a solidus (/) or a negative exponent. *Examples:* 5 mL/h or 5 mL · h^{-1}.
- Symbols should not be combined with spelled-out terms in the same expression. *Examples:* 3 mg/mL, *not* 3 mg/milliliter.
- Plurals of unit names, when spelled out, have an added s. Symbols for units, however, are the same in singular and plural. *Examples:* 5 milliliters or 5 mL, *not* 5 mLs.
- Two symbols exist for microgram: *mcg* (often used in pharmacy practice) and *μ*g (SI).
- The symbol for square meter is m^2; for cubic centimeter, cm^3; and so forth. In pharmacy practice, cm^3 is considered equivalent to milliliter.[2] The symbol cc, for cubic centimeter, is *not* an accepted SI symbol.
- Decimal fractions are used, not common fractions. *Examples:* 5.25 g, *not* 5¼ g.
- A zero should be placed in front of a leading decimal point to prevent medication errors caused by *uncertain* decimal points. *Example:* 0.5 g, *not* .5 g.
  It is *critically important for pharmacists to recognize that a misplaced or misread decimal point can lead to an error in calculation of a minimum of one tenth or ten times the desired quantity.*
- To prevent misreadings and medication errors, "trailing" zeros *should not* be placed following a whole number on prescriptions and medication orders. *Example:* 5 mg, *not* 5.0 mg. However, in some tables (such as those of the SI in this chapter), pharmaceutical formulas, and quantitative results, trailing zeros often are used to indicate exactness to a specific number of decimal places.
- In selecting symbols of unit dimensions, the choice generally is based on selecting the unit that will result in a numeric value between 1 and 1000. *Examples:* 500 g, *rather than* 0.5 kg; 1.96 kg, *rather than* 1960 g; and 750 mL, *rather than* 0.75 L.

Special Considerations of the SI in Pharmacy

Although some remnants of the common systems of measurement (see Appendix A) in pharmacy remain, the use of the SI is nearly total. The system is used to manufacture and label pharmaceutical products (Fig. 2.1); write, fill, and compound prescriptions and institutional medication orders; dose patients; express clinical laboratory test results; and communicate both verbally and through scientific and professional literature.

In the large-scale manufacture of dosage forms, pharmaceutical ingredients are measured in kilogram and kiloliter quantities. In the community and institutional pharmacy, compounding and dispensing in milligram, gram, and milliliter quantities are more common. Drug doses are typically administered in milligram or microgram amounts and prepared in solid dosage forms, such as tablets or capsules, or in a stated volume of a liquid preparation, such as an oral solution (e.g., 30 mg/5 mL) or injection (e.g., 2 mg/mL). Doses for certain drugs are calculated on the basis of body weight and expressed as mg/kg, meaning a certain number of *milligrams of drug per kilogram of body weight*. Clinical laboratory values are in metric units and expressed, for example, as mg/dL, meaning *milligrams of drug per deciliter of body fluid* (such as blood).

Particle Size and Nanotechnology

Drug particle size has long been an important consideration in pharmaceutical technology. Through the milling and reduction of drug materials to micron size, the surface area of particles is increased (Fig. 2.2), and pharmaceutical and clinical benefits often accrue. These benefits may include:[3]

- increased aqueous dissolution rates for poorly soluble substances;
- improved bioavailability, with increased rates of absorption of orally administered drugs;
- lower oral dosage possibilities with enhanced drug absorption; and
- expanded formulation options in the preparation of stable and predictable pharmaceutical suspensions and colloidal dispersions for all routes of administration, including oral, parenteral, respiratory, ophthalmic, and nasal.

▼ FIGURE 2.1 Example of a pharmaceutical product with the label indicating the quantity (10 mL) and strength (5 mg/mL) in SI or metric units. *(Reprinted with permission from Lacher BE.* Pharmaceutical Calculations for the Pharmacy Technician. *Philadelphia: Lippincott Williams & Wilkins, 2007.)*

Total surface area
6 cm^2

Total surface area
12 cm^2

Total surface area
24 cm^2

▼ FIGURE 2.2 Depiction of increased surface area by particle size reduction. *(Adapted from company literature, Nanocrystal, Elan Drug Delivery, Inc.)*

An area of technology with great potential is nanotechnology. ***Nanotechnology*** centers on the understanding and control of matter between approximately 1 and 100 nanometers (nm) in size, referred to as the ***nanoscale*** range.[4] For perspective, a nanometer is one billionth of a meter; about 25,400,000 nm equals 1 in.; the helix of DNA has a diameter of about 2 nm; and a typical bond between two atoms is about 0.15 nm.[5] Nanotechnology has applications for many potential products, including those that integrate chemistry, the biological sciences, medicine, and computer technology.

Measure of Length

The meter is the primary unit of length in the SI
The **table of metric length:**

1 kilometer (km)	=	1000.000 meters
1 hectometer (hm)	=	100.000 meters 1 meter (m)
1 dekameter (dam)	=	10.000 meters
1 decimeter (dm)	=	0.100 meter
1 centimeter (cm)	=	0.010 meter
1 millimeter (mm)	=	0.001 meter
1 micrometer (μm)	=	0.000,001 meter
1 nanometer (nm)	=	0.000,000,001 meter

The table may also be written:

1 meter = 0.001 kilometer
        = 0.01 hectometer
        = 0.1 dekameter
        = 10 decimeters
        = 100 centimeters
        = 1000 millimeters
        = 1,000,000 micrometers
        = 1,000,000,000 nanometers

Equivalencies of the most common length denominations:

1000 millimeters (mm) = 100 centimeters (cm)
100 centimeters (cm)   = 1 meter (m)

A ruler calibrated in millimeter and centimeter units is shown in Figure 2.3.

Distance exercise is undertaken by many people as a component of maintaining good health status and is usually measured by a combination of time and miles or meters. It is useful to understand the relationships shown in Table 2.2.

▼ FIGURE 2.3 Ruler calibrated in millimeter, centimeter, and inch units. *(Courtesy of Schlenker Enterprise, Ltd.)*

Measure of Volume

The *liter* is the primary unit of volume. It represents the volume of the cube of one tenth of a meter, that is, of 1 dm^3.

The **table of metric volume:**

1 kiloliter (kL)	=	1000.000 liters
1 hectoliter (hL)	=	100.000 liters
1 dekaliter (daL)	=	10.000 liters
1 liter (L)	=	1.000 liter
1 deciliter (dL)	=	0.100 liter
1 centiliter (cL)	=	0.010 liter
1 milliliter (mL)	=	0.001 liter
1 microliter (µL)	=	0.000,001 liter

This table may also be written:

1 liter = 0.001 kiloliter
= 0.010 hectoliter
= 0.100 dekaliter
= 10 deciliters
= 100 centiliters
= 1000 milliliters
= 1,000,000 microliters

Although not precisely equivalent, the milliliter is so nearly the same volume as the cubic centimeter (cm^3, cc), *The United States Pharmacopeia—National Formulary*[2] states: "One milliliter (mL) is used herein as the equivalent of 1 cubic centimeter (cc)."

Equivalencies of the most common volume denominations:

1000 milliliters (mL) = 1 liter (L)
100 milliliters (mL) = 1 deciliter (dL)

Examples of metric graduates for measuring volume are shown in Figure 2.4.

Table 2.2 ▼ DEMONSTRATIONS OF LINEAR RELATIONSHIPS

	FEET	YARDS	MILES	METERS	KILOMETERS
1 mile	5280	1760	1	1609.3	1.6093
1 kilometer	3280.8	1093.6	0.62137	1000	1

▼ FIGURE 2.4 Examples of metric-scale cylindrical (**A**) and conical pharmaceutical graduates (**B**). *(Courtesy of Kimble/Kontes Glass.)*

Measure of Weight

The primary unit of weight in the SI is the *gram*, which is the weight of 1 cm³ of water at 4°C, its temperature of greatest density. **For practical purposes, 1 cm³ of water ≈ 1 mL ≈ 1 g of weight.**

The **table of metric weight:**

1 kilogram (kg)	=	1000.000 grams
1 hectogram (hg)	=	100.000 grams
1 dekagram (dag)	=	10.000 grams
1 gram (g)	=	1.000 gram
1 decigram (dg)	=	0.1000 gram
1 centigram (cg)	=	0.010 gram
1 milligram (mg)	=	0.001 gram
1 microgram (µg or mcg)	=	0.000,001 gram
1 nanogram (ng)	=	0.000,000,001 gram
1 picogram (pg)	=	0.000,000,000,001 gram
1 femtogram (fg)	=	0.000,000,000,000,001 gram

This table may also be written:

$$
\begin{aligned}
1 \text{ gram} &= 0.001 \text{ kilogram}\\
&= 0.010 \text{ hectogram}\\
&= 0.100 \text{ dekagram}\\
&= 10 \text{ decigrams}\\
&= 100 \text{ centigrams}\\
&= 1000 \text{ milligrams}\\
&= 1,000,000 \text{ micrograms}\\
&= 1,000,000,000 \text{ nanograms}\\
&= 1,000,000,000,000 \text{ picograms}\\
&= 1,000,000,000,000,000 \text{ femtograms}
\end{aligned}
$$

Equivalencies of the most common weight denominations:

1000 micrograms (μg or mcg)	= 1 milligram (mg)
1000 milligrams (mg)	= 1 gram (g)
1000 grams (g)	= 1 kilogram (kg)

An example of a metric set of weights is shown in Chapter 3.

It should be noted that for *micrograms*, the abbreviation *mcg* and the symbol *μg* are both used in this text. Although the symbol *μg* is used at present in *The United States Pharmacopeia—National Formulary*,[2] the abbreviation *mcg* is widely used in pharmaceutical package labeling and in prescription writing.

Prescription Writing Style Using the SI

Prescriptions written in the SI use Arabic numerals *before* the abbreviations for the denominations (e.g., 6 g). Quantities of weight are usually written as grams and *decimals* of a gram, and volumes as milliliters and *decimals* of a milliliter:

℞	Dextromethorphan HBr	320 mg
	Guaifenesin	3.2 g
	Cherry Syrup, to make	240 mL

Fundamental Computations

Reducing SI Units to Lower or Higher Denominations by Using a Unit-Position Scale

The metric system is based on the decimal system; therefore, conversion from one denomination to another can be done simply by moving the decimal point as demonstrated in Figure 2.5.

To change a metric denomination to the next smaller denomination, move the decimal point one place to the right.

To change a metric denomination to the next larger denomination, move the decimal point one place to the left.

▼ FIGURE 2.5 Position scale of units of weight.

Reduce 1.23 kilograms to grams.

$$1.23 \text{ kg} = 1230 \text{ g, } \textit{answer.}$$

Reduce 9876 milligrams to grams.

$$9876 \text{ mg} = 9.876 \text{ g, } \textit{answer.}$$

In the first example, 1.23 kg are to be converted to grams. On the scale, the gram position is three decimal positions from the kilogram position. Thus, the decimal point is moved three places toward the right. In the second example, the conversion from milligrams also requires the movement of the decimal point three places, but this time to the left.

Reduce 85 micrometers to centimeters.

$$85 \, \mu\text{m} = 0.085 \text{ mm} = 0.0085 \text{ cm, } \textit{answer.}$$

Reduce 2.525 liters to microliters.

$$2.525 \text{ L} = 2525 \text{ mL} = 2,525,000 \, \mu\text{L, } \textit{answer.}$$

The 3-Decimal Point Shift

In pharmacy practice, and health care in general, the denominations most used differ by 1000 or by a factor of 3 decimal places. Thus, on the decimal scale (Fig. 2.5), a 3-place decimal point shift, left to right or right to left, will yield most commonly used denominations.

3-Place Shift for Common Weight Denominations:

kilograms (kg) _ _ _ grams (g) _ _ _ milligrams (mg) _ _ _ micrograms (mcg)

3-Place Shift for Common Volume Denominations:

liters (L) _ _ _ milliliters (mL)

Reducing SI Units to Lower or Higher Denominations by Ratio and Proportion or by Dimensional Analysis

Reduce 1.23 kilograms to grams.
From the table: 1 kg = 1000 g

By ratio and proportion:

$$\frac{1 \text{ kg}}{1000 \text{ g}} = \frac{1.23 \text{ kg}}{\text{x g}}; \text{ x} = 1230 \text{ g, } \textit{answer.}$$

By dimensional analysis:

$$1.23 \text{ kg} \times \frac{1000 \text{ g}}{1 \text{ kg}} = 1230 \text{ g, } \textit{answer.}$$

CALCULATIONS CAPSULE

International System of Units (SI)

- The SI or decimal system of measurement is used in the practice of pharmacy and throughout the pharmaceutical industry.

- The primary SI units for calculating mass or weight (gram), volume (liter), and length (meter) are used along with prefixes to indicate multiples or subdivisions of the primary units.

- To change an SI denomination to the next *smaller* denomination, the decimal point is moved one place to the right:

$$gram(g) > decigram(dg) > centigram(cg) > milligram(mg)$$
$$5.555\,g = 55.55\,dg = 555.5\,cg = 5555\,mg$$

Each value is equivalent.

- To change an SI denomination to the next *larger* denomination, the decimal point is moved one place to the left:

$$kilogram(kg) > hectogram(hg) > dekagram(dg) > gram(g)$$
$$5.555\,kg = 55.55\,hg = 555.5\,dg = 5555\,mg$$

Each value is equivalent.

- A unit position scale (e.g., see Fig 2.5), ratio and proportion, or dimensional analysis may be used to change denominations.
- Only numbers of the same denomination may be added to or subtracted from one another.

Reduce 62,500 mcg to g.
From the table: 1 g = 1,000,000 mcg
By ratio and proportion:

$$\frac{1,000,000 \text{ mcg}}{1 \text{ g}} = \frac{62,500 \text{ mcg}}{x \text{ g}}; \ x = 0.0625 \text{ g, } answer.$$

By dimensional analysis:

$$62,500 \text{ mcg} \times \frac{1 \text{ g}}{1,000,000 \text{ mcg}} = 0.0625 \text{ g, } answer.$$

Recognizing Equivalent Expressions

On occasion, it may be necessary to recognize, or prove by calculation, equivalent expressions. For example, a given quantity expressed in terms of "mg/100 mL" is equivalent to "mg/dL."

Practice problems (# 47 to 50) at the conclusion of this chapter provide exercises to determine equivalent expressions.

Addition and Subtraction

To add or subtract quantities in the SI, reduce them to a *common denomination*, preferably a base unit, and arrange their denominate numbers for addition or subtraction as ordinary decimals.

Add 1 kg, 250 mg, and 7.5 g. Express the total in grams.

$$
\begin{aligned}
1 \text{ kg} &= 1000. & \text{g} \\
250 \text{ mg} &= 0.25 & \text{g} \\
7.5 \text{ g} &= 7.5 & \text{g} \\
\hline
&1007.75 & \text{g or } 1008 \text{ g, } answer.
\end{aligned}
$$

Add 4 L, 375 mL, and 0.75 L. Express the total in milliliters.

$$
\begin{aligned}
4 \text{ L} &= 4000 \text{ mL} \\
375 \text{ mL} &= 375 \text{ mL} \\
0.75 \text{ L} &= 750 \text{ mL} \\
\hline
&5125 \text{ mL, } answer.
\end{aligned}
$$

A capsule contains the following amounts of medicinal substances: 0.075 g, 20 mg, 0.0005 g, 4 mg, and 500 µg. What is the total weight of the substances in the capsule?

$$
\begin{aligned}
0.075 \text{ g} &= 0.075 \text{ g} \\
20 \text{ mg} &= 0.02 \text{g} \\
0.0005 \text{ g} &= 0.0005 \text{ g} \\
4 \text{ mg} &= 0.004 \text{g} \\
500 \text{ µg} &= 0.0005 \text{ g} \\
\hline
&0.1000 \text{ g or } 100 \text{ mg, } answer.
\end{aligned}
$$

Subtract 2.5 mg from 4.85 g.

$$
\begin{aligned}
4.85 \text{ g} &= 4.85 \text{g} \\
2.5 \text{ mg} &= -\,0.0025 \text{ g} \\
\hline
&4.8475 \text{ g or } 4.848 \text{ g, } answer.
\end{aligned}
$$

A prescription calls for 0.06 g of one ingredient, 2.5 mg of another, and enough of a third to make 0.5 g. How many milligrams of the third ingredient should be used?

$$
\begin{aligned}
\text{1st ingredient:} \quad 0.06 \text{ g} &= 0.06 \text{g} \\
\text{2nd ingredient:} \quad 2.5 \text{ mg} &= 0.0025 \text{ g} \\
\hline
&0.0625 \text{ g}
\end{aligned}
$$

$$
\begin{aligned}
\text{Total weight :} & \quad 0.5 \text{ g} \\
\text{Weight of 1st and 2nd :} & \quad -0.0625 \text{ g} \\
\hline
\text{Weight of 3rd :} & \quad 0.4375 \text{ g or } 437.5 \text{ mg, } answer.
\end{aligned}
$$

Multiplication and Division

Because every measurement in the SI is expressed in a single given denomination, problems involving multiplication and division are solved by the methods used for any decimal numbers.

Multiply 820 mL by 12.5 and express the result in liters.

$$820 \text{ mL} \times 12.5 = 10250 \text{ mL} = 10.25 \text{ L}, \textit{answer}.$$

Divide 0.465 g by 15 and express the result in milligrams.

$$0.465 \text{ g} \div 15 = 0.031 \text{ g} = 31 \text{ mg}, \textit{answer}.$$

CASE IN POINT 2.1 A nurse telephones a pharmacy regarding the proper quantity of an injection to administer to a pediatric patient from a 1-mL vial containing 0.1 mg of digoxin. The attending physician had prescribed a dose of 25 mcg. How many milliliters should be the pharmacist's response?

Relation of the SI to Other Systems of Measurement

In addition to the International System of Units, the pharmacy student should be aware of two other systems of measurement: the ***avoirdupois*** and ***apothecaries'*** systems. The avoirdupois system, widely used in the United States in measuring body weight and in selling goods by the ounce or pound, is slowly giving way to the international system. The apothecaries' system, once the predominant pharmacist's system of volumetric and weight measure, has also largely been replaced by the SI. The pharmacist must still appreciate the relationship between the various systems of measurement, however, and deal effectively with them as the need arises.

The avoirdupois and apothecaries' systems of measurement, including all necessary equivalents and methods for intersystem conversion, are presented in Appendix A. The example equivalents presented in Table 2.3 are useful in gaining perspective and in solving certain problems in the text—for example, when there is need to convert fluidounces to milliliters or kilograms to pounds. These equivalents should be committed to memory.

> When quantities in units of the apothecaries' or avoirdupois systems of measurement (see Appendix A) are encountered, it is suggested that they be converted to equivalent quantities in SI units and the required calculation then solved in the usual manner.

Example Problems

An injection contains 5 mg of drug in each 10-mL vial. If the dose of the drug for a patient is determined to be 150 μg, how many milliliters should be administered?

$$150 \text{ }\mu g \times \frac{10 \text{ mL}}{5 \text{ mg}} \times \frac{1 \text{ mg}}{1000 \text{ }\mu g} = 0.3 \text{ mL}, \textit{answer}.$$

Table 2.3 ▼ SOME USEFUL EQUIVALENTS

Equivalents of Length

1 inch	=	2.54 cm
1 meter (m)	=	39.37 in
Equivalents of Volume		
1 fluidounce (fl. oz.)	=	29.57 mL
1 pint (16 fl. oz.)	=	473 mL
1 quart (32 fl. oz.)	=	946 mL
1 gallon, US (128 fl. oz.)	=	3785 mL
1 gallon, UK	=	4545 mL
Equivalents of Weight		
1 pound (lb, Avoirdupois)	=	454 g
1 ounce (oz, Avoirdupois)	=	28.35 g
1 kilogram (kg)	=	2.2 lb

A patient is determined to have a total cholesterol level of 240 mg/dL. What is the equivalent value in mg/100 mL?

1 dL = 100 mL; thus, 240 mg/dL = 240 mg/100 mL, *answer.*

The dose of a drug is 0.5 mg/kg of body weight/day. What is the equivalent dose in μg/lb/day?

0.5 mg = 500 μg
1 kg = 2.2 lb

Thus, 0.5 mg/kg/day = 500 μg/2.2 lb/day = 227.3 μg/lb/day, *answer.*

An oral suspension contains 1.5 g of medication in a pint. Calculate the quantity of medication, in milligrams, present in each 5-mL dose?

$$? \text{ mg} = 5 \text{ mL} \times \frac{1.5 \text{ g}}{1 \text{ pt}} \times \frac{1000 \text{ mg}}{1 \text{ g}} \times \frac{1 \text{ pt}}{473 \text{ mL}} = 15.86 \text{ or } 15.9 \text{ mg, } answer.$$

Or, by ratio and proportion:

1.5 g = 1500 mg
1 pint = 473 mL

$$\frac{1500 \text{ mg}}{473 \text{ mL}} = \frac{x \text{ mg}}{5 \text{ mL}}; \ x = 15.86 \text{ or } 15.9 \text{ mg, } answer.$$

CASE IN POINT 2.2 A hospital pharmacist is asked to prepare an intravenous infusion of dopamine. Based on the patient's weight, the pharmacist calculates a dose of 500 mcg/min for continuous infusion. The concentration of a premixed dopamine infusion is 400 mg/250 mL. What is the concentration of the infusion on a mcg/mL basis? How many milligrams of dopamine is the patient to receive in the first hour of treatment? How long will the infusion last?

PRACTICE PROBLEMS

1. Add 0.5 kg, 50 mg, and 2.5 dg. Reduce the result to grams.

2. Add 7.25 L and 875 cL. Reduce the result to milliliters.

3. Add 0.0025 kg, 1750 mg, 2.25 g, and 825,000 μg, and express the answer in grams.

4. Reduce 1.256 g to micrograms, to milligrams, and to kilograms.

5. Are the terms mcg/mL and mg/L equivalent or not equivalent?

6. A low-strength aspirin tablet contains 81 mg of aspirin per tablet. How many tablets may be prepared from 1 kg of aspirin?

7. Adhesive tape made from fabric has a tensile strength of not less than 20.41 kg/2.54 cm of width. Reduce these quantities to grams and millimeters.

8. A liquid contains 0.25 mg of a substance per milliliter. How many grams of the substance will 3.5 L contain?

9. An inhalation aerosol contains 225 mg of metaproterenol sulfate, which is sufficient for 300 inhalations. How many micrograms of metaproterenol sulfate would be contained in each inhalation?

10. TRIPHASIL-28 birth control tablets are taken sequentially, 1 tablet per day for 28 days, with the tablets containing the following:

    Phase 1—6 tablets, each containing 0.05 mg levonorgestrel and 0.03 mg ethinyl estradiol;
    Phase 2—5 tablets, each containing 0.075 mg levonorgestrel and 0.04 mg ethinyl estradiol;
    Phase 3—10 tablets, each containing 0.125 mg levonorgestrel and 0.03 mg ethinyl estradiol; then, 7 inert tablets (no drug).

    How many total milligrams each of levonorgestrel and ethinyl estradiol are taken during the 28-day period?

11. How many colchicine tablets, each containing 600 mcg, may be prepared from 30 g of colchicine?

12. The following clinical laboratory data are within normal values for an adult. Convert each value to mcg/mL:
    (a) ammonia, 30 mcg/dL
    (b) folate, 18 pg/mL
    (c) serum creatinine, 1.0 mg/dL
    (d) prostate specific antigen (PSA), 3 ng/mL
    (e) cholesterol, total, 150 mg/dL

13. The package insert for DONNATAL EXTENTABS indicates the amount of phenobarbital present in each tablet, in milligrams and in the equivalent weight (3/4 grains) in the Apothecary system. Refer to Appendix A and calculate the milligrams of phenobarbital present in each tablet.

14. Levothyroxine sodium tablets (SYNTHROID) are available in 12 different strengths ranging from 25 to 300 μg. Express this range in (a) mg and (b) ng.

15. Norgestrel and ethinyl estradiol tablets are available containing 0.5 mg of norgestrel and 50 μg of ethinyl estradiol. How many grams of each ingredient would be used in making 10,000 tablets?

16. Approximately 0.02% of a 100-mg dose of the drug miglitol (GLYSET) has been shown to appear in human breast milk. Calculate the quantity of drug detected, in milligrams, following a single dose.

17. How many grams of digoxin (LANOXIN) would be required to make 25,000 tablets each containing 250 mcg of digoxin?

18. Adalimumab (HUMIRA), a recombinant human monoclonal antibody, is available in a prefilled syringe containing 40 mg/0.8 mL of injection.

Calculate the concentration of drug on a mg/ mL basis.

19. If an injectable solution contains 25 µg of a drug substance in each 0.5 mL, how many milliliters would be required to provide a patient with 0.25 mg of the drug substance?

20. A patient is instructed to take one 50 µg tablet of pergolide mesylate (PERMAX) a day for the first two days of treatment; 150 µg/day on the third, fourth, and fifth days of treatment; 250 µg/day on the sixth, seventh, and eighth days; and 350 µg on the ninth day and return to the physician for assessment. During this treatment period, how many milligrams of drug were taken?

21. An oral liquid concentrate of sertraline hydrochloride (ZOLOFT) contains 20 mg/mL of the drug. How many grams of sertraline hydrochloride are in each 60-mL container of the concentrate?

22. Digoxin (LANOXIN) is available for parenteral pediatric use in a concentration of 0.1 mg/mL. How many milliliters would provide a dose of 40 µg?

23. A liquid oral concentrate of morphine sulfate contains 2.4 g of morphine sulfate in a 120-mL bottle. Calculate the concentration of morphine sulfate on a mg/mL basis.

24. The starting dose of sodium oxybate oral solution (XYREM) is 4.5 g/night divided into two equal doses and administered 2.5 to 4 hr apart. How many milliliters of the oral solution containing sodium oxybate, 500 mg/mL, should be administered in each divided dose?

25. An intravenous solution contains 500 µg of a drug substance in each milliliter. How many milligrams of the drug would a patient receive from the intravenous infusion of a liter of the solution?

26. If an intravenous solution containing 123 mg of a drug substance in each 250-mL bottle is to be administered at the rate of 200 µg of drug per minute, how many milliliters of the solution would be given per hour?

27. An oral inhalation (DULERA) to treat asthma provides, in each inhalation, 100 µg of mometasone furoate and 5 µg of formoterol fumarate. The recommended dose is "two inhalations twice daily (morning and evening)." Calculate the quantity of each drug inhaled daily and express the answers in milligrams.

28. One milligram of streptomycin sulfate contains the antibiotic activity of 650 µg of streptomycin base. How many grams of streptomycin sulfate would be the equivalent of 1 g of streptomycin base?

29. A commercial package contains thirty-six 200-mg tablets of ibuprofen. How many kilograms of ibuprofen were used in the manufacture of 1000 packages of the product?

30. A gas chromatographic column measures 1.8 m in length and 3 mm in internal diameter. Convert these measurements to inches.

31. A prefilled syringe contains 20 mg of drug in 2 mL of solution. How many micrograms of drug would be administered by an injection of 0.5 mL of the solution?

32. A vial contains 80 mg of drug in 2 mL of injection. How many milliliters of the injection should be administered to obtain 0.02 g of drug?

33. One-half liter of solution for intravenous infusion contains 2 g of drug. How many milliliters of the solution would contain 0.5 mg of drug?

34. A 125-mL container of amoxicillin contains 600 mg/5 mL. How many milliliters would be used to administer 400 mg of amoxicillin?

35. An effervescent tablet has the following formula:

Acetaminophen	325 mg
Calcium Carbonate	280 mg
Citric Acid	900 mg
Potassium Bicarbonate	300 mg
Sodium Bicarbonate	465 mg

    (a) Calculate the total weight, in grams, of the ingredients in each tablet.

    (b) How many tablets could be made with a supply of 5 kg of acetaminophen?

36. A new analytic instrument is capable of detecting picogram quantities of a chemical substance. How many times more capable is this instrument than one that can detect nanogram quantities of the same chemical?

37. The dimensions of a nicotine transdermal patch system are 4.7 cm by 4.8 cm. Express these dimensions in corresponding inches if 1 inch is equivalent to 25.4 mm.

38. If an albuterol inhaler contains 18 mg of albuterol, how many inhalation-doses can be delivered if each inhalation-dose contains 90 μg?

39. Acetaminophen, in amounts greater than 4 g per day, has been associated with liver toxicity. What is the maximum number of 500-mg tablets of acetaminophen that a person may take daily and not reach the toxic level?

40. Prochlorperazine (COMPAZINE) for injection is available in 10-mL multiple dose vials containing 5 mg/mL. How many 2-mg doses can be withdrawn from the vial?

41. The recommended dose for a brand of nicotine patch is one 21-mg dose per day for 6 weeks, followed by 14 mg per day for 2 weeks, and then 7 mg per day for 2 more weeks. What total quantity, in grams, would a patient receive during this course of treatment?

42. A medical device is sterilized by gamma radiation at 2.5 megarads (Mrad). Express the equivalent quantity in rads.

43. A round transdermal patch measures 4.3 cm in diameter. Convert this dimension to inches and millimeters.

44. A solution for direct IV bolus injection contains 125 mg of drug in each 25 mL of injection. What is the concentration of drug in terms of $\mu g/\mu L$?

45. The total number of human genomic characters is 3.5 billion. Express this quantity numerically without using a decimal point.

46. Conjugated estrogens tablets (PREMARIN) are available in strengths of 0.3 mg, 0.45 mg, 0.625 mg, 0.9 mg, and 1.25 mg. If patient "A" took one tablet daily of the lowest dose and patient "B" took one tablet daily of the highest dose, what is the difference in the total quantities taken between patients "A" and "B" over a period of 30 days?
    (a) 2.85 mg
    (b) 2850 mcg
    (c) 2.85 cg
    (d) 2.85 dg

47. Teratogenic studies of insulin glargine were undertaken in rats at doses up to 0.36 mg/kg/day. This is equivalent to which of the following?
    (a) 360 cg/lb/day
    (b) 792 mcg/lb/day
    (c) 360 mg/lb/day
    (d) 163.6 mcg/lb/day

48. Pharmacy students, traveling to attend a national pharmacy meeting, were on an airplane with an average air speed of 414 miles per hour. Which is the closest equivalent air speed?
    (a) 6 mi/min
    (b) 257 km/h
    (c) 666 km/h
    (d) 180 m/sec

49. The product of biotechnology, filgrastim (NEUPOGEN), is available in vials containing 0.3 mg of drug in each milliliter. Which choice is equivalent in concentration?
    (a) 0.03 mg/0.1 dL
    (b) 300 mcg/0.01 dL
    (c) 3 mcg/0.01 cL
    (d) 300 mcg/10 cL

50. In a clinical study of finasteride (PROSCAR), a single oral dose of 5 mg resulted in an average blood concentration of 37 ng of drug per milliliter (37 ng/mL) of blood plasma. This is equivalent to which of the following?
    (a) 37,000 mcg/mL
    (b) 0.037 mcg/mL
    (c) 0.000037 mg/cL
    (d) 0.0037 mcg/dL

CALCQUIZ

2.A. A health-news story that received widespread attention in recent years involved the successful premature birth of octuplets. The eight babies ranged in weight from 1 lb 8 oz to 3 lb 4 oz. Using the equivalents for the Avoirdupois System given in this chapter, calculate the babies' range in weight, in grams and in kilograms.

2.B. Levothyroxine sodium tablets are available in 11 different strengths, ranging from 0.025 mg to 200 μg. Calculate the difference, in micrograms, between these two strengths.

2.C. An inhalation aerosol contains 0.03 g of albuterol sulfate per canister and is labeled to deliver 200 full inhalations. If each inhalation contains 108 μg of albuterol sulfate, how many milligrams of drug would remain in the canister?

2.D. A 0.5-mL container of an investigational ophthalmic solution contains a drug in a concentration of 0.01 mg/mL. How many micrograms of drug would be administered in a 50-μL drop?

2.E. A long-acting formulation of leuprolide acetate requires injection only once every 3 months. Clinical studies revealed that 4 hours following a single injection, the mean blood plasma level of leuprolide was 36.3 ng/mL and dropped over the next month to a steady level of 23.9 ng/mL. Express the difference between these the two values in μg/dL.

ANSWERS TO "CASE IN POINT" AND PRACTICE PROBLEMS

Case in Point 2.1

0.1 mg/mL = 100 mcg/mL

$$25 \text{ mcg} \times \frac{1 \text{ mL}}{100 \text{ mcg}} = \frac{1}{4} \text{ mL}$$

or 0.25 mL, *answer*.

Case in Point 2.2

Concentration of infusion, mcg/mL:

$$\frac{400 \text{ mg}}{250 \text{ mL}} = \frac{400,000 \text{ mcg}}{250 \text{ mL}}$$

$$= 1600 \text{ mcg/mL}, \text{ } answer.$$

mg, dopamine, first hour:

$$\frac{500 \text{ mcg}}{1 \text{ min}} \times \frac{60 \text{ min}}{1 \text{ h}} \times \frac{1 \text{ mg}}{1000 \text{ mcg}}$$

$$= 30 \text{ mg/h, } answer.$$

Infusion duration:

$$400 \text{ mg} \times \frac{1 \text{ min}}{500 \text{ mcg}} \times \frac{1000 \text{ mcg}}{1 \text{ mg}}$$

$$= 800 \text{ min} = 13 \text{ h, } 20 \text{ min, } answer.$$

Practice Problems

1. 500.3 g
2. 16,000 mL
3. 7.325 g
4. 1,256,000 mcg
   1256 mg
   0.001256 kg
5. equivalent
6. 12,345 tablets
7. 20,410 g/25.4 mm
8. 0.875 g
9. 750 mcg metaproterenol sulfate
10. 1.925 mg levonorgestrel
    0.68 mg ethinyl estradiol
11. 50,000 tablets
12. (a) ammonia, 0.3 mcg/mL
    (b) folate, 0.000018 mcg/mL
    (c) serum creatinine, 10 mcg/mL
    (d) prostate specific antigen (PSA), 0.003 mcg/mL
    (e) cholesterol, 1500 mcg/mL
13. 48.75 mg phenobarbital
14. (a) 0.025 to 0.3 mg and (b) 25,000 to 30,000 ng levothyroxine sodium
15. 5 g norgestrel
    0.5 g ethinyl estradiol
16. 0.02 mg miglitol
17. 6.25 g digoxin

18. 50 mg/mL
19. 5 mL
20. 1.65 mg pergolide mesylate
21. 1.2 g sertraline hydrochloride
22. 0.4 mL
23. 20 mg/mL morphine sulfate
24. 4.5 mL oxybate oral solution
25. 500 mg
26. 24.39 mL
27. 0.4 mg mometasone furoate, and 0.02 mg formoterol fumarate
28. 1.538 g streptomycin sulfate
29. 7.2 kg
30. 70.866 or 70.9 inches
    0.118 or 0.12 inches
31. 5000 mcg
32. 0.5 mL
33. 0.125 mL
34. 3.33 mL
35. (a) 2.27 g
    (b) 15,384 tablets
36. 1000 times
37. 1.85 inches × 1.89 inches
38. 200 doses
39. 8 tablets
40. 25 doses
41. 1.176 g nicotine
42. 2,500,000 rads
43. 1.69 inches and 43 mm
44. 5 µg/µL
45. 3,500,000,000 or 35×10^8
46. (c) 2.85 cg
47. (d) 163.6 mcg/lb/day
48. (c) 666 km/h
49. (b) 300 mcg/0.01 dL
50. (b) 0.037 mcg/mL

References

1. U.S. Metric Association. Correct SI-metric usage. Available at: http://lamar.colostate.edu/~hillger/correct. htm. Accessed September 4, 2008.
2. United States Pharmacopeia 32 National Formulary 27. Rockville, MD: United States Pharmacopeial Convention, 2009;1:9.
3. Available at: http//:www.Nanocrystal.com.html. Accessed September 4, 2008.
4. National Nanotechnology Initiative. *What is nanotechnology*. Available at: www.nano.gov/html/facts/ whatIsNano/html. Accessed March 6, 2011.
5. Seeman NC. Nanotechnology and the double helix. *Scientific American* 2004;290:64–75.

Pharmaceutical Measurement 3

Objectives

Upon successful completion of this chapter, the student will be able to:

- Describe instruments for volumetric measurement and characterize their differences in application and accuracy.
- Describe the correct procedure when using a pharmaceutical balance.
- Define *sensitivity requirement* and apply it in calculations.
- Perform calculations by the aliquot method.
- Demonstrate an understanding of *percentage of error* in pharmaceutical measurement.

Pharmaceutical measurement is an important part of pharmacy practice. It is employed in community and institutional pharmacies, in pharmaceutical research, in the development and manufacture of pharmaceuticals, in chemical and product analysis, and in quality control. This chapter focuses on the equipment and methods used in the accurate measurement of therapeutic and pharmaceutical materials in the community and institutional practice of pharmacy.

The expertise of pharmacists in accurately weighing and measuring materials is a historical and unique skill, acquired through professional education and training. Moreover, this capability is an *expectation* of other health professionals and the patient community being served. It is not an overstatement to say that *patients' lives depend on it.*

The role of the pharmacist in providing pharmaceutical care includes the ability and responsibility to **compound**—that is, to accurately weigh, measure volume, and combine individual therapeutic and pharmaceutical components in the formulation and preparation of prescriptions and medication orders.

Measurement of Volume

Common instruments for the pharmaceutical measurement of volume range from micropipets and burettes used in analytic procedures to large, industrial-size calibrated vessels. The selection of measuring instrument should be based on the level of precision required. In pharmacy practice, the most common instruments for measuring volume are cylindric and conical (cone-shaped) graduates (Fig. 3.1). For the measurement of small volumes, however, the pharmacist often uses a calibrated syringe or, when required, a pipette.

Whereas cylindric graduates are calibrated in SI or metric units, conical graduates are usually dual-scale, that is, calibrated in both metric and apothecary units of volume. (*Note*: metric units of volume are described in Chapter 2, and apothecaries' units are described in Appendix A.) Both glass and plastic graduates are commercially available in a number of capacities, ranging from 5 to 1000 milliliters and greater.

As a general rule, it is best to select the graduate with a capacity equal to or just exceeding the volume to be measured. Measurement of small volumes in large graduates increases the

▼ FIGURE 3.1 Examples of conical and cylindric graduates, a pipet, and a pipet-filling bulb for volumetric measurement.

potential for error. The design of a volumetric apparatus is an important factor in measurement accuracy; the narrower the bore or chamber, the lesser the error in reading the meniscus and the more accurate the measurement (Fig. 3.2). According to the *United States Pharmacopeia*, a deviation of ± 1 mm in the reading of the meniscus when using a 100-mL cylindrical graduate results in an error of approximately 0.5 mL, and 1.8 mL at the 100-mL mark when using a 125-mL conical graduate.[1]

It is essential for the pharmacist to select the proper type and capacity of instrument for volumetric measure and to carefully observe the meniscus at eye level to achieve the desired measurement.

Measurement of Weight

There is a wide range of weights, balances, and scales available for pharmaceutical measurement. The proper selection depends upon the particular task at hand. Standard prescription balances and highly sensitive electronic balances generally suffice in traditional pharmaceutical compounding, whereas large-capacity scales are used in the industrial manufacture of pharmaceutical products. Whichever instrument is used, however, it must meet established standards for sensitivity, accuracy, and capacity.

Class A prescription balances (Fig. 3.3) are designed for the weighing of medicinal or pharmaceutical substances required in the filling of prescriptions or in small-scale compounding. Some prescription balances have a weighbeam and rider, and others a dial, to add up to 1 gram of weight. As required, additional external weights may be added to the

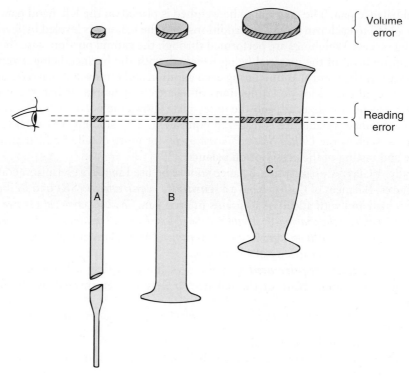

▼ FIGURE 3.2 Volume error differentials due to instrument diameters. **(A)**, volumetric pipet; **(B)**, cylindric graduate; and **(C)**, conical graduate.

▼ FIGURE 3.3 Torbal torsion balance and Ohaus electronic balance. *(Courtesy of Total Pharmacy Supply, Inc.)*

right-hand balance pan. The material to be weighed is placed on the left-hand pan. Powder papers are added to each pan before any additions, and the balance is leveled by leveling feet or balancing screws. Weighings are performed through the careful portion-wise (by spatula) addition and removal of the material being weighed, with the balance being *arrested* (pans locked in place by the control knob) during each addition and removal of material, and *un*arrested with the lid closed for determinations of balance rest points. When the unarrested pans neither ascend nor descend, and the index plate shows the needle is in the center, the material and balance weights are considered equivalent. The student may wish to refer to other sources, such as the *United States Pharmacopeia*, for more detailed information on the proper use and testing of the prescription balance.[1]

Minimally, a Class A prescription balance should be used in all prescription compounding procedures. Balances of this type have a ***sensitivity requirement (SR)*** of 6 milligrams or less with no load and with a load of 10 grams in each pan. *To avoid errors of greater than 5% when using this balance, the pharmacist should not weigh less than 120 milligrams of material (i.e., a 5% error in a weighing of 120 milligrams = 6 milligrams)*. Most commercially available Class A balances have a maximum capacity of 120 grams.

The term ***sensitivity requirement*** is defined as the load that will cause a change of one division on the index plate of the balance. It may be determined by the following procedure:

1. Level the balance.
2. Determine the rest point of the balance.
3. Determine the smallest weight that causes the rest point to shift one division on the index plate.

For greater accuracy than a Class A prescription balance allows, many pharmacies utilize high-precision electronic analytical balances to weigh very small quantities (Fig. 3.4). Many of these balances are capable of weighing accurately 0.1 milligram, are self-calibrating, and

▼ FIGURE 3.4 Sartorious BasicLite analytical balance. *(Courtesy of Sartorius Corporation.)*

▼ FIGURE 3.5 Set of metric weights. *(Courtesy of Mettler-Toledo, Inc.)*

are equipped with convenient digital readout features. The usual maximum capacities for balances of this precision range from about 60 grams to 210 grams depending upon the model. A set of metric weights that may be used to weigh materials on a prescription balance and/or used to calibrate an analytical balance is shown in Figure 3.5.

Aliquot Method of Weighing and Measuring

When a degree of precision in measurement that is beyond the capacity of the instrument at hand is required, the pharmacist may achieve the desired precision by calculating and measuring in terms of aliquot parts. An **aliquot** is a fraction, portion, or part that is contained an exact number of times in another.

Weighing by the Aliquot Method

The *aliquot method of weighing* is a method by which small quantities of a substance may be obtained within the desired degree of accuracy by weighing a larger-than-needed portion of the substance, diluting it with an inert material, and then weighing a portion (aliquot) of the mixture calculated to contain the desired amount of the needed substance. A stepwise description of the procedure is depicted in Figure 3.6 and is described as follows:

Step 1	Step 2	Step 3
5 mg × 25 = 125 mg [drug [multiple [quantity needed] factor] actually weighed]	Add 2875 mg = 3000 mg mixture [diluent] [125 mg drug + 2875 mg diluent]	Weigh 1/25 of 3000 mg = 120 mg [5 mg drug + 115 mg diluent]

▼ FIGURE 3.6 Depiction of the aliquot method of weighing using the example described on the next page.

Preliminary Step. **Calculate the smallest quantity of a substance that can be weighed on the balance with the desired precision.**

The equation used:

$$\frac{100\% \times \text{Sensitivity Requirement (mg)}}{\text{Acceptable Error (\%)}} = \text{Smallest Quantity (mg)}$$

On a balance with an SR of 6 mg, and with an acceptable error of no greater than 5%, a quantity of not less than 120 mg must be weighed.

$$\frac{100\% \times 6 \text{ mg}}{5\%} = 120 \text{ mg}$$

Step 1. **Select a multiple of the desired quantity that can be weighed with the required precision.**

- If the quantity of a required substance is *less than* the minimum weighable amount, select a "multiple" of the required quantity that will yield an amount equal to or greater than the minimum weighable amount. (A larger-than-necessary multiple may be used to exceed the minimum accuracy desired.)
- *Example:*
  *If the balance in the example in the preliminary step is used, and if 5 mg of a drug substance is required on a prescription, then a quantity at least **25 times** (the multiple) the desired amount, or 125 mg (5 mg × 25), must be weighed for the desired accuracy. (If a larger multiple is used, say 30, and 150 mg of the substance is weighed [5 mg × 30], then a weighing error of only 4% would result.)*

Step 2. **Dilute the multiple quantity with an inert substance.**

- *The amount of inert diluent* to use is determined by the fact that the aliquot portion of the drug-diluent mixture weighed in *Step 3* must be equal to or greater than the minimum weighable quantity previously determined.
- By multiplying the amount of the aliquot portion to weigh in *Step 3* by the multiple selected in *Step 1*, the total quantity of the mixture to prepare is determined.
- *Example:*
  According to the preliminary step, 120 milligrams or more must be weighed for the desired accuracy. If we decide on 120 mg for the aliquot portion in Step 3, and multiply it by the multiple selected in Step 1 (i.e., 25), we arrive at 3000 mg for the total quantity of the drug-diluent mixture to prepare. Subtracting the 125 mg of drug weighed in Step 1, we must add 2875 mg of diluent to prepare the 3000 mg of drug-diluent mixture.

Step 3. **Weigh the aliquot portion of the dilution that contains the desired quantity.**

- Since **25 times** the needed amount of drug substance was weighed (*Step 1*), an aliquot part equal to $\frac{1}{25}$ of the 3000-mg drug-diluent mixture, or 120 mg, will contain the required quantity of drug substance.

- *Proof:* $\frac{1}{25} \times 125 \text{ mg}$ (drug substance weighed in *Step 1*) = 5 mg

  $\frac{1}{25} \times 2875 \text{ mg}$ (diluent weighed in *Step 2*) = $\dfrac{115 \text{ mg}}{120 \text{ mg}}$ aliquot part

- *Example:*
  A torsion prescription balance has a sensitivity requirement of 6 milligrams. Explain how you would weigh 4 milligrams of atropine sulfate with an accuracy of ± 5%, using lactose as the diluent.

Because 6 milligrams is the potential balance error, 120 milligrams is the smallest amount that should be weighed to achieve the required precision.

If 120 milligrams, or **30** times the desired amount of atropine sulfate, is chosen as the multiple quantity to be weighed in Step 1, and if 150 milligrams is set as the aliquot to be weighed in Step 3, then:

1. Weigh **30** × 4 mg, or   120 mg of atropine sulfate
2. Dilute with   <u>4380</u> mg of lactose
   to make   4500 mg of dilution
3. Weigh $\frac{1}{30}$ of dilution, or 150 mg of dilution, which will contain 4 mg of atropine sulfate, *answer.*

Proof: $\dfrac{4500 \text{ mg (dilution)}}{150 \text{ mg (dilution)}} = \dfrac{120 \text{ mg (atropine sulfate)}}{x \text{ mg (atropine sulfate)}}$

      = 4 mg, *answer.*

In this example, the weight of the aliquot was arbitrarily set as 150 mg, which exceeds the weight of the multiple quantity, as it preferably should. If 120 mg had been set as the aliquot, the multiple quantity should have been diluted with 3480 mg of lactose to get 3600 mg of dilution, and the aliquot of 120 mg would have contained 4 mg of atropine sulfate.

A torsion prescription balance has a sensitivity requirement of 6.5 milligrams. Explain how you would weigh 15 milligrams of atropine sulfate with an accuracy of ± 5%, using lactose as the diluent.

Because 6.5 milligrams is the potential balance error, 130 milligrams (20 × 6.5 milligrams) is the smallest amount that should be weighed to achieve the required accuracy.

If **10** is chosen as the multiple, and if 130 milligrams is set as the weight of the aliquot, then:

1. Weigh **10** × 15 mg or   150 mg of atropine sulfate
2. Dilute with   <u>1150</u> mg of lactose
   to make   1300 mg of dilution
3. Weigh $\frac{1}{10}$ of dilution, or 130 mg, which will contain 15 mg of atropine sulfate, *answer.*

> **NOTE: It is important for the student to recognize that answers to aliquot calculations may vary, but still be correct, depending on the multiple factors arbitrarily chosen for use.**

Measuring Volume by the Aliquot Method

The aliquot method of measuring volume, which is identical in principle to the aliquot method of weighing, may be used when relatively small volumes must be measured with great precision:

   Step 1. Select a multiple of the desired quantity that can be measured with the required precision.
   Step 2. Dilute the multiple quantity with a compatible diluent (usually a solvent for the liquid to be measured) to an amount evenly divisible by the multiple selected.
   Step 3. Measure the aliquot of the dilution that contains the quantity originally desired.

Examples:

A formula calls for 0.5 milliliter of hydrochloric acid. Using a 10-milliliter graduate calibrated from 2 to 10 milliliters in 1-milliliter divisions, explain how you would obtain the desired quantity of hydrochloric acid by the aliquot method.

If **4** is chosen as the multiple, and if 2 milliliters is set as the volume of the aliquot, then:

1. Measure **4** × 0.5 mL, or   2 mL of the acid
2. Dilute with   <u>6 mL</u> of water
    to make   8 mL of dilution
3. Measure ¼ of dilution, or 2 mL of dilution, which will contain 0.5 mL of hydrochloric acid, *answer.*

A prescription calls for 0.2 mL of clove oil. Using a 5-mL graduate calibrated in units of 0.5 mL, how would you obtain the required amount of clove oil using the aliquot method and alcohol as the diluent?

If **5** is chosen as the multiple, then:

1. Measure **5** × 0.2 mL, or   1 mL of clove oil
2. Dilute with   <u>4 mL</u> of alcohol
    to make   5 mL of dilution
3. Measure ⅕ of the dilution, or 1 mL, which contains 0.2 mL of clove oil, *answer.*

Least Weighable Quantity Method of Weighing

This method may be used as an alternative to the aliquot method of weighing to obtain small quantities of a drug substance.

After determining the quantity of drug substance that is desired and the smallest quantity that can be weighed on the balance with the desired degree of accuracy, the procedure is as follows:

Step 1. Weigh an amount of the drug substance that is *equal to or greater than* the least weighable quantity.

CALCULATIONS CAPSULE

Weighing Accuracy

- The sensitivity requirement (SR) of a balance must be known or determined. An SR of 6 mg is usual.

- An error in weighing of ± 5% or less is acceptable.

- The smallest quantity that should be weighed on a prescription balance is determined by the equation:

$$\frac{100\% \times Sensitivity\ Requirement\ (mg)}{Acceptable\ Error\ (\%)} = Smallest\ Quantity\ (mg)$$

That quantity is usually about 120 mg.

- To weigh smaller quantities, an electronic balance or the aliquot method of weighing should be used.

Step 2. Dilute the drug substance with a calculated quantity of inert diluent such that a predetermined quantity of the drug-diluent mixture will contain the desired quantity of drug.

Example:

If 20 milligrams of a drug substance are needed to fill a prescription, explain how you would obtain this amount of drug with an accuracy of ± 5% using a balance with an SR of 6 milligrams. Use lactose as the diluent.

In the example, 20 milligrams is the amount of drug substance needed. The least weighable quantity would be 120 milligrams. The amount of drug substance to be weighed, therefore, must be equal to or greater than 120 milligrams. In solving the problem, 120 milligrams of drug substance is weighed. In calculating the amount of diluent to use, a predetermined quantity of drug-diluent mixture must be selected to contain the desired 20 milligrams of drug substance. The quantity selected must be greater than 120 milligrams because the drug-diluent mixture must be obtained accurately through weighing on the balance. An amount of 150 milligrams may be arbitrarily selected. The total amount of diluent to use may then be determined through the calculation of the following proportion:

$$\frac{20 \text{ mg (drug needed for } \textrm{R})}{150 \text{ mg (drug} - \text{diluent mixture to use in } \textrm{R})} = \frac{120 \text{ mg (total drug substance weighed)}}{x \text{ mg (total amount of drug-diluent mixture prepared)}}$$

x = 900 mg of the drug-diluent mixture to prepare
Hence, 900 mg – 120 mg = 780 mg of diluent (lactose) to use, *answer.*

It should be noted that in this procedure, each weighing, including that of the drug substance, the diluent, and the drug-diluent mixture, must be determined to be equal to or greater than the least weighable quantity as determined for the balance used and accuracy desired.

Percentage of Error

Because measurements in the community pharmacy are never *absolutely* accurate, it is important for the pharmacist to recognize the limitations of the instruments used and the magnitude of the errors that may be incurred. When a pharmacist measures a volume of liquid or weighs a material, two quantities become important: (1) the *apparent* weight or volume measured, and (2) the possible excess or deficiency in the actual quantity obtained.

Percentage of error may be defined as *the maximum potential error multiplied by 100 and divided by the quantity desired.* The calculation may be formulated as follows:

$$\frac{\text{Error} \times 100\%}{\text{Quantity desired}} = \text{Percentage of error}$$

Calculating Percentage of Error in Volumetric Measurement

The percentage of error in a measurement of volume may be calculated from the above equation, relating the volume in error (determined through devices of greater precision) to the volume desired (or apparently measured).

Example:

Using a graduated cylinder, a pharmacist measured 30 milliliters of a liquid. On subsequent examination, using a narrow-gauge burette, it was determined that the pharmacist had actually measured 32 milliliters. What was the percentage of error in the original measurement?

32 milliliters − 30 milliliters = 2 milliliters, the volume of error

$$\frac{2 \text{ mL} \times 100\%}{30 \text{ mL}} = 6.7\%, \ answer.$$

Calculating Percentage of Error in Weighing

The various scales and balances used in pharmaceutical weighing have ascribed to them different degrees of precision. As described previously in this chapter, knowledge of the *sensitivity requirement* of the balance being used is critical in weighing to a specified degree of accuracy. The sensitivity requirement of a balance may be used to determine the percentage of error in a given weighing.

Examples:

When the maximum potential error is ± 4 milligrams in a total of 100 milligrams, what is the percentage of error?

$$\frac{4 \text{ mg} \times 100\%}{100 \text{ mg}} = 4\%, \ answer.$$

A prescription calls for 800 milligrams of a substance. After weighing this amount on a balance, the pharmacist decides to check by weighing it again on a more sensitive balance, which registers only 750 milligrams. Because the first weighing was 50 milligrams short of the desired amount, what was the percentage of error?

$$\frac{50 \text{ mg} \times 100\%}{800 \text{ mg}} = 6.25\%, \ answer.$$

CASE IN POINT 3.1 A pharmacist is asked to compound the following formula for the preparation of 100 capsules:[2]

Estriol	200 mg
Estrone	25 mg
Estradiol	25 mg
Methocel E4M	10 g
Lactose	23.75 g

Using a balance that has an SR of 6 mg, the aliquot method of weighing, lactose as the diluent, and an error in weighing of 4%, show, by calculations, how the correct quantity of estrone can be obtained to accurately compound the formula.

CASE IN POINT 3.2 A physician prescribed 25 4-mg capsules of a drug for a special needs patient, knowing that the dose prescribed was considered "subtherapeutic." The lowest strength commercially available tablets contain 25 mg.

The pharmacist decided to select the minimum required number of 25-mg tablets (4 tablets); reduce them to a powder with a mortar and pestle; weigh the powder (280 mg); and continue the process using the aliquot method. She called upon her pharmacy student intern to calculate (a) the minimum quantity of lactose (diluent) to use in preparing the crushed tablet-diluent mixture and (b) the quantity of the mixture to use to fill each capsule.

The prescription balance had a SR of 6 mg and a weighing error of 5% was acceptable.

Show your calculations for (a) and (b), and (c) prove that your answer to (b) is correct by demonstrating that each capsule would indeed contain 4 mg of drug.

PRACTICE PROBLEMS

Calculations of Aliquot Parts by Weighing

1. A prescription calls for 50 milligrams of chlorpheniramine maleate. Using a prescription balance with a sensitivity requirement of 6 milligrams, explain how you would obtain the required amount of chlorpheniramine maleate with an error not greater than 5%.

2. A prescription balance has a sensitivity requirement of 0.006 gram. Explain how you would weigh 0.012 gram of a drug with an error not greater than 5%, using lactose as the diluent.

3. A torsion prescription balance has a sensitivity requirement of 4 milligrams. Explain how you would weigh 5 milligrams of hydromorphone hydrochloride with an error not greater than 5%. Use lactose as the diluent.

4. A torsion prescription balance has a sensitivity requirement of 0.004 gram. Explain how you would weigh 0.008 gram of a substance with an error not greater than 5%.

5. A prescription balance has a sensitivity requirement of 6.5 milligrams. Explain how you would weigh 20 milligrams of a substance with an error not greater than 2%.

Calculations of Aliquot Parts by Measuring Volume

6. ℞ Sodium Citrate   5 g
     Tartar Emetic   0.015 g
     Cherry Syrup ad   120 mL

   Using a balance with a sensitivity of 4 mg, an acceptable weighing error of 5% and cherry syrup as the solvent for tartar emetic, how could you obtain the correct quantity of tartar emetic to fill the prescription?

7. A formula calls for 0.6 milliliter of a coloring solution. Using a 10-milliliter graduate calibrated from 2 to 10 milliliters in 1-milliliter units, how could you obtain the desired quantity of the coloring solution by the aliquot method? Use water as the diluent.

8. Using a 10-milliliter graduate calibrated in 1-milliliter units, explain how you would measure 1.25 milliliters of a dye solution by the aliquot method. Use water as the diluent.

9. The formula for 100 milliliters of pentobarbital sodium elixir calls for 0.75 milliliter of orange oil. Using alcohol as a diluent and a 10-milliliter graduate calibrated in 1-milliliter units, how could you obtain the desired quantity of orange oil?

Calculations of Percentage of Error

10. A pharmacist attempts to weigh 120 milligrams of codeine sulfate on a balance with a sensitivity requirement of 6 milligrams. Calculate the maximum potential error in terms of percentage.

11. In compounding a prescription, a pharmacist weighed 0.05 gram of a substance on a balance insensitive to quantities smaller than 0.004 gram. What was the maximum potential error in terms of percentage?

12. A pharmacist weighed 475 milligrams of a substance on a balance of dubious accuracy. When checked on a balance of high accuracy, the weight was found to be 445 milligrams. Calculate the percentage of error in the first weighing.

13. A 10-milliliter graduate weighs 42.745 grams. When 5 milliliters of distilled water are measured in it, the combined weight of graduate and water is 47.675 grams. By definition, 5 milliliters of water should weigh 5 grams. Calculate the weight of the measured water and express any deviation from 5 grams as percentage of error.

14. A graduate weighs 35.825 grams. When 10 milliliters of water are measured in it, the weight of the graduate and water is 45.835 grams. Calculate the weight of the water and express any deviation from 10 grams as percentage of error.

15. A pharmacist attempts to weigh 0.375 gram of morphine sulfate on a balance of dubious accuracy. When checked on a highly accurate balance, the weight is found to be 0.400 gram. Calculate the percentage of error in the first weighing.

CALCQUIZ

3.A. A pharmacist receives a prescription for ear drops, calling for 0.05 mL of glacial acetic acid, 2 mL of glycerin, and 8 mL of purified water. Using a 10-mL graduated cylinder calibrated in 0.5-mL units, explain how the required quantity of glacial acetic acid could be obtained.

3.B. A pharmacist quizzes a pharmacy intern on the aliquot method in the preparation of 12 capsules each to contain 80 mg of morphine sulfate and 3.2 mg of naltrexone hydrochloride. Lactose is to be used as a diluent, a prescription balance with a sensitivity of 6 mg is proposed, and a 4% error is acceptable. Provide the relevant calculations.

3.C. The aliquot method was used to obtain 8 mg of a drug with a prescription balance having a sensitivity of 6 mg. A weighing error of 5% was accepted. If 140 mg of the drug were weighed, added to 2.1 g of lactose, and 120 mg of the mixture used to provide the required quantity of drug, were the calculations correct or incorrect?

3.D. In preparing a zinc oxide ointment, 28.35 g of zinc oxide were used rather than the correct quantity, 31.1 g. What percentage error was incurred?

ANSWERS TO "CASE IN POINT" AND PRACTICE PROBLEMS

Case in Point 3.1

The smallest quantity that should be weighed on the balance:

$$\frac{100\% \times 6 \text{ mg}}{4\%} = 150 \text{ mg}$$

Quantity desired (estrone): 25 mg
Multiple factor selected: 6
Aliquot portion selected: 150 mg

Estrone (25 × 6)	150 mg
Lactose	750 mg
Aliquot mixture	900 mg
Aliquot portion (900 mg ÷ 6)	150 mg of mixture will provide 25 mg estrone, *answer*

Case in Point 3.2

The smallest quantity that should be weighed on the balance:

$$\frac{100\% \times 6 \text{ mg}}{5\%} = 120 \text{ mg}$$

(a) Quantity of mixture required to prepare 25 capsules each containing the weighable quantity of 120 mg:

120 mg × 25 (capsules) = 3000 mg

Quantity of lactose required equals the quantity of mixture required less the weight of the crushed tablets:

3000 mg – 280 mg = 2720 mg or 2.72 g of lactose required, *answer*.

(b) Quantity of mixture to fill each capsule:

3000 mg ÷ 25 (capsules) = 120 mg, *answer*.

(c) Proof of 4 mg of drug per capsule:
Amount of drug in mixture:

4 mg (per tablet) × 25 (tablets) = 100 mg

Amount of drug per capsule:

100 mg ÷ 25 (capsules) = 4 mg, *answer*.

or,

$$\frac{100 \text{ mg } (drug)}{3000 \text{ mg } (mixture)} = \frac{x}{120 \text{ mg } (mixture)}$$
= 4 mg, *answer*.

Practice Problems

Aliquot Parts by Weighing

1. Weigh — 150 mg chlorpheniramine maleate
   Dilute with — 450 mg
   to make — 600 mg
   Weigh — 200 mg

2. Weigh — 120 mg drug
   Dilute with — 1380 mg
   to make — 1500 mg
   Weigh — 150 mg

3. Weigh — 80 mg hydromorphone hydrochloride
   Dilute with — 1520 mg
   to make — 1600 mg
   Weigh — 100 mg

4. Weigh — 160 mg
   Dilute with — 3840 mg
   to make — 4000 mg
   Weigh — 200 mg

5. Weigh — 400 mg
   Dilute with — 7600 mg
   to make — 8000 mg
   Weigh — 400 mg

Aliquot Parts by Measuring Volume

6. Weigh — 90 mg
   Dilute to — 12 mL
   Measure — 2 mL

7. Measure — 3 mL
   Dilute to — 10 mL
   Measure — 2 mL

8. Measure   5 mL
    Dilute to   8 mL
    Measure   2 mL

9. Measure   3 mL orange oil
    Dilute to   8 mL
    Measure   2 mL

Percentage of Error

10. 5%
11. 8%
12. 6.32%
13. 1.4%
14. 0.1%
15. 6.67%

References

1. Prescription balances and volumetric apparatus. *United States Pharmacopeia, 32—National Formulary, 27.* Rockville, MD: United States Pharmacopeial Convention, 2009;1:691–692.
2. Hormone replacement therapy. *Secundum Artem* 8(1):4. Available at: http://paddocklabs.com. Accessed June 6, 2012.

Interpretation of Prescriptions and Medication Orders

4

Objectives

Upon successful completion of this chapter, the student will be able to:

- Demonstrate an understanding of the format and components of a typical prescription.
- Demonstrate an understanding of the format and components of a typical institutional medication order.
- Interpret correctly standard abbreviations and symbols used on prescriptions and medication orders.
- Apply calculations to indicate medication adherence.

By definition, a *prescription* is an order for medication issued by a physician, dentist, or other properly licensed medical practitioner. A prescription designates a specific medication and dosage to be prepared and dispensed by a pharmacist and administered to a particular patient.

A prescription is usually written on preprinted forms containing the traditional symbol ℞ (meaning "recipe," "take thou," or "you take"), name, address, telephone number, and other pertinent information regarding the physician or other prescriber. In addition, blank spaces are used by the prescriber to provide information about the patient, the medication desired, and the directions for use. The information generally found on a completed prescription is shown in Figure 4.1. A prescription written by a veterinarian generally includes the animal species and/or the pet's name and the name of the owner.

A written prescription may be presented at the pharmacy by the patient or caregiver, or it may be transmitted from the prescriber by telephone, FAX, or computer (e-prescription).

In hospitals and other institutions, the forms are somewhat different and are referred to as *medication orders*. A typical medication order sheet is shown in Figure 4.2.

A prescription or medication order for an infant, child, or an elderly person may also include the age, weight, and/or body surface area (BSA) of the patient (as discussed in Chapter 8). This information is sometimes necessary in calculating the appropriate medication dosage. An example of a prescription written for a pediatric patient is shown in Figure 4.3.

It is important to recognize two broad categories of prescriptions: (1) those written for a single component or prefabricated product and *not requiring compounding* or admixture by the pharmacist, and (2) those written for more than a single component and *requiring compounding.*[a] A prescription may include the chemical or nonproprietary (generic) name of

---

[a]The extemporaneous compounding of prescriptions is an activity for which pharmacists are uniquely qualified by virtue of their education, training, and experience. By definition, *pharmacy compounding* involves the mixing, assembling, packaging, and labeling of a medication on receipt of a prescription order for a specific patient. In addition to the compounding of individual prescriptions as received, guidelines of the Food and Drug Administration permit the advance preparation of very limited quantities of compounded products *in anticipation* of prescriptions for specific patients, based on regularly observed prescribing patterns. Unless licensed as a manufacturer, however, pharmacies may not engage in the large-scale production or *manufacturing* of drugs for other pharmacies or for other entities for distribution or resale.[1]

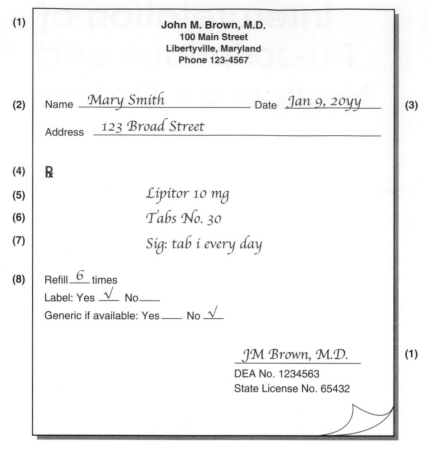

▼ FIGURE 4.1 Components of a typical prescription. Parts labeled are as follows:
(1) Prescriber information and signature
(2) Patient information
(3) Date prescription was written
(4) ℞ symbol (the Superscription), meaning "take thou," "you take," or "recipe"
(5) Medication prescribed (the Inscription)
(6) Dispensing instructions to the pharmacist (the Subscription)
(7) Directions to the patient (the Signa)
(8) Special instructions. It is important to note that for any Medicaid or Medicare prescription and according to individual state laws, a handwritten language by the prescriber, such as "Brand necessary," may be required to disallow generic substitution.
NOTE: When filling the prescription, the pharmacist adds a prescription number for identification.

the substance or the manufacturer's brand or trademark name (shown in all capital letters in this text). Prescriptions requiring compounding contain the quantities of each ingredient required. Medications are prepared into various types of *dosage forms* (e.g., *tablets, syrups, injections*) and *drug delivery systems* (e.g., *transdermal patches*) to ensure that the medication is administered accurately and appropriately. Examples are shown for prescriptions calling for trade-name products (Fig. 4.1 and Fig. 4.3), a generic drug (Fig. 4.4), and compounding (Fig. 4.5). Definitions and descriptions of dosage forms and drug delivery systems are presented in Appendix B.

CITY HOSPITAL
Athens, GA 30600

PATIENT NAME:	Thompson, Linda
ADDRESS:	2345 Oak Circle
CITY, STATE:	Athens, GA
AGE/SEX:	35y/Female
PHYSICIAN:	J. Hardmer
HOSP.NO:	900612345
SERVICE:	Medicine
ROOM:	220 East

PHYSICIAN'S ORDER

DATE	TIME	ORDERS
02/01/yy	1200	1. Propranolol 40 mg po QID
		2. Furosemide 20 mg po q AM
		3. Flurazepam 30 mg at HS prn sleep
		4. D-5-W + 20 mEq kcl/L at 84 mL/hr
		Hardmer, MD

Unless "No substitution permitted" is clearly written after the order, a generic or therapeutic equivalent drug may be dispensed according to the Formulary policies of this hospital.

▼ FIGURE 4.2 Typical hospital medication order sheet.

Mary M. Brown, M.D.
Pediatric Clinic
110 Main Street
Libertyville, Maryland
Phone 456-1234

Name _Suzie Smith_____ Age _5___ Weight _39.4_ lb

Address _123 Broad Street____ Date _Jan 9, 20yy___

℞   *Omnicef Oral Suspension*
     125 mg/5 mL
     Disp. 100 mL
     Give 14 mg/kg/day x 10 days

   Sig: _____ *tsp q 12 h*

Refill _0_ times
Label: Yes _✓_ No ___
Generic if available: Yes ___ No _✓_

                    Mary Brown, M.D.
                    DEA No. MB5555555
                    State License No. 23456

▼ FIGURE 4.3 Example of a prescription for a pediatric patient.

John M. Brown, M.D.
100 Main Street
Libertyville, Maryland
Phone 123-4567

Name _Brad Smith_   Date _Jan 9, 20yy_

Address _123 Broad Street_

RX 1234576

℞

  Amoxicillin 250 mg/5 mL
  Disp. 100 mL
  Sig: two tsp. every 12 hours
  until gone

Refill _0_ times
Label: Yes _✓_ No ___
Generic if available: Yes ___ No ___

  JM Brown, M.D.
  DEA No. CB1234563
  State License No. 65432

▼ FIGURE 4.4 Example of a prescription written for a generic drug.

Tamper-Resistant Prescription Pads

To prevent the unauthorized copying, modification, or counterfeiting of prescriptions, *tamper-resistant prescription pads* have been developed. Their use is mandated for hand-written prescriptions for outpatient drugs covered by Medicaid.[2,3] The tamper-resistant qualities of these prescription forms is accomplished through the use of security paper, erase-resistant paper, thermochromatic ink (which results in the appearance of the word "VOID" on photocopies), and/or imbedded holograms.

e-prescribing/e-prescriptions

Electronic prescribing (e-prescribing) is the computer-to-computer transfer of prescription information between authorized prescribers, pharmacies, intermediaries, and payers under nationally accepted standards.[4] In the inpatient or outpatient setting, a medication order, for a patient is entered into an automated data entry system as a personal computer or a hand-held device loaded with *e-prescribing* software and sent to a pharmacy as an *e-prescription*. When received, a pharmacist prints out the prescription, which appears as the illustration shown in Figure 4.6.

Among the advantages cited for *e-prescriptions* over traditional paper prescriptions are: reduced errors due to prescription legibility; concurrent software screens for drug interactions; reduced incidence of altered or forged prescriptions; efficiency for both prescriber and pharmacist; and, convenience to the patient, whose prescription would likely be ready for pick-up upon arrival at the pharmacy.[5,6]

```
                        John M. Brown, M.D.
                           100 Main Street
                        Libertyville, Maryland
                          Phone 123-4567


     Name  Neil Smith                    Date  Jan 9, 20yy

     Address  123 Broad Street


     R      Metoclopramide HCL      10 g
            Methylparaben           50 mg
            Propylparaben           20 mg
            Sodium Chloride         800 mg
            Purified Water, qs ad   100 mL

            M. ft. nasal spray

            Sig: Nasal spray for chemotherapy-
            induced emesis. Use as directed.
            Discard after 60 days.

     Refill  0  times
     Label: Yes  √  No  ____
     Generic if available: Yes ____ No ____

                                JM Brown, M.D.
                                _____
                                DEA No. CB1234563
                                State License No. 65432
```

▼ FIGURE 4.5 Example of a prescription requiring compounding.

Hospital and Other Institutional Medication Order Forms

As noted previously, a typical *medication order form* used in the hospital setting is shown in Figure 4.2. In addition, other forms may be used within a hospital by specialized units such as infectious disease, cardiac care, pediatrics, obstetrics, orthopedics, and others.[7] Drug-specific forms also may be used, as for heparin dosing, electrolyte infusions, and morphine sulfate in patient-controlled anesthesia. An example of the latter is shown in Figure 4.7.

Many different types of health care institutions, as acute care facilities, outpatient clinics, intermediate- and long-term care facilities (Fig. 4.8), cancer treatment centers, and a host of others utilize medication order forms designed to meet their specific requirements.

Military Time

Military time is used not only in the military but in civilian life as well, such as in hospitals, law enforcement, and emergency services. Its use provides an unambiguous expression of time. In health care institutions, military time may be used to record the time of a patient's admission, when a medication was administered, the time of surgery, and so forth.

```
┌─────────────────────────────────────────────────────────────┐
│                    XYZ PHARMACY SYSTEM                         │
│           Electronically Transmitted to Smith Pharmacy        │
│                      1234 Broad Street                        │
│                      Anytown, State, Zip                      │
│       Date: 10/20/20yy                                         │
│       Rx # 9876543        ID # 11223344                       │
│                                                               │
│                      Patient Information                      │
│       Last Name:   Jones                                      │
│       First Name:  Mary                                       │
│       DOB:         10/18/YY Phone: (XXX)-888-7777             │
│       Sex:         F                                          │
│       Address:     567 King Street                            │
│                    Anytown, State, Zip                        │
│                                                               │
│                  Drug, SIG, and Refill Information            │
│       Drug Name: Gabapentin                                   │
│       Strength:    100 mg                                     │
│       Quantity:    60        Dose Form: capsules              │
│       SIG:         Take 1 capsule at bedtime                  │
│       Refills:     6                                          │
│       Label:       yes                                        │
│                                                               │
│       Prescriber Information                                   │
│       Last Name: Brown                                        │
│       First Name: James M                                     │
│       Address:    100 Main Street                             │
│                   Anytown, State, Zip                         │
│       DEA:        CB1234XXX                                   │
│       NPI:        9876543XXX                                  │
└─────────────────────────────────────────────────────────────┘
```

▼ FIGURE 4.6 Illustration of an electronically transmitted prescription as received by a pharmacy. DEA stands for Drug Enforcement Administration and NPI for National Provider Identifier.

Table 4.1 compares the expressions of military time and regular time. Military time is verbalized, as for example "twenty-three hundred hours." Colons may be used to separate hours and minutes, as 1331 or 13:31 hours (31 minutes past 1 o'clock in the afternoon) and when desired seconds, as 1331:42 or 13:31:42.

Range of Prescription and Medication Order Calculations

This chapter introduces the form, content, and interpretation of prescriptions and institutional medication orders and, as such, *provides the framework for the majority of the calculations that follow in this text, including calculations of the following:*

- *Doses:* including the quantity of a prescribed dose, the total number of doses prescribed, and the number of days the prescribed medication will last.
- *Medication Adherence*: the patient's or caregiver's adherence or compliance with all aspects of prescribed medication treatment, as dose, dosing frequency, and schedule.
- *Drug concentration:* the quantity of an active therapeutic ingredient to use to achieve the desired drug concentration.

City Hospital
Patient Controlled Anesthesia (PCA) Orders
<u>MORPHINE SULFATE INJECTION, 1 mg/mL</u>

Patient Information (Label)

Physician:

Date: Time:

1. Mode (check) ☐PCA ☐Continuous ☐PCA & Continuous	
	DOSING GUIDELINES
2. PCA Dose = _____ mL (mg)	1 mL (1 mg)
3. Period between Injections = _____ minutes	10 minutes
4. Basal (Continuous) Rate = _____ mL (mg)/hr	1 mL (1 mg)/hr
5. One-Hour Limit = _____ mL (mg)	7 mL (7 mg)
6. Initial Loading Dose = _____ mL (mg)	2-5 mL (2-5 mg)

7. Additional Instructions:

Physician's Signature _____

▼ FIGURE 4.7 Example of a hospital form for prescribing a specific drug treatment: Patient-Controlled Anesthesia. *(Adapted with permission from www.hospital-forms.com.[6])*

MEDICATION ORDER FORM
CITY NURSING HOME
Physician's Orders

Attending Physician:			Order Number: (preprinted)		
Resident's Name:				Room Number:	

DRUG	QUANTITY	DOSE AND ROUTE	FREQUENCY	DIAGNOSIS	ADMINISTRATION TIMES
1.					____AM ____PM ____AM ____PM
2.					____AM ____PM ____AM ____PM
3.					____AM ____PM ____AM ____PM
4.					____AM ____PM ____AM ____PM

Physician's Signature:	Time/Date Ordered:
Signature of Nurse Receiving Order:	Time/Date Ordered:
Ordered from Pharmacy, Time/Date:	Received from Pharmacy, Time/Date:

▼ FIGURE 4.8 Example of a nursing home medication order form.

Table 4.1 ▼ COMPARATIVE EXPRESSIONS OF REGULAR AND MILITARY TIME

REGULAR TIME	MILITARY TIME	REGULAR TIME	MILITARY TIME
Midnight	0000	Noon	1200
1:00 A.M.	0100	1:00 P.M.	1300
2:00 A.M.	0200	2:00 P.M.	1400
3:00 A.M.	0300	3:00 P.M.	1500
4:00 A.M.	0400	4:00 P.M.	1600
5:00 A.M.	0500	5:00 P.M.	1700
6:00 A.M.	0600	6:00 P.M.	1800
7:00 A.M.	0700	7:00 P.M.	1900
8:00 A.M.	0800	8:00 P.M.	2000
9:00 A.M.	0900	9:00 P.M.	2100
10:00 A.M.	1000	10:00 P.M.	2200
11:00 A.M.	1100	11:00 P.M.	2300

- *Rate of drug administration:* the quantity of drug administered per unit of time to meet prescribed dosing schedule (e.g., mg/min, drops/minute, or mL/hr for the administration of an intravenous fluid).
- *Compounding:* the quantities of active and inactive ingredients to use in the compounding of a prescription or medication order.
- *Chemical-physical factors:* including calculations to make solutions isotonic, iso-osmotic, equimolar, or buffered.
- *Pharmacoeconomics:* including medication costs, cost-benefit analysis, cost-effectiveness analysis, alternative treatment plans, and medication pricing.

The quantities of ingredients designated on prescriptions and medication orders are almost always expressed in SI metric units. Occasionally, units of the Apothecaries' system may be used (see Appendix A).

In prescription writing, the decimal point may be replaced by a vertical line to designate whole or decimal fractions of grams or milliliters. If the designations "g" or "mL" are absent, as in the second illustration which follows, they are presumed. Unless otherwise noted, solid materials are presumed to be indicated in grams and liquids in milliliters.

Illustration of prescriptions written in SI metric units:

℞ Acetylsalicylic Acid   4 g
Phenacetin   0.8 g
Codeine Sulfate   0.5 g
Mix and make capsules no. 20
Sig. One capsule every 4 hours.

℞ Dextromethorphan   0 | 18
Guaifenesin Syrup   1 | 2
Alcohol   2 | 1
Flavored Syrup ad   60 |
Sig. 5 mL as needed for cough.

Prescription and Medication Order Accuracy and Verification

It is the responsibility of the pharmacist to ensure that each prescription and medication order received is correct in its form and content; is appropriate for the patient being treated; and is subsequently filled, labeled, dispensed, and administered accurately. In essence, each medication should be:

- therapeutically appropriate for the patient;
- prescribed at the correct dose;
- dispensed in the correct strength and dosage form;
- correctly labeled with complete instructions for the patient or caregiver; and
- for the patient in a hospital or other health care facility, each medication must be administered to the correct patient, at the correct time, and by the correct rate and route of administration.

Medication verification is the term used when there is a process in place to assure the above bullet points. It is performed initially through the careful reading, filling (including calculations), checking, and dispensing of the prescription or medication order. The process often is enhanced by technologies, as the computer-matching of a drug package barcode with the prescription order and/or by matching the drug's barcode to a patient's coded wrist band in a patient-care facility (termed *bedside medication verification*).

Errors and Omissions

To ensure such accuracy, the pharmacist is obliged to review each prescription and medication order in a step-by-step manner to detect errors and omissions.

Among the items that the pharmacist should check for the correct reading and interpretation of a prescription or medication order are:

- prescriber information, including address and telephone number, Drug Enforcement Administration (DEA) number (for authority to prescribe schedule drugs including narcotics), state license number and/or the National Provider Identifier (NPI), an identification number for participating health care providers, and signature;
- date of the order and its currency to the request for filling;
- patient identification information and, if pertinent to dose determination, the patient's age, weight, and/or other parameters;
- drug prescribed, including dose, preparation strength, dosage form, and quantity;
- clarity of any abbreviations, symbols, and/or units of measure;
- clarity and completeness of directions for use by the patient or caregiver;
- refill and/or generic substitution authorization;
- need for special labeling, such as expiration date, conditions for storage, and foods and/or other medications not to take concomitantly; and
- a listing of the ingredients and quantities for orders to be compounded.

Once the prescription or medication order is filled and the label prepared, before dispensing, the pharmacist should make certain of the following:

- The filled prescription or medication order contains the correct drug, strength, dosage form, and quantity. Placing a medication's indication (use) on the prescription label has been shown to be of benefit in understanding of the use of their medication for some patients, particularly older patients and those taking multiple medications.[8] The bar-coding of pharmaceutical products used in hospital settings is required by the

▼ FIGURE 4.9 Example of a Pharmaceutical Bar Code used in hospitals and other health-care settings for positive drug identification to reduce medication errors. *(Courtesy of Baxter Healthcare Corporation.)*

federal Food and Drug Administration (FDA) as an added protection to ensure accurate product dispensing and administration (see Fig. 4.9).

- The pharmacy-imprinted serial number on the label matches that on the order.
- The label has the name of the correct patient and physician; the correct drug name, quantity, and strength; the name or initials of the pharmacist who filled the order; and the number of refills remaining. Additional label information and/or auxiliary labels may be required.

It is important that the instructions for use by the patient be clearly understood. This may require that the pharmacist add words of clarity to the labeled instructions. For example, instead of "Take two tablets daily," the directions might state "Swallow one tablet with breakfast and another tablet with dinner." In addition, if the patient or caregiver has difficulty with the language, verbal reinforcement may be required.

Example:

Refer to the prescription shown in Figure 4.4 to identify any errors and/or omissions in the following prescription label.

Main Street Pharmacy
150 Main Street
Libertyville, Maryland
Phone 456-1432

℞ 1234576   Jan 10, 20yy
Brad Smith   Dr. J. M. Brown

Take 2 teaspoonfuls every 12 hours.

Ampicillin 250 mg/5 mL   100 mL
Refills: 0   Pharmacist: AB

Error: Drug name incorrect.
Omission: Directions incomplete.

Note: There would be a serious question of whether the patient received the correct medication.

Additional examples of errors and omissions are presented in the practice problems at the end of the chapter.

Use of Roman Numerals on Prescriptions

Roman numerals commonly are used in prescription writing to designate *quantities*, as the: (1) quantity of medication to be dispensed and/or (2) quantity of medication to be taken by the patient per dose.

The student may recall the eight letters of fixed values used in the Roman system:

ss	=	½	L or l	=	50
i or j	=	1	C or c	=	100
V or v	=	5	D or d	=	500
X or x	=	10	M or m	=	1000

The student also may recall that the following rules apply in the use of Roman numerals:

1. A letter repeated once or more, repeats its value (e.g., xx = 20; xxx = 30).
2. One or more letters placed *after* a letter of greater value *increases* the value of the greater letter (e.g., vi = 6; xij = 12; lx = 60).
3. A letter placed *before* a letter of greater value *decreases* the value of the greater letter (e.g., iv = 4; xl = 40).

Capital or lower case letters may be used. Dotting the lowercase "i" and/or placement of a horizontal line above the "i" with the dot atop serves to avoid misinterpretation. A "j" may be used as the final "i" in a sequence (e.g., viij).

When Roman numerals are used, the tradition of placing the numerals after the term or symbol generally is followed (e.g., capsules no. xxiv; fluidounces xij).

Use of Abbreviations and Symbols

The use of abbreviations is common on prescriptions and medication orders. Some are derived from the Latin through its historical use in medicine and pharmacy, whereas others have evolved through prescribers' use of writing shortcuts. A list of some of these abbreviations is presented in Table 4.2. Unfortunately, medication errors can result from the misuse, misinterpretation, and illegible writing of abbreviations, and through the use of *ad hoc*, or made-up, abbreviations. The use of a controlled vocabulary, a reduction in the use of abbreviations, care in the writing of decimal points, and the proper use of leading and terminal zeros have been urged to help reduce medication errors.[9–11] It should be emphasized that a misplaced or misread decimal point represents a minimum of a 10-fold error.

Among the specific recommendations to help reduce medication errors arising from poorly written, illegible, or misinterpreted prescriptions and medication orders are the following:[9–11]

- *A whole number should be shown without a decimal point and without a terminal zero (e.g., express 4 milligrams as 4 mg and not as 4.0 mg).*

Table 4.2 ▼ SELECTED ABBREVIATIONS, ACRONYMS, AND SYMBOLS USED IN PRESCRIPTIONS AND MEDICATION ORDERS[a,b]

ABBREVIATION (LATIN ORIGIN[c])	MEANING	ABBREVIATION (LATIN ORIGIN[c])	MEANING
Prescription Filling Directions		pt.	pint
		qt.	quart
aa. (*ana*)	of each	ss or $\overline{ss}$ (*semissem*)	one half
ad (*ad*)	up to; to make	**tbsp.**	tablespoonful
disp. (*dispensatur*)	dispense	**tsp.**	teaspoonful
div. (*dividatur*)	divide		
d.t.d. (*dentur tales doses*)	give of such doses	**Signa/Patient Instructions**	
ft (*fiat*)	make	**a.c.** (*ante cibos*)	before meals
M. (*mice*)	mix	ad lib. (*ad libitum*)	at pleasure, freely
No. (*numero*)	number	admin	administer
non rep. or NR (*non repatatur*)	do not repeat	A.M. (*ante meridiem*)	morning
q.s. (*quantum sufficit*)	a sufficient quantity	aq. (*aqua*)	water
		ATC	around the clock
q.s. ad (*quantum sufficiat ad*)	a sufficient quantity to make	**b.i.d.** (*bis in die*)	twice a day
		c or $\overline{c}$ (*cum*)	with
Sig. (*Signa*)	write (directions on label)	**d** (*die*)	day
		dil. (*dilutus*)	dilute
		et	and
Quantities and Measurement		**h. or hr.** (*hora*)	hour
BSA	body surface area	**h.s.** (*hora somni*)	at bedtime
cm³	cubic centimeter or milliliter (mL)	i.c. (*inter cibos*)	between meals
		min. (*minutum*)	minute
f or fl (*fluidus*)	fluid	m&n	morning and night
fl₃ or f₃[d]	fluid dram	N&V	nausea and vomiting
fl₃ss or f₃ss[d]	half-fluidounce	noct. (*nocte*)	night
g	gram	NPO (*non per os*)	nothing by month
gal	gallon	**p.c.** (*post cibos*)	after meals
gtt (*gutta*)	drop	**P.M.** (*post meridiem*)	afternoon; evening
I.U. or IU[b]	international unit(s)		
lb (*libra*)	pound	**p.o.** (*per os*)	by mouth (orally)
kg	kilogram	p.r.n. (*pro re nata*)	as needed
L	liter	q (*quaque*)	every
m² or M²	square meter	qAM	every morning
mcg	microgram	**q4h, q8h,** etc.	every __ hours
mEq	milliequivalent	**q.i.d.** (*quarter in die*)	four times a day
mg	milligram	rep. (*repetatur*)	repeat
mg/kg	milligrams (of drug) per kilogram (of body weight)	s (*sine*)	without
		s.i.d. (*semel in die*)	once a day
		s.o.s. (*si opus sit*)	if there is need; as needed
mg/m²	milligrams (of drug) per square meter (of body surface area)	**stat.** (*stamin*)	immediately
		t.i.d. (*ter in die*)	three times a day
MIU[b]	million international units	ut dict. (*ut dictum*)	as directed
mL	milliliter	wk.	week
mL/h	milliliters (of drug administered) per hour (as through intravenous administration)		
		Medications	
		APAP	acetaminophen
mOsm or mOsmol	milliosmoles	ASA	aspirin
oz.	ounce	AZT	zidovudine

Table 4.2 ▼ SELECTED ABBREVIATIONS, ACRONYMS, AND SYMBOLS USED IN PRESCRIPTIONS AND MEDICATION ORDERS[a,b]
(Continued)

ABBREVIATION (LATIN ORIGIN[c])	MEANING	ABBREVIATION (LATIN ORIGIN[c])	MEANING
EES	erythromycin ethylsuc-cinate	D5NS	dextrose 5% in normal saline (0.9% sodium chloride)
HC	hydrocortisone		
HCTZ	hydrochlorothiazide	D5W	dextrose 5% in water
MTX	methotrexate	D10W	dextrose 10% in water
NTG	nitroglycerin	elix.	elixir
Clinical		inj.	injection
		NS	normal saline
BM	bowel movement	½NS	half-strength normal saline
BP	blood pressure		
BS	blood sugar	**oint** or ungt. (*unguentum*)	ointment
CHD	coronary heart disease		
CHF	congestive heart failure	pulv. (*pulvis*)	powder
GERD	gastrointestinal reflux disease	RL, R/L or LR	Ringer's Lactate or Lactated Ringer's
GI	gastrointestinal	**sol.** (*solutio*)	solution
GFR	glomerular filtration rate	**supp.** (*suppositorium*)	suppository
GU	genitourinary	**susp.**	suspension
HA	headache	**syr.** (*syrupus*)	syrup
HBP	high blood pressure	**tab.** (*tabletta*)	tablet
HRT	hormone replacement therapy		
HT or HTN	hypertension	**Routes of Administration**	
IOP	intraocular pressure	CIVI	continuous (24 hour) intravenous infusion
MI	myocardial ischemia/infarction		
		ID	intradermal
OA	osteoarthritis	IM	intramuscular
Pt	patient	IT	intrathecal
SOB	shortness of breath	IV	intravenous
TPN	total parenteral nutrition	IVB	intravenous bolus
URI	upper respiratory infection	IV Drip	intravenous infusion
		IVP	intravenous push
UTI	urinary tract infection	IVPB	intravenous piggy back
Dosage Forms/Vehicles		NGT	nasogastric tube
amp.	ampul	**p.o.** or PO (*per os*)	by mouth
cap.	capsule	rect.	rectal or rectum
D5LR	dextrose 5% in lactated Ringer's	SL	sublingual
		SubQ or SC	subcutaneously
		Top.	topically
		V or PV	vaginally

[a]The abbreviations set in **boldface type** are considered most likely to appear on prescriptions. It is suggested that these be learned first.

[b]In practice, periods and/or capital letters may or may not be used with the abbreviations. Some abbreviations, acronyms, and symbols have medication-error risks associated with their use. Therefore, the Institute for Safe Medication Practices (ISMP) and the Joint Commission on Accreditation of Healthcare Organizations (JCAHO) have issued a list of items prohibited from use and others considered for prohibition (see text).[9] These designated items are not included in Table 4.2, with the exception of *hs, I.U., MIU, subQ, AZT,* and *HCTZ*, which are included for instructional purpose due to their remaining use in practice.

[c]Muldoon HC. *Pharmaceutical Latin.* 4th Ed. New York: John Wiley & Sons, 1952.

[d]A fluid dram is 1/8th of a fluid ounce (29.57 mL) or ≈ 3.69 mL; however, when the dram symbol is written in the *signa* portion of a prescription, the prescriber may intend the interpretation to be "teaspoonful." Similarly, when a half-ounce symbol is indicated in the *signa*, a "tablespoon" or 15 mL may be intended.

- *A quantity smaller than one should be shown with a zero preceding the decimal point (e.g., express two tenths of a milligram as 0.2 mg and not as .2 mg).*
- *Leave a space between a number and the unit (e.g., 10 mg and not 10mg).*
- *Use whole numbers when possible and not equivalent decimal fractions (e.g., use 100 mg and not 0.1 g).*
- *Use the full names of drugs and not abbreviations (e.g., use phenobarbital and not PB).*
- *Use USP designations for units of measure (e.g., for grams, use g and not Gm or gms; for milligrams, use mg and not mgs or mgm).*
- *Spell out "units" (e.g., use 100 units and not 100 u or 100 U since an illegible U may be misread as a zero, resulting in a 10-fold error, i.e., 1000). The abbreviation I.U., which stands for "International Units," should also be spelled out so it is not interpreted as I.V., meaning "intravenous."*
- *Certain abbreviations that could be mistaken for other abbreviations should be written out (e.g., write "right eye" or "left eye" rather than use o.d. or o.l., and spell out "right ear" and "left ear" rather than use a.d. or a.l.).*
- *Spell out "every day," rather than use q.d.; "every other day," rather than q.o.d; "four times a day," rather than q.i.d; and "three times a week," rather than t.i.w. to avoid misinterpretation.*
- *Avoid using d for "day" or "dose" because of the profound difference between terms, as in mg/kg/day versus mg/kg/dose.*
- *Integrate capital or "tall man" letters to distinguish between "look alike" drug names, such as AggreSTAT and AggreNOX; hydrOXYZINE and hydrALAZINE; and DIGoxin and DESoxyn.*
- *Amplify the prescriber's directions on the prescription label when needed for clarity (e.g., use "Swallow one (1) capsule with water in the morning" rather than "one cap in a.m.").*

The Institute for Safe Medication Practices (ISMP) regularly publishes a list of abbreviations, symbols, and dose designations that it recommends for consideration for discontinuance of use.[9]

The portions of the prescription presenting directions to the pharmacist (the Subscription) and the directions to the patient (the Signa) commonly contain abbreviated forms of English or Latin terms as well as Arabic and Roman numerals. The correct interpretation of these abbreviations and prescription notations plays an important part in pharmaceutical calculations and thus in the accurate filling and dispensing of medication.

Although described fully in Chapter 7, it should be noted here that when appearing in the Signa, the symbol ʒi, *5 mL*, and the abbreviation *tsp.* are each taken to mean "one teaspoonful," and the symbol ʒ ss, *15 mL*, and the abbreviation *tbsp.* are each taken to mean "one tablespoonful."

Examples of prescription directions to the pharmacist:
(a) *M. ft. ung.*
Mix and make an ointment.
(b) *Ft. sup. no xii*
Make 12 suppositories.
(c) *M. ft. cap. d.t.d. no. xxiv*
Mix and make capsules. Give 24 such doses.

Examples of prescription directions to the patient:
(a) *Caps. i. q.i.d. p.c. et h.s.*
Take one (1) capsule four (4) times a day after each meal and at bedtime.
(b) *gtt. ii rt.eye every a.m.*
Instill two (2) drops in the right eye every morning.
(c) *tab. ii stat tab. 1 q. 6 h. × 7 d.*
Take two (2) tablets immediately, then take one (1) tablet every 6 hours for 7 days.

CASE IN POINT 4.1 A pharmacist received the following prescription, which requires the correct interpretation of abbreviations prior to engaging in calculations, compounding, labeling, and dispensing.

℞

Lisinopril	
Hydrochlorothiazide aa.	10 mg
Calcium Phosphate	40 mg
Lactose q.s. ad	300 mg
M.ft. cap. i D.T.D. # 30	
Sig: cap. i AM a.c.	

(a) How many milligrams each of lisinopril and hydrochlorothiazide are required to fill the prescription?
(b) What is the weight of lactose required?
(c) Translate the label directions to the patient.

Medication Scheduling and Medication Adherence

Medication scheduling may be defined as the frequency (i.e., times per day) and duration (i.e., length of treatment) of a drug's prescribed or recommended use. Some medications, because of their physical, chemical, or biological characteristics or their dosage formulations, may be taken just once daily for optimum benefit, whereas other drug products must be taken two, three, four, or more times daily for the desired effect. Frequency of medication scheduling is also influenced by the patient's physical condition and the nature and severity of the illness or condition being treated. Some conditions, such as indigestion, may require a single dose of medication for correction. Other conditions, such as a systemic infection, may require multiple daily, around-the-clock dosing for 10 days or more. Long-term maintenance therapy for conditions such as diabetes and high blood pressure may require daily dosing for life.

For optimum benefit of the medications prescribed, it is incumbent on the patient to adhere to the prescribed dosage regimen.

Medication adherence (formerly referred to as *compliance*) indicates a patient's following of the instructions for taking the medication prescribed, including the correct dose, dosing frequency, and duration of treatment. *Medication nonadherence* is a patient's failure to adhere or comply with the instructions.

Patient nonadherence may result from a number of factors, including unclear or misunderstood directions, undesired side effects of the drug that discourage use, lack of patient confidence in the drug and/or prescriber, discontinued use because the patient feels better or worse, economic reasons based on the cost of the medication, absence of patient counseling and understanding of the need for and means of compliance, confusion over taking multiple medications, and other factors. Frequently, patients forget whether they have taken their medications. Special compliance aids are available to assist patients in their proper scheduling of medications. These devices include medication calendars, reminder charts, and special containers.

Patient nonadherence is not entirely the problem of ambulatory or noninstitutionalized patients. Patients in hospitals, nursing homes, and other inpatient settings are generally more compliant because of the efforts of health care personnel who are assigned the responsibility of issuing and administering medication on a prescribed schedule. Even in these settings, however, a scheduled dose of medication may be omitted or administered incorrectly or in an untimely fashion because of human error or oversight.

The consequences of patient nonadherence may include worsening of the condition, the requirement of additional and perhaps more expensive and extensive treatment methods or surgical procedures, otherwise unnecessary hospitalization, and increased total health care cost. Students interested in additional information on medication adherence are referred to other sources of information.[12–16]

Medication nonadherence has been measured in a number of ways, including by biological sample (i.e., determining medication blood levels), patient surveys, monitoring the on-time refilling of prescriptions, examining prescription drug-claim (insurance) data, and by other means.

Consider the following illustrations.

℞   Hydrochlorothiazide   50 mg
       Tablets No. XC
       Sig. i q AM for HBP

If the prescription was filled initially on April 15, on about what date should the patient return to have the prescription refilled?

Answer: 90 tablets, taken 1 per day, should last 90 days, or approximately 3 months, and the patient should return to the pharmacy on or shortly before July 15 of the same year.

℞   Penicillin V Potassium Oral Solution   125 mg/5 mL
       Disp. _____mL
       Sig. 5 mL q 6h ATC × 10 d

How many milliliters of medicine should be dispensed?

Answer: 5 mL times 4 (doses per day) equals 20 mL times 10 (days) equals 200 mL.

A pharmacist may calculate a patient's percent compliance rate as follows:

$$\% \text{ Compliance rate} = \frac{\text{Number of days supply of medication}}{\text{Number of days since last Rx refill}} \times 100$$

What is the percent compliance rate if a patient received a 30-day supply of medicine and returned in 45 days for a refill?

$$\% \text{ Compliance rate} = \frac{30 \text{ days}}{45 \text{ days}} \times 100 = 66.6\%, \textit{answer.}$$

In determining the patient's actual (rather than apparent) compliance rate, it is important to determine if the patient had available and used extra days' dosage from some previous filling of the prescription.

CASE IN POINT 4.2 A 72-year-old male who is diabetic is admitted to the emergency room with shortness of breath and general weakness. Tests reveal anemia, hypotension, atrial fibrillation, and coronary artery blockage. During 2 weeks of hospitalization, the patient receives intravenous infusions, oral medications, and blood transfusions; four cardiovascular stents are inserted; and the patient is discharged with the following prescriptions:

> PLAVIX (clopidogrel bisulfate) tablets, 75 mg, 1 tab q.d.
> ACTOS (pioglitazone hydrochloride) tablets, 15 mg, 1 tab q.d.
> PROTONIX (pantoprazole sodium) tablets, 40 mg, 1 tab b.i.d.
> ZOCOR (simvastatin) tablets 40 mg, 1 tab q.d. h.s.
> HUMULIN 70/30, inject 35 Units q.d. AM and 45 Units q.d. P.M.
> COREG (carvedilol) tablets, 3.125 mg 1 tab b.i.d. × 2 wk; then 6.25 mg 1 tab b.i.d.
> CORDARONE (amiodarone hydrochloride) tablets, 200 mg, 2 tabs b.i.d. × 7 d; then 1 tab b.i.d. × 7 d; then 1 tab q.d.
> CYMBALTA (duloxetine hydrochloride) capsules, 30 mg, 1 cap q.d. × 7 d; then 1 cap b.i.d.

(a) How many total tablets and capsules would the patient initially be taking daily?

(b) If HUMULIN contains 100 units per milliliter, how many milliliters would be administered each morning and each evening?

(c) How many CORDARONE tablets would constitute a 30-day supply?

(d) If 60 CYMBALTA capsules were initially dispensed and the patient requested a refill after 17 days, is *medication nonadherence* and thus the patient's well-being a reasonable concern? Show calculations.

PRACTICE PROBLEMS

1. Interpret each of the following *Subscriptions* (directions to the pharmacist) taken from prescriptions:

   (a) Disp. supp. rect. no. xii

   (b) M. ft. iso. sol. Disp. 120 mL.

   (c) M. et div. in pulv. no. xl

   (d) DTD vi. Non rep.

   (e) M. et ft. ung. Disp. 10 g

   (f) M. et ft. caps. DTD xlviii

   (g) M. et ft. susp. 1 g/tbsp. Disp. 60 mL.

   (h) Ft. cap. #1. DTD no.xxxvi N.R.

   (i) M. et ft. pulv. DTD #C

   (j) M. et ft. I.V. inj.

   (k) Label: hydrocortisone, 20 mg tabs.

2. Interpret each of the following *Signas* (directions to the patient) taken from prescriptions:

   (a) Gtt. ii each eye q. 4 h. p.r.n. pain.

   (b) Tbsp. i in ⅓ gl. aq. q. 6 h.

   (c) Appl. a.m. & p.m. for pain prn.

   (d) Gtt. iv right ear m. & n.

   (e) Tsp. i ex aq. q. 4 or 5 h. p.r.n. pain.

   (f) Appl. ung. left eye ad lib.

   (g) Caps i c̄ aq. h.s. N.R.

   (h) Gtt. v each ear 3 × d. s.o.s.

   (i) Tab. i sublingually, rep. p.r.n.

   (j) Instill gtt. ii each eye of neonate.

   (k) Dil. c̄ = vol. aq. and use as gargle q. 5 h.

(l) Cap. ii 1 h. prior to departure, then cap. i after 12 h.

(m) Tab i p.r.n. SOB

(n) Tab i qAM HBP

(o) Tab ii q 6h ATC UTI

(p) ℥ii 4 × d p.c. & h.s.

(q) ℥ss a.c. t.i.d.

(r) Add crushed tablet to pet's food s.i.d.

3. Interpret each of the following taken from medication orders:

(a) AMBIEN 10 mg p.o. qhs × 5 d

(b) 1000 mL D5W q. 8 h. IV $\bar{c}$ 20 mEq KC1 to every third bottle.

(c) Admin. Prochlorperazine 10 mg IM q. 3h. prn N&V

(d) Minocycline HCl susp. 1 tsp p.o. q.i.d. DC after 5 d.

(e) Propranolol HCl 10 mg p.o. t.i.d. a.c. & h.s.

(f) NPH U-100 insulin 40 Units subc every day A.M.

(g) Cefamandole nafate 250 mg IM q. 12 h.

(h) Potassium chloride 15 mEq p.o. b.i.d. p.c.

(i) Vincristine sulfate 1 mg/m² pt. BSA.

(j) Flurazepam 30 mg at HS prn sleep.

(k) D5W + 20 mEq KCl/L at 84 mL/ hour.

(l) 2.5 g/kg/day amino acids TPN.

(m) PROCRIT (epoetin alpha) stat. 150 units/kg subQ. 3 × wk. × 3–4 wks.

(n) MTX 2.5 mg tab t.i.d. 1 ×/wk.

(o) HCTZ tabs 12.5 mg q.d. AM

4. (a) If a 10-mL vial of insulin contains 100 units of insulin per milliliter, and a patient is to administer 20 units daily, how many days will the product last the patient? (b) If the patient returned to the pharmacy in exactly 7 weeks for another vial of insulin, was the patient compliant as indicated by the percent compliance rate?

5. A prescription is to be taken as follows: 1 tablet q.i.d. the first day; 1 tablet t.i.d. the second day; 1 tablet b.i.d. × 5 d; and 1 tablet q.d. thereafter. How many tablets should be dispensed to equal a 30-day supply?

6. In preparing the prescription in Figure 4.3, the pharmacist calculated and labeled the dose as "1 teaspoonful every 12 hours." Is this correct or in error?

7. Refer to Figure 4.1 and identify any errors or omissions in the following prescription label:

Patient: Mary Smith   Dr. JM Brown Date: Jan 9, 20yy Take 1 capsule every day in the morning Refills: 5

8. Refer to Figure 4.4 and identify any errors or omissions in the following prescription label:

Patient: Brad Smith   Dr. JM Brown Date: Jan 9, 20yy Take two (2) teaspoonfuls every twelve (12) hours until all of the medicine is gone Amoxicillin 250 mL/5 mL Refills: 0

9. Refer to Figure 4.5 and identify any errors or omissions in the following prescription label:

Patient: Brad Smith   Dr. JM Brown Date: Jan 9, 20yy Nasal spray for chemotherapy-induced emesis. Use as directed. Discard after 60 days. Metoclopramide HCl 10 g/100 mL Nasal Spray Refills: 0

10. Refer to Figure 4.2 and identify any errors or omissions in a transcribed order for the first three drugs in the medication order.

    (1) Propranolol, 40 mg orally every day

    (2) Flutamide, 20 mg orally every morning

    (3) Flurazepam, 30 mg at bedtime as needed for sleep

11. Refer to Figure 4.6 and identify any errors in the following prescription label:

Patient: Mary Jones   Dr. JM Brown
Date: Oct 20, 20yy
Swallow one (1) capsule at bedtime.
Gabapentin 100 mg
Rx: 9876543   Refills: 6

CALCQUIZ

4.A. Interpret the underlined portions taken directly from current product references:[17]

   (a) Dose of ritonavir when coadministered with fluconazole: <u>200 mg q6h × 4d.</u>
   (b) Dose of epoetin alpha: <u>150 units/kg SC TIW.</u>
   (c) Dose of acetylcysteine: for patients <u>>20 to <40 kg, 150 mg/kg.</u>
   (d) Pediatric dose of cefuroxime axetil: <u>30 mg/kg/day, divided dose (b.i.d.).</u>
   (e) Dose of ciprofloxacin hydrochloride: <u>750 mg tablet q12h or 400 mg IV q8h.</u>
   (f) Dose of interferon alpha-2b: <u>30 MIU/m² TIW.</u>
   (g) Infusion rate, rocuronium bromide: <u>4 mg/kg/min.</u>
   (h) Dose of enoxaparin sodium injection: <u>1.5 mg/kg q.d. SC.</u>
   (i) Dose of voriconazole: <u>200 mg po q12h × 8 d.</u>
   (j) Dose of certolizumab pegol: <u>200 mg + MTX q2 wk.</u>

4.B. The following are hospital medication orders, and in parenthesis, the product available in the pharmacy:

   (a) Furosemide 40 mg IV qd (10 mg/mL in 2-mL syringes)
   (b) Erythromycin 750 mg IV q6h (500 mg/vial)
   (c) Acyclovir 350 mg IV q8h (500 mg/vial)
   (d) MEGACE 40 mg PO tid (40 mg/mL oral suspension)
   (e) FORTAZ 2 g IV q8h (500 mg/vial)

For each, indicate the quantity to be provided daily by the pharmacy.

ANSWERS TO "CASE IN POINT" PRACTICE PROBLEMS

Case in Point 4.1

(a) Since aa. means "of each," 10 mg lisinopril and 10 mg hydrochlorothiazide are needed for each capsule. And since D.T.D. means "give of such doses," 30 capsules are to be prepared. Thus,

10 mg lisinopril × 30 (capsules) = 300 mg lisinopril and

10 mg hydrochlorothiazide × 30 (capsules) = 300 mg hydrochlorothiazide are needed to fill the prescription.

(b) Since q.s. ad means "a sufficient quantity to make," the total in each capsule is 300 mg. The amount of lactose per capsule would equal 300 mg *less* the quantity of the other ingredients (10 mg + 10 mg + 40 mg), or 240 mg. Thus,

240 mg lactose/capsule × 30 (capsules) = 7200 mg = 7.2 g lactose.

(c) Take one (1) capsule in the morning before breakfast.

Case in Point 4.2

(a) 12 total tablets and capsules.

(b) $? \text{mL} = \dfrac{1\,\text{mL}}{100\,\text{units}} \times \dfrac{35\,\text{units}}{\text{AM}}$
$= 0.35\,\text{mL in the AM}$

$? \text{mL} = \dfrac{1\,\text{mL}}{100\,\text{units}} \times \dfrac{45\,\text{Units}}{\text{PM}}$
$= 0.45\,\text{mL in the PM}$

(c) First 7 days: 2 tablets × 2 (twice daily) × 7 days = 28 tablets;
Next 7 days: 1 tablet × 2 (twice daily) × 7 days = 14 tablets;
Next 16 days: 1 tablet (daily) = 16 tablets;
28 + 14 + 16 = 58 tablets.

(d) 1 capsule daily × 7 days = 7 capsules;
1 capsule × 2 (twice daily) × (next) 10 days = 20 capsules;
7 + 20 = 27 capsules taken with 33 capsules remaining.
Thus, nonadherence *would be* a concern.

Practice Problems

1. (a) Dispense 12 rectal suppositories.
(b) Mix and make an isotonic solution. Dispense 120 mL.
(c) Mix and divide into 40 powders.
(d) Dispense six such doses. Do not repeat.
(e) Mix and make ointment. Dispense 10 grams.
(f) Mix and make capsules. Dispense 48 such doses.
(g) Mix and make a suspension containing 1 gram per tablespoon. Dispense 60 milliliters.
(h) Make one capsule. Dispense 36 such doses. Do not repeat.
(i) Mix and make powder. Divide into 100 such doses.
(j) Mix and make an intravenous injection.
(k) Label: hydrocortisone, 20 mg tabs.

2. (a) Instill 2 drops in each eye every four (4) hours as needed for pain.
(b) Take 1 tablespoonful in one-third glass of water every 6 hours.
(c) Apply morning and night as needed for pain.
(d) Instill 4 drops into the right ear morning and night.
(e) Take 1 teaspoonful in water every 4 or 5 hours as needed for pain.
(f) Apply ointment to the left eye as needed.
(g) Take 1 capsule with water at bedtime. Do not repeat.
(h) Instill 5 drops into each ear 3 times a day as needed.
(i) Place 1 tablet under the tongue, repeat if needed.
(j) Instill 2 drops into each eye of the newborn.
(k) Dilute with an equal volume of water and use as gargle every 5 hours.
(l) Take 2 capsules 1 hour prior to departure, then 1 capsule after 12 hours.
(m) Take 1 tablet as needed for shortness of breath.
(n) Take 1 tablet every morning for high blood pressure.
(o) Take 2 tablets every 6 hours around the clock for urinary tract infection.
(p) Take 2 teaspoonfuls 4 times a day after meals and at bedtime.

(q) Take 1 tablespoonful before meals 3 times a day.

(r) Add crushed tablet to pet's food once a day.

3. (a) AMBIEN 10 milligrams by mouth at every bedtime for 5 days.

(b) 1000 milliliters of 5% dextrose in water every 8 hours intravenously with 20 milliequivalents of potassium chloride added to every third bottle.

(c) Administer 10 milligrams of prochlorperazine intramuscularly every 3 hours, if there is need, for nausea and vomiting.

(d) One teaspoonful of minocycline hydrochloride suspension by mouth four times a day. Discontinue after 5 days.

(e) 10 milligrams of propranolol hydrochloride by mouth three times a day before meals and at bedtime.

(f) 40 units of NPH 100-Unit insulin subcutaneously every day in the morning.

(g) 250 milligrams of cefamandole nafate intramuscularly every 12 hours.

(h) 15 milliequivalents of potassium chloride by mouth twice a day after meals.

(i) 1 milligram of vincristine sulfate per square meter of patient's body surface area.

(j) Administer 30 mg of flurazepam at bedtime as needed for sleep.

(k) Administer 20 milliequivalents of potassium chloride per liter in D5W (5% dextrose in water) at the rate of 84 milliliters per hour.

(l) Administer 2.5 grams per kilogram of body weight per day of amino acids in total parenteral nutrition.

(m) Start epoetin alpha (PROCRIT) immediately at 150 units per kilogram of body weight subcutaneously and then 3 times a week for 3 to 4 weeks.

(n) Methotrexate tablets, 2.5 mg each, to be taken 3 times a day one day a week.

(o) Hydrochlorothiazide tablets, 12.5 mg, to be taken once each day in the morning.

4. (a) 50 days

(b) yes

5. (a) 40 tablets

6. (a) correct

7. ℞ calls for *tablets* but label indicates *capsules*.

Sig: "in the morning" has been added, which may be correct if that is the prescriber's usual directive.

Refill "5" times is incorrect; the original filling of a prescription does not count as a refill.

℞ calls for drug name/strength on label; an omission.

It should be noted that after filling the prescription, the pharmacist would have added a prescription number, which would also appear on the label.

8. The words "all of the medicine" have been added and the numbers enhanced; this clarifies the directions and thus is positive. 250 *mL* should be 250 *mg*.

The prescription number should appear on the label.

9. Patient's name is incorrect. The active drug name *only* on the label is proper for a compounded prescription. The other ingredients are "pharmaceutic."

It should be noted that after filling the prescription, the pharmacist would have added a prescription number, which would also appear on the label.

10. (1) "QID" means 4 times a day.

(2) Drug name is incorrect.

(3) Correct.

11. Correct label.

References

1. Manual of Compliance Policy Guides. *U.S. Food and Drug Administration.* Available at: http://www.fda.gov/ICECI/ComplianceManuals/CompliancePolicyGuidanceManual/ucm074398.htm. Accessed March 6, 2011.
2. http://www.aphanet.org. Accessed August 31, 2007.
3. Jamgochian H. *Pharmacy Today* 2007;13(9):44.
4. NCPDP Electronic Prescribing Standards. *National Council for Prescription Programs.* Available at: http://www.ncpdp.org/pdf/NCPDP_101.pdf. Accessed March 6, 2011.
5. Kilbridge P. E-Prescribing. California HealthCare Foundation. 2001. Available at: http://www.chcf.org/documents/EPrescribing.pdf. Accessed August 20, 2007.
6. American College of Physicians. Statement, June 26, 2006. Available at: http://www.acponline.org/hpp/dea-218n.pdf. Accessed August 20, 2007.
7. http://www.hospital-forms.com. Accessed September 5, 2008.
8. Burnside NL, Bardo JA, Bretz CJ, et al. Effects of including medication indications on prescription labels. *Journal of the American Pharmacists Association* 2007;47:756–758.
9. Institute for Safe Medication Practices. Available at: http:www.ismp.org/tools/errorprone abbreviations.pdf. Accessed February 2, 2011.
10. Davis NM. A controlled vocabulary for reducing medication errors. *Hospital Pharmacy* 2000;35:227–228.
11. The Official "Do Not Use" List of Abbreviations. *The Joint Commission.* Available at: http://www.jointcommission.org/Do_Not_Use_List_of_Abbreviations/. Accessed March 6, 2011.
12. Bond WS, Hussar DA. Detection methods and strategies for improving medication compliance. *American Journal of Hospital Pharmacy* 1991;48:1978.
13. Mackowiak JI. *Enhancing Patient Compliance.* Ridgefield, CT: Boehringer Ingelheim Pharmaceuticals, 1990.
14. Osterberg L, Blaschke T. Adherence to medication. *The New England Journal of Medicine* 2005;353(5):487–497.
15. Fleming WK. Pharmacy management strategies for improving drug adherence. *Supplement to Journal of Managed Care Pharmacy* 2008;14(6):16–20.
16. Bubalo J, *et al.* Medication adherence: pharmacist perspective. *Journal of the American Pharmacists Association* 2010;50(3):394–406.
17. *Physicians' Desk Reference.* Montvale, NJ. PDR Network 2011:65.

Density and Specific Gravity 5

Objectives

Upon successful completion of this chapter, the student will be able to:

- Define *density* and *specific gravity*, and determine each through appropriate calculations.
- Calculate specific gravity from data derived from the use of a pycnometer.
- Apply specific gravity correctly in converting weight to volume and volume to weight.

Density

Density (*d*) is mass per unit volume of a substance. It is *usually* expressed as *grams per cubic centimeter* (*g/cc*). Because the *gram* is defined as the mass of 1 cc of water at 4°C, the density of water is *1 g/cc*. For our purposes, because the *United States Pharmacopeia*[1] states that 1 mL may be used as the equivalent of 1 cc, the density of water may be expressed as *1 g/mL*.

Density may be calculated by dividing mass by volume, that is:

$$\text{Density} = \frac{\text{Mass}}{\text{Volume}}$$

Thus, if 10 mL of sulfuric acid weighs 18 g, its density is:

$$\text{Density} = \frac{18 \ (g)}{10 \ (mL)} = 1.8 \text{ grams per milliliter}$$

Specific Gravity

Specific gravity (*sp gr*) is a ratio, *expressed decimally*, of the weight of a substance to the weight of an equal volume of a substance chosen as a standard, both substances at the same temperature. It is useful to understand specific gravity as being a *relative value*; that is, the weight of a substance *relative* to the weight of a standard.

Water is used as the standard for the specific gravities of liquids and solids; the most useful standard for gases is hydrogen.

Specific gravity may be calculated by dividing the weight of a given substance by the weight of an equal volume of water, that is:

$$\text{Specific gravity} = \frac{\text{Weight of substance}}{\text{Weight of equal volume of water}}$$

Thus, if 10 mL of sulfuric acid weighs 18 g, and 10 mL of water, under similar conditions, weighs 10 g, the specific gravity of the acid is:

Table 5.1 ▼ SOME REPRESENTATIVE
           SPECIFIC GRAVITIES AT 25°C

AGENT	SP GR
Ether (at 20°C)	0.71
Isopropyl alcohol	0.78
Acetone	0.79
Alcohol	0.81
Liquid petrolatum	0.87
Peppermint oil	0.90
Olive oil	0.91
Peanut oil	0.92
Cod liver oil	0.92
Castor oil	0.96
Water	**1.00**
Propylene glycol	1.03
Clove oil	1.04
Liquefied phenol	1.07
Polysorbate 80	1.08
Polyethylene glycol 400	1.13
Glycerin	1.25
Syrup	1.31
Hydrochloric acid	1.37
Nitric acid	1.42
Chloroform	1.47
Nitroglycerin	1.59
Phosphoric acid	1.70
Mercury	13.6

$$\text{Specific gravity} = \frac{18 \ (g)}{10 \ (g)} = 1.8$$

- *Substances that have a specific gravity less than 1 are lighter than water.*
- *Substances that have a specific gravity greater than 1 are heavier than water.*

Table 5.1 presents some representative specific gravities. Figure 5.1 depicts the layering of immiscible liquids due to their relative weights.

   Although specific gravities may be expressed to as many decimal places as the accuracy of their determination warrants, in pharmacy practice, expressions to two decimal places generally suffice. In the *United States Pharmacopeia*, specific gravities are based on data from temperatures of 25°C, with the exception of that for alcohol that is based on 15.56°C by government regulation.[2]

Density Versus Specific Gravity

The density of a substance is a concrete number (*1.8 g/mL* in the example), whereas specific gravity, being a ratio of like quantities, is an abstract number (*1.8* in the example). Whereas density varies with the units of measure used, specific gravity has no dimension and is therefore a constant value for each substance. Thus, whereas the density of water may be variously expressed as *1 g/mL, 1000 g/L,* or *62½ lb/cu ft*, the specific gravity of water is always 1.

Mineral oil
(sp gr 0.89)

Water
(sp gr 1.00)

Chloroform
(sp gr 1.47)

▼ FIGURE 5.1 Depiction of layering of immiscible liquids in a test tube, mineral oil being lighter than water and chloroform being heavier.

Calculating the Specific Gravity of Liquids

Known Weight and Volume

The specific gravity of a liquid of known weight and volume may be calculated by the equation:

$$\text{Specific gravity} = \frac{\text{Weight of substance}}{\text{Weight of equal volume of water}}$$

If 54.96 mL of an oil weighs 52.78 g, what is the specific gravity of the oil?

54.96 mL of water weighs 54.96 g

$$\text{Specific gravity of oil} = \frac{52.78 \ (g)}{54.96 \ (g)} = 0.9603, \ answer.$$

If a pint of a certain liquid weighs 601 g, what is the specific gravity of the liquid?

1 pint = 16 fl. oz.
16 fl. oz. of water weighs 473 g

$$\text{Specific gravity of liquid} = \frac{601 \ (g)}{473 \ (g)} = 1.27, \ answer.$$

Pycnometer or Specific Gravity Bottle

A *pycnometer* is a special glass bottle used to determine specific gravity (Fig. 5.2). Pycnometers are generally available for laboratory use in volumes ranging from 1 mL to 50 mL. Pycnometers have fitted glass stoppers with a capillary opening to allow trapped air and excess fluid to escape. Some pycnometers have thermometers affixed in order to relate the specific gravity, as determined, with temperature.

In using a pycnometer, it is first weighed empty and then weighed again when filled to capacity with water. The weight of the water is calculated by difference. Since 1 g of water equals 1 mL, the exact volume of the pycnometer becomes known. Then, when any other

▼ FIGURE 5.2 Examples of *pycnometers* used to determine the specific gravity of liquids. Shown are 1-mL and 25-mL sizes. See text for description of their use. *(Courtesy of Thomas Scientific.)*

liquid subsequently is placed in the pycnometer, it is of *equal volume* to the water, and its specific gravity may be determined.

A 50 mL pycnometer is found to weigh 120 g when empty, 171 g when filled with water, and 160 g when filled with an unknown liquid. Calculate the specific gravity of the unknown liquid.

Weight of water: 171 g – 120 g = 51 g
Weight of unknown liquid: 160 g – 120 g = 40 g

$$\text{Specific gravity} = \frac{\text{Weight of substance}}{\text{Weight of equal volume of water}}$$

$$\text{Specific gravity of unknown liquid} = \frac{40\ (g)}{51\ (g)} = 0.78,\ answer.$$

A specific gravity bottle weighs 23.66 g. When filled with water, it weighs 72.95 g; when filled with another liquid, it weighs 73.56 g. What is the specific gravity of the liquid?

73.56 g – 23.66 g = 49.90 g of liquid
72.95 g – 23.66 g = 49.29 g of water

$$\text{Specific gravity of liquid} = \frac{49.90\ (g)}{49.29\ (g)} = 1.012,\ answer.$$

There are additional methods for determining specific gravity, which may be found in earlier editions of this textbook.

Use of Specific Gravity in Calculations of Weight and Volume

When *specific gravity is used as a factor in a calculation, the result should contain no more significant figures than the number in the factor.*

It is important to remember that specific gravity is a *factor* that expresses how much heavier or lighter a substance is than water, the standard with a specific gravity of 1.0. For example, a liquid with a specific gravity of 1.25 is 1.25 times as heavy as water, and a liquid with a specific gravity of 0.85 is 0.85 times as heavy as water.

Thus, if we had 50 mL of a liquid with a specific gravity of 1.2, it would weigh 1.2 times as much as an equivalent volume of water. An equivalent volume of water, 50 mL, would weigh 50 g, and therefore the liquid would weigh 1.2 times that, or 60 g.

Calculating Weight, Knowing the Volume and Specific Gravity

Based on the explanation in the previous paragraphs, we can derive the following equation:

$$\text{Grams} = \text{Milliliters} \times \text{Specific gravity}$$

Although it is both obvious and true that one cannot multiply milliliters by specific gravity and have a product in grams, the equation "works" because the volume of the liquid in question is assumed to be the same volume as water for which milliliters equal grams. So, in essence, the true equation would be:

$$\text{Grams (other liquid)} = \text{Grams (of equal volume of water)}$$
$$\times \text{Specific gravity (other liquid)}$$

What is the weight, in grams, of 3620 mL of alcohol with a specific gravity of 0.82?

$$3620 \text{ mL of water weigh } 3620 \text{ g}$$
$$3620 \text{ g} \times 0.82 = 2968 \text{ g, } \textit{answer.}$$

What is the weight, in grams, of 2 fl. oz. of a liquid having a specific gravity of 1.118?

In this type of problem, it is best to convert the given volume to its metric equivalent first and then solve the problem in the metric system.

$$2 \times 29.57 \text{ mL} = 59.14 \text{ mL}$$
$$59.14 \text{ mL of water weigh } 59.14 \text{ g}$$
$$59.14 \text{ g} \times 1.118 = 66.12 \text{ g, } \textit{answer.}$$

Calculating Volume, Knowing the Weight and Specific Gravity

By rearranging the previous equation, we can calculate the volume of a liquid using the equation:

$$\text{Milliliters} = \frac{\text{Grams}}{\text{Specific gravity}}$$

What is the volume, in milliliters, of 492 g of nitric acid with a specific gravity of 1.40?

492 g of water measure 492 mL

$$\frac{492 \text{ mL}}{1.40} = 351 \text{ mL, } \textit{answer.}$$

What is the volume, in milliliters, of 1 lb of methyl salicylate with a specific gravity of 1.185?

1 lb = 454 g

454 g of water measure 454 mL

$$\frac{454 \text{ mL}}{1.185} = 383.1 \text{ mL, } \textit{answer.}$$

What is the volume, in pints, of 50 lb of glycerin having a specific gravity of 1.25?

50 lb = 454 g × 50 = 22,700 g
22,700 g of water measure 22,700 mL and 1 pint = 473 mL

$$\frac{22,700 \text{ mL}}{1.25} = 18,160 \text{ mL} \div 473 \text{ mL} = 38.4 \text{ pints, } answer.$$

What is the cost of 1000 mL of glycerin, specific gravity 1.25, bought at $5.43 per pound?

1000 mL of water weigh 1000 g
Weight of 1000 mL of glycerin = 1000 g × 1.25 = 1250 g
1 lb = 454 g

$$\$5.43 \times \frac{1250\,\text{g}}{454\,\text{g}} = \$14.95, \, answer.$$

What is the cost of 1 pint of chloroform, specific gravity 1.475, bought at $25.25 per pound?

1 pint = 473 mL
473 mL of water weigh 473 g
Weight of 473 mL of chloroform = 473 g × 1.475 = 697.7 g
1 lb = 454 g

$$\$25.25 \times \frac{697.7\,\text{g}}{454\,\text{g}} = \$38.80, \, answer.$$

Special Considerations of Specific Gravity

Pharmaceutical Applications

As described previously, specific gravity is employed when a pharmacist wishes to convert the weight of an ingredient or preparation to volume or vice versa. In practice, liquid materials are usually the objects of the conversions.

Another application of specific gravity is in automated pharmaceutical equipment used by pharmacists to prepare total parenteral nutrition (TPN) admixtures. In these *automated compounders*, the purpose of the specific gravity of the large-volume liquids being mixed is to determine the weights of components (e.g., dextrose, amino acids, and water). The component weights are automatically calculated, based on the specific gravity, volume, and percentage concentration of the solutions used (e.g., 70% dextrose injection) in the admixture. The automatic compounder then uses the *weight* to make the correct mixture rather than the *volume* of the solution being measured.

Clinical Application

Specific gravity is an important factor in urinalysis. In normal adults, the specific gravity of urine is usually within the range of 1.020 and 1.028 with a normal fluid intake (this range may vary with the reference source).[3]

Specific gravity is an indicator of both the concentration of particles in the urine and a patient's degree of hydration. A higher-than-normal specific gravity indicates that the urine is concentrated. This may be due to the presence of excess waste products or electrolytes in the urine, the presence of glucose (glucosuria) or protein (proteinuria), excessive water loss, decreased fluid intake, or other factors. A low specific gravity indicates that the urine is dilute, which may be a result of diabetes insipidus, renal disease (by virtue of the kidney's reduced ability to concentrate urine), increased fluid intake, intravenous hydration, or other factors.[4]

In the modern clinical laboratory, the specific gravity of urine is determined (using the refractive index method) as a component of a comprehensive urinalysis performed by sophisticated, fully automated equipment that determines, in seconds, urine chemistry, specific gravity, pH, color, and clarity.[5]

CASE IN POINT 5.1[8]

℞ Lactic Acid
    Salicylic Acid aa.   1.5 g
    Flexible Collodion qs ad   15 mL
    Sig: Apply one drop to wart twice a day.
    Label: Wart remover. For external use only.

Lactic acid is available as a liquid containing 85 g of the acid in 100 g of solution (sp.gr. 1.21). Calculate the quantity of this solution, in milliliters, needed to fill the prescription.

CALCULATIONS CAPSULE

Specific Gravity

The specific gravity (sp gr) of a substance or a pharmaceutical preparation may be determined by the following equation:

$$Specific\ gravity = \frac{Weight\ of\ substance\ (g)}{Weight\ of\ equal\ volume\ of\ water\ (g)}$$

The following equation may be used to convert the volume of a substance or pharmaceutical preparation to its weight:*

$$Weight\ of\ substance = Volume\ of\ substance \times Specific\ gravity$$

Or simply,

$$\mathbf{g = mL \times sp\ gr}$$

The following equation may be used to convert the weight of a substance or pharmaceutical preparation to its volume:*

$$Volume\ of\ substance = \frac{Weight\ of\ substance}{Specific\ gravity}$$

Or simply,

$$\mathbf{mL = \frac{g}{sp\ gr}}$$

*The full explanation on why these equations work may be found in the section "Use of Specific Gravity in Calculations of Weight and Volume."

PRACTICE PROBLEMS

Calculations of Density

1. If 250 mL of alcohol weighs 203 g, what is its density?

2. A piece of copper metal weighs 53.6 g, and has a volume of 6 mL. Calculate its density.

Calculations of Specific Gravity

3. If 150 mL of a sorbitol solution weigh 170 g, what is its specific gravity?

4. If a liter of a cough syrup weighs 1285 g, what is its specific gravity?

5. If 500 mL of ferric chloride solution weighs 650 g, what is its specific gravity?

6. If 2 fl. oz. of glycerol weighs 74.1 g, what is its specific gravity?

7. Five pints of diluted hydrochloric acid weighs 2.79 kg. Calculate its specific gravity.

8. A pycnometer weighs 21.62 g. Filled with water, it weighs 46.71 g; filled with another liquid, it weighs 43.28 g. Calculate the specific gravity of the liquid.

9. A modified Ringer's Irrigation has the following formula:

Sodium chloride	8.6	g
Potassium chloride	0.3	g
Calcium chloride	0.33	g
PEG 3350	60	g
Water for injection ad	1000	mL

Assuming that 980 mL of water is used in preparing the irrigation, calculate its specific gravity.

Calculations of Weight or Volume Using Specific Gravity

Note: Use the information in Table 5.1 if necessary.

10. Calculate the weight, in grams, of 100 mL of each of the following:

   (a) acetone
   (b) liquid petrolatum
   (c) syrup
   (d) nitroglycerin
   (e) mercury

11. What is the weight, in kilograms, of 5 liters of sulfuric acid with a specific gravity of 1.84?

12. What is the weight, in pounds, of 5 pints of nitric acid?

13. What is the weight, in kilograms, of 1 gallon of sorbitol solution having a specific gravity of 1.285?

14. If 500 mL of mineral oil are used to prepare a liter of mineral oil emulsion, how many grams of the oil, having a specific gravity of 0.87, would be used in the preparation of 1 gallon of the emulsion?

15. Calculate the volume, in milliliters, of 100 g of each of the following:

   (a) peanut oil
   (b) castor oil
   (c) polysorbate 80
   (d) phosphoric acid
   (e) mercury

16. What is the volume, in milliliters, of 1 lb of benzyl benzoate having a specific gravity of 1.12?

17. What is the volume, in milliliters, of 1 kg of sulfuric acid with a specific gravity of 1.83?

18. Calculate the corresponding weights of liquefied phenol and propylene glycol needed to prepare 24 15-mL bottles of the following formula for a cold sore topical liquid:

Liquefied phenol	0.4 mL
Camphor	0.5 g
Benzocaine	2.2 g
Ethanol	65 mL
Propylene glycol	17 mL
Purified water ad	100 mL

19. Calculate the total weight of the following formula for a pediatric chewable gummy gel base for medication.[7]

Gelatin	43.4 g
Glycerin	155 mL
Purified Water	21.6 mL

20. Calculate the number of milliliters of polysorbate 80 required to prepare 48 100-g tubes of the following formula for a progesterone vaginal cream.[8]

Progesterone, micronized	3 g
Polysorbate 80	1 g
Methylcellulose 2% Gel	96 g

21. If fifty glycerin suppositories are made from the following formula, how many milliliters of glycerin, having a specific gravity of 1.25, would be used in the preparation of 96 suppositories?

Glycerin	91 g
Sodium stearate	9 g
Purified water	5 g

22. Two 10-mL samples of urine have specific gravities of 1.003 and 1.030. What is the difference in weight, in milligrams, between the two samples?

23. R[9]
Testosterone propionate	2 g
Mineral Oil, light	10 g
Polysorbate 80	1 g
Methylcellulose 2% gel	87 g

    The specific gravity of light mineral oil is 0.85 and that of polysorbate 80 is 1.08. Calculate the milliliters of each needed to fill the prescription.

24. A formula for an anesthetic ointment is:

Benzocaine	200 g
Polyethylene glycol 400	600 g
Polyethylene glycol 3350	ad 1000 g

    Polyethylene glycol 400 is a liquid, sp.gr. 1.13, benzocaine and polyethylene glycol 3350 are powders. How many milliliters of polyethylene glycol would be used in the formula?

Calculations of Drug Costs Using Specific Gravity

25. The formula for 1000 g of polyethylene glycol ointment calls for 600 g polyethylene glycol 400. At $19.15 per pint, what is the cost of the polyethylene glycol 400, specific gravity 1.140, needed to prepare 4000 g of the ointment?

CALCQUIZ

5.A. Syrup, USP is prepared by dissolving 850 g of sucrose in sufficient purified water to make 1000 mL of syrup. Syrup has a specific gravity of 1.31. How many milliliters of water are used to prepare a liter of syrup?

5.B. A saturated solution of potassium iodide contains, in each 100 mL, 100 g of potassium iodide. The solubility of potassium iodide is 1 g in 0.7 mL of water. Calculate the specific gravity of the saturated solution.

5.C. Cocoa butter (theobroma oil) is used as a suppository base. It is a solid at room temperature, melts at 34°C, and has a specific gravity of 0.86. If a formula for medicated suppositories calls for 48 mL of theobroma oil, how many grams are equivalent?

ANSWERS TO "CASE IN POINT" AND PRACTICE PROBLEMS

Case in Point 5.1

Quantity of lactic acid needed to fill ℞:
1.5 g
Source of lactic acid: liquid containing
85 g/100 g; or, by using specific gravity:

100 g ÷ 1.21 = 82.64 mL

Thus, 85 g of lactic acid are in 82.64 mL of the source liquid.
By proportion:

$$\frac{85\,g}{82.64\,mL} = \frac{1.5\,g}{x\,mL}; x = 1.46\ mL,\ answer.$$

Practice Problems

1. 0.812 g/mL
2. 8.933 g/mL
3. 1.133
4. 1.285
5. 1.30
6. 1.25
7. 1.18
8. 0.86
9. 1.05
10. (a) 79 g acetone
    (b) 87 g liquid petrolatum
    (c) 131 g syrup
    (d) 159 g nitroglycerin
    (e) 1360 g mercury
11. 9.2 kg sulfuric acid
12. 7.397 or 7.4 lb nitric acid
13. 4.86 kg sorbitol solution
14. 1646.5 g mineral oil
15. (a) 108.7 mL peanut oil
    (b) 104.17 mL castor oil
    (c) 92.59 mL polysorbate 80
    (d) 58.82 mL phosphoric acid
    (e) 7.35 mL mercury
16. 405.36 mL benzyl benzoate
17. 546.45 mL sulfuric acid
18. 1.54 g liquefied phenol
    63.04 g camphor
19. 258.75 g
20. 44.44 mL polysorbate 80
21. 139.78 mL glycerin
22. 270 mg
23. 11.76 mL light mineral oil
    0.93 mL polysorbate 80
24. 530.97 mL polyethylene glycol 400
25. $85.23

References

1. United States Pharmacopeial Convention. *United States Pharmacopeia 32 National Formulary 27*. Rockville, MD: United States Pharmacopeial Convention, 2009;1:9.
2. United States Pharmacopeial Convention. *United States Pharmacopeia 32 National Formulary 27*. Rockville, MD: United States Pharmacopeial Convention, 2009;1:8–9.
3. Urine specific gravity. MedlinePlus. Available at: http://www.nlm.nih.gov/medlineplus/ency/article/003587. htm. Accessed March 6, 2011.
4. The Internet Pathology Laboratory for Medical Education. Urinalysis tutorial. Available at: http://library. med.utah.edu/WebPath/TUTORIAL/URINE/URINE.html. Accessed January 18, 2011.
5. CLINITEK AUWi System [product information]. Deerfield, IL: Siemens Healthcare Diagnostics, Inc.
6. Prince SJ. Calculations. *International Journal of Pharmaceutical Compounding* 1998;2:310.
7. *International Journal of Pharmaceutical Compounding* 1997;1:106.
8. *International Journal of Pharmaceutical Compounding* 1998;2:58.
9. *International Journal of Pharmaceutical Compounding* 1998;2:67.

Percentage, Ratio Strength, and Other Expressions of Concentration

Objectives

Upon successful completion of this chapter, the student will be able to:

- Perform calculations based on *percent weight-in-volume*, *percent volume-in-volume*, and *percent weight-in-weight*.
- Perform calculations based on *ratio strength*.
- Convert percent strength to ratio strength and ratio strength to percent strength.

Percent/Percentage

The term *percent* and the corresponding "%" sign indicate the number of *parts in a hundred*. The quantity also may be expressed as a common or decimal fraction. Thus, 50%, 50/100, and 0.5 are equivalent. The term *percentage* refers to the *rate per hundred*.

For the purposes of computation, percents are usually changed to equivalent decimal fractions. This change is made by dropping the percent sign (%) and dividing the expressed numerator by 100. Thus, $12.5\% = \dfrac{12.5}{100}$, or 0.125 and $0.05\% = \dfrac{0.05}{100}$, or 0.0005. We must not forget that in the reverse process (changing a decimal to a percent), the decimal is multiplied by 100 and the percent sign (%) is affixed.

Percent is an essential component of pharmaceutical calculations. It is used to (a) *express the strength* of a component in a pharmaceutical preparation as well as to (b) *determine the quantity* of a component to use when a certain percent strength is desired.

Percentage Preparations

The percentage concentrations of active and inactive constituents in various types of pharmaceutical preparations are defined as follows by the *United States Pharmacopeia*[1]:

Percent weight-in-volume (w/v) expresses the number of *grams* of a constituent in *100 mL* of solution or liquid preparation and is used regardless of whether water or another liquid is the solvent or vehicle. Expressed as: _____% w/v.

Percent volume-in-volume (v/v) expresses the number of *milliliters* of a constituent in *100 mL* of solution or liquid preparation. Expressed as: _____% v/v.

Percent weight-in-weight (w/w) expresses the number of *grams* of a constituent in *100 g* of solution or preparation. Expressed as: _____ % w/w.

The term *percent*, or the symbol %, when used *without qualification* means:

* for solutions or suspensions of solids in liquids, *percent weight-in-volume*;
* for solutions of liquids in liquids, *percent volume-in-volume*;
* for mixtures of solids or semisolids, *percent weight-in-weight*; and
* for solutions of gases in liquids, *percent weight-in-volume*.

Special Considerations in Percentage Calculations

In general, the physical nature of the ingredients in a pharmaceutical preparation determines the basis of the calculation. That is, a powdered substance dissolved or suspended in a liquid vehicle would generally be calculated on a *weight-in-volume* basis; and a powdered substance mixed with a solid or semisolid, such as an ointment base, would generally be calculated on a *weight-in-weight* basis; and, a liquid component in a liquid preparation would be calculated on a *volume-in-volume* basis. *If the designation of the term of a calculation (e.g., w/v, w/w, or v/v) is not included in a problem, the appropriate assumption must be made.*

The use of *percent* to indicate the strength of a product generally is limited nowadays to certain topical products, such as ointments, creams, and eye drops. However, there are some notable exceptions, such as 5% dextrose injection, used in intravenous infusions. In most other instances, product strengths are expressed in specific quantitative terms, such as 10-mg tablets and 2 mg/mL injections. [*The problems in this chapter take certain liberties from this standard practice in order to afford a broad experience in the calculations process.*]

Percentage Weight-in-Volume

In a *true* expression of *percentage (i.e., parts per 100 parts)*, the percentage of a liquid preparation (e.g., solution, suspension, lotion) would represent the *grams* of solute or constituent in *100 g* of the liquid preparation. However, in practice, the pharmacist most frequently uses a different definition of percentage for solutions and for other liquid preparations, one in which the *parts* of the percentage represent *grams* of a solute or constituent in *100 mL* of solution or liquid preparation.

Indeed, in weight-in-volume expressions, the "correct" strength of a 1% (w/v) solution or other liquid preparation is defined as containing 1 g of constituent in 100 mL of product. This variance to the definition of *true percentage* is based on an assumption that the *solution/ liquid preparation has a specific gravity of 1, as if it were water*. It is on this assumption that each 100 mL of solution/liquid preparation is presumed to weigh 100 g and thus is used as the basis for calculating percentage weight-in-volume (e.g., 1% w/v = 1% of [100 mL, taken to be] 100 g = 1 g in 100 mL).

Taking water to represent any solvent or vehicle, we may prepare weight-in-volume percentage solutions or liquid preparations by the SI metric system if we use the following rule.

Multiply the required number of milliliters by the percentage strength, expressed as a decimal, to obtain the number of grams of solute or constituent in the solution or liquid preparation. *The volume, in milliliters, represents the weight in grams of the solution or liquid preparation as if it were pure water.*

Volume (mL, representing grams) × % (expressed as a decimal) = grams (g) of solute or constituent

Examples of Weight-in-Volume Calculations

How many grams of dextrose are required to prepare 4000 mL of a 5% solution?

4000 mL represents 4000 g of solution
5% = 0.05
4000 g × 0.05 = 200 g, *answer*.

Or, solving by dimensional analysis:

$$\frac{5\text{ g}}{100\text{ mL}} \times 4000\text{ mL} = 200\text{ g dextrose, } answer.$$

How many grams of potassium permanganate should be used in compounding the following prescription?

℞   Potassium Permanganate   0.02%
     Purified Water ad   250 mL
     Sig. as directed.
250 mL represents 250 g of solution
        0.02% = 0.0002
250 g × 0.0002 = 0.05 g potassium permanganate, *answer*.

A cyclosporine ophthalmic emulsion (RESTASIS) contains 0.05% w/v cyclosporine in 0.4 mL vials. Calculate the content of cyclosporine, in milligrams, per vial.

0.4 mL × 0.05% w/v = 0.0002 mL (equivalent in a w/v problem to 0.0002 g)
            0.0002 g = 0.2 mg cyclosporine, *answer*.

The topical antibacterial solution HIBICLENS contains 4% w/v chlorhexidine gluconate in 4-fluidounce containers. Calculate the content of chlorhexidine gluconate, in grams.

4 (fluidounces) × 29.57 mL = 118.28 mL
118.28 mL × 4% w/v = 4.73 g chlorhexidine gluconate, *answer*.

Bimatoprost ophthalmic solution (LUMIGAN) contains 0.03% w/v of drug in each 2.5 mL. Calculate the micrograms of bimatoprost in a container of solution.

2.5 mL × 0.03% w/v = 0.00075 g = 0.75 mg = 750 μg bimatoprost, *answer*.

An ophthalmic solution contains 0.1 mg of travoprost in 2.5 mL containers. Calculate the percentage strength of travoprost in the solution.

0.1 mg = 0.0001 g
$$\frac{0.0001\text{g}}{2.5\text{g}} \times 100\% = 0.004\% \text{ w/v, travoprost, } answer.$$

Percentage Volume-in-Volume

Liquids are usually measured by volume, and the percentage strength indicates the number of parts by volume of an ingredient contained in the total volume of the liquid preparation considered as 100 parts by volume.

Examples of Volume-in-Volume Calculations

How many milliliters of liquefied phenol should be used in compounding the following prescription?

℞	Liquefied Phenol	2.5%
	Calamine Lotion ad	240 mL
	Sig. For external use.	

Volume (mL) × % (expressed as a decimal) = milliliters of active ingredient

240 mL × 0.025 = 6 mL, *answer.*

Or, solving by dimensional analysis:

$$\frac{2.5 \text{ mL}}{100 \text{ mL}} \times 240 \text{ mL} = 6 \text{ mL, liquefied phenol, } answer.$$

In preparing 250 mL of a certain lotion, a pharmacist used 4 mL of liquefied phenol. What was the percentage (v/v) of liquefied phenol in the lotion?

$$\frac{250 \text{ (mL)}}{4 \text{ (mL)}} = \frac{100 \text{ (\%)}}{\text{x (\%)}}$$

$$x = 1.6\%, \text{ } answer.$$

What is the percentage strength v/v of a solution of 800 g of a liquid with a specific gravity of 0.8 in enough water to make 4000 mL?

800 g of water measures 800 mL
800 mL ÷ 0.8 = 1000 mL of active ingredient

$$\frac{4000 \text{ (mL)}}{1000 \text{ (mL)}} = \frac{100 \text{ (\%)}}{\text{x (\%)}}$$

$$x = 25\%, \text{ } answer.$$

Or, solving by dimensional analysis:

$$\frac{800 \text{ mL}}{0.8} \times \frac{1}{4000 \text{ mL}} \times 100\% = 25\%, \text{ } answer.$$

Peppermint spirit contains 10% v/v of peppermint oil. What volume of the spirit will contain 75 mL of peppermint oil?

$$\frac{10 \text{ (\%)}}{100 \text{ (\%)}} = \frac{75 \text{ (mL)}}{\text{x (mL)}}$$

$$x = 750 \text{ mL, } answer.$$

If a veterinary liniment contains 30% v/v of dimethyl sulfoxide, how many milliliters of the liniment can be prepared from 1 lb of dimethyl sulfoxide (sp gr 1.10)?

1 lb = 454 g
454 g of water measures 454 mL
454 mL ÷ 1.10 = 412.7 mL of dimethyl sulfoxide

$$\frac{30 \text{ (\%)}}{100 \text{ (\%)}} = \frac{412.7 \text{ (mL)}}{\text{x (mL)}}$$

$$x = 1375.7 \text{ or } 1376 \text{ mL, } answer.$$

Or, solving by dimensional analysis:

$$\frac{1\,\text{lb}}{30\%} \times \frac{454\,\text{g}}{1\,\text{lb}} \times \frac{1\,\text{mL}}{1\,\text{g}} \times \frac{1}{1.10} \times 100\% = 1375.7 \text{ or } 1376 \text{ mL, } \textit{answer.}$$

Percentage Weight-in-Weight

Percentage weight-in-weight indicates the number of parts by weight of active ingredient contained in the total weight of the preparation.

Examples of Weight-in-Weight Calculations

How many grams of phenol should be used to prepare 240 g of a 5% (w/w) solution in water?

Weight of solution (g) × % (expressed as a decimal) = g of solute

240 g × 0.05 = 12 g, *answer.*

How many grams of a drug substance are required to make 120 mL of a 20% (w/w) solution having a specific gravity of 1.15?

120 mL of water weighs 120 g
120 g × 1.15 = 138 g, weight of 120 mL of solution
138 g × 0.20 = 27.6 g plus enough water to make 120 mL, *answer.*

Or, solving by dimensional analysis:

$$120 \text{ mL} \times \frac{1.15\,\text{g}}{1\,\text{mL}} \times \frac{20\%}{100\%} = 27.6 \text{ g, } \textit{answer.}$$

Sometimes in a weight-in-weight calculation, the weight of one component is known but *not* the total weight of the intended preparation. This type of calculation is performed as demonstrated by the following example.

How many grams of a drug substance should be added to 240 mL of water to make a 4% (w/w) solution?

100% − 4% = 96% (by weight) of water
240 mL of water weighs 240 g

$$\frac{96\,(\%)}{4\,(\%)} = \frac{240\,(\text{g})}{\text{x}\,(\text{g})}$$

$$\text{x} = 10 \text{ g, } \textit{answer.}$$

It is usually impossible to prepare a specified *volume* of a solution or liquid preparation of given weight-in-weight percentage strength because the volume displaced by the active ingredient cannot be known in advance. If an excess is acceptable, we may make a volume somewhat more than that specified by taking the given volume to refer to the solvent or vehicle and from this quantity calculating the weight of the solvent or vehicle (the specific gravity of the solvent or vehicle must be known). Using this weight, we may follow the method just described to calculate the corresponding weight of the active ingredient needed.

How should you prepare 100 mL of a 2% (w/w) solution of a drug substance in a solvent having a specific gravity of 1.25?

100 mL of water weighs 100 g
100 g × 1.25 = 125 g, weight of 100 mL of solvent
100% − 2% = 98% (by weight) of solvent

$$\frac{98\,(\%)}{2\,(\%)} = \frac{125\,(g)}{x\,(g)}$$

$$x = 2.55\;g$$

Therefore, dissolve 2.55 g of drug substance in 125 g (or 100 mL) of solvent, *answer.*

Calculating Percentage Strength Weight-in-Weight

If 1500 g of a solution contains 75 g of a drug substance, what is the percentage strength (w/w) of the solution?

$$\frac{1500\,(g)}{75\,(g)} = \frac{100\,(\%)}{x\,(\%)}$$

$$x = 5\%,\ answer.$$

Or, solving by dimensional analysis:

$$\frac{75\;g}{1500\;g} \times 100\% = 5\%,\ answer.$$

If 5 g of boric acid are added to 100 mL of water, what is the percentage strength (w/w) of the solution?

100 mL of water weighs 100 g
100 g + 5 g = 105 g, weight of solution

$$\frac{105\,(g)}{5\,(g)} = \frac{100\,(\%)}{x\,(\%)}$$

$$x = 4.76\%,\ answer.$$

If 1000 mL of syrup with a specific gravity of 1.313 contains 850 g of sucrose, what is its percentage strength (w/w)?

1000 mL of water weigh 1000 g
1000 g × 1.313 = 1313 g, weight of 1000 mL of syrup

$$\frac{1313\,(g)}{850\,(g)} = \frac{100\,(\%)}{x\,(\%)}$$

$$x = 64.7\%,\ answer.$$

A 60-g tube of DESONATE gel contains 0.05% w/w desonide. Calculate the concentration of desonide on a mg/g basis.

1 g × 0.05% w/w = 0.0005 g = 0.5 mg/g desonide, *answer.*

DIPROLENE lotion contains 0.05% w/w betamethasone dipropionate. If the specific gravity of the lotion is 0.96, how many milligrams of betamethasone dipropionate would be present in a 60-mL container of the lotion?

60 mL × 0.96 = 57.6 g

57.6 g × 0.05% = 0.0288 or 0.029 g = 29 mg betamethasone dipropionate, *answer*.

Weight-in-Weight Calculations in Compounding

Weight-in-weight calculations are used in the following types of manufacturing and compounding problems.

What weight of a 5% (w/w) solution can be prepared from 2 g of active ingredient?

$$\frac{5\,(\%)}{100\,(\%)} = \frac{2\,(g)}{x\,(g)}$$

$$x = 40 \text{ g, } answer.$$

How many milligrams of hydrocortisone should be used in compounding the following prescription?

℞	Hydrocortisone	⅛%
	Hydrophilic Ointment ad	10 g
	Sig. Apply.	

⅛% = 0.125%

10 g × 0.00125 = 0.0125 g or 12.5 mg hydrocortisone, *answer*.

How many grams of benzocaine should be used in compounding the following prescription?

℞	Benzocaine	2%
	Polyethylene Glycol Base ad	2 g
	Make 24 such suppositories	
	Sig. Insert one as directed.	

2 g × 24 = 48 g, total weight of mixture

48 g × 0.02 = 0.96 g benzocaine, *answer*.

Or, solving by dimensional analysis:

$$24 \text{ supp.} \times \frac{2\text{ g}}{1\text{ supp.}} \times \frac{2\%}{100\%} = 0.96 \text{ g benzocaine, } answer.$$

Use of Percent in Compendial Standards

Percent is used in the *United States Pharmacopeia* to express the degree of tolerance permitted in the purity of single-chemical entities and in the labeled quantities of ingredients in dosage forms. For instance, according to the United States Pharmacopeia,[2] "Aspirin contains not less than 99.5% and not more than 100.5% of $C_9H_8O_4$ (pure chemical aspirin) calculated on the dried basis." Further, "Aspirin Tablets contain not less than 90.0% and not more than 110.0% of the labeled amount of $C_9H_8O_4$." Although dosage forms are formulated with the intent to provide 100% of the quantity of each ingredient declared on the label, some tolerance is permitted to allow for analytic error, unavoidable variations in manufacturing and

CALCULATIONS CAPSULE

Percentage Concentration

The amounts of therapeutically active and/or inactive ingredients in certain types of pharmaceutical preparations are expressed in terms of their percentage concentrations.

Unless otherwise indicated:

(a) Liquid components in liquid preparations have *volume-in-volume* relationships with calculations following the equation:

mL of preparation × % concentration[a] = mL of component

(b) Solid components in liquid preparations have *weight-in-volume* relationships with calculations following the equation:

mL of preparation × % concentration[a] = g of component

The terms of this equation are accepted due to the assumption that the specific gravity of the preparation is 1, as if it were water, and thus each milliliter represents the weight of one gram.

(c) Solid or semisolid components in solid or semisolid preparations have *weight-in-weight* relationships with calculations following the equation:

g of preparation × % concentration[a] = g of component

---

[a]In these equations, "% concentration" is expressed decimally (e.g., 0.05, *not* 5%).

compounding, and for deterioration to an extent considered insignificant under practical conditions.

The following problem demonstrates calculations involving percent in compendial standards.

If ibuprofen tablets are permitted to contain not less than 90% and not more than 110% of the labeled amount of ibuprofen, what would be the permissible range in content of the drug, expressed in milligrams, for ibuprofen tablets labeled 200 mg each?

$$90\% \text{ of } 200 \text{ mg} = 180 \text{ mg}$$
$$110\% \text{ of } 200 \text{ mg} = 220 \text{ mg}$$
$$\text{Range} = 180 \text{ mg to } 220 \text{ mg ibuprofen, } answer.$$

CASE IN POINT 6.1[3] A patient with myasthenia gravis has undergone treatment to separate and remove certain abnormal antibodies and other unwanted elements from the blood (plasmapheresis). The desired red blood cell component is then returned back to the blood, but the patient has lost protein and blood volume.

The patient's physician orders 2000 mL of a 5% w/v solution of albumin in 0.9% w/v sodium chloride injection to replace lost protein and fluid.

In filling the order, the pharmacist decides to use a piece of automated equipment to compound the mixture. The equipment must be programmed with the specific gravities of the solutions being mixed. The pharmacist selects to use a 25% w/v albumin solution as the source of the albumin plus a 0.9% sodium chloride injection.

From the literature, the pharmacist finds that 0.9% sodium chloride has a specific gravity of 1.05. Using a precise 25-mL pycnometer with a tare weight of 28 g, the pharmacist fills it with the 25% w/v albumin solution and determines the weight of the flask and its content to be 58 g.

(a) What is the specific gravity of the albumin solution?
(b) How many milliliters of the 25% w/v albumin solution are needed to make 2000 mL containing 5% w/v albumin?
(c) What is the weight of the 25% albumin solution needed to fill the order?
(d) If the pharmacist mixed the required number of milliliters of the 25% albumin solution with a sufficient 0.9% w/v sodium chloride injection to make the required 2000 mL mixture, what would be the specific gravity of the resultant solution?

CASE IN POINT 6.2[3] A pharmacist receives the following prescription but does not have hydrocortisone powder on hand. However, the pharmacist does have an injection containing 100 mg of hydrocortisone per milliliter of injection. A search of the literature indicates that the injection has a specific gravity of 1.5.

℞   Hydrocortisone   1.5%
       Cold Cream qs   30 g

(a) How many grams of hydrocortisone are needed to fill the prescription?
(b) How many milliliters of the hydrocortisone injection would provide the correct amount of hydrocortisone?
(c) How many grams of cold cream are required?

Ratio Strength

The concentrations of weak solutions are frequently expressed in terms of ratio strength. Because all percentages are a ratio of parts per hundred, ratio strength is merely another way of expressing the percentage strength of solutions or liquid preparations (and, less frequently, of mixtures of solids). For example, *5%* means *5 parts per 100* or *5:100*. Although *5 parts per 100* designates a ratio strength, it is customary to translate this designation into a ratio, the first figure of which is *1*; thus, *5:100 = 1:20*.

When a ratio strength, for example, *1:1000*, is used to designate a concentration, it is to be interpreted as follows:

- *For solids in liquids = 1 g* of solute or constituent in *1000 mL* of solution or liquid preparation.
- *For liquids in liquids = 1 mL* of constituent in *1000 mL* of solution or liquid preparation.
- *For solids in solids = 1 g* of constituent in *1000 g* of mixture.

The ratio and percentage strengths of any solution or mixture of solids are proportional, and either is easily converted to the other by the use of proportion.

Example Calculations Using Ratio Strength

Express 0.02% as a ratio strength.

$$\frac{0.02\,(\%)}{100\,(\%)} = \frac{1\,(\text{part})}{x\,(\text{parts})}$$

$$x = 5000$$

Ratio strength $= 1:5000$, *answer.*

Express 1:4000 as a percentage strength.

$$\frac{4000\,(\text{parts})}{1\,(\text{part})} = \frac{100\,(\%)}{x\,(\%)}$$

$$x = 0.025\%, \textit{answer.}$$

Note: To change ratio strength to percentage strength, it is sometimes convenient to "convert" the last two zeros in a ratio strength to a percent sign (%) and change the remaining ratio first to a common fraction and then to a decimal fraction in expressing percent:

$$
\begin{aligned}
1{:}100 &= \tfrac{1}{1}\% &&= 1\% \\
1{:}200 &= \tfrac{1}{2}\% &&= 0.5\% \\
3{:}500 &= \tfrac{3}{5}\% &&= 0.6\% \\
1{:}2500 &= \tfrac{1}{25}\% &&= 0.04\% \\
1{:}10{,}000 &= \tfrac{1}{100}\% &&= 0.01\%
\end{aligned}
$$

Calculating the ratio strength of a solution or liquid preparation, given the weight of solute or constituent in a specified volume of solution or liquid preparation involves the following.

A certain injectable contains 2 mg of a drug per milliliter of solution. What is the ratio strength (w/v) of the solution?

$$2\ \text{mg} = 0.002\ \text{g}$$

$$\frac{0.002\,(\text{g})}{1\,(\text{g})} = \frac{1\,(\text{mL})}{x\,(\text{mL})}$$

$$x = 500\ \text{mL.}$$

Ratio strength $= 1:500$, *answer.*

What is the ratio strength (w/v) of a solution made by dissolving five tablets, each containing 2.25 g of sodium chloride, in enough water to make 1800 mL?

$$2.25\ \text{g} \times 5 = 11.25\ \text{g of sodium chloride}$$

$$\frac{11.25\,(\text{g})}{1\,(\text{g})} = \frac{1800\,(\text{mL})}{x\,(\text{mL})}$$

$$x = 160\ \text{mL.}$$

Ratio strength $= 1:160$, *answer.*

In solving problems in which the calculations are based on ratio strength, it is sometimes convenient to translate the problem into one based on percentage strength and to solve it accordingly.

How many grams of potassium permanganate should be used in preparing 500 mL of a 1:2500 solution?

$$1:2500 = 0.04\%$$
$$500 \text{ (g)} \times 0.0004 = 0.2 \text{ g potassium permanganate, } answer.$$

Or,

1:2500 means 1 g in 2500 mL of solution

$$\frac{2500 \text{ (mL)}}{500 \text{ (mL)}} = \frac{1 \text{ (g)}}{x \text{ (g)}}$$
$$x = 0.2 \text{ g potassium permanganate, } answer.$$

How many milligrams of gentian violet should be used in preparing the following solution?

℞   Gentian Violet Solution   500 mL
                    1:10,000
      Sig. Instill as directed.

$$1:10,000 = 0.01\%$$
$$500 \text{ (g)} \times 0.0001 = 0.050 \text{ g or 50 mg gentian violet, } answer.$$

Or,

1:10,000 means 1 g of 10,000 mL of solution

$$\frac{10,000 \text{ (mL)}}{500 \text{ (mL)}} = \frac{1 \text{ (g)}}{x \text{ (g)}}$$
$$x = 0.050 \text{ g, or 50 mg gentian violet, } answer.$$

How many milligrams of hexachlorophene should be used in compounding the following prescription?

℞   Hexachlorophene   1:400
      Hydrophilic Ointment ad   10 g
      Sig. Apply.

$$1:400 = 0.25\%$$
$$10 \text{ (g)} \times 0.0025 = 0.025 \text{ g or 25 mg hexachlorophene, } answer.$$
Or,

1:400 means 1 g in 400 g of ointment

$$\frac{400 \text{ (g)}}{10 \text{ (g)}} = \frac{1 \text{ (g)}}{x \text{ (g)}}$$
$$x = 0.025 \text{ g, or 25 mg hexachlorophene, } answer.$$

Simple Conversions of Concentration to "mg/mL"

Occasionally, pharmacists, particularly those practicing in patient care settings, need to *convert rapidly* product concentrations expressed as percentage strength, ratio strength, or as grams per liter (as in IV infusions) *to milligrams per milliliter* (mg/mL). These conversions may be made quickly by using simple techniques. Some suggestions follow.

CALCULATIONS CAPSULE

Ratio Strength

The concentrations of very weak pharmaceutical preparations (usually weight-in-volume solutions) often are expressed in terms of their ratio strengths.

Ratio strength is another way of expressing percentage strength. For example, a 1% w/v solution and a ratio strength of 1:100 w/v are equivalent.

The preferable style of a ratio strength is to have the numeric value of the solute as 1. This is accomplished when calculating a ratio strength, by setting up a proportion from the data as:

$$\frac{g\,(given\,solute)}{mL\,(given\,solution)} = \frac{1}{x}; then,\ 1: value\ of\ x, answer.$$

In using a ratio strength in a calculations problem, there are two options: (a) convert it to a percentage strength and perform calculations in the usual manner, or (2) use the ratio strength directly in a problem-solving proportion.

(a) To convert a ratio strength to a percentage strength; for example, 1:10,000 w/v:

$$\frac{1\,g}{10,000\,mL} = \frac{x\,(g)}{100\,mL}$$

Solving for x yields percent, by definition (parts per hundred).

(b) Problem-solving proportion, for example:

$$\frac{1\,g}{10,000\,mL} = \frac{x\,g}{(given\,quality,\,mL)}; x = g\,in\,given\,mL$$

To convert *product percentage strength to mg/mL*, multiply the percentage strength, expressed as a whole number by 10.

Example:

Convert 4% (w/v) to mg/mL

4×10 = 40 mg/mL, *answer.*
Proof or alternate method: 4% (w/v) = 4 g/100 mL
= 4000 mg/100 mL
= 40 mg/mL

To convert *product ratio strengths to mg/mL*, divide the ratio strength by 1000.

Example:

Convert 1: 10,000 (w/v) to mg/mL

$10,000 \div 1000$ = 1 mg/10 mL, *answer.*
Proof or alternate method: 1:10,000 (w/v) = 1 g/10,000 mL
= 1000 mg/10,000 mL
= 1 mg/10 mL

To convert *product strengths expressed as grams per liter (g/L) to mg/mL*, convert the numerator of milligrams and divide by the number of milliliters in the denominator.

Convert a product concentration of 1 g per 250 mL to mg/mL

$$1000 \div 250 \qquad\qquad\qquad = 4 \text{ mg/mL, } answer.$$
Proof or alternate method: 1 g/250 mL   = 1000 mg/250 mL = 4 mg/mL

Milligrams Percent

The term *milligrams percent* (mg%) expresses the number of milligrams of substance in 100 mL of liquid. It is used occasionally to denote the concentration of a drug or natural substance in a biologic fluid, as in the blood. Thus, the statement that the concentration of nonprotein nitrogen in the blood is 30 mg% means that each 100 mL of blood contains 30 mg of nonprotein nitrogen. However, the concentrations of substances in biologic fluids are more often expressed in milligrams per deciliter (mg/dL) than in mg%.

Parts per Million (PPM) and Parts per Billion (PPB)

The strengths of very dilute solutions are commonly expressed in terms of *parts per million (ppm)* or *parts per billion (ppb)*, i.e., the number of parts of the agent per 1 million or 1 billion parts of the whole. For example, we are all familiar with fluoridated drinking water in which fluoride has been added at levels of between 1 to 4 parts per million (1:1,000,000 to 4:1,000,000) for the purpose of reducing dental caries.

We also are aware of and concerned with the presence of trace amounts of *contaminants* in our drinking water and food which can pose a risk to our health and safety. Many pharmacists serve on community committees and boards which address environmental issues. Although they may not refer to themselves as **environmental pharmacists**, their backgrounds and interest in public health make them invaluable members of such bodies. Pharmacists have a special leadership role in providing guidance in the safe disposal of unused and/or expired medications.[4,5] Federal regulations and guidelines have been established to address this issue.[6,7]

Example Calculations of Parts per Million and Parts per Billion

Express 5 ppm of iron in water in percentage strength and ratio strength.

$$5 \text{ ppm} = 5 \text{ parts in } 1,000,000 \text{ parts} \quad = 1{:}200,000 \text{, ratio strength, } and$$
$$= 0.0005\% \text{, percentage strength, } answers.$$

The concentration of a drug additive in an animal feed is 12.5 ppm. How many milligrams of the drug should be used in preparing 5.2 kg of feed?

12.5 ppm = 12.5 g (drug) in 1,000,000 g (feed)

Thus,

$$\frac{1,000,000 \text{ g}}{12.5 \text{ g}} = \frac{5,200 \text{ g}}{x \text{ g}}$$
$$x = 0.065 \text{ g} = 65 \text{ mg, } answer.$$

The drinking water in a community has detected lead in its drinking water at a level of 2.5 ppb. The EPA's MCL is set at 15 ppb. Express the difference between these two values as a ratio strength.

15 ppb − 2.5 ppb = 12.5 ppb = 12.5:1,000,000,000 = 1:80,000,000, *answer.*

PRACTICE PROBLEMS

Weight-in-Volume Calculations

1. CLOBEX lotion contains 0.05% w/v clobetasol propionate in 118 mL containers. Calculate the content of drug, in milligrams.

2. ℞   Ofloxacin Ophthalmic
        Solution   0.3%
        Disp.   10 mL
        Sig: 2 drops into eyes q 4 hours ×
        2 days; then 2 drops q 6 hours ×
        4 days.

   A pharmacist filled the prescription with OCUFLOX ophthalmic solution. How many milligrams of ofloxacin are contained in the dispensed prescription?

3.[8] ℞   Dexamethasone Sodium
          Phosphate   100 mg
          Sterile Water for Injection
          ad   100 mL
          Sig: 2 drops into eyes q 4 hours ×
          2 days; then 2 drops q 6 hours ×
          4 days.

   Calculate the percent strength of dexamethasone sodium phosphate in the prescription.

4. If 100 mL of a pharmaceutical preparation contains 20 µL of a 50% w/v solution of benzalkonium chloride, what is the percentage strength of that agent in the solution?

5. A tissue plasminogen activator (TPA) ophthalmic solution is prepared to contain 25 µg/100 µL.

   (a) Calculate the percentage concentration of TPA in the solution.
   (b) What volume of a solution containing TPA, 50 mg/ 50 mL, should be used to prepare each 100 µL of the ophthalmic solution?

6. How many milligrams of methylparaben are needed to prepare 8 fluidounces of a solution containing 0.12% (w/v) of methylparaben?

7. A pharmacist emptied the contents of eight capsules, each containing 300 mg of clindamycin phosphate, into a liquid vehicle to prepare 60 mL of a suspension. Calculate the percentage strength of clindamycin phosphate in the preparation.

8. ℞   ACULAR (ketorolac
        tromethamine)
        Ophthalmic Solution   0.5%
        Disp.   5 mL
        Sig: One drop q.i.d. prn allergic
        conjunctivitis

   How many milligrams of the active constituent would be present in each drop of the ophthalmic solution if the dropper service delivers 20 drops per milliliter?

   (a) 0.25 mg
   (b) 25 mg
   (c) 0.025 mg
   (d) 1.25 mg

9. A formula for an antifungal shampoo contains 2% w/v ketoconazole. How many grams of ketoconazole would be needed to prepare 25 liters of the shampoo?

10. The biotechnology drug interferon gamma-1b (ACTIMMUNE) contains 100 mcg/0.5 mL. Calculate the percentage strength of the solution.

11. NEUPOGEN (filgrastim) prefilled syringes contain 480 mcg of active constituent in each 0.8 mL. The equivalent concentration is:

   (a) 0.6%
   (b) 0.384 mg/mL
   (c) 0.06%
   (d) 0.6 g/mL

12. LEVAQUIN (levofloxacin) injection contains 5 mg/mL of levofloxacin and 5% of dextrose. How much of each would be delivered to a patient upon the administration of a 100-mL injection?

    (a) 5 g levofloxacin and 5 g dextrose
    (b) 50 mg levofloxacin and 5 g dextrose
    (c) 500 mg levofloxacin and 500 mg dextrose
    (d) 0.5 g levofloxacin and 5 g dextrose

13. An injection (ARANESP) contains in each milliliter, 60 µg of darbepoetin alpha, 0.05 mg of polysorbate 80, and 8.18 mg of sodium chloride. Calculate the percent of each in the injection.

14. An injection of adalimumab (HUMIRA) contains 40 mg/0.8 mL. Calculate the percentage concentration of the injection.

15.[9] ℞ Erythromycin
    Lactobionate   500 mg
    Dexamethasone Sodium
        Phosphate   100 mg
        Glycerin   2.5 mL
    Sterile Water for
        Injection ad   100 mL
    M. ft. Ophthalmic Solution

    (a) What is the percentage strength of erythromycin lactobionate in the prescription?

    (b) If glycerin has a specific gravity of 1.25, what is its concentration (w/v) in the prescription?

16. How many milliliters of a 0.9% (w/v) solution of sodium chloride can be prepared from 50 tablets, each containing 2.25 g of sodium chloride?

17. The antibacterial agent moxifloxacin hydrochloride is available in 250-mL bags for intravenous infusion containing 400 mg of drug and 0.8% w/v sodium chloride. Calculate (a) the percent strength of moxifloxacin hydrochloride and (b) the quantity of sodium chloride, in grams, in the infusion.

18. A prefilled syringe contains 50 mg of lidocaine hydrochloride per 5 mL of injection. Express the percentage concentration of lidocaine hydrochloride in the injection.

19. A blood volume expansion solution contains 6% (w/v) of hetastarch and 0.9% (w/v) of sodium chloride. How many grams of each agent would be present in 250 mL of the solution?

20. A pharmacist adds 10 mL of a 20% (w/v) solution of a drug to 500 mL of D5W for parenteral infusion. What is the percentage strength of the drug in the infusion solution?

    (a) 2% v/v
    (b) 2% w/v
    (c) 1.96% w/v
    (d) 0.39% w/v

21. Calculate the percentage strength of an injection that contains 2 mg of hydromorphone hydrochloride in each milliliter of injection.

22. VIRAMUNE Oral Suspension contains 1% w/v of nevirapine. Calculate the milligrams of nevirapine present in a 240 mL bottle of the suspension.

23. ℞[10] Misoprostol 200-µg
        tablets   12 tablets
    Lidocaine
        Hydrochloride   1 g
    Glycerin qs ad   100 mL

    Calculate the strength of misoprostol in the prescription.

    (a) 2.4% w/v misoprostol
    (b) 0.0002% w/v misoprostol
    (c) 0.024 mg/mL misoprostol
    (d) 2.4 mcg/mL misoprostol

24. ℞[11] Fentanyl Citrate   20 µg/mL
    Bupivacaine
        Hydrochloride   0.125%
    Sodium Chloride
        (0.9%) Injection ad 100 mL

Calculate the percentage concentration of fentanyl citrate in the prescription.

25. Bepotastine besilate (BEPREVE) ophthalmic solution contains 1.5% w/v of the therapeutic agent. Express this concentration in mg/mL.

26. If 100 mL of a solution for patient-controlled anesthesia contains 200 mg of morphine sulfate and 8 mg of droperidol, calculate the percentage strength of each of these ingredients in the solution.

27. Oxycodone hydrochloride oral concentrate solution (OXYFAST) contains 20 mg/1 mL. If a dose of 0.75 mL is added to 30 mL of juice prior to administration, calculate (a) the milligrams of oxycodone hydrochloride administered, and (b) the percentage concentration (w/v) of oxycodone hydrochloride in the drink.

28. A morphine sulfate extended-release liposome injection (DEPODUR) contains morphine sulfate 10 mg/mL of injection. Calculate the percentage strength of morphine sulfate in the injection.

29. A topical solution contains 3% w/v hydroquinone. How many liters of the solution can be prepared from 30 g of hydroquinone?

Volume-in-Volume Calculations

30. What is the percentage strength (v/v) if 225 g of a liquid having a specific gravity of 0.8 is added to enough water to make 1.5 liters of the solution?

31. How many liters of a mouthwash can be prepared from 100 mL of cinnamon flavor if its concentration is to be 0.5% (v/v)?

32. A lotion vehicle contains 15% (v/v) of glycerin. How much glycerin should be used in preparing 5 gallons of the lotion?

(a) 2271 g glycerin
(b) 3339.7 mL glycerin
(c) 2671.8 g glycerin
(d) 3548.4 g glycerin

33. The formula for 1 liter of an elixir contains 0.25 mL of a flavoring oil. What is the percentage (v/v) of the flavoring oil in the elixir?

34. A dermatologic lotion contains 1.25 mL of liquefied phenol in 500 mL. Calculate the percentage (v/v) of liquefied phenol in the lotion.

Weight-in-Weight Calculations

35. Each gram of LOTRISONE lotion contains 10 mg of clotrimazole and 0.643 mg of betamethasone dipropionate. Calculate the percent concentration of each of these two agents in the lotion.

36. A hemorrhoidal ointment contains, on a weight-in-weight basis, 46.6% mineral oil, 1% pramoxine HCl, and 12.5% zinc oxide in an ointment base. Calculate the grams of each ingredient, including the ointment base, in each 30-g tube.

37. What is the percentage strength (w/w) of a solution made by dissolving 62.5 g of potassium chloride in 187.5 mL of water?

38. If 500 g of dextrose are dissolved in 600 mL of water with a resultant final volume of 1 liter, what is the percentage strength of dextrose in the solution on a w/w basis?

39. Hydromorphone hydrochloride suppositories contain 3 mg of active ingredient and weigh approximately 2 grams each. What is the equivalent percentage strength?

(a) 1.5%
(b) 0.15%
(c) 0.015%
(d) none of the above

40. A metronidazole vaginal gel contains 0.75% of drug in 70-g tubes. An applicator will hold 5 g of gel for each administration. How much drug will be contained in each application?

    (a) 0.0375 mg metronidazole
    (b) 3.75 mg metronidazole
    (c) 37.5 mg metronidazole
    (d) 375 mg metronidazole

41. ℞   ZOVIRAX (acyclovir) 5% Cream
        Lidocaine 4% Cream aa. 15 g

    The percent of acyclovir and quantity of lidocaine in the filled prescription are:

    (a) 3.75% acyclovir, 0.3 g lidocaine
    (b) 5% acyclovir, 1.2 g lidocaine
    (c) 2.5% acyclovir, 0.6 g lidocaine
    (d) 2.5% acyclovir, 1.2 g lidocaine

42. How many grams of hydrocortisone should be used in preparing 120 suppositories, each weighing 2 g and containing 1% of hydrocortisone?

43. If a topical cream contains 1.8% (w/w) of hydrocortisone, which of the following strengths is equivalent?

    (a) 2.7 mg hydrocortisone in 15 g of cream
    (b) 27 mg hydrocortisone in 15 g of cream
    (c) 0.54 g hydrocortisone in 30 g of cream
    (d) 54 mg hydrocortisone in 30 g of cream

44.[12] ℞ Benzoin Tincture   18 mL
        Peru Balsam   10 g
        Cold Cream   70 g
        Sig: cold sore ointment

    If benzoin tincture has a specific gravity of 0.88, calculate its percentage strength (w/w) in the mixture.

    (a) 1.26% w/w
    (b) 25.7% w/w
    (c) 22.5% w/w
    (d) 16.5% w/w

45. Alclometasone dipropionate (ACLO-VATE) ointment contains 0.05% w/w of the drug in 15-g and 45-g tubes. Calculate the difference in the quantity of drug between the two tube sizes.

46. How many grams of azelaic acid (FINACEA) are contained in 50-g tubes of the 15% w/w gel?

47. Tretinoin gel (RETIN-A-MICRO) is available in a 0.04% w/w concentration. Which of the following represents an equivalent strength?

    (a) 30 mg tretinoin/30 g gel
    (b) 0.06 g tretinoin/15 g gel
    (c) 60 mg tretinoin/15 g gel
    (d) 6 mg tretinoin/15 g gel

Mixed Percent Calculations

48.[13] ℞ Progesterone, micronized   4 g
        Glycerin   5 mL
        Methylcellulose (1%)
          Solution   50 mL
        Cherry Syrup ad   100 mL

    (a) What is the percentage concentration (w/v) of progesterone in the prescription?

    (b) What is the percentage concentration (w/v) of methylcellulose in the prescription?

    (c) What is the percentage concentration (v/v and w/v) of glycerin (sp gr 1.25) in the prescription?

49.[14] ℞ Lactic Acid   4 g
        Salicylic Acid   5 g
        Trichloroacetic Acid   2 g
        Flexible Collodion
          q.s. ad   100 g
        Sig: wart remover. Use as directed.

    (a) Flexible collodion contains 20% w/w camphor and 30% w/w castor oil. How many grams of each would be contained in 30 g of the mixture?

    (b) The specific gravity of castor oil is 0.955. How many milliliters of the oil are contained in 30 g of the mixture?

(c) If the specific gravity of the mixture is 0.781, what are the w/v concentrations of lactic acid, salicylic acid, and trichloroacetic acid in the mixture?

Ratio Strength Calculations

50. Express each of the following as a percentage strength:

    (a) 1:1500   (d) 1:400
    (b) 1:10,000   (e) 1:3300
    (c) 1:250   (f) 1:4000

51. Express each of the following as a ratio strength:

    (a) 0.125%   (d) 0.6%
    (b) 2.5%   (e) $^1/_3$%
    (c) 0.80%   (f) $^1/_2$%

52. Express each of the following concentrations as a ratio strength:

    (a) 2 mg of active ingredient in 2 mL of solution
    (b) 0.275 mg of active ingredient in 5 mL of solution
    (c) 2 g of active ingredient in 250 mL of solution
    (d) 1 mg of active ingredient in 0.5 mL of solution

53. A doxycycline calcium syrup is preserved with 0.08% (w/v) of methylparaben, 0.02% (w/v) of propylparaben, and 0.1% (w/v) of sodium metabisulfite. Express these concentrations as ratio strengths.

54. An injection contains 0.5% (w/v) of lidocaine hydrochloride and 1:200,000 (w/v) of epinephrine. Express the concentration of lidocaine hydrochloride as a ratio strength and that of epinephrine as a percentage.

55. A sample of white petrolatum contains 10 mg of tocopherol per kilogram as a preservative. Express the amount of tocopherol as a ratio strength.

56. ℞   Potassium Permanganate
    Tablets   0.2 g
    Disp. #100

Sig: two tablets in 4 pt of water and use as directed.

Express the concentration, as a ratio strength, of the solution prepared according to the directions given in the prescription.

57. A skin test for fire ant allergy involves the intradermal skin prick of 0.05 mL of a 1:1,000,000 (w/v) dilution of fire ant extract. How many micrograms of extract would be administered in this manner?

58. In acute hypersensitivity reactions, 0.5 mL of a 1:1000 (w/v) solution of epinephrine may be administered subcutaneously or intramuscularly. Calculate the milligrams of epinephrine given.

59.[15] ℞ Tetracaine Hydro-
    Chloride   0.75%
    Epinephrine Hydro-
    Chloride   1:4000
    Cocaine Hydro-
    Chloride   3%
    Sodium Chloride, qs
    Sterile Water ad   30 mL

How many milligrams each of tetracaine hydrochloride, epinephrine hydrochloride, and cocaine hydrochloride are needed to fill the prescription?

Parts per Million Calculations

60. Purified water contains not more than 10 ppm of total solids. Express this concentration as a percentage.

61. How many grams of sodium fluoride should be added to 100,000 liters of drinking water containing 0.6 ppm of sodium fluoride to provide a recommended concentration of 1.75 ppm?

62. If a commercially available insulin preparation contains 1 ppm of proinsulin, how many micrograms of proinsulin would be contained in a 10-mL vial of insulin?

CALCQUIZ

6.A. AURALGAN Otic Drops contain:

Antipyrine	5.4%
Benzocaine	1.4%
Acetic acid	0.01%
u-polycosanol 410	0.01%
Glycerin, ad	10 mL

   (a) What would be the content of antipyrine, in mg/mL?

   (b) If a patient used 5 drops of the otic solution, equivalent to 0.25 mL, how many milligrams of benzocaine would have been administered?

   (c) How many μL of acetic acid would be used to prepare the 10 mL of drops?

   (d) What would be the equivalent ratio strength (v/v) of u-polycosanol 410?

6.B. Among its other ingredients, VISINE-A eye drops contain the active ingredients: 0.025% naphazoline hydrochloride and 0.3% pheniramine maleate; and, 1:10,000 benzalkonium chloride as a preservative. Calculate (a) the corresponding percent strength of benzalkonium chloride and (b) the quantities of each of the three ingredients in a 15 mL container.

6.C. An intravenous solution of AVELOX contains 400 mg of moxifloxacin hydrochloride (1.6 mg/mL). Calculate (a) the percent concentration of moxifloxacin hydrochloride and (b) the volume of solution in the product.

6.D. ATROVENT Nasal Spray contains 0.03% of ipratropium bromide in a 30-mL metered dose container. If the container is calibrated to deliver 345 sprays, calculate (a) the volume of each spray, in microliters, and (b) the number of milligrams of ipratropium bromide in each spray.

6.E. A homeopathic teething gel states on its product label that it contains 0.0000003% alkaloid. Express the alkaloid content in ppm.

ANSWERS TO "CASE IN POINT" AND PRACTICE PROBLEMS

Case in Point 6.1

(a) 58 g (weight of filled pycnometer) − 28 g (weight of pycnometer) = 30 g (weight of 25 mL of albumin solution);

   30 g ÷ 25 mL = 1.2, specific gravity of albumin solution, *answer*.

(b) 2000 mL × 0.05 (5%) = 100 g of albumin needed;

$$\frac{25 \text{ g}}{100 \text{ mL}} = \frac{100 \text{ g}}{\text{x mL}}; \text{ x} = 400 \text{ mL},$$

   albumin solution needed, *answer*.

(c) 400 mL × 1.2 (specific gravity) = 480 g, albumin solution needed, *answer*.

(d) 2000 mL (total solution) − 400 mL (albumin solution) = 1600 mL (0.9% sodium chloride solution);

   1600 mL × 1.05 (specific gravity) = 1680 g (weight of 0.9% sodium chloride solution);

   1680 g + 480 g = 2160 g (total weight of the 2000 mL);

   2160 g ÷ 2000 mL = 1.08, specific gravity of the mixture, *answer*.

Case in Point 6.2

(a) 30 g × 0.015 (1.5% w/w) = 0.45 g hydrocortisone needed, *answer*.

(b) $\dfrac{0.1\ g}{1\ mL} = \dfrac{0.45\ g}{x\ mL}$; x = 4.5 mL hydrocortisone injection, *answer*.

(c) 4.5 mL × 1.5 (specific gravity) = 6.75 g (weight of hydrocortisone injection); 30 g − 6.75 g = 23.25 g cold cream needed, *answer*.

Practice Problems

1. 59 mg clobetasol propionate

2. 30 mg ofloxacin

3. 0.1% w/v dexamethasone sodium phosphate

4. 0.01% w/v benzalkonium chloride

5. (a) 0.025% w/v TPA
   (b) 0.025 mL

6. 283.9 mg methylparaben

7. 4 % w/v clindamycin phosphate

8. (a) 0.25 mg ketorolac tromethamine

9. 500 g ketoconazole

10. 0.02% w/v interferon gamma-1b

11. (c) 0.06%

12. (d) 0.5 g levofloxacin and 5 g dextrose

13. 0.006% w/v darbepoetin alpha, 0.005% w/v polysorbate 80, and 0.818% w/v sodium chloride

14. 5% w/v adalimumab

15. (a) 0.5% w/v erythromycin lactobionate
    (b) 3.125% w/v glycerin

16. 12,500 mL

17. (a) 0.16% moxifloxacin hydrochloride
    (b) 2 g sodium chloride

18. 1% w/v lidocaine hydrochloride

19. 15 g hetastarch
    2.25 g sodium chloride

20. (d) 0.39% w/v

21. 0.2% w/v hydromorphone

22. 2400 mg nevirapine

23. (c) 0.024 mg/mL misoprostol

24. 0.002% w/v fentanyl citrate

25. 15 mg bepotastine besilate/mL

26. 0.2% w/v morphine sulfate and 0.008% w/v droperidol

27. (a) 15 mg oxycodone hydrochloride
    (b) 0.049% w/v oxycodone hydro-chloride

28. 1% w/v morphine sulfate

29. 1 liter

30. 18.75% v/v

31. 20 liters

32. (d) 3548.4 g glycerin

33. 0.025% v/v flavoring oil

34. 0.25% v/v liquefied phenol

35. 1% w/w clotrimazole
    0.0643% w/w betamethasone dipro-pionate

36. 13.98 g mineral oil
    0.3 g pramoxine HCl
    3.75 g zinc oxide
    11.97 g ointment base

37. 25% w/w potassium chloride

38. 45.45% w/w dextrose

39. (b) 0.15%

40. (c) 37.5 mg metronidazole

41. (c) 2.5% acyclovir, 0.6 g lidocaine

42. 2.4 g hydrocortisone

43. (c) 0.54g hydrocortisone in 30 g of cream

44. (d) 16.5% w/w

45. 15 mg alclometasone dipropionate

46. 7.5 g azelaic acid

47. (d) 6 mg tretinoin/15 g gel

48. (a) 4% w/v progesterone
    (b) 0.5% w/v methylcellulose
    (c) 5% v/v and 6.25% w/v glycerin

49. (a) 5.34 g camphor and 8.01 g castor oil
    (b) 8.39 mL castor oil
    (c) 3.12% w/v lactic acid, 3.91% w/v salicylic acid, and 1.56% w/v trichloroacetic acid

50. (a) 0.067%
    (b) 0.01%
    (c) 0.4 %
    (d) 0.25%
    (e) 0.03%
    (f) 0.025%

51. (a) 1:800
    (b) 1:40
    (c) 1:125
    (d) 1:166.67 or 1:167
    (e) 1:300
    (f) 1:2000

52. (a) 1:1000
    (b) 1:18,182
    (c) 1:125
    (d) 1:500

53. 1:1250 w/v methylparaben
    1:5000 w/v propylparaben
    1:1000 w/v sodium metabisulfite

54. 1:200 w/v lidocaine hydrochloride
    0.0005% w/v epinephrine

55. 1:100,000 w/w tocopherol

56. 1:4730 w/v potassium permanganate

57. 0.05 µg fire ant extract

58. 0.5 mg epinephrine

59. 225 mg tetracaine hydrochloride
    7.5 mg epinephrine hydrochloride
    900 mg cocaine hydrochloride

60. 0.001% w/v

61. 115 g sodium fluoride

62. 10 µg proinsulin

References

1. United States Pharmacopeial Convention. *United States Pharmacopeia 32 National Formulary 27*. Vol. 1. Rockville, MD: United States Pharmacopeial Convention, 2009:8.
2. United States Pharmacopeial Convention. *United States Pharmacopeia 32 National Formulary 27*. Vol. 2. Rockville, MD: United States Pharmacopeial Convention, 2009:1582.
3. Flynn Warren, Bishop, GA.
4. Johnson MG. Tools based on experiences of a community pharmacy providing destruction services for unwanted medications. *Journal of the American Pharmacists Association* 2010;50(3):388–392.
5. Gray-Winnett MD, Davis CS, Yokley SG, et al. From dispensing to disposal: the role of student pharmacists in medication disposal and implementation of a take-back program. *Journal of the American Pharmacists Association* 2010;50(5):613–618.
6. Office of National Drug Control Policy. *Proper Disposal of Prescription Drugs*. Washington, DC: Office of National Drug Control Policy. October 2009. http://www.whitehousedrugpolicy.gov/publications. Accessed January 22, 2011.
7. Federal Register. *Secure and Responsible Drug Disposal Act of 2010*. Vol. 75. Federal Register; 2010:245.
8. *International Journal of Pharmaceutical Compounding* 1998;2:147.
9. *International Journal of Pharmaceutical Compounding* 2002;6:452.
10. Ford P. *International Journal of Pharmaceutical Compounding* 1999;3:48.
11. *International Journal of Pharmaceutical Compounding* 1997;1:178.
12. *International Journal of Pharmaceutical Compounding* 2002;6:127.
13. *International Journal of Pharmaceutical Compounding* 1998;2:57.
14. Prince SJ. *International Journal of Pharmaceutical Compounding* 2003;7:46.
15. Prince SJ. Calculations. *International Journal of Pharmaceutical Compounding* 2000;4:221.

Calculation of Doses: General Considerations

7

Objectives

Upon successful completion of this chapter, the student will be able to:

- Perform calculations relevant to various drug doses and dosing regimens.
- Perform calculations of doses involving household measures.

Dose Definitions

The *dose* of a drug is the quantitative *amount* administered or taken by a patient for the intended medicinal effect. The dose may be expressed as a *single dose*, the amount taken at one time; a *daily dose*; or a *total dose*, the amount taken during the course of therapy. A daily dose may be subdivided and taken in *divided doses*, two or more times per day depending on the characteristics of the drug and the illness. The schedule of dosing (e.g., *four times per day for 10 days*) is referred to as the *dosage regimen*.

Quantitatively, drug doses vary greatly among drug substances; some drugs have small doses, other drugs have relatively large doses. The dose of a drug is based on its biochemical and pharmacologic activity, its physical and chemical properties, the dosage form used, the route of administration, and various patient factors. The dose of a drug for a particular patient may be determined in part on the basis of the patient's age, weight, body surface area, general physical health, liver and kidney function (for drug metabolism and elimination), and the severity of the illness being treated. Considerations of some specific patient parameters in dosing are presented in Chapter 8 and an introduction to *pharmacokinetic* dosing is presented in Chapter 22. Pharmacokinetic dosing takes into account a patient's ability to metabolize and eliminate drugs from the body due to impaired liver or renal function, which often necessitates a reduction in dosage.

The *usual adult dose* of a drug is the amount that ordinarily produces the medicinal effect intended in the adult patient. The *usual pediatric dose* is similarly defined for the infant or child patient. The "usual" adult and pediatric doses of a drug serve as a guide to physicians

---

CALCULATIONS CAPSULE

Doses

Given two factors in the following equation, by rearrangement, the third may be calculated:

$$\text{Number of doses} = \frac{\text{Total quantity}}{\text{Size of dose}}$$

In using the equation, the total quantity and the size of dose must be in the same unit of measure.

who may select to prescribe that dose initially or vary it depending on the assessed requirements of the particular patient. The **usual dosage range** for a drug indicates the quantitative range or amounts of the drug that may be prescribed within the guidelines of usual medical practice. Drug use and dose information is provided in the package labeling and inserts that accompany manufacturers' pharmaceutical products, as well as in a variety of references, such as *Drug Facts and Compari*sons,[1] *Physicians' Desk Reference*,[2] *Pediatric Dosage Handbook: Including Neonatal Dosing, Drug Administration, & Extemporaneous Preparations*,[3] *Geriatric Dosage Handbook*,[4] and *Drug Information Handbook*.[5]

The dose response of individuals varies as depicted in Figure 7.1 and may require dosage adjustment in a given patient. For certain conditions, as in the treatment of cancer patients, drug dosing is highly specialized and individualized. Frequently, combinations of drugs are used, with the doses of each adjusted according to the patient's response. Many anticancer drugs are administered *cyclically*, usually for 21 to 28 days, with a rest period between dosing cycles to allow recovery from the toxic effects of the drugs. As presented in Chapter 8, anticancer drugs are most commonly dosed on the basis of the patient's body surface area.

The **median effective dose** of a drug is the amount that produces the desired intensity of effect in 50% of the individuals tested. The **median toxic dose** of a drug is the amount that produces toxic effects in 50% of the individuals tested. Drugs intended to produce systemic effects must be absorbed or placed directly into the circulation and distributed in adequate concentrations to the body's cellular sites of action. For certain drugs, a correlation exists between drug dosage, the drug's blood serum concentration after administration, and the presentation and degree of drug effects. An average blood serum concentration of a drug can be measured, and the minimum concentration determined that can be expected to produce the drug's desired effects in a patient. This concentration is referred to as the **minimum effective concentration** (MEC). The base level of blood serum concentration that produces dose-related toxic effects is referred to as the **minimum toxic concentration** (MTC) of the drug.

Optimally, appropriate drug dosage should result in blood serum drug concentrations that are above the MEC and below the MTC for the period of time that drug effects are desired.

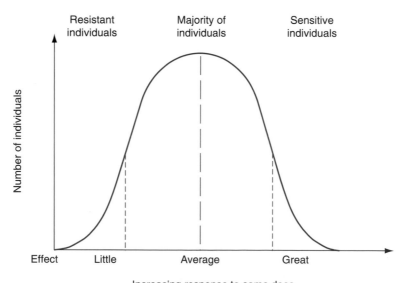

▼ FIGURE 7.1 Drug effect in a population sample.

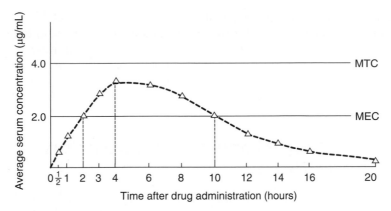

▼ FIGURE 7.2 Example of a blood level curve for a hypothetical drug as a function of the time after oral administration. MEC, minimum effective concentration; MTC, minimum toxic concentration.

As shown in Figure 7.2 for a hypothetical drug, the serum concentration of the drug reaches the MEC 2 hours after its administration, achieves a peak concentration in 4 hours, and falls below the MEC in 10 hours. If it would be desired to maintain the drug serum concentration above the MEC for a longer period, a second dose would be required at about an 8-hour time frame. In some cases, ***incremental dose escalation*** is employed whereby the patient is started on a known low dose of a drug followed by additional doses until the desired effect is achieved.

The *frequency or scheduling* of dosing is dependent on many factors including whether the illness or condition is responsive to short-term or long-term treatment; the physical–chemical and biologic characteristics of the drug substance itself; and features of the product formulation and route of drug administration. A single good example of the variation in the frequency of dosing is the drug ibandronate sodium (BONIVA) which is formulated as once-a-day tablets, monthly-dosed tablets, and a once-every-3-months injection.

For certain drugs, a larger-than-usual initial dose may be required to achieve the desired blood drug level. This dose is referred to as the ***priming*** or ***loading dose***. Subsequent ***maintenance*** doses, similar in amount to usual doses, are then administered according to the dosage regimen to sustain the desired drug blood levels or drug effects. To achieve the desired drug blood level rapidly, the loading dose may be administered as an injection or oral liquid, whereas the subsequent maintenance doses may be administered in other forms, such as tablets or capsules.

As discussed later in this chapter, there are certain instances in which ***low-dose therapy*** or ***high-dose therapy*** is prescribed for a particular patient. And, for certain drugs there may be different doses required depending on whether the use is for ***monotherapy***, that is, as the primary drug treatment, or ***adjunctive therapy***, that is, additional to or supportive of a different primary treatment.

Certain biologic or immunologic products, such as vaccines, may be administered in ***prophylactic doses*** to protect the patient from contracting a specific disease. Other products, such as antitoxins, may be administered in ***therapeutic doses*** to counter a disease after exposure or contraction. The doses of some biologic products, such as insulin, are expressed in ***units of activity***, derived from biologic assay methods. Calculations pertaining to these types of products are presented in Chapter 9.

Prefabricated products prepared on a large scale within the pharmaceutical industry and dispensed in community and institutional pharmacies generally contain the dosage strengths and dosage forms most often used. However, in instances in which the desired strength or dosage form is not available, pharmacists may be called upon to ***compound*** the preparation.

Pharmaceutical products may be prepared to contain one or more therapeutic agents. Products containing more than one therapeutic agent are termed **combination products**.

One of the primary responsibilities of the pharmacist is to check doses specified in prescriptions based on a knowledge of the usual doses, usual dose ranges, and dosage regimens of the medicines prescribed. If an unusual dose is noted, the pharmacist is ethically bound to consult the physician to make certain that the dose as written or interpreted is the dose intended and that it is suitable for the patient and condition being treated.

Routes of Drug/Dose Administration and Dosage Forms

Doses of drugs are administered by a variety of dosage forms and routes of administration, as shown in Table 7.1. In addition to the drug itself, dosage forms contain **pharmaceutical ingredients**, which provide the physical features, stability requirements, and aesthetic characteristics desired for optimal therapeutic effects. Included in the array of pharmaceutical ingredients are solvents, vehicles, preservatives, stabilizers, solubilizers, binders, fillers, disintegrants, flavorants, colorants, and others.

With added pharmaceutical ingredients, the quantity of an active ingredient in a dosage form represents only a portion (often a small portion) of the total weight or volume of a product. For example, a tablet with 10 mg of drug actually could weigh many times that amount because of the added pharmaceutical ingredients.

Definitions of the various dosage forms and drug delivery systems are found in Appendix B.

Dose Measurement

In the institutional setting, doses are measured and administered by professional and paraprofessional personnel. A variety of measuring devices may be used, including calibrated

Table 7.1 ▼ SELECTED ROUTES OF ADMINISTRATION AND REPRESENTATIVE DOSAGE FORMS

ROUTE OF ADMINISTRATION	REPRESENTATIVE DOSAGE FORMS
Oral (mouth, GI tract)	Tablets, capsules, lozenges, solutions, drops, syrups, and suspensions
Sublingual (under the tongue)	Tablets
Parenteral (injection)	Solutions and suspensions
Epicutaneous/ Transdermal (skin)	Ointments, creams, powders, lotions, aerosols, and patches
Conjunctival (eye)	Solutions, suspensions, and ointments
Intranasal (nose)	Solutions, sprays, and ointments
Intrarespiratory (lungs)	Aerosols and inhalant solutions
Rectal (rectum)	Ointments, creams, suppositories, solutions, and suspensions
Vagina (vagina)	Ointments, creams, tablets, suppositories, gels, solutions, and emulsion foams
Urethral (urethra)	Solutions and suppositories

▼ FIGURE 7.3 An example of a calibrated medication cup for admininstering oral liquid medication.

cups and oral syringes for liquid oral medications (Figs. 7.3 and 7.4). For pediatric patients, use of oral syringes is recommended as a means of reducing medication dosing errors.[6] In hospitals, many medications are administered by injection and by intravenous infusion.

In the home setting, the patient, caregiver, or, in the case of a child, the parent generally measures and administers oral medication. Liquids are measured using household measures such as teaspoons and tablespoons (Table 7.2), calibrated spoons or cups, oral syringes, or drops. Patients being treated by home health care personnel may receive medications by all routes of administration including parenteral.

▼ FIGURE 7.4 An example of calibrated Exacta-Med® Oral Dispenser for administering liquid medication to pediatric patients. *(Courtesy of BAXA Corporation.)*

Table 7.2 ▼ USEFUL APPROXIMATE EQUIVALENT OF HOUSEHOLD MEASURE

HOUSEHOLD MEASURE (ABBREVIATION)	OUNCE	METRIC MEASURE
1 teaspoonful (tsp.)	≈1/6 fluidounce ≈	5 mL
1 teaspoonful (tbsp.)	≈1/2 fluidounce ≈	15 mL

Teaspoon and Tablespoon

Household spoons vary greatly in capacities. In approximate terms, the teaspoon is considered to hold 5 mL of volume and the tablespoon 15 mL (Table 7.2).[7] However, due to the variability in capacity, the Food and Drug Administration states that "*a kitchen teaspoon or tablespoon is not an appropriate measuring device for giving medicines to children.*"[8] It urges the use of a measuring device that either accompanies the product or is obtained separately *and* is calibrated to deliver the recommended dose. A calibrated oral syringe is a good option.

Occasionally, a prescriber will indicate a teaspoonful dose by using the fluidram symbol (*fl ʒ*) in the *Signa* portion of a prescription, and the pharmacist interprets it accordingly.[a] A half-teaspoonful would be indicated by *ʒss*. However, once again, a more accurate measuring device than a household spoon should be used.

The Drop as a Unit of Measure

Occasionally, the *drop* (abbreviated *gtt*) is used as a measure for small volumes of liquid medications. A drop does not represent a definite quantity, because drops of different liquids issued from different droppers vary greatly. In an attempt to standardize the drop as a unit of volume, the *United States Pharmacopeia* defines the official medicine dropper as being constricted at the delivery end to a round opening with an external diameter of about 3 mm.[9] The dropper, when held vertically, delivers water in drops, each of which weighs between 45 and 55 mg. Accordingly, the official dropper is calibrated to deliver approximately 20 drops of water per milliliter (i.e., 1 mL of water = 1 gram or 1000 mg ÷ 50 mg [ave.]/drop ≅ 20 drops).

It should be kept in mind, that few medicinal liquids have the same surface and flow characteristics as water, and therefore the size of drops varies materially from one liquid to another. The drop should not be used as a measure for a specific liquid medication until the volume that the drop represents has been determined for that liquid. This determination is made by *calibrating* the dispensing dropper. Most manufacturers include a specially calibrated dropper along with their prepackaged medications for use by patients in measuring dosage. Examples of calibrated droppers are shown in Figure 7.5.

A dropper may be calibrated by counting the drops of a liquid as they fall into a graduate until a measurable volume is obtained. The number of drops per unit volume is then established (e.g., 20 drops/mL).

If a pharmacist counted 40 drops of a medication in filling a graduate cylinder to the 2.5-mL mark, how many drops per milliliter did the dropper deliver?

---

[a] The *fluidram* is a quantity in the Apothecaries' system as presented in Appendix A.

▼ FIGURE 7.5 Examples of calibrated droppers used in the administration of pediatric medications.

$$\frac{40\,(\text{drops})}{x\,(\text{drops})} = \frac{2.5\,(\text{mL})}{1\,(\text{mL})}$$

$$x = 16\,\text{drops mL},\, \textit{answer.}$$

CASE IN POINT 7.1 A physician asks a pharmacist to calculate the dose of a cough syrup so that it may be safely administered dropwise to a child. The cough syrup contains the active ingredient dextromethorphan HBr, 30 mg/15 mL, in a 120-mL bottle.

Based on the child's weight and literature references, the pharmacist determines the dose of dextromethorphan HBr to be 1.5 mg for the child.

The medicine dropper to be dispensed with the medication is calibrated by the pharmacist and shown to deliver 20 drops of the cough syrup per 1 mL.

Calculate the dose, in drops, for the child.

General Dose Calculations

A pharmacist often needs to calculate the size of a dose, the number of doses, or the total quantity of medication to dispense. For these calculations the following equation is useful *with the terms rearranged depending on the answer required.* In using the equation, the units of weight or volume must be the same for the total quantity and size of the dose.

$$\textbf{Number of doses} = \frac{\textbf{Total quantity}}{\textbf{Size of dose}}$$

Example Calculations of the Number of Doses

If the dose of a drug is 200 mg, how many doses are contained in 10 g?

$$10\,\text{g} = 10{,}000\,\text{mg}$$

$$\text{Number of doses} = \frac{10{,}000\,(\text{mg})}{200\,(\text{mg})} = 50\,\text{doses},\, \textit{answer.}$$

Or, solving by dimensional analysis:

$$\frac{1\,\text{dose}}{200\,\text{mg}} \times \frac{1000\,\text{mg}}{1\,\text{g}} \times 10\,\text{g} = 50\,\text{doses},\, \textit{answer.}$$

If 1 tablespoon is prescribed as the dose, approximately how many doses will be contained in 1 pint of the medicine?

$$1 \text{ tablespoon} = \quad 15 \text{ mL}$$
$$1 \text{ pint} \qquad = \ 473 \text{ mL}$$

$$\text{Number of doses} = \frac{473 \text{ mL}}{15 \text{ mL}} = 31.5 \text{ or } 31 \text{ doses}, \textit{answer}.$$

If the dose of a drug is 50 μg, how many doses are contained in 0.02 g?

$$0.02 \text{ g} = 20 \text{ mg}$$
$$50 \,\mu g \ = 0.05 \text{ mg}$$

$$\text{Number of doses} = \frac{20 \,(\text{mg})}{0.05 \,(\text{mg})} = 400 \text{ doses}, \textit{answer}.$$

Example Calculations of the Size of a Dose

$$\textbf{Size of dose} = \frac{\textbf{Total quantity}}{\textbf{Number of doses}}$$

The *size of the dose* is expressed in whatever denomination is chosen for measuring the given total quantity.

How many teaspoonfuls would be prescribed in each dose of an elixir if 180 mL contained 18 doses?

$$\text{Size of dose} = \frac{180 \text{ mL}}{18} = 10 \text{ mL} = 2 \text{ teaspoonfuls}, \textit{answer}.$$

How many drops would be prescribed in each dose of a liquid medicine if 15 mL contained 60 doses? The dispensing dropper calibrates 32 drops/mL.

$$15 \text{ mL} = 15 \times 32 \text{ drops} = 480 \text{ drops}$$

$$\text{Size of dose} = \frac{480 \,(\text{drops})}{60} = 8 \text{ drops}, \textit{answer}.$$

Or, solving by dimensional analysis:

$$\frac{32 \text{ drops}}{1 \text{ mL}} \times \frac{1}{60 \text{ doses}} \times 15 \text{ mL} = 8 \text{ drops/dose}, \textit{answer}.$$

Example Calculations of the Total Quantity of Product

$$\textbf{Total quantity = number of doses} \times \textbf{size of dose}$$

It is convenient first to convert the given dose to the denomination in which the total quantity is to be expressed.

How many milliliters of a liquid medicine would provide a patient with 2 tablespoonfuls twice a day for 8 days?

$$\text{Number of doses} \ = 16$$
$$\text{Size of dose} \qquad = 2 \text{ tablespoonfuls or 30 mL}$$
$$\text{Total quantity} \qquad = 16 \times 30 \text{ mL} = 480 \text{ mL}, \textit{answer}.$$

How many milliliters of a mixture would provide a patient with a teaspoonful dose to be taken three times a day for 16 days?

Number of tsp doses $= 16 \times 3 = 48$ tsp
Total quantity $\qquad = 48 \times 5$ mL $= 240$ mL, *answer*.

How many grams of a drug will be needed to prepare 72 dosage forms if each is to contain 30 mg?

Number of doses $\quad = 72$
Size of dose $\qquad = 30$ mg
Total quantity $\qquad = 72 \times 30$ mg $= 2160$ mg $= 2.16$ g, *answer*.

It takes approximately 4 g of ointment to cover an adult patient's leg. If a physician prescribes an ointment for a patient with total leg eczema to be applied twice a day for 1 week, which of the following product sizes should be dispensed: 15 g, 30 g, or 60 g?

Number of doses $\quad = 2$ per day $\times 7$ days $= 14$
Size of dose $\qquad = 4$ g
Total quantity $\qquad = 14 \times 4$ g $= 56$ g; thus, 60 g product size, *answer*.

Additional Examples of Calculations of Dose

If 0.05 g of a substance is used in preparing 125 tablets, how many micrograms are represented in each tablet?

$$0.05 \text{ g} = 50 \text{ mg} = 50,000 \text{ } \mu g$$
$$\frac{50,000 \text{ } (\mu g)}{125} = 400 \text{ } \mu g, \textit{answer}.$$

Or, solving by dimensional analysis:

$$\frac{1,000,000 \text{ } \mu g}{1 \text{ g}} \times \frac{1}{125 \text{ tablets}} \times 0.05 \text{ g} = 400 \text{ } \mu g/\text{tablet}, \textit{answer}.$$

If a preparation contains 5 g of a drug in 500 mL, how many grams are contained in each table-spoonful dose?

$$1 \text{ tablespoonful} = 15 \text{ mL}$$
$$\frac{500 \text{ (mL)}}{15 \text{ (mL)}} = \frac{5 \text{ (g)}}{x}$$
$$x = 0.15 \text{ g}, \textit{answer}.$$

A cough mixture contains 48 mg of hydromorphone hydrochloride in 8 fl. oz. How many milligrams of hydromorphone hydrochloride are in each 2-teaspoonful dose?

$$1 \text{ fl. oz.} \quad = \quad 6 \text{ tsp.}$$
$$8 \text{ fl. oz.} \quad = 48 \text{ tsp.}$$
$$48 \text{ tsp} \div 2 \quad = 24 \text{ doses}$$
$$48 \text{ mg} \div 24 \quad = \quad 2 \text{ mg}, \textit{answer}.$$

Or,

$$\frac{48 \text{ (tsp.)}}{2 \text{ (tsp.)}} = \frac{48 \text{ (mg)}}{x \text{ (mg)}}$$
$$x = 2 \text{ mg}, \textit{answer}.$$

How many milligrams each of hydrocodone bitartrate and guaifenesin will be contained in each dose of the following prescription?

℞   Hydrocodone Bitartrate   0.12 g
     Guaifenesin   2.4 g
     Cherry Syrup ad   120 mL
     Sig. Teaspoonful for cough.
     1 teaspoonful = 5 mL
     120 ÷ 5 = 24 doses
     0.12 g ÷ 24 = 0.005 g = 5 mg hydrocodone bitartrate, *and*
     2.4 g ÷ 24 = 0.1 g = 100 mg guaifenesin, *answers.*

How many grams of a drug substance are required to make 120 mL of a solution each teaspoonful of which contains 3 mg of the drug substance?

$$1 \text{ teaspoonful} = 5 \text{ mL}$$

$$\frac{5\,(\text{mL})}{120\,(\text{mL})} = \frac{3\,(\text{mg})}{x\,(\text{mg})}$$

$$x = 72 \text{ mg or } 0.072 \text{ g}, answer.$$

Or, solving by dimensional analysis:

$$\frac{1\,\text{g}}{1000\,\text{mg}} \times \frac{3\,\text{mg}}{5\,\text{mL}} \times 120 \text{ mL} = 0.072 \text{ g}, answer.$$

A physician ordered 500-mg capsules of tetracycline to be taken twice a day for 10 days. How many total grams of tetracycline would be prescribed?

Size of dose   = 500 mg
Total number of doses = 2 (a day) × 10 (days) = 20 doses
Total quantity   = 500 mg × 20 (doses) = 10,000 mg = 10 g, *answer.*

Dosing Options

Low-Dose and High-Dose Therapies

The administration of doses that are much smaller or much larger than the *usual dose* of a drug is referred to as *low-dose* or *high-dose* therapy, respectively. This terminology is different in intent from the normal variation in a standard dose based on a patient's age, weight, renal function, or other specific parameter.

The most common example of low-dose therapy is the use of aspirin in 81-mg amounts (rather than the usual dose of 325 mg) to lower the risk of heart attack and clot-related stroke. Other examples are low-dose oral contraceptive use[10] and low-dose postmenopausal hormone therapy.[11]

High-dose therapy is commonly associated with the chemotherapeutic treatment of cancer, in which there is an attempt, through increased dose intensity, to kill tumor cells.[9] Other examples are the high-dose use of progestin in the treatment of endometriosis[12] and the high-dose influenza vaccination of the elderly.[13]

Pharmacists must be aware of the use of high-dose therapies while remaining vigilant in protecting patients against unintended high doses and consequent drug overdose.

Example Calculations of Low-Dose and High-Dose Therapies

If a patient is changed from a daily standard-dose postmenopausal product containing 0.625 mg of conjugated estrogens (CE) to a low-dose formulation containing 0.35 mg CE, how many milligrams less of CE would the patient take per week?

$$0.625 \text{ mg} - 0.35 \text{ mg} = 0.275 \text{ mg} \times 7 \text{ (days)} = 1.925 \text{ mg conjugated estrogens, } answer.$$

To reduce the inflammation of an optic nerve, a patient is administered high-dose prednisone, 900 mg/day for 5 days by intravenous infusion. The usual daily dose of prednisone is 5 to 60 mg/day, depending on the condition being treated. Calculate the dose that the patient received, as a multiple of the highest usual daily dose.

$$\frac{900 \text{ mg}}{60 \text{ mg}} = 15, \text{ multiple of the highest usual dose, } answer.$$

Fixed-Dose Combination Products

A variety of prescription and nonprescription products are available containing two or more therapeutic agents in fixed-dose combinations. An advantage of combination products is that two or more needed drugs may be taken in a single dose, which may be more convenient, enhance compliance, and be less expensive for the patient than taking the same drugs individually. A disadvantage is the relative inflexibility in dosing compared with individual drug dosing.

Whether the fixed-dose combination is a liquid (e.g., a syrup) or a solid (e.g., a tablet) dosage form, when a dose is taken, the component drugs are taken in a fixed-dose ratio. To provide some options in dosing, many combinations of prescription drugs are formulated into different strengths. For example, capsules containing amlodipine and benazepril HCl (LOTREL), two drugs used in the treatment of hypertension, are available in strengths of 2.5 mg/10 mg, 5 mg/10 mg, 5 mg/20 mg, 5 mg/40 mg, 10 mg/20 mg, and 10 mg/40 mg. The prescriber can select the desired combination.

Example Calculation Based on Fixed-Dose Combination Products

Valsartan and hydrochlorothiazide tablets are available separately or in combination in strengths of 80 mg/12.5 mg, 160 mg/12.5 mg, 160 mg/25 mg and 320 mg/12.5 mg. If a patient was receiving the lowest-dose combination product and the physician wished to double the dose of hydrochlorothiazide, what is the option?

An additional prescription for 12.5 mg of hydrochlorothiazide or individual prescriptions for 80 mg of valsartan and 25 mg of hydrochlorothiazide may be written, *answer.*

Tablet Splitting and Crushing

A number of tablets are *scored*, or grooved, to allow breaking into approximately equal pieces (usually halves). This allows dosage flexibility, particularly when a patient is started at a half dose and then is titrated up to a full dosage level. It also enables a patient to take a product at a strength that is not otherwise available.

Some patients use tablet-splitting devices to cut scored or unscored tablets for economic reasons. For some medications, the price of tablets of twice the strength required is similar to the lower-strength tablets, and the patient can double his or her supply by tablet splitting. Unfortunately, this practice often results in unequal portions of tablets and thus in uneven doses.[14–17] *Tablet splitting should be performed as carefully as possible and only for drugs for which the clinical outcomes are not compromised.*[18] Additionally, patients may not be aware that many solid dosage forms should not be cut or crushed but must remain intact for proper drug absorption. Listings of drug products that should not be crushed are readily available from a number of sources, including that of the reference indicated.[19] However, for tablets that *can* be crushed without destroying desired absorption characteristics, *tablet crushing* is a commonly employed practice for home- or institutional-patients who are unable to swallow

▼ FIGURE 7.6 An example of a tablet crusher. A tablet is placed in a paper cup, covered with a second cup, and then placed in the crusher. When the handles are gently squeezed, the pressure reduces the tablet to particles that may then be mixed with food or drink for administration. The device is used in patient-care facilities and wherever a patient may have difficulty swallowing whole dosage units. (Courtesy of Creative Living Medical, Brainerd, MN.)

intact solid dosage forms. In these instances, mortars and pestles or specially designed tablet crushers are used (Fig. 7.6). After crushing, the resulting particles may be suspended in a beverage or mixed with a foodstuff as applesauce or yogurt prior to administration.

Example Calculation Based on Tablet Splitting

A patient attempted to split in half 20-mg unscored tablets of a drug, resulting in "half-tablets" differing by 1.5 mg in drug content. Assuming a whole tablet was uniform in drug content, calculate the amount of drug in each "half tablet."

If L = larger "half" and S = smaller "half,"
$$\begin{aligned} \text{then } L + S &= 20 \text{ mg} \\ \underline{L - S} &= \underline{1.5 \text{ mg}} \\ 2L &= 21.5 \text{ mg} \end{aligned}$$

L = 10.75 mg and
S = 20 mg − 10.75 mg = 9.25 mg, *answers.*

Proof: 10.75 mg − 9.25 mg = 1.5 mg difference in drug content and
10.75 mg + 9.25 mg = 20 mg total drug content

Special Dosing Regimens

Certain drugs have unique dosing regimens. Among them are chemotherapeutic agents (discussed in Chapter 8) and oral contraceptives. In the case of the latter, the prescribed regimen is based on a 28-day dosing cycle of 21 consecutive days of tablets containing a combination of estrogenic and progestational drugs followed by 7 consecutive days of tablets containing nondrug material. One tablet is taken daily, preferably at approximately the same time. The tablets generally are color coded and packaged in special dispensers to facilitate compliance.

Example Calculation Based on Special Dosing Regimen

The ORTHO TRI-CYCLEN LO 28-day regimen consists of norgestimate (N), ethinyl estradiol (EE), and nonmedicated tablets as follows:

7 white tablets containing 0.18 mg (N) + 0.025 mg (EE);
7 light blue tablets containing 0.215 mg (N) + 0.025 mg (EE);
7 dark blue tablets containing 0.25 mg (N) + 0.025 mg (EE);
7 green tablets containing 0 mg (N) + 0 mg (EE).

How many milligrams each of norgestimate and ethinyl estradiol are taken during each 28-day cycle?

$$\text{Norgestimate: } \begin{aligned} 0.18 \text{ mg} \times 7 &= 1.26 \text{ mg} \\ 0.215 \text{ mg} \times 7 &= 1.505 \text{ mg} \\ 0.25 \text{ mg} \times 7 &= \underline{1.75 \text{ mg}} \\ & \quad 4.515 \text{ mg norgestimate and} \end{aligned}$$

$$\text{Ethinyl estradiol: } \begin{aligned} 0.025 \text{ mg} \times 7 &= 0.175 \text{ mg} \\ 0.025 \text{ mg} \times 7 &= 0.175 \text{ mg} \\ 0.025 \text{ mg} \times 7 &= \underline{0.175 \text{ mg}} \\ & \quad 0.525 \text{ mg ethinyl estradiol, } \textit{answers.} \end{aligned}$$

PRACTICE PROBLEMS

Doses: Solid Dosage Forms

1. How many capsules, each containing a 150-mcg dose of a drug may be prepared from 0.12 g of the drug?

2. The following regimen for oral prednisone is prescribed for a patient: 50 mg/day × 10 days; 25 mg/day × 10 days; 12.5 mg/day × 10 days; 5 mg/day × 10 weeks. How many scored 25-mg tablets and how many 5-mg tablets should be dispensed to meet the dosing requirements?

3. A physician reduces a patient's once-daily dose of conjugated estrogen (PREMARIN) from tablets containing 0.625 mg to tablets containing 0.45 mg. What is the total reduction in conjugated estrogens taken, in milligrams, during a 30-day month?

4. A fixed-dose combination product contains amlodipine besylate and atorvastatin calcium (CADUET) for the treatment of both hypertension and hypercholesterolemia. If a physician starts a patient on a 5-mg/10-mg dose for 14 days and then raises the dose to 10 mg /20 mg, how many milligrams of each drug will the patient take during the first 30 days?

5. A patient cuts 100-mg scored tablets to take his 50-mg prescribed daily dose. A prescription for thirty 100-mg tablets costs $45, and a prescription for thirty 50-mg tablets costs $40. The patient asked the pharmacist to weigh an uncut tablet on an electronic balance into two "halves." The uncut tablet was found to weigh 240 mg, and the cut "halves" weighed 125 mg and 115 mg, respectively. (a) How much money did the patient save on a monthly basis by dosing with half tablets? (b) What was the percentage error in the weight of the cut tablets compared with "exact halves"?

6. The recommended dose of memantine HCl (NAMENDA) is:

   Week 1, 5 mg/day
   Week 2, 10 mg/day (5 mg, b.i.d.)
   Week 3, 15 mg/day (10 mg a.m., 5 mg p.m.)
   Week 4, 20 mg/day (10 mg b.i.d.)

   How many 5-mg tablets must be dispensed for a 4-week supply of the medication?

7. Prior to a colonoscopy, a patient is instructed to take OSMOPREP tablets each of which contains 1.102 g sodium phosphate monobasic monohydrate

and 0.398 g sodium phosphate dibasic anhydrous. The dose is:

- *The evening before the procedure:* 4 tablets with 8 ounces of clear liquids every 15 minutes for 5 cycles, and
- *Starting 3 hours before the procedure:* 4 tablets with 8 ounces of clear liquids every 15 minutes for 3 cycles.

How many tablets, how much liquid, and how much total sodium phosphates are taken?

- (a) 8 tablets, 16 ounces liquid, 2 g sodium phosphates
- (b) 16 tablets, 1000 mL liquid, 32 g sodium phosphates
- (c) 32 tablets, 1 quart liquid, 40 g sodium phosphates
- (d) 32 tablets, 0.5 gallon liquid, 48 g sodium phosphates

8. CHANTIX (varenicline tartrate), for smoking cessation, is available in two strengths, 0.5-mg and 1-mg tablets. The dose is:

- *Days 1 to 3*: 0.5 mg once daily;
- *Days 4 to 7*: 0.5 mg twice daily (A.M. and P.M.); and
- Days 8 to end of treatment: 1 mg twice daily (A.M. and P.M.).

The treatment period is 12 weeks. How many 0.5-mg tablets and 1-mg tablets should be dispensed?

- (a) 7 0.5-mg tablets and 11 1-mg tablets
- (b) 8 0.5-mg tablets and 84 1-mg tablets
- (c) 10 0.5-mg tablets and 84 1-mg tablets
- (d) 11 0.5-mg tablets and 154 1-mg tablets

Doses: Drops

9. A ciprofloxacin otic solution contains 0.5 mg of ciprofloxacin in a 0.25 mL single-dose package. Based on 20 drops/mL: (a) how many drops would be administered and (b) how many micrograms of ciprofloxacin would be in each drop?

10. ℞ Acetaminophen Oral Drops
    Disp. 15 mL
    Sig. 0.5 mL t.i.d.

- (a) If acetaminophen oral drops contain 1.5 g of acetaminophen per 15-mL container, how many milligrams are there in each prescribed dose?
- (b) If the dropper is calibrated to deliver 22 drops/mL, how many drops should be administered per dose?

11. RESTASIS Ophthalmic Emulsion contains 0.05% w/v cyclosporin. If a dose of one drop measures 28 µL, how many micrograms of cyclosporin are present?

12.[20] The oral dose of a drug is 2.5 mg. If a solution contains 0.5% w/v of the drug in a dropper bottle that delivers 12 drops/mL, how many drops would supply the dose?

13. Infants' MYLICON anti-gas drops contain 2 g of simethicone in a 30-mL container. (a) How many milligrams of simethicone are contained in each 0.3-mL dose and if 12 doses per day are not to be exceeded, calculate the corresponding 12-dose (b) volume and (c) simethicone content.

Doses: Oral Liquids

14. Rimantadine HCl syrup contains 2.4 g of rimantadine HCl in each 240 mL of syrup. How many milligrams of rimantadine HCl would there be in 2.5 mL delivered by oral dispenser?

15. If a liquid medicine is to be taken three times daily, and if 180 mL are to be taken in 4 days, how many tablespoonfuls should be prescribed for each dose?

16. If a cough syrup contains 0.18 g of dextromethorphan HBr in 120 mL, how many milligrams of the drug are contained in each teaspoonful dose?

17. A cough syrup contains 0.09 g of dextromethorphan HBr in each fluidounce. How many milligrams of this agent would be present in each teaspoonful dose?

18. A physician prescribes tetracycline HCl syrup for a patient who is to take 2 teaspoonfuls four times per day for 4 days, and then 1 teaspoonful four times per day for 2 days. How many milliliters of the syrup should be dispensed to provide the quantity for the prescribed dosage regimen?

19. Ipecac oral solution has the following formula:

Powdered Ipecac	70 g
Glycerin	100 mL
Syrup ad	1000 mL

Powdered ipecac contains 2 grams of the combined alkaloids emetine and cephaeline in each 100 grams of powder. Calculate the quantity of these alkaloids, in milligrams, in each 5-mL dose of ipecac oral solution.

20. A dose of digoxin for rapid digitalization is a total of 1 mg, divided into two or more portions at intervals of 6 to 8 hours. How many milliliters of digoxin elixir containing 50 μg/mL would provide the 1 mg dose?

21. Ciprofloxacin (CIPRO) oral suspension contains 250 mg of ciprofloxacin per 5 mL. A physician prescribed 125 mg of ciprofloxacin q.i.d. × 10 days. (a) How many doses are needed? (b) How many milliliters should be given per dose? (c) How many milliliters of ciprofloxacin oral suspension containing 250 mg per 5 mL should be dispensed?

22. A patient has been instructed to take 15 mL of alumina and magnesium oral suspension every other hour for four doses daily. How many days will two 12-fl. oz. bottles of the suspension last?

23.　　 Dextromethorphan HBr 50 mg/tsp.
　　　 Guaifenesin Syrup ad 120 mL
　　　 Sig. ℥i q.i.d. a.c. & h.s.

How many grams of dextromethorphan HBr would be needed to fill the prescription?

24. The dose of AUGMENTIN oral suspension for a patient is 5-mL b.i.d. Each 5 mL of suspension contains 400 mg of amoxicillin and 57 mg of clavulanic acid. If the suspension is to be taken for 10 days and is available in 50-mL, 75-mL, and 100-mL containers, calculate (a) the least wasteful package size to dispense and (b) total quantity of amoxicillin taken during the treatment period.

Doses: Injections

25. A physician ordered 20 mg of MEPERGAN and 0.3 mg of atropine sulfate to be administered preoperatively to a patient. MEPERGAN is available in a syringe containing 25 mg/mL, and atropine sulfate is in an ampul containing 0.4 mg per 0.5 mL. How many milliliters of each should be used in filling the medication order?

26. How many milliliters of an injection containing 250 mg of aminophylline in each 10 mL should be used in filling a medication order calling for 15 mg of aminophylline?

27.[21] Pediatric LANOXIN injection contains digoxin, 100 mcg/mL. What volume must be administered to provide a dose of 0.04 mg?

Doses: Other Dosage Forms

28. The recommended maintenance dose of BECLOVENT (beclomethasone dipropionate), an aerosolized inhalant, is 100 mcg administered twice daily. The commercial inhaler delivers 50 mcg per metered inhalation and contains 200 inhalations. How many inhalers should be dispensed to a patient if a 60-day supply is prescribed?

29. A 16-week regimen for a brand of a nicotine patch calls for a patient to wear a 21-mg patch each day for the first 6 weeks, followed by a 14-mg patch each day for the next 2 weeks, and then a 7-mg patch for the next 2 weeks to conclude the treatment regimen. In all, how many milligrams of nicotine are administered?

30. A transdermal patch contains 5 mg of fentanyl and has a drug-release rate of 50 mcg/hour. The patch is worn for 72 hours. Calculate (a) the milligrams of fentanyl delivered daily, (b) the milligrams of fentanyl remaining in the patch when it is removed, and (c) the percentage of drug remaining in the patch when it is removed.

31. If a VENTOLIN inhaler contains 20 mg of albuterol, how many inhalation-doses can be delivered if each inhalation-dose contains 90 mcg?

32. FLONASE Nasal Spray contains 50 mcg of fluticasone propionate per actuation spray in each 100 mg of formulation. Each container provides 120 metered sprays. How many milligrams of fluticasone propionate are contained in each container?

33. The dose of VOLTAREN (diclofenac sodium) GEL, when applied to the hands in the treatment of arthritic pain, is 2 g four times a day. The gel contains diclofenac sodium 1% and is available in 100-g tubes. How many grams of the drug diclofenac sodium would be administered per day and how many days of treatment would be available per tube of gel?
    (a) 8 g diclofenac sodium per day for 8 days
    (b) 8 g diclofenac sodium per day for 12.5 days
    (c) 80 mg diclofenac sodium per day for 8 days
    (d) 0.08 g diclofenac sodium per day for 12.5 days

34. SYMBICORT 80/4.5 is an oral inhalation product containing 80 mcg of budesonide and 4.5 mcg of formoterol fumarate per inhalation. The dose is stated as "two inhalations twice daily." How much of *each drug* would be administered daily?
    (a) 160 mcg budesonide and 9 mcg formoterol fumarate
    (b) 0.32 mg budesonide and 0.18 mg formoterol fumarate
    (c) 320 mcg budesonide and 0.18 mg formoterol fumarate
    (d) 0.32 mg budesonide and 0.018 mg formoterol fumarate

CALCQUIZ

7.A. The ophthalmic solution ALPHAGAN P contains 0.15% brimonidine tartrate in 10-mL containers. The recommended dose is one drop in the affected eye(s) three times daily. If a glaucoma patient doses each eye, and the dropper used delivers 20 drops/mL, calculate the quantity, in milligrams, of brimonidine tartrate administered each day.

7.B. The starting dose of sodium oxybate oral solution (XYREM) is 4.5 g/night divided into two equal doses and administered 2.5 to 4 hours apart. How many milliliters of the oral solution containing sodium oxybate, 500 mg/mL, should be administered in each divided dose?

7.C. A pediatric stool softener contains 393.3 mg of docusate sodium in each four fluid ounce (118 mL) container. If the labeled dose is two tablespoonsful for a 5-year-old child, how many milligrams of docusate sodium would be contained per dose?

7.D. An oral inhalation (DULERA) to treat asthma, provides in each inhalation, 100 μg of mometasone furoate and 5 μg of formoterol fumarate. The recommended dose is "two inhalations twice daily (morning and evening)." Calculate the quantity, in milligrams, of each drug inhaled daily.

7.E. In an experiment of tablet-splitting effectiveness, a pharmacist had a pharmacy student split a previously weighed lisinopril tablet containing 20 mg of drug. On an electronic balance, the whole tablet weighed 111.62 mg. After splitting, one "half tablet" weighed 51.21 mg and the other "half," 58.49 mg. There was residue powder remaining. Calculate (a) the percent of lost tablet (residue), (b) the percent accuracy in actual weight (to ideal weight) for each "half-tablet," and (c) the *supposed* quantity of drug, in milligrams, (not assayed, of course) in each "half-tablet."

ANSWERS TO "CASE IN POINT" AND PRACTICE PROBLEMS

Case in Point 7.1

First calculate the volume of cough syrup containing the child's dose of 1.5 mg of dextromethorphan HBr:

$$\frac{30\,mg}{15\,mL} = \frac{1.5\,mg}{x\,mL}; x = 0.75\,mL$$

Then determine the number of drops of cough syrup that will provide the 0.75-mL dose:

$$\frac{1\,mL}{20\,drops} = \frac{0.75\,mL}{x\,drops};$$

$$x = 15 \text{ drops of cough syrup, } answer.$$

Practice Problems

1. 800 capsules
2. thirty-five 25-mg tablets and seventy 5-mg tablets

3. 5.25 mg conjugated estrogen
4. 230 mg amlodipine besylate and 460 mg atorvastatin calcium
5. (a) $17.50
   (b) 4.2%
6. 70 tablets
7. (d) 32 tablets, 0.5 gallon liquid, 48 g sodium phosphates
8. (d) 11 0.5-mg tablets and 154 1-mg tablets
9. (a) 5 drops ciprofloxacin otic solution
   (b) 100-μg ciprofloxacin/drop
10. (a) 50 mg acetaminophen
    (b) 11 drops
11. 14 mcg cyclosporine
12. 6 drops

13. (a) 20-mg simethicone
    (b) 3.6 mL of Infants' MYLICON drops
    (c) 240-mg simethicone
14. 25 mg rimantadine HCl
15. 1 tablespoonful
16. 7.5 mg dextromethorphan HBr
17. 15.2 mg dextromethorphan HBr
18. 200 mL tetracycline HCl syrup
19. 7 mg alkaloids
20. 20 mL digoxin elixir
21. (a) 40 doses
    (b) 2.5 mL/dose
    (c) 100 mL ciprofloxacin oral suspension
22. 11⁺ days
23. 1.2 g dextromethorphan HBr

24. (a) 100-mL package
    (b) 8000 mg or 8 g of amoxicillin
25. 0.8 mL MEPERGAN and 0.375 mL atropine sulfate injections
26. 0.6 mL aminophylline injection
27. 0.4 mL LANOXIN injection
28. 2 inhalers
29. 1176 mg nicotine
30. (a) 1.2 mg fentanyl
    (b) 1.4 mg fentanyl
    (c) 28%
31. 222 doses
32. 6 mg fluticasone propionate
33. (d) 0.08 g diclofenac sodium per day for 12.5 days
34. (d) 0.32 mg budesonide and 0.018 mg formoterol fumarate

References

1. *Drug Facts and Comparisons*. St. Louis, MO: Wolters Kluwer Health, 2011.
2. *Physicians' Desk Reference*. Montvale, NJ: Medical Economics, 65:2011.
3. Taketomo CK, Hodding JH, Kraus DM. *Pediatric Dosage Handbook: Including Neonatal Dosing, Drug Administration, & Extemporaneous Preparations*. 15th Ed. Hudson, OH: Lexi-Comp, 2010.
4. Semla TP, Beizer JL, Higbee MD. *Geriatric Dosage Handbook*. 15th Ed. Hudson, OH: Lexi-Comp, 2010.
5. Lacy CF, Armstrong LL, Goldman MP, et al. *Drug Information Handbook*. 19th Ed. Hudson, OH: Lexi-Comp, 2010.
6. The Joint Commission. Available at: http://www.jointcommission.org/assets/1/18/SEA_39.PDF. Accessed April 4, 2011.
7. United States Pharmacopeial Convention. *United States Pharmacopeia 32 National Formulary 27*. Rockville, MD: United States Pharmacopeial Convention, 2009;1:728.
8. Available at: http://www.fda.gov/Drugs/DrugSafety/DrugSafetyPodcasts/ucm077929.htm. Accessed April 4, 2011.
9. United States Pharmacopeial Convention. *United States Pharmacopeia 32 National Formulary 27*. Rockville, MD: United States Pharmacopeial Convention, 2009;1:604.
10. Warner Chilcott Company, LO LOESTRIN FE, product information, Accessed November 2010.
11. Postmenopausal hormone therapy: An endocrine society scientific statement. *The Journal of Clinical Endocrinology and Metabolism* 2010;95:S1–S66.
12. Available at: http://www.women.webmd.com/endometriosis/high-dose-progestin-for-endometriosis. Accessed September 5, 2008.
13. Foster SL, Moore WP. High-dose influenza vaccination in the elderly. *Journal of the American Pharmacists Association* 2010;50:546–547.
14. Rashed SM, Nolly RJ, Robinson L, et al. Weight variability of scored and unscored split psychotropic drug tablets. *Hospital Pharmacy* 2003;38:930–934.
15. Hill SW, Varker AS, Karlage K, et al. Analysis of drug content and weight uniformity for half-tablets of 6 commonly split medications. *Journal of Managed Care Pharmacy* 2009;15:253–261.
16. Verrue C, Mehuys E, Boussery K, et al. Tablet-splitting: a common yet not so innocent practice. *Journal of Advanced Nursing* 2010;67:26–32.
17. Green G, Berg C, Polli JE, et al. Pharmacopeial standards for the subdivision characteristics of scored tablets. *Pharmacopeial Forum* 2009;35:1598.
18. Navarro RP. Tablet splitting. *Journal of Managed Care Pharmacy* 2009;15:272–274.
19. Physicians' Desk Reference. *Drugs that should not be crushed*. Montvale, NJ: Medical Economics, 2011;65:323.
20. Prince S. *International Journal of Pharmaceutical Compounding* 2003;7:212.
21. Beach W. *College of Pharmacy*. Athens, GA: The University of Georgia, 2004.

Calculation of Doses: Patient Parameters

8

Objectives

Upon successful completion of this chapter, the student will be able to:

- Calculate doses based on factors of age, body weight, and body surface area.
- Utilize dosing tables and nomograms in calculations.
- Calculate doses for single and combination chemotherapy regimens.

As noted in the previous chapter, the *usual dose* of a drug is the amount that ordinarily produces the desired therapeutic response in the majority of patients in a general, or otherwise defined, population group. The drug's *usual dosage range* is the range of dosage determined to be safe and effective in that same population group. This provides the prescriber with dosing guidelines in initially selecting a drug dose for a particular patient and the flexibility to change that dose as the patient's clinical response warrants. Usual doses and dosage regimens are based on the results of clinical studies conducted during the drug development process as well as on clinical information gathered following the initial approval and marketing of the drug (*postmarketing surveillance/postmarketing studies*).

For certain drugs and for certain patients, drug dosage is determined on the basis of specific patient parameters. These parameters include the patient's age, weight, body surface area, and nutritional and functional status. Among patients requiring individualized dosage are neonates and other pediatric patients, elderly patients with diminished biologic functions, individuals of all age groups with compromised liver and/or kidney function (and thus reduced ability to metabolize and eliminate drug substances), critically ill patients, and patients being treated with highly toxic chemotherapeutic agents. Certain drugs with a narrow therapeutic window often require individualized dosing based on blood level determinations and therapeutic monitoring. Digoxin, for example, at a blood level of 0.9 to 2 ng/mL is considered therapeutic, but above 2 ng/mL it is toxic.[1]

Since age, body weight, and body surface area are often-used factors in determining the doses of drugs for pediatric and elderly patients, these parameters represent the majority of the calculations presented in this chapter. The dosing of chemotherapeutic agents also is included because it represents a unique dosing regimen compared with most other categories of drugs.

Pediatric Patients

Pediatrics is the branch of medicine that deals with disease in children from birth through adolescence. Because of the range in age and bodily development in this patient population, the inclusive groups are defined further as follows: *neonate* (newborn), from birth to 1 month; *infant*, 1 month to 1 year; *early childhood*, 1 year through 5 years; *late childhood*, 6 years through 12 years; and *adolescence*, 13 years through 17 years of age.[2] A neonate is considered *premature* if born at less than 37 weeks' gestation.

Proper drug dosing of the pediatric patient depends on a number of factors, including the patient's age and weight, overall health status, the condition of such biologic functions as respiration and circulation, and the stage of development of body systems for drug metabolism (e.g., liver enzymes) and drug elimination (e.g., renal system). In the neonate, these biologic functions and systems are underdeveloped. Renal function, for example, develops over the span of the first 2 years of life. This fact is particularly important because the most commonly used drugs in neonates, infants, and young children are antimicrobial agents, which are eliminated primarily through the kidneys. If the rate of drug elimination is not properly considered, drug accumulation in the body could occur, leading to drug overdosage and toxicity. Thus, the use of *pharmacokinetic* data (i.e., the rates and extent of drug absorption, distribution, metabolism, and elimination; see Chapter 22), together with individual patient factors and therapeutic response, provides a rational approach to pediatric drug dosage calculations.[2]

Special Considerations in Dose Determinations for Pediatric Patients

The majority of medications commercially available are formulated and labeled for adult use. When used for the pediatric patient, appropriate dosage calculations must be made, and often, so must adjustments to the concentration of the medication.

Among the special considerations in pediatric dosing are:[3]

- Doses should be based on accepted clinical studies as reported in the literature.
- Doses should be age appropriate and generally based on body weight or body surface area.
- Pediatric patients should be weighed as closely as possible to the time of admittance to a health care facility and that weight recorded in kilograms.
- As available, pediatric formulations rather than those intended for adults should be administered.
- All calculations of dose should be double-checked by a second health professional.
- All caregivers should be properly advised with regard to dosage, dose administration, and important clinical signs to observe.
- Calibrated oral syringes should be used to measure and administer oral liquids.

Doses of drugs used in pediatrics, including neonatology, may be found in individual drug product literature as well as in references, such as those listed at the conclusion of this chapter.[4,5]

CASE IN POINT 8.1 A hospital pharmacist is asked to determine the dose of clindamycin for a 3-day-old neonate weighing 3 lb. 7 oz. In checking the literature, the pharmacist determines that the dose is listed as follows:[4]

> <1200 g: 10 mg/kg/day divided q12h.
> <2000 g and 0–7 days old: 10 mg/kg/day divided q12h.
> <2000 g and >7 days old: 15 mg/kg/day divided q8h.
> >2000 g and 0–7 days old: 15 mg/kg/day divided q8h.
> >2000 g and >7 days old: 20–30 mg/kg/day divided q12h.

Each divided dose is to be added to an intravenous infusion at the scheduled hour and infused over a period of 20 minutes.

Clindamycin is available in an IV bag containing 600 mg/50 mL of injectable solution. How many milliliters of this solution should be given for each divided dose?

> **CASE IN POINT 8.2** A pediatric patient is being administered enalaprilat (VASOTEC IV) every 12 hours by intravenous injection to manage hypertension and possible heart failure.[4] Based on a dose of 5 mcg/kg, the patient is receiving 55 mcg of enalaprilat per dose. The physician wishes to convert the patient to oral enalapril at a dosage of 100 mcg/kg as a single daily dose. The standard procedure is to crush a 2.5-mg tablet of enalapril, mix with sterile water to make 12.5 mL, and administer the appropriate dose using a calibrated oral dispenser. Calculate the dose, in milliliters, to be administered to this patient.

Geriatric Patients

Although the term *elderly* is subject to varying definitions with regard to chronologic age, it is clear that the functional capacities of most organ systems decline throughout adulthood, and important changes in drug response occur with advancing age. *Geriatric medicine* or *geriatrics* is the field that encompasses the management of illness in the elderly.

In addition to medical conditions affecting all age groups, some conditions are particularly common in the elderly, including degenerative osteoarthritis, congestive heart failure, venous and arterial insufficiency, stroke, urinary incontinence, prostatic carcinoma, parkinsonism, and Alzheimer's disease. Many elderly patients have coexisting pathologies that require multiple-drug therapies.

Most age-related physiologic functions peak before age 30 years, with subsequent gradual linear decline.[2] Reductions in physiologic capacity and function are cumulative, becoming more profound with age. Kidney function is a major consideration in drug dosing in the elderly because reduced function results in reduced drug elimination.

Because reduced kidney function increases the possibility of toxic drug levels in the body and adverse drug effects, initial drug dosing in the elderly patient often reflects a downward variance from the usual adult dose. There is also a frequent need for dosage adjustment or medication change due to adverse effects or otherwise unsatisfactory therapeutic outcomes.

There are a number of other common features of medication use in the elderly, including the long-term use of maintenance drugs; the need for multidrug therapy, with the attendant increased possibility of drug interactions and adverse drug effects; and difficulties in patient adherence. The latter is often due to impaired cognition, confusion over the various dosing schedules of multiple medications, and economic reasons in not being able to afford the prescribed medication.

Special Considerations in Dose Determinations for Elderly Patients

Dose determinations for elderly patients frequently require consideration of some or all of the following:

- Therapy is often initiated with a lower-than-usual adult dose.
- Dose adjustment may be required based on the therapeutic response.
- The patient's physical condition may determine the drug dose and the route of administration employed.

- The dose may be determined, in part, on the patient's weight, body surface area, health and disease status, and pharmacokinetic factors.
- Concomitant drug therapy may affect drug/dose effectiveness.
- A drug's dose may produce undesired adverse effects and may affect patient adherence.
- Complex dosage regimens of multiple drug therapy may affect patient adherence.

Example:

The adult dose of a drug is 500 mg every eight hours. For an elderly patient with impaired renal function, the dose is reduced to 250 mg every 6 hours. Calculate the reduction in the daily dose, in milligrams.

Daily doses: 500 mg × 3 (every 8 hours) = 1500 mg
250 mg × 4 (every 6 hours) = 1000 mg
1500 mg − 1000 mg = 500 mg, *answer.*

Dosage Forms Applicable to Pediatric and Geriatric Patients

In the general population, solid dosage forms, such as tablets and capsules, are preferred for the oral administration of drugs because of their convenience, precise dose, ease of administration, ready identification, transportation, and lower cost per dose relative to other dosage forms. However, solid dosage forms are often difficult or impossible for the pediatric, geriatric, or infirm patient to swallow. In these instances, liquid forms are preferred, such as oral solutions, syrups, suspensions, and drops. With liquid forms, the dose can be adjusted by changing the volume administered. When necessary, liquid forms of medication may be administered by oral feeding tube. Pharmacists are sometimes asked to compound an oral liquid from a counterpart solid dosage form when a liquid product is not available. Chewable tablets and solid gel forms (medicated "gummy bears") that disintegrate or dissolve in the mouth are often used for pediatric and geriatric patients. In addition, and as noted in the previous chapter, *tablet splitting* and *tablet crushing* are options for individuals unable to swallow whole tablets.

For systemic effects, injections may be used rather than the oral route of administration when needed for pediatric and elderly patients, with the dose or strength of the preparation adjusted to meet the requirements of the individual patient.

Drug Dosage Based on Age

For reasons stated earlier, the young and the elderly require special dosing considerations based on factors characteristic of these groups.

Before the physiologic differences between adult and pediatric patients were clarified, the latter were treated with drugs as if they were merely miniature adults. Various rules of dosage in which the pediatric dose was a fraction of the adult dose, based on relative age, were created for youngsters (e.g., *Young's rule*). *Today these rules are not in general use because age alone is no longer considered a singularly valid criterion in the determination of accurate dosage for a child, especially when calculated from the usual adult dose, which itself provides*

Table 8.1 ▼ CALCULATION OF PEDIATRIC
DOSAGES OF DIGOXIN
BASED ON AGE AND WEIGHT

AGE	DIGOXIN DOST (μg/kg)
Premature	15 to 25
Full term	20 to 30
1 to 24 months	30 to 50
2 to 5 years	25 to 35
5 to 10 years	15 to 30
Over 10 years	8 to 12

wide clinical variations in response. Some of these rules are presented in the footnote for perspective and historical purposes.[a]

Currently, when age *is* considered in determining dosage of a *potent* therapeutic agent, it is used generally in conjunction with another factor, such as weight. This is exemplified in Table 8.1, in which the dose of the drug digoxin is determined by a combination of the patient's age and weight.

Example Calculations of Dose Based on Age

An over-the-counter cough remedy contains 120 mg of dextromethorphan in a 60-mL bottle of product. The label states the dose as $1^1/2$ teaspoonfuls for a child 6 years of age. How many milligrams of dextromethorphan are contained in the child's dose?

$$1\tfrac{1}{2} \text{ teaspoonfuls} = 7.5 \text{ mL}$$

$$\frac{60 \text{ mL}}{120 \text{ mg}} = \frac{7.5 \text{ mL}}{\text{x mg}}$$

$$\text{x} = 15 \text{ mg dextromethorphan, } \textit{answer}.$$

The dose of a drug for an adolescent is acceptable as either 10 mg/kg or 300 mg. Calculate the difference in these alternative doses for a 9-year-old child weighing 70 lb.

---

[a] Young's rule, based on age:

$$\frac{\text{Age}}{\text{Age} + 12} \times \text{Adult dose} = \text{Dose for child}$$

Cowling's rule:

$$\frac{\text{Age at next birthday (in years)} \times \text{Adult dose}}{24} = \text{Dose for child}$$

Fried's rule for infants:

$$\frac{\text{Age (in months)} \times \text{Adult dose}}{150} = \text{Dose for infant}$$

Clark's rule, based on weight:

$$\frac{\text{Weight (in lb)} \times \text{Adult dose}}{150 \,(\text{average weight of adult in lb.})} = \text{Dose for child}$$

Note: The value of 150 in Fried's rule was an estimate of the age (12.5 years or 150 months) of an individual who would normally receive an adult dose, and the number 150 in Clark's rule was an estimate of the weight of an individual who likewise would receive an adult dose.

Dose at 10 mg/kg: 70 lb ÷ 2.2 lb/kg = 31.8 kg; 31.8 kg × 10 mg/kg = 318.2 mg
Difference in dose = 318.2 mg − 300 mg = 18.2 mg, *answer.*

From the data in Table 8.1, calculate the dosage range for digoxin for a 20-month-old infant weighing 6.8 kg.

$$\frac{30 \ \mu g}{x \ \mu g} = \frac{1 \ kg}{6.8 \ kg} \qquad \frac{50 \ \mu g}{x \ \mu g} = \frac{1 \ kg}{6.8 \ kg}$$

$$x = 204 \ \mu g; \qquad x = 340 \ \mu g$$

Dose range, 204 to 340 μg digoxin, *answer.*

In contrast to the preceding example of dose determination for a potent prescription drug, over-the-counter medications purchased for self-medication include labeling instructions that provide guidelines for safe and effective dosing. For pediatric use, doses generally are based on age groupings; for example, 2 to 6 years old, 6 to 12 years old, and over 12 years of age. For children 2 years of age or younger, the label recommendation generally states "consult your physician."

Drug Dosage Based on Body Weight

Drug doses based on weight are expressed as a specific quantity of drug per unit of patient weight, such as *milligrams of drug per kilogram of body weight* (abbreviated [*mg/kg*]). Dosing in this manner makes the quantity of drug administered specific to the weight of the patient being treated.

Example Calculations of Dose Based on Body Weight

A useful equation for the calculation of dose based on body weight is:

$$\text{Patient's dose (mg)} = \text{Patient's weight (kg)} \times \frac{\text{Drug dose (mg)}}{1 \text{ (kg)}}$$

This equation is based on a drug dose in mg/kg and the patient's weight in kilograms. When different units are given or desired, other units may be substituted in the equation as long as the terms used are consistently applied.

The usual initial dose of chlorambucil is 150 mcg/kg of body weight. How many milligrams should be administered to a person weighing 154 lb.?

CALCULATIONS CAPSULE

Dose Based on Body Weight

A useful equation for the calculation of dose based on body weight is:

$$\text{Patient's dose (mg)} = \text{Patient's weight (kg)} \times \frac{\text{Drug dose (mg)}}{1 \text{ (kg)}}$$

This equation is based on a drug dose in mg/kg and patient's weight in kilograms. When different units are given or desired, other units may be substituted in the equation as long as the terms used are consistently applied.

Solving by the equation:
150 mcg = 0.15 mg

$$\text{Patient's dose (mg)} = 154 \text{ lb.} \times \frac{0.15 \text{ mg}}{2.2 \text{ lb}} = 10.5 \text{ mg chlorambucil, } \textit{answer.}$$

Or, solving by ratio and proportion:
150 mcg = 0.15 mg   1 kg = 2.2 lb.

$$\frac{2.2 \text{ lb}}{154 \text{ lb}} = \frac{0.15 \text{ mg}}{x \text{ mg}}; x = 10.5 \text{ mg chlorambucil, } \textit{answer.}$$

Or, solving by dimensional analysis:

$$\frac{1 \text{ mg}}{1000 \text{ mcg}} \times \frac{150 \text{ mcg}}{1 \text{ kg}} \times \frac{1 \text{ kg}}{2.2 \text{ lb}} \times \frac{154 \text{ lb.}}{1} = 10.5 \text{ mg chlorambucil, } \textit{answer.}$$

The usual dose of sulfisoxazole for infants over 2 months of age and children is 60 to 75 mg/kg of body weight. What would be the usual range for a child weighing 44 lb.?

1 kg	= 2.2 lb
20 kg	= 44 lb
60 mg/kg × 20 kg	= 1200 mg
75 mg/kg × 20 kg	= 1500 mg

Thus, the dosage range would be 1200 to 1500 mg, *answer.*

The dose of minocycline to treat acne vulgaris is given as 1 mg/kg/day × 12 weeks. Tablet strengths available include 45 mg, 55 mg, 65 mg, 80 mg, 90 mg, 105 mg, and 115 mg of mino-cycline. What strength tablet and how many tablets should be prescribed for the entire course of treatment for a 100-lb patient?

100 lb ÷ 2.2 lb/kg = 45.5 kg
1 mg/kg/day × 45.5 kg = 45.5 mg/day ≈ 45-mg minocycline tablets, and
12 wk × 7 day/wk = 84 days; thus, 84 tablets required, *answers.*

A dose of enoxaparin sodium injection (LOVENOX) is "1 mg/kg q12h SC." If a graduated prefilled syringe containing 80 mg/0.8 mL is used, how many milliliters should be administered per dose to a 154-lb patient?

154 lb ÷ 2.2 lb/kg = 70 kg
1 mg/kg × 70 kg = 70 mg

$$0.8 \text{ mL} \times \frac{70 \text{ mg}}{80 \text{ mg}} = 0.7 \text{ mL enoxaparin sodium injection, } \textit{answer.}$$

CASE IN POINT 8.3 A hospital pharmacist is called to a pediatric nursing station to calculate the quantity of an injection to administer to a pediatric patient. The daily dose of the injection for the child's weight is stated as 15 mg/kg/day, divided into three equal portions. The child weighs 10 kg. The injection contains 5 mg/mL of the prescribed drug.

How many milliliters of injection should be administered?

Dosing Tables Based on Body Weight

For some drugs dosed according to body weight or body surface area, dosing tables appear in product literature to assist the physician and pharmacist. An example is presented in Table 8.2.

Using Table 8.2 and a daily dose of 0.5 mg/kg, how many 20-mg capsules of the drug product should be dispensed to a patient weighing 176 lb if the dosage regimen calls for 15 weeks of therapy?

$$2 \text{ capsules/day} \times 7 \text{ days/week} \times 15 \text{ weeks} = 210 \text{ capsules, } answer.$$

A pharmacist compounds a suspension from oseltamivir phosphate capsules to contain 15 mg of drug per milliliter. Using Table 8.3, calculate the single dose in milliliters for a pediatric patient weighing 40 lb.

From Table 8.3, the dose for the pediatric patient is 45 mg.

$$45 \text{ mg} \times \frac{1 \text{ mL}}{15 \text{ mL}} = 3 \text{ mL, dose of oseltamivir phosphate suspension, } answer.$$

Drug Dosage Based on Body Surface Area

The *body surface area (BSA)* method of calculating drug doses is widely used for two types of patient groups: cancer patients receiving chemotherapy and pediatric patients.

Table 8.4 shows the *approximate* relation between body weight and body surface area, in square meters (m^2), based on average body dimensions. The average adult is considered to have a BSA of 1.73 m^2. Thus, in reading Table 8.4, a person with a BSA of 1.30 (or about 75% of that of the average adult) would receive about 75% of the adult dose.

Example Calculations of Dose Based on Body Surface Area

A useful equation for the calculation of dose based on BSA is:

$$\text{Patient's dose} = \frac{\text{Patient's BSA (m}^2)}{1.73 \text{ m}^2} \times \text{Drug dose (mg)}$$

If the adult dose of a drug is 100 mg, calculate the approximate dose for a child with a BSA of 0.83 m^2, using (a) the equation and (b) Table 8.4.

(a)   Child's dose $= \dfrac{0.83 \text{ m}^2}{1.73 \text{ m}^2} \times 100 \text{ mg} = 47.97 \text{ or } 48 \text{ mg, } answer.$

(b)   According to Table 8.4, a BSA of 0.83 m^2 represents 48% of the average adult BSA of 1.73 m^2; thus, the child dose would be 48% of the average adult dose:

$$100 \text{ mg} \times 0.48 = 48\text{-mg dose for child, } answer.$$

Dosing Tables Based on Body Surface Area

For certain drugs, dosing tables may be provided to determine the approximate dose based on a patient's body surface area. Table 8.5 presents an example for a hypothetical drug.

Using Table 8.5, find the dose of the hypothetical drug at a dose level of 300 mg/m^2 for a child determined to have a BSA of 1.25 m^2. Calculate to verify.

Table 8.2 ▼ **DOSING BY BODY WEIGHT FOR A HYPOTHETICAL DRUG**

BODY WEIGHT		TOTAL mg/DAY		
KILOGRAMS	POUNDS	0.5 mg/kg	1 mg/kg	2 mg/kg
40	88	20	40	80
50	110	25	50	100
60	132	30	60	120
70	154	35	70	140
80	176	40	80	160
90	198	45	90	180
100	220	50	100	200

From Table 8.5, the dose = 375 mg, *answer*.
From calculations: 300 mg/m^2 × 1.25 m^2 = 375 mg dose, *answer*.

Nomograms for Determining Body Surface Area

Most BSA calculations use a standard *nomogram*, which includes both weight and height. Nomograms for children and adults are shown in Figures 8.1 and 8.2. The BSA of an individual is determined by drawing a straight line connecting the person's height and weight. The point at which the line intersects the center column indicates the person's BSA in square meters. In the example shown in Figure 8.1, a child weighing 15 kg and measuring 100 cm in height has a BSA of 0.64 m^2.

If the adult dose of a drug is 75 mg, what would be the dose for a child weighing 40 lb, and measuring 32 in. in height using the BSA nomogram?

From the nomogram, the BSA = 0.60 m^2

$$\frac{0.60 \text{ m}^2}{1.73 \text{ m}^2} \times 75 \text{ mg} = 26 \text{ mg}, answer.$$

The usual pediatric dose of a drug is stated as 25 mg/m^2. Using the nomogram, calculate the dose for a child weighing 18 kg and measuring 82 cm in height.

From the nomogram, the BSA = 0.60 m^2

$$25 \text{ mg} \times 0.60 = 15 \text{ mg}, answer.$$

Table 8.3 ▼ **DOSING OF OSELTAMIVIR PHOSPHATE IN THE TREATMENT OF INFLUENZA IN PEDIATRIC PATIENTS[a]**

BODY WEIGHT		
KILOGRAMS	POUNDS	RECOMMENDED DOSE FOR 5 DAYS
≤15 kg	≤33 lbs	30 mg twice daily
>16 kg to 23 kg	>35 to 51 lbs	45 mg twice daily
>24 to 40 kg	>53 lbs to 88 lbs	60 mg twice daily
≥41 kg	≥90 lbs	75 mg twice daily

[a]Adapted from product literature for oseltamivir phosphate (TAMIFLU), Roche Laboratories, 2008.

Table 8.4 ▾ APPROXIMATE RELATION OF SURFACE AREA
AND WEIGHTS OF INDIVIDUALS OF AVERAGE
BODY DIMENSION

KILOGRAMS	POUNDS	SURFACE AREA IN SQUARE METERS	PERCENTAGE OF ADULT DOSE*
2	4.4	0.15	9
3	6.6	0.20	11.5
4	8.8	0.25	14
5	11.0	0.29	16.5
6	13.2	0.33	19
7	15.4	0.37	21
8	17.6	0.40	23
9	19.8	0.43	25
10	22.0	0.46	27
15	33.0	0.63	36
20	44.0	0.83	48
25	55.0	0.95	55
30	66.0	1.08	62
35	77.0	1.20	69
40	88.0	1.30	75
45	99.0	1.40	81
50	110.0	1.51	87
55	121.0	1.58	91

*Based on average adult surface area of 1.73 square meters.
Adapted from Martin EW et al., *Techniques of Medication*, J. B. Lippincott, 1969:31, who adapted it from
Modell's Drugs of Choice (Mosby).

The nomogram in Figure 8.2 designed specifically for determining the BSA of *adults* may be used in the same manner as the one previously described. The adult dose is then calculated as follows:

$$\frac{\text{BSA of adult (m}^2)}{1.73 \text{ m}^2} \times \text{Usual adult dose} = \text{Dose for adult}$$

Table 8.5 ▾ PEDIATRIC DOSING GUIDELINE FOR A
HYPOTHETICAL DRUG BASED ON BSA

PATIENT'S BSA (m²)	DOSE LEVEL			
	250 mg/m² DOSE	*300 mg/m²* DOSE	*350 mg/m²* DOSE	*400 mg/m²* DOSE
0.25	62.5 mg	75 mg	87.5 mg	100 mg
0.50	125 mg	150 mg	175 mg	200 mg
1.00	250 mg	300 mg	350 mg	400 mg
1.25	312.5 mg	375 mg	437.5 mg	500 mg
1.50	375 mg	450 mg	525 mg	600 mg

Nomogram for Determination of Body Surface Area From Height and Weight

Example:

BSA for a
15-kg. child,
100 cm. tall =
0.64 M²

From the formula of Du Bots and Du Bots, *Arch Intern Med* 17, 863 (1916): $S = W^{0.425} \times H^{0.725} \times 71.84$, or log S = log $W \times 0.425$ + log $H \times 0.725$ + 1.8564 (S = body surface in cm², W = weight in kg, H = height in cm).

▼ FIGURE 8.1 Body surface area of children. (*From Diem K, Lentner C, Geigy JR*. Scientific Tables. *7th Ed. Basel, Switzerland: JR Geigy, 1970:538.*)

Nomogram for Determination of Body Surface Area from Height and Weight

Height	Body surface area	Weight
cm 200 — 79 in	2.80 m²	kg 150 — 330 lb
78	2.70	145 — 320
195 — 77		140 — 310
76	2.60	135 — 300
190 — 75	2.50	130 — 290
74		280
185 — 73	2.40	125 — 270
72		120 — 260
180 — 71	2.30	
70		115 — 250
175 — 69	2.20	110 — 240
68		105 — 230
170 — 67	2.10	
66		100 — 220
165 — 65	2.00	95 — 210
64	1.95	
160 — 63	1.90	90 — 200
62	1.85	190
155 — 61	1.80	85 — 180
60	1.75	80 —
150 — 59	1.70	170
58	1.65	75 — 160
145 — 57	1.60	70 —
56	1.55	150
140 — 55	1.50	65 — 140
54	1.45	
135 — 53	1.40	60 — 130
52	1.35	55 —
130 — 51	1.30	120
50		
125 — 49	1.25	50 — 110
48	1.20	105
120 — 47	1.15	45 — 100
46	1.10	95
115 — 45		90
44	1.05	40 — 85
110 — 43	1.00	80
42	0.95	35 — 75
105 — 41		
40	0.90	70
cm 100 — 39 in	0.86 m²	kg 30 — 66 lb

From the formula of Du Bots and Du Bots, *Arch Intern Med* 17, 863 (1916): $S = W^{0.425} \times H^{0.725} \times 71.84$, or $\log S = \log W \times 0.425 + \log H \times 0.725 + 1.8564$ (S = body surface in cm², W = weight in kg, H = height in cm).

▼ FIGURE 8.2 Body surface area of adults. (*From Diem K, Lentner C, Geigy JR*. Scientific Tables. *7th Ed. Basel, Switzerland: JR Geigy, 1970:538.*)

CALCULATIONS CAPSULE

Dose Based on Body Surface Area

A useful equation for the calculation of dose based on body surface area is:

$$Patient's\ dose = \frac{Patient's\ BSA\ (m^2)}{1.73\ m^2} \times Drug\ dose\ (mg)$$

If there is need to determine a patient's BSA, a nomogram, or the following equation may be used:

$$Patient's\ BSA\ (m^2) = \sqrt{\frac{Patient's\ height\ (cm) \times Patient's\ weight\ (kg)}{3600}}$$

If the usual adult dose of a drug is 120 mg, what would be the dose based on BSA for a person measuring 6 ft tall and weight 200 lb?

$$BSA\ (from\ the\ nomogram) = 2.13\ m^2$$

$$\frac{2.13\ m^2}{1.73\ m^2} \times 120\ mg = 147.75\ mg\ or\ 148\ mg,\ answer.$$

If the dose of a drug is 5 mg/m², what would be the dose for a patient with a BSA of 1.9 m²?

$$5\ mg \times 1.9 = 9.5\ mg,\ answer.$$

BSA Equation

In addition to the use of the nomogram, BSA may be determined through use of the following Mosteller Formula:[6]

$$BSA,\ m^2 = \sqrt{\frac{Ht\ (cm) \times Wt\ (kg)}{3600}}$$

Calculate the BSA for a patient measuring 165 cm in height and weighing 65 kg.

$$BSA,\ m^2 = \sqrt{\frac{165\ (cm) \times 65\ (kg)}{3600}}$$

$$BSA = 1.73\ m^2,\ answer.$$

Note: For the sake of comparison, check Figure 8.2 to derive the BSA for the same patient using the nomogram.

Dosage Based on the Medical Condition to be Treated

In addition to the factors previously discussed that might be used to determine a drug's dose, the medical condition to be treated and the severity of that condition must also be considered.

Table 8.6 presents an example of a dosage schedule for a drug based both on a patient's age and the medical condition to be treated.

By using Table 8.6, calculate the IV drug dose for a 3-pound 3-ounce neonate.

$$3 \text{ pounds } = 3 \times 454 \text{ g} = 1362 \text{ g}$$
$$3 \text{ ounces } = 3 \times 28.35 \text{ g} = 85 \text{ g}$$
$$\text{Weight of neonate } = 1362 \text{ g} + 85 \text{ g} = 1447 \text{ g}$$
$$1447 \text{ g}/1000 = 1.447 \text{ kg}$$
$$30 \text{ mg/kg} \times 1.447 \text{ kg} = 43.4 \text{ mg every 12 hours, } answer.$$

By using Table 8.6, calculate the daily IV dose of the drug in the treatment of a lung infection for a patient weighing 160 lb.

$$160 \text{ lb} \div 2.2 \text{ lb/kg} = 72.72 \text{ kg}$$
$$72.72 \text{ kg} \times 40 \text{ mg/kg/dose} = 2909 \text{ mg/dose (every 8 h)}$$
$$2909 \text{ mg} \times 3 \text{ doses per day} = 8727 \text{ mg or 8.73 g daily dose.}$$

Special Dosing Considerations in Cancer Chemotherapy

The term *chemotherapy* applies to the treatment of disease with chemical drugs or *chemotherapeutic agents*. Chemotherapy is primarily associated with the treatment of cancer patients and is considered the mainstay of such treatment in that it is effective in widespread or metastatic cancer, whereas treatments such as surgery and radiation therapy are limited to specific body sites. Chemotherapeutic agents most often are administered orally, by intravenous injection, or by continuous intravenous infusion.

Although a single anticancer drug may be used in a patient's treatment plan, *combination chemotherapy* perhaps is more usual. By using combinations of drugs having different mechanisms of action against the target cancer cells, the effectiveness of treatment may be enhanced, lower doses used, and side effects reduced. The combination chemotherapy plans often include *two-agent regimens*, *three-agent regimens*, and *four-agent regimens*.[7-11]

Cancer chemotherapy is unique in the following ways:

• It may involve single or multiple drugs of well-established drug therapy regimens or protocols, or it may involve the use of investigational drugs as a part of a clinical trial.
• Combinations of drugs may be given by the same or different routes of administration, most often oral and/or intravenous.

Table 8.6 ▼ PARENTERAL DOSAGE SCHEDULE FOR A HYPOTHETICAL ANTI-INFECTIVE DRUG BASED ON PATIENT AGE AND CONDITION BEING TREATED

	DOSE	ROUTE	FREQUENCY
Adults			
Urinary tract infection	250 mg	IV or IM	q12h
Bone and joint infections	2 g	IV	q12h
Pneumonia	500 mg–1g	IV or IM	q8h
Mild skin infections	500 mg–1g	IV or IM	q8h
Life-threatening infections	2 g	IV	q8h
Lung infections (normal kidney function)	40 mg/kg (NMT 6 g/day)	IV	q8h
Neonates (up to 1 month)	30 mg/kg	IV	q12h
Infants and Children (1 month to 12 years)	30–50 mg/kg (NMT 6 g/day)	IV	q8h

- The drugs may be administered concomitantly or alternately on the same or different days during a prescribed treatment cycle (e.g., 28 days). The days of treatment generally follow a prescribed format of written instructions, with D for "day," followed by the day(s) of treatment during a cycle, with a dash (–) meaning "to" and a comma (,) meaning "and." Thus, *D 1–4* means "days 1 to 4," and *D1,4* means "days 1 and 4."[9]
- The drugs used in combination chemotherapy often fit into a standard drug/dosage regimen identified by abbreviations or *acronyms*. For example, a treatment for bladder cancer referred to as MVAC consists of methotrexate + vinblastine + doxorubicin (or actinomycin) + cisplatin; a treatment for colorectal cancer called FU/LU consists of fluorouracil + leucovorin; a treatment for lung cancer called PC consists of paclitaxel + carboplatin; and one for ovarian cancer called CHAD consists of cyclophosphamide + hexamethylmelamine + Adriamycin + diamminedichloroplatinum (cisplatin).
- In addition to the use of abbreviations for the drug therapy regimens, the drugs themselves are commonly abbreviated in medication orders, such as MTX for "methotrexate," DOX, for "doxorubicin," VLB, for "vinblastine," and CDDP for "cisplatin." Tables of standard chemotherapy treatments, dosing regimens, and abbreviations of the drugs and treatment regimens may be found in the indicated references.[7–11]
- For systemic action, chemotherapeutic agents are usually dosed based either on body weight or on body surface area. Often, the drug doses stated in standard regimens must be reduced, based on a particular patient's diminished kidney or liver function and, thus, his or her ability to metabolize and eliminate the drug(s) from the body.
- For certain patients, high-dose chemotherapy is undertaken in an effort to kill tumor cells.

To help prevent errors in chemotherapy, pharmacists must correctly interpret medication orders for the chemotherapeutic agents prescribed, follow the individualized dosing regimens, calculate the doses of each medication prescribed, and dispense the appropriate dosage forms and quantities/strengths required.[12]

Example Calculations of Chemotherapy Dosage Regimens

Regimen: VC[11]
Cycle: 28 d; repeat for 2–8 cycles
Vinorelbine, 25 mg/m², IV, D 1,8,15,22
Cisplatin, 100 mg/m², IV, D 1.

For each of vinorelbine and cisplatin, calculate the total intravenous dose per cycle for a patient measuring 5 ft. 11 in. in height and weighing 175 lb.

From the nomogram for determining BSA (a) find the patient's BSA and (b) calculate the quantity of each drug in the regimen.

(a) BSA = 2.00 m², *answer*
(b) Vinorelbine: 25 mg × 2.00 (BSA) × 4 (days of treatment) = 200 mg,
Cisplatin: 100 mg × 2.00 (BSA) × 1 = 200 mg, *answers.*

Regimen: CMF[11]
Cycle: 28 d
Cyclophosphamide, 100 mg/m²/d po, D 1–14.
Methotrexate, 40 mg/m², IV, D 2,8.
Fluorouracil, 600 mg/m², IV, D 1,8.

Table 8.7 ▼ EXAMPLES OF DOSAGE REGIMENS IN CANCER CHEMOTHERAPY[a]

TYPE OF CANCER[b]	ABBREVIATION	DRUG/DOSE	ROUTE	DAY(S) OF ADMINISTRATION PER TREATMENT CYCLE[c]
Bladder	MVAC	methotrexate, 30 mg/m²	I.V.	days 1, 15, and 22
		vinblastine, 3 mg/m²	I.V.	days 2, 15, and 22
		doxorubicin (Adriamycin), 30 mg/m²	I.V.	day 2
		cisplatin, 70 mg/m²	I.V.	day 2
Breast	AC	doxorubicin (Adriamycin), 60 mg/m²	I.V.	day 1
		cyclophosphamide, 600 mg/m²	I.V.	day 1
Esophagus	DCF	docetaxel, 75 mg/m²	I.V.	day 1
		cisplatin, 75 mg/m²	I.V.	day 1
		5-fluorouracil, 750 mg/m²/day	I.V.	days 1–5
Lung	CAE	cyclophosphamide, 1000 mg/m²	I.V.	day 1
		doxorubicin, 45 mg/m²	I.V.	day 1
		etoposide, 100 mg/m²	I.V.	days 1–3
Stomach	ELF	etoposide, 120 mg/m²	I.V.	days 1–3
		leucovorin, 150 mg/m²	I.V.	days 1–3
		5-fluorouracil, 500 mg/m²	I.V.	days 1–3

[a]Table from references.[8–11]
[b]Types of cancer are stated broadly and not differentiated by sub-classifications.
[c]The frequency and number of treatment cycles vary according to the specific protocols employed.

Calculate the total cycle dose for cyclophosphamide, methotrexate, and fluorouracil for a patient having a BSA of 1.5 m².

Cyclophosphamide:	100 mg × 1.5 (BSA) × 14 (days)	= 2100 mg	= 2.1 g,
Methotrexate:	40 mg × 1.5 × 2	= 120 mg,	
Fluorouracil:	600 mg × 1.5 × 2	= 1800 mg	= 1.8 g, *answers.*

Using Table 8.7 as a reference, calculate the quantities of doxorubicin and cyclophosphamide administered per treatment cycle to a woman measuring 5 ft 4 in. in height and weighing 142 lb during the "AC" protocol for breast cancer.

BSA (from Table 8.2) = 1.70 m²
1.70 m² × 60 mg/m² doxorubicin = 102 mg doxorubicin, and
1.70 m² × 600 mg/m² cyclophosphamide = 1,020 mg cyclophosphamide, *answers.*

A variation of the "AC" protocol, referred to as "AC→T," follows four cycles of the AC protocol with paclitaxel (TAXOL), 175 mg/m² by intravenous infusion every 14 to 21 days for four cycles.[11] Calculate the total quantity of paclitaxel, in milligrams, that the patient in the previous problem would receive during this treatment plan.

BSA = 1.70 m²
1.70 m² × 175 mg/m² paclitaxel = 297.5 mg (per cycle) × 4 (cycles)
= 1190 mg paclitaxel, *answer.*

If an injection is available containing paclitaxel, 6 mg/mL, calculate the volume required per cycle to treat the patient in the previous problem.

297.5 mg ÷ 6 mg/mL = 49.6 mL paclitaxel injection, *answer.*

CASE IN POINT 8.4[13] In treating a 54-year-old female patient, an oncologist selects the drug temozolomide, an antitumor agent used in the treatment of refractory astrocytoma (brain tumor). The drug is used as part of a 28-day regimen, during which the first five days of treatment include temozolomide at a once-daily dose of 150 mg/m²/day. The patient's medical chart indicates that she measures 5 ft. in height and weighs 117 lb. The physician asks the pharmacist to determine the proper combination of available capsules to use in dosing the patient. The drug is available in capsules containing 5, 20, 100, and 250 mg of temozolomide. What combination of capsules would provide the daily dose of this drug?

PRACTICE PROBLEMS

Calculations Based on Body Weight

1. The dose of a drug is 500 mcg/kg of body weight. How many milligrams should be given to a child weighing 55 lb.?

2. The dose of gentamicin for premature and full-term neonates is 2.5 mg/kg administered every 12 hours. What would be the daily dose for a newborn weighing 5.6 lb.?

3. The dose of gentamicin for patients with impaired renal function is adjusted to ensure therapeutically optimal dosage. If the normal daily dose of the drug for adults is 3 mg/kg/day, administered in three divided doses, what would be the single (8-hour) dose for a patient weighing 165 lb. and scheduled to receive only 40% of the usual dose, based on renal impairment?

4. A patient weighing 120 lb. was administered 2.1 g of a drug supposed to be dosed at 30 mg/kg. Was the dose administered *correct*, or was it an *overdose*, or was it an *underdose*?

5. In a clinical trial of ciprofloxacin (CIPRO), pediatric patients were initiated on 6 to 10 mg/kg intravenously every 8 hours and converted to oral therapy, 10 to 20 mg/kg, every 12 hours. Calculate the ranges of the total daily amounts of ciprofloxacin that would have been administered intravenously and orally to a 40-lb. child.

6. ℞ Erythromycin 400 mg/5 mL
   Ethylsuccinate
   Disp. 100 mL
   Sig. _____ tsp. q.i.d. until all medication is taken.

   If the dose of erythromycin ethylsuccinate is given as 40 mg/kg per day,

   (a) What would be the proper dose of the medication in the Signa, if the prescription is for a 44 lb. child?
   (b) How many days will the prescribed medication last?

7. If the pediatric dosage of chlorothiazide (DIURIL) is 10 to 20 mg/kg of body weight per day in a single dose or two divided doses, not to exceed 375 mg per day, calculate the *daily dosage range* of an oral suspension containing 250 mg chlorothiazide per 5 mL that should be administered to a 48-lb child.

8. Cyclosporine is an immunosuppressive agent administered before and after organ transplantation at a single dose of 15 mg/kg. How many milliliters of a 50-mL bottle containing 100 mg of cyclosporine per milliliter would be administered to a 140-lb. kidney transplant patient?

9. The adult dose of a liquid medication is 0.1 mL/kg of body weight. How many teaspoonfuls should be administered to a person weighing 220 lb.?

10. A hospitalist prescribed dimenhydrinate to treat a 48-lb child. The labeled dose of the drug is 1.125 mg/kg. The available oral solution contains dimenhydrinate, 12.5 mg/5 mL. Prior to administering the solution, the floor nurse decides to check her calculated dose of 9.8 mL with the hospital pharmacist. Were her calculations correct?

11. ℞ Fluconazole tabs   100 mg
       Disp. ___ tabs
       Sig: tab ii stat, then 3 mg/kg b.i.d. × 7 d thereafter.

    Calculate the number of tablets to dispense to a patient weighing 147 lb.

12. A physician desires a dose of 40 mcg/kg of digoxin for an 8-lb. newborn child. How many milliliters of an injection containing 0.25 mg of digoxin per milliliter should be given?

13. Intravenous digitalizing doses of digoxin in children are 80% of oral digitalizing doses. Calculate the intravenous dose for a 5-year-old child weighing 40 lb. if the oral dose is determined to be 20 mcg/kg.

14. An intratracheal suspension for breathing enhancement in premature infants is dosed at 2.5 mL/kg of birth weight. How many milliliters of the suspension should be administered to a neonate weighing 3 lb.?

15. A 142-lb. patient was receiving filgrastim (NEUPOGEN) in doses of 10 mcg/kg/day when, as a result of successful blood tests, the dose was lowered to 6 mcg/kg/day. Using an injection containing 0.3 mg filgrastim per 0.5 mL, calculate the previous and new dose to be administered.

(a) 17.7 mL and 64.6 mL
(b) 5.23 mL and 3.14 mL
(c) 1.08 mL and 0.65 mL
(d) 3.87 mL and 2.3 mL

16. A 25-lb. child is to receive 4 mg of phenytoin per kilogram of body weight daily as an anticonvulsant. How many milliliters of pediatric phenytoin suspension containing 30 mg per 5 mL should the child receive?

17. The loading dose of digoxin in premature infants with a birth weight of less than 1.5 kg is 20 mcg/kg administered in three *un*equally divided doses (½, ¼, ¼) at 8-hour intervals. What would be the initial dose for an infant weighing 1.2 kg?

18. The pediatric dose of cefadroxil is 30 mg/kg/day. If a child was given a daily dose of 2 teaspoonfuls of a pediatric suspension containing 125 mg of cefadroxil per 5 mL, what was the weight, in pounds, of the child?

19. How many milliliters of an injection containing 1 mg of drug per milliliter of injection should be administered to a 6-month-old child weighing 16 lb. to achieve a dose of 0.01 mg/kg?

20. Prior to hip replacement surgery, a patient receives an injection of an anticoagulant-drug at a dose of 30 mg. Following the patient's surgery, the drug is injected at 1 mg/kg. For a 140-lb. patient, calculate the total of the pre- and postsurgical doses.

21. Using Table 8.2 and a daily dose of 2 mg/kg, how many 20-mg capsules would a 176-lb. patient be instructed to take per dose if the daily dose is to be taken in divided doses, q.i.d.?

22. For a 22-lb pediatric patient, the dose of cefdinir (OMNICEF) was determined to be 7 mg/kg. What quantity of an oral suspension containing

125 mg of cefdinir in each 5 mL should be administered?

(a) 2.8 mL
(b) 5.6 mL
(c) 8.9 mL
(d) 13.6 mL

23. How many capsules, each containing 250 mg of clarithromycin, are needed to provide 50 mg/kg/day for 10 days for a person weighing 176 lb.?

24. If the pediatric dose of dactinomycin is 15 mcg/kg/day for 5 days, how many micrograms should be administered to a 40-lb. child over the course of treatment?

25. If the administration of gentamicin at a dose of 1.75 mg/kg is determined to result in peak blood serum levels of 4 mcg/mL, calculate the dose, in milligrams, for a 120-lb. patient that may be expected to result in a blood serum gentamicin level of 4.5 mcg/mL.

26. A medication order calls for tobramycin sulfate, 1 mg/kg of body weight, to be administered by IM injection to a patient weighing 220 lb. Tobramycin sulfate is available in a vial containing 80 mg per 2 mL. How many milliliters of the injection should the patient receive?

27. The usual pediatric dose of acyclovir is 20 mg/kg administered by infusion and repeated every 8 hours. What would be the single dose, in milligrams, for a child weighing 33 lb.?

28. If the recommended dose of tobramycin for a premature infant is 4 mg/kg/day, divided into two equal doses administered every 12 hours, how many milligrams of the drug should be given every 12 hours to a 2.2-lb. infant?

29. If a 3-year-old child weighing 35 lb. accidentally ingested twenty 81-mg aspirin tablets, how much aspirin did the child ingest on a milligram per kilogram basis?

30. The recommended pediatric dose of epinephrine for allergic emergencies is 0.01 mg/kg. If a physician, utilizing this dose, administered 0.15 mg, what was the weight of the patient in pounds?

31. The initial maintenance dose of vancomycin for infants less than 1 week old is 15 mg/kg every 18 hours.

(a) What would be the dose, in milligrams, for an infant weighing 2500 g?
(b) How many milliliters of an injection containing 500 mg per 25 mL should be administered to obtain this dose?

32. The loading dose of indomethacin in neonates is 0.2 mg/kg of body weight by intravenous infusion.

(a) What would be the dose for a neonate weighing 6 lb., 4 oz.?
(b) How many milliliters of an injection containing 1 mg of indomethacin per 0.5 mL should be administered to obtain this dose?

33. ℞[13] Jimmy Jones   Age: 8 years
    Wt: 88 pounds
    Metronidazole Suspension
    7.5 mg/kg/day
    M.ft. dose = 5 mL
    Sig: 5 mL bid × 10 days

(a) How many milligrams of metronidazole will the patient receive per dose?
(b) How many milliliters of the prescription should be prepared and dispensed?
(c) If metronidazole is available in 250-mg tablets, how many tablets will be needed to fill the prescription?

34. ℞[13] Betty Smith   Age: 4 years
       Weight: 52.8 pounds
       Erythromycin Ethyl Succinate
       (EES) 200 mg/5 mL
       Disp. 300 mL
       Sig: _____ mL qid until gone
    (a) If the dose of EES is 50 mg/kg/
        day, how many milliliters would
        provide each dose?
    (b) How many days would the pre-
        scription last the patient?

Calculations Based on Body Surface Area

Note: As needed, refer to the BSA nomograms, Mosteller Formula, and/or tables
in this chapter.

35. If the daily dose of a drug is given
    in the literature as 8 mg/kg of body
    weight or 350 mg/m², calculate the
    dose on each basis for a patient
    weighing 150 lb. and measuring 5 ft.
    8 in. in height.

36. If the dose of a drug is 10 mg/m² per
    day, what would be the daily dose,
    in milligrams, for a child weighing
    30 lb. and measuring 26 in. in height?

37. The dose of mitomycin injection
    is 20 mg/m² per day. Determine
    the daily dose for a patient who
    weighs 144 lb. and measures 68 in.
    in height.

38. The pediatric starting dose of rito-
    navir (NORVIR) is 250 mg/m² by
    mouth twice daily. The available oral
    solution contains 600 mg of ritona-
    vir in each 7.5 mL of solution. The
    correct volume and corresponding
    quantity of ritonavir to be adminis-
    tered to a child with a body surface
    area of 0.75 m² per dose is:
    (a) 5.6 mL (450.4 mg)
    (b) 2.8 mL (450.4 mg)
    (c) 2.8 mL (225.2 mg)
    (d) 2.3 mL (187.5 mg)

39. Calculate the dose for a child 4 years
    of age, 39 in. in height, and weighing
    32 lb. for a drug with an adult dose
    of 100 mg, using the following: (a)
    Young's rule, (b) Cowling's rule, (c)
    Clark's rule, and (d) BSA (use the
    BSA equation).

40. The daily dose of diphenhydramine
    HCl for a child may be determined
    on the basis of 5 mg/kg of body
    weight or on the basis of 150 mg/m².
    Calculate the dose on each basis for a
    child weighing 55 lb. and measuring
    40 in. in height.

Calculations of Chemotherapeutic Regimens

41. The drug cabazitaxel is used treating
    prostate cancer in doses of 25 mg/m².
    Calculate the dose for a patient mea-
    suring 73 in. in height and weighing
    190 lb.

42. Calculate the quantities of each drug
    administered to a patient on day 2 of
    the ELF protocol if the patient's BSA
    is 1.64 m².

43. If the dose of etoposide for a patient
    on the CAE protocol is increased to
    120 mg/m², calculate the increase
    in the dose, in milligrams, if the
    patient measures 150 cm and weighs
    48 kg.

44. The drug carboplatin for ovarian
    carcinoma is administered intrave-
    nously at a dose of 360 mg/m² except
    in patients with impaired kidney
    function, in which case the dose is
    reduced by 30%. How many mil-
    ligrams of the drug should be admin-
    istered to a renally impaired patient
    measuring 5 ft. 2 in. and weighing
    110 lb.?

45. A high-dose treatment of osteosar-
    coma includes the use of methotrex-
    ate at a starting dose of 12 g/m² as

a 4-hour intravenous infusion. For a patient having a BSA of 1.7 m^2 and weighing 162 lb., calculate the dose on the basis of mg/kg/min.

46. A two-agent dosage regimen, termed MP, for the treatment of multiple myeloma is as follows:[11]

    Melphalan 0.25 mg/kg, PO,
             D1–4/week × 6 weeks
    Prednisone 2 mg/kg, PO,
             D1–4/week × 6 weeks

    (a) Calculate the total milligrams each of melphalan and prednisone taken per week by a patient who weighs 165 lb.
    (b) If melphalan is available in 2-mg tablets, how many tablets are required to dose this patient for the entire treatment cycle?
    (c) If the patient prefers prednisone oral solution to prednisone tablets, how many milliliters of the solution (5 mg/mL) should be dispensed weekly?

47. A three-agent dosage regimen, termed VAD, for the treatment of multiple myeloma includes the following drugs taken over a 28-day cycle:[11]

    Vincristine   0.4 mg/d, CIVI, D 1–4
    Doxorubicin   9 mg/m^2/d, CIVI, D 1–4
    Dexamethasone 40 mg/d, PO, D 1–4, 9–12, 17–20

    Calculate the total quantity of each drug administered over the course of the treatment cycle for a patient with a BSA of 1.65 m^2.

48. A four-agent dosage regimen, termed MOPP, for the treatment of Hodgkin lymphoma includes the following drugs taken over a 28-day cycle:[11]

    Mechlorethamine 6 mg/m^2, I.V., D 1,8
    Vincristine   1.4 mg/m^2, I.V., D 1,8
    Procarbazine   100 mg/m^2/d, p.o., D 1–14
    Prednisone   40 mg/m^2/d, p.o., D 1–14

    Calculate the total number of 20-mg tablets of prednisone and 50-mg tablets of procarbazine to dispense to treat a patient with a BSA of 1.5 m^2 during the course of one treatment cycle.

49. The oncolytic agent lapatinib (TYKERB) is administered in the treatment of breast cancer in daily doses of 1250 mg for 21 consecutive days in combination with the drug capecitabine (XELODA), which is administered in doses of 1000 mg/m^2/day during days 1 to 14 of the 21-day treatment cycle. Calculate the total quantity of *each drug* to be administered during the treatment cycle to a 5′2″ woman weighing 110 pounds.

50. Among the single chemotherapeutic agents for breast cancer is docetaxel (TAXOTERE), which is administered @ 60 mg/m^2 IV every 3 weeks. Calculate the dose for a 5 ft 4 in. patient who weighs 160 lb.

51. Based on the dose calculated in the above problem, how many milliliters of an injection containing 80 mg/2 mL docetaxel would be administered per dose?

52. The chemotherapy regimen "CAF" during a 21-day cycle is:[11]

    Cyclophosphamide 500 mg/m^2, D-1
    Doxorubicin   50 mg/m^2, D-1
      (Adriamycin)
    5-Fluorouracil   500 mg/m^2, D-1, 8

    Calculate the dose of each drug/cycle for a patient with a BSA of 1.9 m^2.

CALCQUIZ

8.A. The drug eribulin mesylate is used in late-stage metastatic breast cancer at an intravenous dose of 1.4 mg/m². It is administered on days 1 and 8 of a 21-day cycle. The dose is reduced by 20 percentage for patients with moderate renal impairment. Calculate the reduced dose, in (a) mg/m², (b) mg/kg, and (c) the treatment-day dose, in milligrams, for a 110-lb patient measuring 5 ft 2 in. in height.

8.B. A parent takes her 5- and 7-year-old boys to the pediatrician, both with pharyngitis. The boys weigh 40 and 50 lb, respectively. The doctor prescribes an oral suspension of cefuroxime axetil (CEFTIN) at a dose of 20 mg/kg/day divided b.i.d. × 10 days. The suspension has a cefuroxime axetil concentration of 125 mg/mL. How many milliliters of suspension will be needed during the course of treatment?

8.C. The first-day loading dose of a drug is 70 mg/m² followed by a dose of 50 mg/m² daily thereafter. Irrespective of the patient's BSA, a dose is not to exceed 70 mg. For a 5-ft 8-in. 150-lb patient, calculate the (a) BSA using the Mosteller Formula, (b) loading dose, (c) maintenance dose, and indicate whether each dose is within the safe limit.

8.D. The pediatric oral dose of ciprofloxacin is given as 10 to 20 mg/kg every 8 hours, not to exceed a single dose of 400 mg irrespective of body weight. If a child weighing 55 lb is prescribed a one-teaspoonful dose of a 5% ciprofloxacin oral suspension every 8 hours, calculate whether or not the dose prescribed is within the therapeutic range.

8.E. The drug peginterferon alpha-2b is sometimes administered according to a "step-down" protocol from a starting dose of 1.5 mcg/kg/wk, to 1 mcg/kg/wk, to 0.5 mcg/kg/wk. Calculate the three doses for a 5-ft 5-in, 132-lb patient (a) in micrograms and (b) on a mcg/m² basis.

ANSWERS TO "CASE IN POINT" AND PRACTICE PROBLEMS

Case in Point 8.1

The metric weight of a 3 lb. 7 oz. neonate is calculated:

1 lb. = 454 g; 1 oz. = 28.35 g
3 lb. × 454 g/lb. = 1362 g
7 oz. × 28.35 g/oz. = 198.45 g
1362 g + 198.45 g = 1560.45 g, weight of the neonate

According to the dosing table, the dose for a 3-day-old neonate weighing less than 2000 g is 10 mg/kg/day divided every 12 hours.

The dose, in mg, may be calculated by dimensional analysis:

$$\frac{1\ kg}{1000\ g} \times \frac{10\ mg}{1\ kg/day} \times 1560.45\ g$$

= 15.6 mg clindamycin/day

Since the daily dose is administered in two divided doses, each divided dose is:

$$\frac{15.6\ mg}{2}$$

= 7.8 mg clindamycin every 12 hours.

The volume of injectable solution is then calculated:

$$\frac{50\ mL}{600\ mg} \times 7.8\ g = 0.65\ mL,\ answer.$$

Case in Point 8.2

To calculate the oral dose of enalapril for the patient, it is necessary to know the patient's weight. This may be calculated from the intravenous dose:

$$\frac{1\ kg}{5\ mcg} \times 55\ mcg$$

= 11 kg, the weight of the patient

Then the oral dose may be calculated:

$$\frac{100 \text{ mcg}}{1 \text{ kg}} \times 11 \text{ kg} = 1100 \text{ mcg} = 1.1 \text{ mg}$$

By crushing and mixing the 2.5-mg enalapril tablet with sterile water to make 12.5 mL, the oral dose may be calculated:

$$\frac{2.5 \text{ mg}}{12.5 \text{ mL}} = \frac{1.1 \text{ mg}}{\text{x mL}}; x = 5.5 \text{ mL}, \textit{answer}.$$

Case in Point 8.3

Daily dose: 15 mg/kg × 10 kg = 150 mg
Single dose: 150 mg ÷ 3 = 50 mg

Quantity of injection: $50 \text{ mg} \times \dfrac{1 \text{ mL}}{5 \text{ mg}} = 10$

mL, *answer*.

Case in Point 8.4

To calculate the dose for the patient, the pharmacist must first determine the patient's body surface area. The pharmacist elects to use the following equation:

$$\text{BSA, m}^2 = \sqrt{\frac{\text{Ht (cm)} \times \text{Wt (kg)}}{3600}}$$

To use this equation, the patient's weight and height are converted to metric units:

Height = 5 ft. = 60 in. × 2.54 cm/in.
$\qquad$ = 152.4 cm
Weight = 117 lb. ÷ 2.2 lb./kg = 53.2 kg

Solving the equation:

$$\text{BSA, (m}^2) = \sqrt{\frac{152.4 \times 53.2}{3600}} = 1.50 \text{ m}^2$$

The daily dose is calculated as 150 mg/m² × 1.50 m² = 225 mg

To obtain 225 mg, the patient may take two 100-mg capsules, one 20-mg capsule, and one 5-mg capsule daily, *answer*.

Practice Problems

1. 12.5 mg
2. 12.73 mg gentamicin
3. 30 mg gentamicin

4. overdose
5. I.V.: 327.3–545.5 mg ciprofloxacin
   Oral: 363.6–727.3 mg ciprofloxacin
6. (a) ½ tsp. (2.5 mL) erythromycin ethylsuccinate
   (b) 10 days
7. 4.4–7.5 mL chlorothiazide oral suspension
8. 9.55 mL cyclosporin
9. 2 tsp.
10. Yes, calculations were correct.
11. 30 tablets
12. 0.58 mL digoxin injection
13. 290.9 or 291 mcg digoxin
14. 3.41 mL
15. (c) 1.08 mL and 0.65 mL filgrastim injection
16. 7.58 mL phenytoin suspension
17. 12 mcg digoxin
18. 18.33 lb.
19. 0.073 mL
20. 93.64 or 94 mg
21. 2 capsules
22. (a) 2.8 mL cefdinir oral suspension
23. 160 clarithromycin capsules
24. 1364 mcg dactinomycin
25. 107.39 mg gentamicin
26. 2.5 mL tobramycin injection
27. 300 mg acyclovir
28. 2 mg tobramycin
29. 101.83 mg/kg aspirin
30. 33 pounds
31. (a) 37.5 g vancomycin
    (b) 1.875 mL vancomycin injection
32. (a) 0.57 mg indomethacin
    (b) 0.28 mL indomethacin injection
33. (a) 150 mg metronidazole
    (b) 100 mL
    (c) 12 metronidazole tablets
34. (a) 7.5 mL
    (b) 10 days
35. 545.5 mg and 630 mg

36. 4.5 mg

37. 35.4 mg mitomycin

38. 2.3 mL (187.5 mg) ritonavir

39. (a) 25 mg
    (b) 20.83 mg
    (c) 21.33 mg
    (d) 36.57 mg

40. (a) 125 mg diphenhydramine HCl
    (b) 120 mg diphenhydramine HCl

41. 52.7 mg cabazitaxel

42. 196.8 mg etoposide
    246 mg leucovorin
    820 mg 5-fluorouracil

43. 29.7 mg etoposide

44. 372.96 mg carboplatin

45. 1.15 mg/kg/min methotrexate

46. (a) 75 mg melphalan and 600 mg prednisone
    (b) 225 tablets
    (c) 120 mL prednisone oral solution

47. 1.6 mg vincristine
    59.4 mg doxorubicin
    480 mg dexamethasone

48. 42 procarbazine tablets
    42 prednisone tablets

49. 26.25 g lapatinib and 20.72 g capecitabine

50. 108.7 mg docetaxel

51. 2.7 mL docetaxel injection

52. 1900 mg 5-fluorouracil
    95 mg doxorubicin
    950 mg cyclophosphamide

References

1. Ferri FF. *Practical Guide to the Care of the Medical Patient.* 8th ed. Maryland Heights, MO: Elsevier, 2011.
2. Berkow R, Ed. *The Merck Manual.* 16th Ed. Rahway, NJ: Merck Research Laboratories, 1992.
3. The Joint Commission. Available at: http://www.jointcommission.org/sentinelEvents/ sentinelEventAlert/ sea_39.htm. Accessed February 9, 2011.
4. Gomella TL, ed. *Neonatology: Management, Procedures, On-Call Problems, Diseases, and Drugs.* 6th Ed. New York: McGraw-Hill, 2009.
5. Taketomo CK, Hodding JH, Kraus DM. *Pediatric Dosage Handbook.* 16th Ed. Hudson, OH: Lexi-Comp, 2009.
6. Mosteller Formula: Mosteller RD. Simplified calculation of body surface area. *New England Journal of Medicine* 1987;317:1098.
7. American Cancer Society. Available at: http://www.cancer.org/Treatment/ TreatmentsandSideEffects/ TreatmentTypes/index. Accessed February 10, 2011.
8. OncologyStat. Available at: http://oncologystat.com/drugs_and_regimens/index.html. Accessed February 10, 2011.
9. Medicine Online. Available at: http://www.meds.com/DoseCalc/dcintro.html. Accessed February 10, 2011.
10. OncologyStat. Available at: http://oncologystat.com/drugs_and_regimens/chemo_regimens/ new/Cisplatin_ vinorelbine_NSCLC.html. Accessed February 12, 2011.
11. Chemoregimen.com. Available at: http://chemoregimen.com/index.php. Accessed February 16, 2011.
12. Schwarz LR. Delivering cytotoxic chemotherapy safely in a community hospital. *Hospital Pharmacy* 1996;31:1108–1118.
13. Beach W. College of Pharmacy. Athens GA: The University of Georgia, 2004.

Some Calculations Involving "Units," "μg/mg," and Other Measures of Potency

Objectives

Upon successful completion of this chapter, the student will be able to:

• Perform calculations involving units of activity and other measures of potency.

The potencies of some antibiotics, endocrine products, vitamins, products derived through biotechnology, and biologics (e.g., vaccines) are based on their *activity* and are expressed in terms of *units* (of activity), in *micrograms per milligram* (*μg/mg*), or in other standardized terms of measurement. These measures of potency meet standards approved by the Food and Drug Administration and are set forth in the *United States Pharmacopeia* (USP).[1] Further, the World Health Organization (WHO), provides internationally agreed upon reference standards for biological preparations, which define potency or activity, as expressed in *International Units (I.U. or IU)*.[2]

Degrees of activity are determined by comparison against a suitable working standard, generally a USP Reference Standard. Reference standards are authentic specimens used as comparison standards in compendial tests and assays. The number of USP Units of an antibiotic, for example, is based on a comparison of activity of a sample of that antibiotic on a milligram basis to the corresponding USP Reference Standard. For instance, there are 1590 USP Units of penicillin G sodium per milligram of the USP Reference Standard of the antibiotic. Pharmaceutical products and preparations are allowed specific variances in potency; for example, the USP monograph for sterile penicillin G sodium specifies a potency of not less than 1500 Penicillin G Units and not more than 1750 Penicillin G Units per milligram.[3] The activity or potency of antibiotics is determined by their inhibitory effect on microorganisms. *No relationship exists between the unit of potency of one drug and the unit of potency of another drug.*

The potency of some drugs and their respective weight equivalents are given in Table 9.1.

Just as potencies of certain drugs are designated in units, so too are their doses. Of the drugs for which potency is expressed in units, insulin is perhaps the most common. In the case of insulin, although the commercially available types vary according to time of onset of action, time of peak action, and duration of action, all products are standardized to contain either 100 or 500 insulin units per milliliter of solution or suspension. These strengths are designated as U-100 and U-500 as shown in Figure 9.1. As noted earlier in this text, dispensing errors can occur when a medication order abbreviates the term *units* with a *U* and places it *after* the number of units, since a poorly written *U* can be mistaken for a zero; for example, "100U" could be mistaken for 1000 units. Thus, it is good practice to spell out the term *units* when used following the designated number. Special syringes are available for measuring units of insulin (Fig. 9.2).

CALCULATIONS CAPSULE

Units of Activity

The potency of many pharmaceutical products derived from biological sources is based on *units of activity*. Units of activity are determined against specific biologic standards and vary between products. Generally, there is an established relationship between a product's units of activity and a measurable quantity (e.g., units per milligram; units per milliliter). This relationship may be used in a ratio and proportion to determine either the number of units of activity or the weight or volume containing a specified number of units:

$$\frac{Units\, of\, activity\, (given)}{Weight\, or\, volume\, (given)} = \frac{Units\, of\, activity\, (given\, or\, desired)}{Weight\, or\, volume\, (given\, or\, desired)}$$

Biologics are preparations produced from a living source. They include vaccines, toxoids, and immune sera, used for the development of *immunity*, or resistance to disease; certain antitoxins and antivenins, used as treatment against specific antigens; and, toxins and skin antigens, used as diagnostic aids. Biologics are prepared from human serum (e.g., immune globulin), horse serum (e.g., tetanus antitoxin), chick cell culture (e.g., measles virus vaccine), and other such animate media.

The strengths of the various biologic products are expressed in a number of ways. The strength of a bacterial vaccine commonly is expressed in terms of micrograms (μg) or units of antigen per milliliter. The strength of a viral vaccine is expressed most commonly in terms of the *tissue culture infectious dose* ($TCID_{50}$), which is the quantity of virus estimated to infect 50% of inoculated cultures. Viral vaccines may also be described in terms of units, micrograms of antigen, or number or organisms per milliliter. The strength of a toxoid is generally expressed in terms of *flocculating units (Lf Unit)*, with 1 Lf Unit having the capacity to flocculate or precipitate one unit of standard antitoxin.

Vaccines are available for a large number of diseases, including cervical cancer (human papillomavirus), hepatitis A and B, influenza, measles, mumps, pneumococcal, shingles (herpes zoster), smallpox, and tuberculosis. In addition, many additional vaccines are in various stages of development. The National Institute of Allergy and Infectious Diseases (NIAID) of the National Institutes of Health (NIH), lists all vaccines licensed for use in the United States as well as the status of vaccines in current research and development.[4] The Centers for Disease Control and Prevention (CDC) offers current guidelines for vaccine use in different population groups, as infants, children, adults, and pregnant women.[5]

Specific examples of the *potency* of vaccines expressed in terms other than weight are:

Hepatitis A Vaccine, Inactivated, 1440 EL.U (ELISA units) per 1-mL dose

Influenza Virus Vaccine, Live (intranasal), $10^{6.5-7.5}$ FFU (fluorescent focus units per 0.2 mL dose

Measles Virus Vaccine, Live NLT 1000 $TCID_{50}$ (50% tissue culture infectious dose) in each 0.5-mL dose

Zoster Vaccine, Live, 19,400 PFU (plaque-forming units) per 0.65-mL dose

Table 9.1 ▼ EXAMPLES OF DRUG POTENCY EQUIVALENTS

DRUG	UNITS OR μg OF POTENCY PER WEIGHT EQUIVALENT[a]
Alteplase	580,000 USP Alteplase Units per mg of protein
Bacitracin Zinc	NLT 65 Bacitracin Units per mg
Cefdinir	NLT 960 μg and NMT 1020 μg of cefdinir per mg
Clindamycin Hydrochloride	NLT 800 μg of clindamycin per mg
Cod Liver Oil	In each gram: NLT 180 μg (600 USP Units) and NMT 750 μg (2500 USP Units) of Vitamin A and NLT 1.5 μg (60 USP Units) and NMT 6.25 μg (250 USP Units) of Vitamin D
Erythromycin Estolate	NLT 600 μg of erythromycin per mg
Gentamicin Sulfate	NLT 590 μg of gentamicin per mg
Heparin Sodium	NLT 140 USP Heparin Units per mg
Insulin	NLT 26.5 USP Insulin Units per mg
Insulin Glargine	27.5 units/mg
Insulin Glulisine	28.7 units/mg
Insulin Human	NLT 27.5 USP Insulin Human Units per mg
Insulin Lispro	NLT 27 USP Insulin Lispro Units per mg
Interferon alfa-2b	2.6×10^8 international units per mg
Interferon alfa-n3	2×10^8 international units per mg
Interferon beta-1b	3.2×10^7 international units per mg
Neomycin Sulfate	NLT 600 μg of neomycin per mg
Nystatin	NLT 4400 USP Nystatin Units per mg
Penicillin G Benzathine	NLT 1090 and NMT 1272 Penicillin G Units per mg
Penicillin G Potassium	NLT 1440 and NMT 1680 Penicillin G Units per mg
Penicillin V Potassium	NLT 1380 and NMT 1610 Penicillin V Units per mg
Polymyxin B Sulfate	NLT 6000 Polymyxin B Units per mg
Somatropin	3 international units per mg
Tobramycin	NLT 900 μg of tobramycin per mg
Vancomycin	NLT 900 μg vancomycin per mg
Vasopressin	NLT 300 Vasopressin Units per mg
Vitamin A	1 USP Vitamin A Unit equals the biologic activity of 0.3 μg of the all-*trans* isomer of retinol
Vitamin D	40 units per μg

[a]Data taken or derived from various literature sources including the United States Pharmacopeia 32 National Formulary 27:2009.

Pharmacy-Based Immunizations

Pharmacy-based immunization programs are commonplace nowadays. Many colleges of pharmacy and pharmacy organizations have developed pharmacy immunization training programs and states permit pharmacists to administer immunizations under established guidelines and protocols.[6]

▼ FIGURE 9.1 Example of a pharmaceutical product standardized in units of activity.

Example Calculations of Measures of Activity or Potency

Determinations of the activity or potency of a biologic material considered in this chapter may be performed through the use of ratio and proportion or dimensional analysis, as demonstrated by the following examples.

Units of Activity. Calculations involving units of activity are exemplified as follows.

How many milliliters of U-100 insulin should be used to obtain 40 units of insulin?
U-100 insulin contains 100 units/mL

$$\frac{100 \text{ (units)}}{40 \text{ (units)}} = \frac{1 \text{ (mL)}}{x \text{ (mL)}}$$

$$x = 0.4 \text{ mL U-100 insulin, } \textit{answer.}$$

Or, solving by dimensional analysis:

$$40 \text{ units} \times \frac{1 \text{ mL}}{100 \text{ units}} = 0.4 \text{ mL U-100 insulin, } \textit{answer.}$$

▼ FIGURE 9.2 Example of an insulin syringe calibrated in Units. *(Courtesy of Becton, Dickinson and Company.)*

A physician prescribed 100 units of insulin to be added to 500 mL of D5W in treating a patient with severe diabetic acidosis. How many milliliters of insulin injection concentrate, U-500, should be used?

U-500 insulin contains 500 units/mL

$$\frac{500 \ (\text{units})}{100 \ (\text{units})} = \frac{1 \ (\text{mL})}{x \ (\text{mL})}$$

$$x = 0.2 \, \text{mL U-500 insulin, } answer.$$

Or, solving by dimensional analysis:

$$100 \ \text{units} \times \frac{1 \ \text{mL}}{500 \ \text{units}} = 0.2 \ \text{mL U-500 insulin, } answer.$$

How many milliliters of a heparin sodium injection containing 200,000 units in 10 mL should be used to obtain 5,000 Heparin Sodium Units that are to be added to an intravenous dextrose solution?

$$\frac{200,000 \ (\text{units})}{5,000 \ (\text{units})} = \frac{10 \ (\text{mL})}{x \ (\text{mL})}$$

$$x = 0.25 \ \text{mL heparin sodium injection, } answer.$$

If a 2.5-mL vial contains 100 units of onabotulinumtoxinA (BOTOX), and 0.1 mL is injected into each of five sites during a procedure, how many units of drug would remain in the vial?

Used in procedure: 0.1 mL × 5 (sites) = 0.5 mL
Remaining in vial: 2.5 mL − 0.5 mL = 2 mL

$$\frac{100 \ \text{units} \times 2 \ \text{mL}}{2.5 \ \text{mL}} = 80 \ \text{units onabotulinumtoxin A, } answer.$$

Activity Based on Weight. Calculations involving the determination of activity per unit of weight are exemplified as follows.

If neomycin sulfate has a potency of 600 μg of neomycin per milligram, how many milligrams of neomycin sulfate would be equivalent in potency to 1 mg of neomycin?

$$\frac{600 \ (\mu\text{g of neomycin})}{1,000 \ (\mu\text{g of neomycin})} = \frac{1 \ (\text{mg of neomycin sulfate})}{x \ (\text{mg of neomycin sulfate})}$$

$$x = 1.67 \ \text{mg neomycin sulfate, } answer.$$

Dose or Antigen Content of a Biologic Based on Potency. Calculations of the dose or the antigen content of a biologic product are exemplified as follows.

A biologic contains 50 Lf Units of diphtheria toxoid in each 2.5 mL of product. If a pediatric patient is to receive 10 Lf Units, how many milliliters of product should be administered?

$$\frac{50 \ (\text{Lf Units})}{10 \ (\text{Lf Units})} = \frac{2.5 \ (\text{mL})}{x \ (\text{mL})}$$

$$x = 0.5 \ \text{mL, } answer.$$

CASE IN POINT 9.1[a] A pharmacist is asked to assist in determining the correct dose of epoetin alpha injection (PROCRIT) for a 76-year-old, 165-lb male patient suffering from anemia, in part due to chronic renal failure. The patient's initial hemoglobin is 9.2 g/dL.

The literature states the starting adult dose of epoetin alpha to be "50–100 units/kg SC TIW" to stimulate red blood cell production. Firstly, (a) what would be the correct interpretation of this dosage statement?[b]

The literature further states that the dose is to be *reduced* by 25% when the patient's hemoglobin reaches a level suitable to avoid transfusion or increases >1 g/dL in any 2-week period. The dose is to be *increased* to "300 units/kg TIW" after 2–4 weeks if the hemoglobin response is insufficient or if transfusions are still required.

Using epoetin alpha injection, 10,000 units/mL, and the minimal starting dose, calculate (b) the number of milliliters required for the initial dose and (c) the total number of milliliters to be administered during the first week of treatment. If the patient's hemoglobin increases to 10.5 g/dL after 2 weeks of treatment, what would be the new dose in (d) units of epoetin alpha and in (e) milliliters of injection?

[a]Case in Point courtesy of Flynn Warren, Bishop, GA.
[b]If unsure of the abbreviations, refer to Chapter 4 for guidance.

Measles Virus Vaccine Live is prepared to contain 1000 TCID$_{50}$ per 0.5-mL dose. What is the TCID$_{50}$ content of a 50-mL multiple dose vial of the vaccine?

$$\frac{1000 \ (\text{TCID}_{50})}{x \ (\text{TCID}_{50})} = \frac{0.5 \ (\text{mL})}{50 \ (\text{mL})}$$

$$x = 100,000 \ \text{TCID}_{50}, \ answer.$$

PRACTICE PROBLEMS

Units of Activity Calculations

1. How many milliliters of U-100 insulin zinc suspension should be used to obtain 18 units of insulin?

2. If a diabetic patient injects 20 Units of insulin twice daily, how many days will a 10-mL vial of the U-100 product last the patient?

3. The biotechnology-derived product interferon beta-1b contains 32 million international units per milligram. Calculate the number of international units present in a vial containing 0.3 mg of interferon beta-1b.

4. ALFERON N injection contains 5 million international units of interferon alpha-n3 per milliliter. How many units will an injection of 0.05 mL deliver?

5. Insulin glargine (LANTUS) injection is available in 10-mL vials containing 100 units/mL. How many milliliters would a patient administer for (a) a starting dose of 10 units and (b) a maintenance dose of 4 units?

6. The content of a vial of penicillin G potassium weighs 600 mg and represents 1 million units. How many milligrams are needed to prepare 15 g of an ointment that is to contain 15,000 units of penicillin G potassium per gram?

7. HUMALOG contains 100 units of insulin lispro (rDNA origin) per milliliter. How many complete days will a 3-mL HUMALOG PEN last a patient whose dose is 35 units b.i.d?

8. A physician prescribes 2.5 million units of penicillin G potassium daily for 1 week. If 1 unit of penicillin G potassium equals 0.6 μg, how many tablets, each containing 250 mg, will provide the prescribed dosage regimen?

9. ℞ Penicillin G
   Potassium   5000 units
                       per mL
   Isotonic Sodium
      Chloride Solution ad 15 mL
   Sig. Nose drops.

   Using soluble penicillin tablets, each containing 200,000 units of crystalline penicillin G potassium, explain how you would obtain the penicillin G potassium needed in compounding the prescription.

10. FOSAMAX PLUS D contains 70 mg alendronate and 140 mcg of vitamin D_3, the latter equivalent to 5600 international units of vitamin D. At a once-a-week dose, calculate the daily intake of vitamin D_3 in milligrams and units.

11. A vial for preparation of 100 mL of injection of the drug alteplase (ACTIVASE) contains 100 mg of drug equivalent to 58 million international units to be administered by intravenous infusion. Calculate (a) the units administered to a 176-lb. patient at a dose of 0.9 mg/kg and (b) the milliliters of injection to use.

12. Calcitonin is available as an injection containing 200 international units per milliliter. Adult doses of up to 32 units per kilogram have produced no adverse effects. On this basis, if a 120-lb. patient were administered 0.75 mL of injection, would adverse effects be anticipated?

13. A physician's hospital medication order calls for a patient to receive 1 unit of insulin injection subcutaneously for every 10 mg/dL of blood sugar over 175 mg/dL, with blood sugar levels and injections performed twice daily in the morning and evening. The patient's blood sugar was 200 mg/dL in the morning and 320 mg/dL in the evening. How many total units of insulin injection were administered?

14. A physician's hospital medication order calls for isophane insulin suspension to be administered to a 136-lb. patient on the basis of 1 unit/kg per 24 hours. How many units of isophane insulin suspension should be administered daily?

15. Somatropin (NUTROPIN) contains 5 mg of drug equivalent to approximately 15 international units of drug in a vial to prepare 10 mL of injection. If the starting adult dose is 0.006 mg/kg, calculate the dose (a) in units and (b) in milliliters for a 132-lb. patient.

16. Cod liver oil is available in capsules containing 0.6 mL per capsule. Using Table 9.1, calculate the amounts, in units, each of vitamins A and D in each capsule. The specific gravity of cod liver oil is 0.92.

17. A hepatitis B immune globulin contains 312 international units per milliliter. If the dose is 0.06 mL/kg for certain at-risk persons, calculate the dose (a) in units and (b) in milliliters for a 132-lb. person.

18. If a 5-mL vial of HUMATROPE, a biosynthetic somatropin of rDNA origin, contains 5 mg of somatotropin equivalent to 13 international units, how many milligrams of somatotropin and how many international units would be administered in a 0.6-mL dose?

19. EPOGEN injection is available containing in each milliliter, 2000, 3000, 4000, or 10,000 units of epoetin alfa. If the staring dose for a 160-lb. patient is prescribed at 50 units/kg, which of the following would provide that dose?
    (a) 4 mL of 2000 units/mL
    (b) 1 mL of 3000 units/mL
    (c) 0.9 mL of 4000 units/mL
    (d) 0.8 mL of 10,000 units/mL

20. The prophylactic dose of tetanus anti-toxin is 1500 units for persons weighing less than 65 lb. and 3000 to 5000 units for persons weighing more than 65 lb. The antitoxin is available in dose vials of 1500 units, 3000 units, 5000 units, and 20,000 units. Which vial should a pharmacist provide for administration to a patient weighing 25 kg?

Additional Calculations of Potency

21. Using Table 9.1, calculate the clindamycin potency equivalence, in milligrams per milliliter, of a solution containing 1 g of clindamycin hydrochloride in 10 mL of solution.

22. Each 1-mL adult dose of hepatitis A vaccine contains 1440 EL.U. of viral antigen. What would be the pediatric dose of this vaccine if 360 EL.U. of viral antigen are to be administered?

   (a) 0.8 mL
   (b) 0.25 mL

   (c) 4 mL
   (d) 0.4 mL

23. Each 0.01 mL of a mumps vaccine contains 400 $TCID_{50}$ of the mumps virus. If the usual dose contains 20,000 $TCID_{50}$, how many milliliters of vaccine should be administered?

24. If a biologic product contains 7.5 Lf Units of diphtheria toxoid per 0.5 mL, how many flocculating units would be present in a 7.5-mL multiple dose vial?

25. Zoster Vaccine Live (ZOSTAVAX) contains about 29,850 plaque-forming units (PFU) of attenuated virus per 0.1 cL. Approximately how many PFUs would be contained in each 0.65-mL dose?

   (a) 45,900 PFU
   (b) 4590 PFU
   (c) 1940 PFU
   (d) 19,400 PFU

CALCQUIZ

9.A. If a 5-mL quantity of a nystatin oral suspension is prepared to contain 500,000 USP Nystatin Units, using Table 9.1, calculate (a) the concentration of nystatin in the suspension in mg/mL. If a child's dose is 2 mL four times a day, how many (b) nystatin units and (c) milligrams of nystatin would be administered daily?

9.B. The drug dalteparin sodium (FRAGMIN) is administered by subcutaneous injection in patients with unstable angina or myocardial infarction at doses of 120 units/kg but not to exceed 10,000 units. Prefilled calibrated syringes are available with the following strengths (units/mL): 2500/0.2 mL, 5000/0.2 mL, 7500/0.3 mL, 10,000/0.4 mL, 12,500/0.5 mL, and 15,000/0.6 mL. Calculate: (a) the most efficient product strength to use to dose a patient weighing 148 lb, (b) the volume of that injection to administer, and (c) the weight of a hypothetical patient, in pounds, to reach the maximum dose of 10,000 units.

9.C. An injection contains 5 million International Units (MIU) of interferon alpha n3 (ALFERON N) proteins per milliliter. The recommended dose is 0.05 mL. The literature states that the activity of interferon alpha-n3 is approximately equal to 2.6×10^8 international units/mg of protein. Calculate: (a) the number of international units and (b) the micrograms of interferon alfa-n3 proteins administered per dose.

9.D. One general guideline for the maintenance dosing of heparin in pediatric patients is 100 units/kg every 4 hours, or, 20,000 units/m^2/24 h administered continuously. The available injection for use by intravenous infusion contains 1000 USP Heparin units/mL. For a 44-lb child, measuring 42 in. in height, calculate the *difference* between the quantities of heparin administered over a 24-hour period in (a) heparin units, (b) milligrams of heparin (sodium), and (c) in milliliters of heparin injection.

ANSWERS TO "CASE IN POINT" AND PRACTICE PROBLEMS

Case in Point 9.1

(a) TIW = three times a week (*it should be noted that although this abbreviation appears in the literature, it is considered error-prone and thus its use is not approved by the Institute of Safe Medication Practices.*)

(b) 165 lb ÷ 2.2 lb/kg = 75 kg, weight of patient
Minimal starting dose = 50 units/kg; thus, 50 units × 75 (kg) = 3750 units
3750 units ÷ 10,000 units/mL = 0.375 mL of epoetin alpha injection.

(c) 0.375 mL/dose × 3 (times per week) = 1.125 mL epoetin alpha injection.

(d) Dose reduced by 25% or 937.5 units; thus 3750 − 937.5 = 2812.5 units epoetin alpha.

(e) 2812.5 units ÷ 10,000 units/mL = 0.28 mL epoetin alpha injection.

Practice Problems

1. 0.18 mL U-100 insulin zinc suspension

2. 25 days

3. 9,600,000 units interferon beta 1-b

4. 250,000 international units

5. (a) 0.1 mL insulin glargine
   (b) 0.04 mL insulin glargine

6. 135 mg penicillin G potassium

7. 4 days

8. 42 penicillin G potassium tablets

9. Dissolve 1 tablet in enough isotonic sodium chloride solution to make 8 mL, and take 3 mL of the dilution.

10. 800 units and 0.02 mg/day

11. (a) 41.76 million units alteplase
    (b) 72 mL alteplase injection

12. No

13. 17 units insulin

14. 61.82 units isophane insulin

15. (a) 1.08 units somatropin
    (b) 0.72 mL somatropin injection

16. 331.2 to 1380 units of vitamin A
    33.12 to 138 units of vitamin D

17. (a) 1123.2 IU hepatitis B immune globulin
    (b) 3.6 mL hepatitis B immune globulin

18. 0.6 mg, and 1.56 or 1.6 IU somatropin

19. (c) 0.9 mL of 4000 units/mL

20. 1500-unit vial

21. 80 mg/mL clindamycin

22. (b) 0.25 mL

23. 0.5 mL mumps vaccine

24. 112.5 Lf Units diphtheria toxoid

25. (d) 19,400 PFU

References

1. *United States Pharmacopeia 32 National Formulary 27.* Rockville, MD: The United States Pharmacopeial Convention, 2009;1:5,419–420.
2. World Health Organization (WHO). Available at: http://www.who.int/biologicals/reference_preparations/en/. Accessed February 20, 2011.
3. *United States Pharmacopeia 32 National Formulary 27.* Rockville, MD: The United States Pharmacopeial Convention, 2009;3:3238.
4. National Institute of Allergy and Infectious Diseases. Available at: http://www.niaid.nih.gov/labsandresources/labs/aboutlabs/Pages/default.aspx. Accessed February 20, 2011.
5. Centers for Disease Control and Prevention. Available at: http://www.cdc.gov/vaccines/. Accessed February 20, 2011.
6. Goad JA. Collaborative practice for pharmacy-based immunization. *Pharmacy Today* 2007;13:77.

Selected Clinical Calculations

10

Objectives

Upon successful completion of this chapter, the student will be able to:

- Calculate heparin doses from medication orders and standardized protocols.
- Calculate ideal body weight and apply in dose determinations.
- Calculate estimated creatinine clearance rates and apply in dose determinations.
- Calculate various cholesterol ratios and cholesterol reduction percent from clinical laboratory data.
- Convert blood serum chemistry values from *mg/dL* to *mmol/L* (international system).

Heparin-Dosing Calculations

Heparin is a heterogenous group of mucopolysaccharides that have anticoagulant properties. Heparin slows clotting time. It is derived from the intestinal mucosa or other suitable tissues of domestic animals (often porcine) used for food by man. Salt forms of heparin, such as heparin sodium, are standardized to contain 140 USP Heparin Units in each milligram. Heparin salts are administered as sterile aqueous solutions by intravenous infusion, intermittent intravenous injection, or deep subcutaneous injection for the prophylaxis and treatment of venous thrombosis. The commercial preparations, available in single-use syringes and multiple-dose vials, indicate on their labeling the number of USP Heparin Units of activity contained per milliliter.

Heparin is the fundamental treatment in acute venous thromboembolism; however, its use carries with it, the risk of hemorrhage. Patients especially at risk include elderly patients, post-surgical patients, patients with a history of peptic ulcers, severe renal or hepatic failure, and patients who recently have taken other medications that affect blood clotting time.[1]

When heparin sodium is administered in therapeutic amounts, its dosage is adjusted according to the results of tests measuring the patient's level of blood coagulation, or partial thromboplastin time (PTT). These tests are performed before each intravenous injection and approximately every 4 to 6 hours when administered by intravenous infusion or subcutaneously. In general, the PTT value should be maintained at 1.5 to 2 times the patient's pretreatment PTT value or, when the whole blood-clotting time is evaluated, approximately 2 to 3 times the control value.

The dose varies depending on the circumstances. Bolus doses, given by direct intravenous injection, may be followed by intravenous infusion as a heparin drip.

Low-dose heparin administration provides effective prophylaxis (rather than therapeutic effects) in a variety of surgical procedures. Patients receive 5000 units given by deep subcutaneous injection 2 hours before surgery and an additional 5000 units every 8 to 12 hours thereafter as required.[2]

Medium-dose heparin, indicated for patients with active phlebitis, with pulmonary emboli, and in hip replacement surgery, has a dosage range of 20,000 to 60,000 units per day, generally by intravenous infusion.[2]

High-dose heparin is indicated in patients with massive pulmonary embolism. Doses of 60,000 to 120,000 units are given by continuous intravenous infusion for the first day and then decreased to medium-dose heparin after 24 hours.[2]

In pediatric use, the initial dose may be 50 units/kg by intravenous drip, followed by maintenance doses of 100 units/kg every 4 hours or 20,000 units/m²/24 hours, infused continuously.[3]

Figure 10.1 presents a hospital form for an adult weight-based heparin protocol. The form allows physicians' orders for bolus doses, as well as protocols for low-dose and high-dose intravenous heparin infusions. The values given in this figure may differ from heparin protocols at other institutions. Pharmacists must follow those used within their institutions of practice.

It is important to note that a variety of low-molecular-weight heparins are also used as antithrombotic agents: for example, enoxaparin sodium (LOVENOX) and dalteparin sodium (FRAGMIN). Heparin has a molecular weight ranging from 3000 to 30,000 daltons whereas low molecular-weight heparins are fragments of heparin with mean molecular weights of 4000 to 6000 daltons.[4] These shorter compounds may be administered subcutaneously (rather than intravenously, as is heparin), they interfere less with platelet function, and they generally have a more predictable anticoagulant response that does not require monitoring of clotting times.

Special Considerations in Heparin Management

Heparin is a very useful but potentially dangerous agent. It is administered only when necessary and with extreme caution. Hemorrhage is a distinct risk with heparin use, requiring patients to be closely monitored. Pediatric patients and seniors are among those who require particular care in dosing. Heparin dosing errors can result from miscommunication (as with the use of the abbreviation "u" for units), from miscalculation of the appropriate dose, or from the administration of a product of incorrect strength. To reduce the likelihood of the latter, products are available in which the strengths are made distinctive by use of stark color-coding and bold, tall-letter labeling.

Example Calculations of Heparin Dosing

An intravenous infusion contained 20,000 units of heparin sodium in 1000 mL of D5W. The rate of infusion was set at 1600 units per hour for a 160-lb. patient. Calculate (a) the concentration of heparin sodium in the infusion, in units/mL; (b) the length of time the infusion would run, in hours; and (c) the dose of heparin sodium administered to the patient, on a unit/kg/minute basis.

(a) $\dfrac{20,000 \text{ units}}{1000 \text{ mL}} = 20 \text{ units/mL}, \text{ and}$

(b) $\dfrac{20,000 \text{ units}}{1600 \text{ units/hour}} = 12.5 \text{ hours}, \text{ and}$

CITY HOSPITAL

ADULT WEIGHT-BASED HEPARIN PROTOCOL

Standard Heparin IV Premixed Solution is 25,000 units in 250 mL (100 units per mL)
Initial laboratory tests (draw before starting heparin): PTT, PT, CBC with platelet count
Day 2 and every 3 days thereafter. CBC with platelet count
PTT six (6) hours after heparin drip is started
PTT six (6) hours after every change in heparin administration rate or bolus dose of heparin
Once a therapeutic PTT level is reached, do a PTT six (6) hours later
After two (2) consecutive therapeutic PTT levels are obtained, do a PTT daily at 0600
Discontinue all IM medications and other IM injections

Patient _____ MAY _____ MAY NOT receive drugs containing aspirin.

Patient _____ MAY _____ MAY NOT receive drugs containing non-steroidal antiinflammatory agents.

_____ For a PTT Value of 50 to 70 seconds (LOW-DOSE HEPARIN PROTOCOL)	
_____ No Bolus Dose	Start heparin drip at a rate of
_____ Bolus with 70 units of heparin per kg (limit 10,000 units)	_____ 15 units per kg per hr
_____ Bolus with _____ units of heparin	or _____ units per kg per hr

PTT Value	Heparin Dose Adjustments
<35 seconds	Bolus with 70 units per kg and increase infusion rate by 4 units per kg per hour
35 to 49 seconds	Bolus with 40 units per kg and increase infusion rate by 2 units per kg per hour
50 to 70 seconds	No change in heparin infusion rate
71 to 99 seconds	Decrease infusion rate by 1 unit per kg per hour
100 to 120 seconds	Decrease infusion rate by 2 units per kg per hour
>120 seconds	Hold heparin infusion for 1 hour; when restarted, decrease heparin infusion rate by 3 units per kg per hour

_____ For a PTT Value of 70 to 99 seconds (HIGH-DOSE HEPARIN PROTOCOL)	
_____ No Bolus Dose	Start heparin drip at a rate of
_____ Bolus with 70 units of heparin per kg (limit 10,000 units)	_____ 18 units per kg per hr
_____ Bolus with _____ units of heparin	or _____ units per kg per hr

PTT Value	Heparin Dose Adjustments
<35 seconds	Bolus with 70 units per kg and increase infusion rate by 4 units per kg per hour
35 to 49 seconds	Bolus with 40 units per kg and increase infusion rate by 3 units per kg per hour
50 to 70 seconds	Increase infusion rate by 2 units per kg per hour
71 to 99 seconds	No change in heparin infusion rate
100 to 120 seconds	Decrease infusion rate by 1 unit per kg per hour
>120 seconds	Hold heparin infusion for 1 hour; when restarted, decrease heparin infusion rate by 2 units per kg per hour
DATE	TIME
	M.D.

▼ FIGURE 10.1 Example of hospital form for audit weight-based heparin protocol. *(Courtesy of Flynn Warren, Bishop, GA.)*

(c) 160 pounds = 72.7 kg

12.5 hours = 750 minutes

$$\frac{20,000\ units}{750\ minutes} = 26.67\ units/minute$$

$$\frac{26.67\ units/minute}{72.7\ kg} = 0.37\ units/kg/minute, \textit{answers.}$$

A patient weighing 80 kg was given an initial bolus dose of heparin and a heparin drip for the first 6 hours. Using Figure 10.1 and the low-dose heparin protocol, what was the total amount of heparin administered in this period?[5]

Bolus dose [70 units/kg]: 70 units × 80 (kg) = 5600 units
Heparin drip [15 units/kg/hr]: 15 units × 80 (kg) × 6 (hours) = 7200 units
Thus, 5600 units + 7200 units = 12,800 units, *answer.*

Heparin sodium may be administered to children by intermittent intravenous infusion every 4 hours at doses ranging from 50 to 100 units/kg of body weight. Using an injection containing heparin, 5000 units/mL, calculate the daily dosage range, in milliliters, for a 50-lb child.

Child's weight in kg = 50 lb ÷ 2.2 lb/kg = 22.7 kg
Dosage range for the child = 50 to 100 units/kg × 22.7 kg = 1135 to 2270 units
Daily dosage range in units = 1135 to 2270 units × 6 (doses per day) = 6810 to 13,620 units
Daily dosage range in mL = 6810 units ÷ 5000 units/mL = 1.36 mL, and
13,620 units ÷ 5000 units/mL = 2.72 mL; thus
1.36 mL to 2.72 mL heparin sodium injection, *answer.*

The pediatric maintenance dose of heparin sodium is stated in the literature as 20,000 units/ m²/24 hours. Using the BSA nomogram in Chapter 8, and a heparin sodium injection containing heparin sodium, 1000 units/mL, calculate the daily volume of injection to administer to a 25-lb child measuring 22 in. in height.

BSA = 0.37 m²
20,000 units × 0.37 m² = 7400 units
7400 units ÷ 1000 units/mL = 7.4 mL heparin sodium injection, *answer.*

Example Calculations of Low-Molecular-Weight Heparin Dosing

The recommended dose of dalteparin sodium (FRAGMIN) for patients undergoing hip replacement surgery is 2500 international units within 2 hours before surgery, 2500 units 4 to 8 hours after surgery, and 5000 units daily × 5 to 10 days, starting on the postoperative day. How many milliliters from a vial containing 10,000 units/mL should be administered (a) before surgery, (b) after surgery, and (c) the day following surgery?

(a) $\dfrac{1\ mL}{10,000\ units} \times 2500\ units = 0.25\ mL,$

(b) same as (a) = 0.25 mL

(c) $\dfrac{1\ mL}{10,000\ units} \times 5000\ units = 0.5\ mL, \textit{answer.}$

CASE IN POINT 10.1[a] A 198-lb hospitalized patient is placed on a high-dose heparin protocol. The patient requires a bolus injection followed by a heparin infusion. The hospital follows the protocol shown in Figure 10.1.

The hospital pharmacist has heparin available for bolus doses containing 5000 units per milliliter in 5-mL vials and heparin for intravenous infusion in 250-mL infusion bags each containing 25,000 units of heparin.

(a) How many milliliters of the 5000 units/mL injection should the pharmacist recommend as a bolus dose?

(b) How many milliliters per hour of the heparin infusion should the pharmacist instruct the nurse to deliver, based on the standard drip protocol?

(c) If the intravenous set is programmed to deliver 60 drops per milliliter, what should be the flow rate, in drops per minute, to deliver the mL/hr required in answer (b)?

(d) How long will the 250-mL infusion bag last, in hours?

[a]Case in Point courtesy of Flynn Warren, Bishop, GA.

Dosage Calculations Based on Creatinine Clearance

Dose of a Drug. The two major mechanisms by which drugs are eliminated from the body are through hepatic (liver) metabolism and renal (kidney) excretion. When renal excretion is the major route, a loss of kidney function will dramatically affect the rate at which the drug is cleared from the body.

With many drugs, it is important to reach and maintain a specific drug concentration in the blood to realize the proper therapeutic effect. The initial blood concentration attained from a specific dose depends, in part, on the weight of the patient and the volume of body fluids in which the drug is distributed.

The ideal body weight (IBW) provides an excellent estimation of the distribution volume, particularly for some polar drugs that are not well distributed in adipose (fat) tissue. The IBW may be calculated readily through the use of the following formulas based on the patient's height and sex.

For males:
IBW = 50 kg + 2.3 kg for each inch of patient's height over 5 feet
or, in pounds
110 lb. + 5 lb. for each inch over 5 feet

For females:
IBW = 45.5 kg + 2.3 kg for each inch of patient height over 5 feet
or, in pounds
100 lb. + 5 lb. for each inch over 5 feet

Example Calculations of Ideal Body Weight

Calculate the ideal body weight for a male patient weighing 164 lb. and measuring 5 ft. 8 in. in height.

IBW = 110 lb. + (8 + 5 lb.)
110 lb. + 40 lb. = 150 lb, *answer.*

Calculate the ideal body weight for a female patient weighing 60 kg and measuring 160 cm in height.

160 cm = 63 in. = 5 ft. 3 in.
IBW = 45.5 kg + (3 × 2.3 kg)
45.5 kg + 6.9 kg = 52.4 kg, *answer*.

Note: In instances in which the IBW is determined to be greater than the actual body weight, the latter is used in dosage calculations.

The kidneys receive about 20% of the cardiac output (blood flow) and filter approximately 125 mL per minute of plasma. As kidney function is lost, the quantity of plasma filtered per minute decreases, with an accompanying decrease in drug clearance. The filtration rate of the kidney can be estimated by a number of methods. One of the most useful, however, is the estimation of the creatinine clearance rate (CrCl) through the use of the following empiric formulas based on the patient's age, weight, and serum creatinine (S_{cr}) value. Creatine, which is a break-down product of muscle metabolism, is generally produced at a constant rate and in quantities that depend on the muscle mass of the patient. Females usually have a lower serum creatinine than males due to less muscle mass. Because creatinine is eliminated from the body essentially through renal filtration, reduced kidney performance results in a reduced creatinine clearance rate. The normal adult value of serum creatinine is 0.6 to 1.3 mg/dL (the range varies with the laboratory used as the reference source). The creatinine clearance rate represents the volume of blood plasma that is cleared of creatinine by kidney filtration per minute. It is expressed in milliliters per minute.

By the Jelliffe equation:[5,6]
For males:

$$CrCl = \frac{98 - 0.8 \times (\text{Patient's age in years} - 20)}{\text{Serum creatinine in mg/dL}}$$

For females:

$$CrCl = 0.9 \times CrCl \text{ determined using formula for males}$$

By the Cockcroft-Gault equation:[7]
For males:

$$CrCl = \frac{(140 - \text{Patient's age in years}) \times \text{Body weight in kg}}{72 \times \text{Serum creatinine in mg/dL}}$$

For females:

$$CrCl = 0.85 \times CrCl \text{ determined using formula for males}$$

Example Calculations of Creatinine Clearance

Determine the creatinine clearance rate for an 80-year-old male patient weighing 70 kg and having a serum creatinine of 2 mg/dL. Use both the Jelliffe and Cockcroft-Gault equations.

By the Jelliffe equation:

$$CrCl = \frac{98 - 0.8 \times (80 - 20)}{2 \text{ (mg/dL)}}$$
$$= \frac{98 - (0.8 \times 60)}{2 \text{ (mg/dL)}} = \frac{98 - 48}{2 \text{ (mg/dL)}} = \frac{50}{2 \text{ (mg/dL)}}$$
$$= 25 \text{ mL/min, } answer.$$

By the Cockcroft-Gault equation:

$$CrCl = \frac{(140 - 80) \times 70}{72 \times 2 \ (mg/dL)}$$

$$= \frac{60 \times 70}{144}$$

$$= \frac{4200}{144}$$

$$= 29.2 \ mL/min, \ answer.$$

A 70-year-old gentleman and his 68-year-old wife have their annual physical exams. He weighs 160 lb and she, 126 lb. His blood work reveals a serum creatinine of 1.3 mg/dL and hers is 1.1 mg/dL. Using the Cockcroft-Gault equation, calculate their respective creatinine clearance rates.

$$His \ CrCl = \frac{(140 - 70) \times 72.7}{72 \times 1.3} = 54.4 \ mL/min \ and$$

$$Her \ CrCl = 0.85 \times \frac{(140 - 68) \times 57.3}{72 \times 1.1} = 44.3 \ mL/min, \ answers.$$

In addition to the Jelliffe and Cockcroft-Gault equations, other equations are used to estimate creatinine clearance, including the Sanaka equation, for select patients over 60 years of age, and the Schwartz equation, for pediatric and adolescent patients from neonates to 17 years of age.[8]

Sanaka equation:
For males:

$$CrCl = \frac{Patient's \ weight \ (kg) \times [19 \times Plasma \ albumin \ (g/dL) + 32]}{100 \times Serum \ creatinine \ (mg/dL)}$$

For females:

Substitute in the equation: [13 Plasma albumin (g/dL) + 29]

Schwartz equation:

$$CrCl = \frac{k \times Patient's \ height \ (cm)}{Serum \ creatinine \ (mg/dL)}$$

where k is a proportionality constant with a value ranging from 0.33 (for neonates) to 0.70 (for adolescent males).

Adjusting Creatinine Clearance for Body Surface Area. It is sometimes desirable to adjust the calculated creatinine clearance for body surface area to account for this possible variable in determining drug dosage. This adjustment is accomplished through the use of a nomogram of body surface area (BSA), as described previously in Chapter 8, and the following formula:

$$\frac{BSA}{1.73} \times CrCl = Adjusted \ CrCl$$

If a patient weighing 120 lb. and measuring 60 in. in height has a calculated creatinine clearance of 40 mL per minute, adjust the CrCl based on body surface area.

Using the nomogram in Chapter 8, the patient's BSA is determined to be 1.50 m². Thus,

$$\frac{1.50 \ m^2}{1.73 \ m^2} \times 40 \ mL/min = 3.47 \ mL/min, \ adjusted \ CrCl, \ answer.$$

Normal creatinine clearance rate may be considered 100 mL per minute. Thus, in the preceding example, the patient would exhibit about 35% of normal creatinine clearance.

The creatinine clearance rate method for determining drug dose is used with various categories of drugs in which renal function is a factor. Such dosing is routine, for example, for aminoglycoside antibiotics including gentamicin, tobramycin, and amikacin.

Once the creatinine clearance rate and the ideal body weight have been calculated, the *loading dose* (initial dose) required to reach a certain drug concentration in the patient and the *maintenance dose* needed to maintain the specified concentration can be calculated.

The loading dose is based solely on the ideal body weight of the patient (except in obese patients), whereas the maintenance dose is based on the ideal body weight *and* the renal clearance rate of the drug.

*To calculate the **loading dose (LD)**, perform the following:*

LD = IBW in kg or lb. × Drug dose per kg or lb.

*To calculate the **maintenance dose (MD)**, perform the following:*

For the "normal" patient:

$$MD = IBW \ (kg) \times Dose \ per \ kg \ per \ dosing \ interval$$

For the renally impaired patient:

$$MD = \frac{CrCl \ (patient)}{CrCl \ (normal)} \times Dose \ for \ "normal" \ patient$$

Determine the loading and maintenance doses of gentamicin for a 76-year-old male patient weighing 190 lb. with a height of 6 feet and having a serum creatinine of 2.4 mg/dL. The physician desires a loading dose of 1.5 mg/kg of ideal body weight and a maintenance dose of 1 mg/kg of ideal body weight to be administered every 8 hours after the initial dose.

$$
\begin{aligned}
IBW &= 110 \ lb. + (5 \ lb. \times 12) \\
&= 110 \ lb. + 60 \ lb. \\
&= 170 \ lb. \ or \ 77.3 \ kg
\end{aligned}
$$

$$
\begin{aligned}
CrCl &= \frac{98 - 0.8 \times (76 - 20)}{2.4 \ (mg/dL)} \\
&= \frac{98 - 44.8}{2.4 \ (mg/dL)} = \frac{53.2}{2.4 \ (mg/dL)} = 22.2 \ mL \ per \ minute
\end{aligned}
$$

LD = 77.3 kg × 1.5 mg/kg = 116 mg gentamicin, *answer.*

MD for "normal" patient:

$$
\begin{aligned}
&= 77.3 \ kg \times 1 \ mg/kg \ every \ 8 \ hours \\
&= 77.3 \ mg \ every \ 8 \ hours
\end{aligned}
$$

MD for renally impaired patient:

$$= \frac{22.2 \ mL \ per \ minute}{100 \ mL \ per \ minute} \times 77.3 \ mg$$

$$= 17.2 \ mg \ gentamicin \ every \ 8 \ hours, \ answer.$$

Use of Creatinine Clearance Dosage Tables. For certain drugs, tables of dosage guidelines may be presented in the labeling/literature to adjust for impaired renal function. For

Table 10.1 ▼ CREATININE CLEARANCE DOSING GUIDELINES FOR CEFTAZIDIME (IV OR IM)[a]

RENAL FUNCTION	CREATININE CLEARANCE (mL/min/1.73m²)	DOSE	FREQUENCY
Normal to mild impairment	100–51	1 g	q8–12h
Moderate impairment	50–31	1g	q12h
Severe impairment	30–16	1g	q24h
Very severe impairment	15–6	500 mg	q24h
Essentially none	<5	500 mg	q48h

[a]Table modified from product literature for FORTAZ (ceftazidime), GlaxoSmithKline, Research Triangle Park, NC, through *Physicians' Desk Reference.* Montvale, NJ: PDR Network 2011;65:1386–1391.

example, the usual dose of the anti-infective drug ceftazidime is 1 g every 8 to 12 hours, with dosage adjusted based on the location and severity of the infection and the patient's renal function. For adult patients with impaired renal function, guidelines for dosage based on creatinine clearance with adjustment for body surface area are given in Table 10.1.

CALCULATIONS CAPSULE

Creatinine Clearance Equations[5–8]

Jelliffe equation

For males:

$$CrCl = \frac{98 - 0.8 \times (\text{patient's age in years} - 20)}{\text{Serum creatinine in mg/dL}}$$

For females:

$$CrCl = 0.9 \times CrCl \text{ determined by equation for males}$$

Cockcroft-Gault equation

For males:

$$CrCl = \frac{(140 - \text{Patient's age in years}) \times \text{pt. wt., kg}}{72 \times \text{Serum creatinine in mg/dL}}$$

For females:

$$CrCl = 0.85 \times CrCl \text{ determined using formula for males}$$

Adjusting CrCl for body surface area

$$\frac{BSA}{1.73} \times CrCl = \text{Adjusted } CrCl$$

Schwartz equation

For pediatric and adolescent patients:

$$CrCl = \frac{k \times \text{Patient's height (cm)}}{\text{Serum creatinine (mg/dL)}}$$

Where k is a proportionality constant ranging from 0.33 (for neonates) to 0.70 (for adolescent males)

Using the table of dosage guidelines for ceftazidime and adjusting for body surface area, determine the dose and daily dose schedule for a patient weighing 70 kg, measuring 70 in. in height, and having a creatinine clearance (CrCl) of 48 mL per minute.

Using the nomogram in Chapter 8, the patient is determined to have a BSA of 1.87 m^2. Applying the formula for the adjustment of CrCl based on BSA, the patient's CrCl is then determined:

$$\frac{1.87\,m^2}{1.73\,m^2} \times 48\,mL/min = 51.9 \text{ or } 52\,mL/min$$

The dosage table and the adjusted CrCl indicate a dosage of:
1 g every 8 to 12 hours, *answer.*

CASE IN POINT 10.2[a] A 35-year-old male patient weighing 180 lb. and standing 5 ft. 8 in. tall has been diagnosed with AIDS. His physician prescribes lamivudine (EPIVIR) as a component of his treatment program and knows that the dose of the drug must be adjusted based on the patient's renal function. Laboratory tests indicate that the patient's serum creatinine is 2.6 mg/dL and has held at the same level for 5 days.

(a) Calculate the patient's ideal body weight (IBW) and use in subsequent calculations if the IBW is lower than the patient's actual weight.
(b) Calculate the patient's CrCl by the Cockcroft-Gault equation.
(c) Select the appropriate dose of lamivudine from the dosing schedule:

Creatinine Clearance	Initial Dose	Maintenance Dose
<5 mL/min	50 mg	25 mg once daily
5–14 mL/min	150 mg	50 mg once daily
15–29 mL/min	150 mg	100 mg once daily
30–49 mL/min	150 mg	150 mg once daily

[a]Case in Point courtesy of Flynn Warren, Bishop, GA.

Clinical Laboratory Tests

It is common practice in assessing health status to analyze biologic fluids, especially blood and urine, for specific chemical content. The clinical laboratory tests used, known as *chemistries*, analyze samples for such chemicals as glucose, cholesterol, total lipids, creatinine, blood urea nitrogen, bilirubin, potassium, sodium, calcium, carbon dioxide, and other substances, including drugs following their administration. Blood chemistries are performed on plasma (the fluid part of the blood) or serum (the watery portion of clotted blood). Depending on the laboratory equipment used as well as patient factors (such as age and gender), the "usual" amount of each chemical substance varies, with no single "normal" value, but rather a common range. For example, the reference range of glucose in serum is, by some laboratories, 65 to 99 mg/dL and that for creatinine is 0.6 to 1.3 mg/dL.

Table 10.2 presents examples of the normal ranges of serum chemistry values for some commonly analyzed blood components. The "conversion factors" shown are used to convert the units most often used in the United States to those of the international system.

Table 10.2 ▼ EXAMPLES OF NORMAL RANGES OF SERUM CHEMISTRY VALUES[a]

LABORATORY TEST	NORMAL VALUES (RANGE, IN US UNITS)	CONVERSION FACTOR (MULTIPLY)		INTERNATIONAL SYSTEM[b]
Albumin	3.6–5.1 g/dL	10	=	36–51 g/L
Calcium	8.6–10.3 mg/dL	0.25	=	2.2–2.6 mmol/L
Cholesterol, total	125–200 mg/dL	0.026	=	3.25–5.2 mmol/L
HDL cholesterol	> or = 40 mg/dL	0.026	=	> or = 1.04 mmol/L
LDL cholesterol	<130 mg/dL	0.026	=	<3.38 mmol/L
Glucose	65–99 mg/dL	0.055	=	3.58–5.45 mmol/L
Triglycerides	<150 mg/dL	0.011	=	<1.65 mmol/L
Creatinine	0.6–1.3 mg/dL	88.4	=	53.0–114.9 µmol/L
Urea Nitrogen (BUN)	7–25 mg/dL	0.357	=	2.50–8.93 mmol/L

[a]Normal values shown may vary between test laboratories and may be referred to as "reference," "healthy," or "goal" values.
[b]The International system is generally expressed in mmol (or other units) per liter.

For example, a cholesterol reading of 180 (mg/dL) may be recorded as 4.65 millimoles per liter (mmol/L). Low-density lipoprotein cholesterol (LDL-C), high-density lipoprotein (HDL-C), and total cholesterol (TC) are each measured in assessing a patient's risk for atherosclerosis.[9] The greatest risk comes from the non–high-density lipoprotein cholesterol (non–HDL-C), particularly in patients with high serum levels of triglycerides (TG or TGR). In addition, certain accompanying patient factors are considered added risk factors and affect the LDL-C goal for a particular patient. These include personal and/or familial history of coronary heart disease, atherosclerotic disease, diabetes, hypertension, and cigarette smoking.

Table 10.3 presents categories of cholesterol and triglyceride blood levels.

In calculating total cholesterol (TC), the triglyceride level is divided by five and that result added to the value of the HDL and LDL levels.

There are a number of "cholesterol ratios" that are considered clinically relevant to risk assessment. One is the ratio of total cholesterol to HDL cholesterol, the target being 5:1 or less, with 3.5:1 considered optimal. In addition, other ratios calculated to assess risk are LDL:HDL and HDL:LDL. Greater proportions of HDL are considered to lower risk of cardiovascular disease.

Example Calculations Involving Clinical Laboratory Tests

If a patient is determined to have a serum cholesterol level of 200 mg/dL, what is the equivalent value expressed in terms of millimoles (mmol) per liter?

Molecular Weight (m.w. of cholesterol) = 387
1 mmol cholesterol = 387 mg
200 mg/dL = 2000 mg/L

$$\frac{387 \text{ (mg)}}{2000 \text{ (mg)}} = \frac{1 \text{ (millimole)}}{x \text{ (millimoles)}}$$

$$x = 5.17 \text{ mmol/L}, answer.$$

Table 10.3 ▼ CATEGORIES OF CHOLESTEROL AND TRIGLYCERIDE BLOOD LEVELS[a]

BLOOD LEVEL (FASTING)	CLINICAL CATEGORY
Total Cholesterol (TC) Levels:	
Less than 200 mg/dL	Desirable
200–239 mg/dL	Borderline high
240 mg/dL and above	High
Low-Density Cholesterol (LDL):	
Less than 100 mg/dL	Optimal
100–129 mg/dL	Near optimal
130–159 mg/dL	Borderline high
160–189 mg/dL	High
190 mg/dL and above	Very high
High-Density Cholesterol (HDL):	
Less than 40 mg/dL	Low level/increased risk
40–50 mg/dL (men); 50–59 mg/dL (women)	Average level/average risk
60 mg/dL and above	High level/less than average risk
Triglycerides (TRG):	
Less than 150 mg/dL	Desirable
150–199 mg/dL	Borderline high
200–499 mg/dL	High
500 mg/dL and above	Very high

[a]National Heart, Lung and Blood Institute, National Institutes of Health, Public Health Service, U.S. Department of Health and Human Services. NIH Publication No. 05-3290. Available at: http://www.nhlbi.nih.gov/health/public/heart/chol/wyntk.htm. Accessed March 2, 2011.

Calculate the TC:HDL ratio when the total cholesterol is 240 mg/dL and the HDL cholesterol is 60 mg/dL.

240 mg/dL:60 mg/dL = 4:1, *answer.*

In order to achieve a goal-level of LDL cholesterol, the percent reduction required may be calculated.

If 160 mg/dL is a patient's current LDL level and the desired level is 100 mg/dL, calculate the percent reduction required.

The percent reduction is the difference in values as a percent of the current level:

Difference in values: 160 mg/dL – 100 mg/dL = 60 mg/dL

Difference as a percent of current level: $\dfrac{60 \text{ mg/dL}}{160 \text{ mg/dL}} \times 100\% = 37.5\%$, *answer.*

Therapeutic Drug Monitoring

Also termed ***drug therapy monitoring***, this process often includes the analysis of blood serum samples to ensure optimum drug therapy. This is especially important for categories of drugs in which the margin between safe and toxic levels is narrow. Data are available indicating these levels.[10]

Drug-Specific Clinical Equations

For certain clinical conditions, there are equations that are useful for determining patient requirements. For example, the following is used in determining the amount of iron required to bring hemoglobin (Hb) values to normal levels:

$$\text{Iron required (mg)} =$$
$$\text{Body weight (lb.)} \times 0.3 \times \left[100 - \frac{\text{Hb (g/dL)} \times 100}{14.8 \text{ g/dL}} \right]$$

In the equation, 14.8 g/dL is the normal value of hemoglobin in adults and the factor 0.3 is its iron content (percent).

Example:

Using the equation for determining iron deficiency, calculate the number of milliliters of an iron dextran solution containing 50 mg/mL of iron to be administered to a 150-lb. patient with a hemoglobin value of 10 g/dL.

$$\text{Iron required (mg)} = 150 \times 0.3 \times \left[100 - \frac{10 \times 100}{14.8} \right]$$
$$= 150 \times 0.3 \times 32.4$$
$$= 1458 \text{ mg}$$

$$\text{by proportion,} \quad \frac{50 \text{ mg}}{1458 \text{ mg}} = \frac{1 \text{ mL}}{\text{x mL}}$$
$$\text{x} = 29 \text{ mL iron dextran solution, } \textit{answer.}$$

PRACTICE PROBLEMS

Heparin-Dosing Calculations

1. A hospital pharmacy order calls for 5000 units of heparin to be administered to a patient, twice daily, subcutaneously, for the prevention of thrombi. The pharmacist has on hand a vial containing 10,000 Heparin Units/mL. How many milliliters of the injection should be administered for each dose?

2. A physician orders 1500 units of heparin to be administered by intravenous infusion per hour. The pharmacy provides a heparin intravenous bag containing 25,000 units of heparin in 250 mL of D5W. How many milliliters should be administered per minute?

3.[11] A male patient weighing 76 kg is placed on heparin therapy for the prevention of deep vein thrombosis after surgery.

(a) How many milliliters of a heparin injection containing 5000 units/mL should be administered for a loading dose of 80 units/kg?

(b) What should be the infusion rate, in mL/hr, using a solution that contains heparin 25,000 units/500 mL, to administer 18 units/kg/hr?

(c) Six hours after heparin therapy is initiated, the patient's PTT is found to be 60 seconds. Adjust the infusion rate, in mL/hr, according to the high-dose heparin protocol (Fig. 10.1).

4.[11] A blood sample taken from a 113-lb. patient 6 hours after heparin therapy is initiated shows a PTT of 24 seconds. Calculate (a) the bolus dose and (b) the infusion rate, in mL/hr, according to the high-dose heparin protocol (Fig. 10.1).

5. Enoxaparin sodium (LOVENOX) injection, a low-molecular-weight heparin, contains 150 mg/mL in 0.8-mL prefilled syringes. The recommended dose for knee replacement surgery is 30 mg every 12 hours. How many milliliters of the injection should be administered per dose?

Creatinine Clearance Calculations

6. The usual adult dose of levofloxacin is a 500-mg initial dose followed by subsequent doses of 250 mg every 24 hours for 10 days. For patients with a CrCl of less than 19 mL/min, doses following the initial dose are administered every 48 hours. How many 250-mg levofloxacin tablets should be dispensed to a 75-year-old, 160 pound male patient with a serum creatinine of 1.32?

7. Determine the loading and maintenance doses of tobramycin for a 72-year-old female patient weighing 187 lb. and measuring 5 ft. 3 in. in height with a serum creatinine of 2.8 mg/dL. The loading dose desired is 1.0 mg/kg of ideal body weight and 1.66 mg/kg of ideal body weight every 8 hours as the maintenance dose (adjusted for renal impairment).

8. Determine the loading and maintenance doses of amikacin for a 42-year-old female patient weighing 210 lb. and measuring 5 ft. in height with a serum creatinine of 1.8 mg/dL. The physician requests a loading dose of 7.5 mg/kg of ideal body weight and a maintenance dose of 5 mg/kg of ideal body weight (adjusted for renal impairment) to be administered continually at intervals of 8 hours.

9. Calculate the creatinine clearance rate for a 20-year-old male patient weighing 70 kg with a serum creatinine of 1 mg/dL. If a patient is 5 ft. 8 in. tall, adjust the creatinine clearance based on body surface area.

10. Using the creatinine clearance dosing table in this chapter and the nomogram for body surface area in Chapter 8, what would be the dose and dosage schedule of ceftazidime for a patient weighing 50 kg, measuring 66 in. in height, and having a creatinine clearance (unadjusted for BSA) of 31 mL per minute?

Clinical Laboratory Test Calculations

11. If a serum sample is determined to contain 270 mg/dL of cholesterol, what is the concentration of cholesterol (m.w. 386) in terms of millimoles per liter?

12. Among clinical recommendations to prevent cardiovascular disease in women is the maintenance of lipid levels as follows: low-density lipoproteins (LDL) <100 mg/dL; high-density lipoproteins (HDL) >50 mg/dL; and triglycerides (TG) <150 mg/dL.[12] Which of the following meet these criteria?

   (a) LDL <2.6 mmol/L
   (b) HDL >1.3 mmol/L
   (c) TG <1.65 mmol/L
   (d) all of the above

13. If a patient is instructed by her physician to reduce her LDL cholesterol level from 130 mg/dL to 100 mg/dL, calculate the percent reduction required.

14. A patient has an HDL of 50 mg/dL, an LDL of 150 mg/dL, and a TG of 85 mg/dL. Calculate the (a) TC:HDL ratio and (b) LDL percent reduction required for a goal of 100 mg/dL.

15. On the basis of the information in Table 10.2, calculate the mmol/L of glucose equivalent to a value of 140 mg/dL.

   (a) 7.7 mmol/L
   (b) 2.5 mmol/L
   (c) 5.4 mmol/L
   (d) 6.2 mmol/L

CALCQUIZ

10.A. When a PTT was performed on the patient described in "Case in Point 10.1," the patient's value was 40 seconds. Based on the high-dose protocol (Fig. 10.1), calculate (a) the needed bolus dose, in units, and (b) the new infusion rate, in mL/hr, using heparin injection, 25,000 units/250 mL.

10.B. The dose of a drug for patients with normal renal function is stated as 500 mg every 12 hours. The dose is to be reduced in frequency to every 24 hours for patients with a creatinine clearance of 6–30 mL/min and to every 48 hours if the creatinine clearance is ≤5. What should be the dosing frequency for a 65-year-old male patient weighing 165 pounds measuring 68 in. in height, with a serum creatinine of 1.5 mg/dL?

10.C. The dose of cefuroxime in severe infections is 1.5 g every 8 hours by infusion. The dose is reduced to 750 mg every 12 hours for patients with CrCl of 10 to 20 mL/min and 750 mg every 24 hours if the CrCl is below 10 mL/min. How many milliliters per hour of an infusion containing cefuroxime, 15 mg/mL, would constitute the dose for a 56-year-old female patient weighing 140 lb, measuring 62 in. in height, and with a S_{cr} of 3.5 mg/100 mL?

10.D. Based on creatinine clearance, the dose of a drug is

CrCl = 8–10 mL/min; dose = 2.43 mg/kg every 24 hours, divided into two doses
CrCl = 11–20 mL/min; dose = 3.58 mg/kg every 24 hours, divided into two doses
CrCl = 21–40 mL/min; dose = 5.87 mg/kg every 24 hours as a single dose.

For a 52-year-old male patient weighing 155 lb and measuring 69 in. with a serum creatinine of 2.6, calculate the per-dose volume to administer of an injection containing drug, 80 mg/mL.

10.E. Calculate the total cholesterol in a patient with a HDL of 87 mg/dL, LDL of 152 mg/dL, and a TRG of 50 mg/dL. Also, which of the following are correct?
(a) HDL:LDL ratio ≈ 1:1.7
(b) TC:HDL ratio ~ 2.9:1
(c) HDL = high risk
(d) LDL = low risk
(e) TRG = low risk
(f) After being placed on a statin drug, the patient's LDL dropped to 106 mg/dL, equivalent to a 30% reduction.

ANSWERS TO "CASE IN POINT" AND PRACTICE PROBLEMS

Case in Point 10.1

(a) Patient's weight in kg:

$$198 \text{ lb.} \times \frac{1 \text{ kg}}{2.2 \text{ lb}} = 90 \text{ kg}$$

High-dose protocol, bolus dose: 70 units heparin/kg

70 units × 90 (kg) = 6300 units

$$6300 \text{ units} \times \frac{1 \text{ mL}}{500 \text{ units}}$$

= 1.26 mL, *answer*

(b) High-dose protocol, infusion rate: 18 units/kg/hr

18 units/kg/hr × 90 (kg)
= 1620 units/hr

$$\frac{250 \text{ mL}}{25,000 \text{ units}} \times \frac{1620 \text{ units}}{1 \text{ hr}}$$

= 16.2 mL/hr, *answer*.

(c) $\dfrac{16.2 \text{ mL}}{1 \text{ hr}} \times \dfrac{60 \text{ drops}}{1 \text{ mL}} \times \dfrac{1 \text{ hr}}{60 \text{ min}}$

= 16.2 or 16 drops/min, *answer*.

(d) $250 \text{ mL} \times \dfrac{1 \text{ hr}}{16.2 \text{ mL}} = 15.43 \text{ hr}$, *answer*.

Case in Point 10.2

(a) $\text{IBW} = 50 \text{ kg} + (2.3 \times 8 \text{ in})$
$= 68.4 \text{ kg}$, *answer*.

Patient's actual weight $= 180 \text{ lb.} \div 2.2$
$\text{lb./kg} = 81.8 \text{ kg}$

(b) $\text{CrCl} = \dfrac{[(140 - 35) \times 68.4 \text{ kg}]}{72 \times 2.6 \text{ mg/dL}}$

$= \dfrac{7182}{187.2} = 38.37 \text{ mL/min}$,
answer.

(c) Dose = 150 mg initially and 150 mg maintenance dose once daily, *answer*.

Practice Problems

1. 0.5 mL heparin injection
2. 0.25 mL/min
3. (a) 1.2 mL heparin injection

(b) 27.36 or 27 mL/hr
(c) 30.4 or 30 mL/hr
4. (a) 3595 units
(b) 11.3 mL/hr
5. 0.2 mL enoxaparin sodium injection
6. 12 levofloxacin tablets
7. 52.3 mg tobramycin (loading dose) 15.7 mg tobramycin (maintenance dose)
8. 340.9 mg amikacin (loading dose) 91.3 mg amikacin (maintenance dose)
9. 117 mL/min 123.8 mL/min
10. 1 g ceftazidime every 24 hours
11. 6.99 mmol/L
12. (d) all of the above
13. 23%
14. (a) 4.34:1= TC:HDL ratio
(b) 33.3%
15. (a) 7.7 mmol/L

References

1. Heparin dosing. Available at: http://www.rxkinetics.com/heparin.html. Accessed March 2, 2011.
2. Berkow R, ed. *The Merck Manual*. 24th Ed. Rahway, NJ: Merck Sharpe & Dohme Research Laboratories, 1982:2404–2405.
3. Heparin Sodium Injection, USP. Available at: http://www.hospira.com/Files/heparin_sodium_injection.pdf. Accessed March 2, 2011.
4. Bontempo FA, Hassett AC. Low molecular weight heparin. Available at: http://www.itxm.org/tmu/tmu1996/tmu6-96.htm. Accessed February 26, 2011.
5. Jelliffe RW. Estimations of creatinine clearance when urine cannot be collected. *Lancet* 1971;1:975.
6. Jelliffe RW. Creatinine clearance bedside estimate. *Annals of Internal Medicine* 1973;79:604.
7. Cockcroft DW, Gault MH. Prediction of creatinine clearance from serum creatinine. *Nephron* 1976;16:31.
8. Anaizi N. Estimation of creatinine clearance. Drug Monitor. Available at: http://www.thedrugmonitor.com/clcreqs.html. Accessed March 1, 2011.
9. National Cholesterol Education program report. *Circulation* 2004;110:227–239. Available at: http://www.circulationa ha.org. Accessed March 1, 2011.
10. Pagana KD, Pagana TJ. *Mosby's Diagnostic and Laboratory Test Reference*. 6th Ed. Philadelphia: Mosby, 2003.
11. Ansel HC, Prince SJ. Pharmaceutical calculations. In: *The Pharmacist's Handbook*. Baltimore, MD: Lippincott Williams & Wilkins, 2004:236–240.
12. Women's health: What's hot. *Pharmacy Today* 2007;13(9):28.

Isotonic and Buffer Solutions

11

Objectives

Upon successful completion of this chapter, the student will be able to:

- Calculate the dissociation factor (i) of a chemical agent.
- Calculate the sodium chloride equivalent (*E-factor*) of a chemical agent.
- Demonstrate by calculation whether a solution is hypotonic, isotonic, or hypertonic.
- Perform calculations required in the preparation of isotonic solutions.
- Apply the buffer equation in pharmaceutical calculations.

When a solvent passes through a semipermeable membrane from a dilute solution into a more concentrated one, the concentrations become equalized and the phenomenon is known as *osmosis*. The pressure responsible for this phenomenon is termed *osmotic pressure* and varies with the nature of the solute.

If the solute is a nonelectrolyte, its solution contains only molecules and the osmotic pressure varies with the concentration of the solute. If the solute is an electrolyte, its solution contains ions and the osmotic pressure varies with both the concentration of the solute and its degree of dissociation. Thus, solutes that dissociate present a greater number of particles in solution and exert a greater osmotic pressure than *un*dissociated molecules.

Two solutions that have the same osmotic pressure are termed *isosmotic*. Many solutions intended to be mixed with body fluids are designed to have the same osmotic pressure for greater patient comfort, efficacy, and safety. A solution having the same osmotic pressure as a *specific* body fluid is termed *isotonic* (meaning of equal tone) with *that* specific body fluid.

Solutions of *lower* osmotic pressure than that of a body fluid are termed *hypotonic*, whereas those having a *higher* osmotic pressure are termed *hypertonic*. Pharmaceutical dosage forms intended to be added directly to the blood or mixed with biological fluids of the eye, nose, and bowel are of principal concern to the pharmacist in their preparation and clinical application.

Special Clinical Considerations of Tonicity

It is generally accepted that for ophthalmic and parenteral administration, isotonic solutions are better tolerated by the patient than those at the extremes of hypo- and hypertonicity. With the administration of an isotonic solution, there is a homeostasis with the body's intracellular fluids. Thus, *in most instances*, preparations that are isotonic, or nearly so, are preferred. However, there are exceptions, as in instances in which hypertonic solutions are used to "draw" fluids out of edematous tissues and into the administered solution.

Most ophthalmic preparations are formulated to be isotonic, or approximately isotonic, to duplicate ophthalmic tears for the comfort of the patient. These solutions are also prepared and buffered at an appropriate pH, both to reduce the likelihood of irritation to the eye's tissues and to maintain the stability of the preparations.

Injections that are not isotonic should be administered slowly and in small quantities to minimize tissue irritation, pain, and cell fluid imbalance. The tonicity of small-volume injections is generally inconsequential when added to large-volume parenteral infusions because of the presence of tonic substances, such as sodium chloride or dextrose in the large-volume infusion, which serve to adjust the tonicity of the smaller added volume.[1]

Intravenous infusions, which are hypotonic or hypertonic, can have profound adverse effects because they generally are administered in large volumes.[1] Large volumes of *hypertonic* infusions containing dextrose, for example, can result in hyperglycemia, osmotic diuresis, and excessive loss of electrolytes. Excess infusions of *hypotonic* fluids can result in the osmotic hemolysis of red blood cells and surpass the upper limits of the body's capacity to safely absorb excessive fluids. Even isotonic fluids, when infused intravenously in excessive volumes or at excessive rates, can be deleterious due to an overload of fluids placed into the body's circulatory system.

Physical/Chemical Considerations in the Preparation of Isotonic Solutions

The calculations involved in preparing isotonic solutions may be made in terms of data relating to the colligative properties of solutions. Theoretically, any one of these properties may be used as a basis for determining tonicity. Practically and most conveniently, a comparison of freezing points is used for this purpose. It is generally accepted that −0.52°C is the freezing point of both blood serum and lacrimal fluid.

When one gram molecular weight of any nonelectrolyte, that is, a substance with negligible dissociation, such as boric acid, is dissolved in 1000 g of water, the freezing point of the solution is about 1.86°C below the freezing point of pure water. By simple proportion, therefore, we can calculate the weight of any nonelectrolyte that should be dissolved in each 1000 g of water if the solution is to be isotonic with body fluids.

Boric acid, for example, has a molecular weight of 61.8; thus (in theory), 61.8 g in 1000 g of water should produce a freezing point of −1.86°C. Therefore:

$$\frac{1.86 \ (°C)}{0.52 \ (°C)} = \frac{61.8 \ (g)}{x \ (g)}$$
$$x = 17.3 \ g$$

In short, 17.3 g of boric acid in 1000 g of water, having a weight-in-volume strength of approximately 1.73%, should make a solution isotonic with lacrimal fluid.

With electrolytes, the problem is not so simple. Because osmotic pressure depends more on the number than on the kind of particles, substances that dissociate have a tonic effect that increases with the degree of dissociation; the greater the dissociation, the smaller the quantity required to produce any given osmotic pressure. If we assume that sodium chloride in weak solutions is about 80% dissociated, then each 100 molecules yields 180 particles, or 1.8 times as many particles as are yielded by 100 molecules of a nonelectrolyte. This dissociation factor, commonly symbolized by the letter i, must be included in the proportion when we seek to determine the strength of an isotonic solution of sodium chloride (m.w. 58.5):

$$\frac{1.86 \ (°C) \times 1.8}{0.52 \ (°C)} = \frac{58.5 \ (g)}{x \ (g)}$$
$$x = 9.09 \ g$$

Hence, 9.09 g of sodium chloride in 1000 g of water should make a solution isotonic with blood or lacrimal fluid. In practice, a 0.9% w/v sodium chloride solution is considered isotonic with body fluids.

Simple isotonic solutions may then be calculated by using this formula:

$$\frac{0.52 \times \text{molecular weight}}{1.86 \times \text{dissociation } (i)} = \text{g of solute per 1000 g of water}$$

The value of *i* for many a medicinal salt has not been experimentally determined. Some salts (such as zinc sulfate, with only some 40% dissociation and an *i* value therefore of 1.4) are exceptional, but most medicinal salts approximate the dissociation of sodium chloride in weak solutions. If the number of ions is known, we may use the following values, lacking better information:

Nonelectrolytes and substances of slight dissociation: 1.0
Substances that dissociate into 2 ions: 1.8
Substances that dissociate into 3 ions: 2.6
Substances that dissociate into 4 ions: 3.4
Substances that dissociate into 5 ions: 4.2

A special problem arises when a prescription directs us to make a solution isotonic by adding the proper amount of some substance other than the active ingredient or ingredients. Given a 0.5% w/v solution of sodium chloride, we may easily calculate that 0.9 g − 0.5 g = 0.4 g of additional sodium chloride that should be contained in each 100 mL if the solution is to be made isotonic with a body fluid. But how much sodium chloride should be used in preparing 100 mL of a 1% w/v solution of atropine sulfate, which is to be made isotonic with lacrimal fluid? The answer depends on *how much sodium chloride is in effect represented by the atropine sulfate.*

The relative tonic effect of two substances—that is, the quantity of one that is the equivalent in tonic effects to a given quantity of the other—may be calculated if the quantity of one having a certain effect in a specified quantity of solvent is divided by the quantity of the other having the same effect in the same quantity of solvent. For example, we calculated that 17.3 g of boric acid per 1000 g of water and 9.09 g of sodium chloride per 1000 g of water are both instrumental in making an aqueous solution isotonic with lacrimal fluid. If, however, 17.3 g of boric acid are equivalent in tonicity to 9.09 g of sodium chloride, then 1 g of boric acid must be the equivalent of 9.09 g ÷ 17.3 g or 0.52 g of sodium chloride. Similarly, 1 g of sodium chloride must be the "tonicic equivalent" of 17.3 g ÷ 9.09 g or 1.9 g of boric acid.

We have seen that one quantity of any substance should in theory have a constant tonic effect if dissolved in 1000 g of water: 1 g molecular weight of the substance divided by its *i* or dissociation value. Hence, the relative quantity of sodium chloride that is the tonicic equivalent of a quantity of boric acid may be calculated by these ratios:

$$\frac{58.5 \div 1.8}{61.8 \div 1.0} \quad \text{or} \quad \frac{58.5 \times 1.0}{61.8 \times 1.8}$$

and we can formulate a convenient rule: *quantities of two substances that are tonicic equivalents are proportional to the molecular weights of each multiplied by the* i *value of the other.*

To return to the problem involving 1 g of atropine sulfate in 100 mL of solution:

Molecular weight of sodium chloride   = 58.5; *i* = 1.8
Molecular weight of atropine sulfate   = 695; *i* = 2.6

$$\frac{695 \times 1.8}{58.5 \times 2.6} = \frac{1 \,(g)}{x \,(g)}$$

x = 0.12 g of sodium chloride represented by
1 g of atropine sulfate

Because a solution isotonic with lacrimal fluid should contain the equivalent of 0.9 g of sodium chloride in each 100 mL of solution, the difference to be added must be 0.9 g − 0.12 g = 0.78 g of sodium chloride.

Table 11.1 gives the *sodium chloride equivalents* (E-values) of each of the substances listed. These values were calculated according to the rule stated previously. ***If the number of grams of a substance included in a prescription is multiplied by its sodium chloride equivalent, the amount of sodium chloride represented by that substance is determined.***

The procedure for the *calculation of isotonic solutions with sodium chloride equivalents* may be outlined as follows:

Step 1. Calculate the amount (in grams) of sodium chloride *represented* by each ingredient in a prescription by multiplying the amount (in grams) of each ingredient by its sodium chloride equivalent.

Step 2. Calculate the amount (in grams) of sodium chloride, alone, that would be contained in an isotonic solution of the volume specified in the prescription, namely, *the amount of sodium chloride in a 0.9% solution of the specified volume.*

Step 3. Subtract the amount of sodium chloride represented by the ingredients in the prescription (Step 1) from the amount of sodium chloride, alone, that would be represented in the specific volume of an isotonic solution (Step 2). The answer represents the amount (in grams) of sodium chloride to be added to make the solution isotonic.

Step 4. If an agent other than sodium chloride, such as boric acid, dextrose, or potassium nitrate, is to be used to make a solution isotonic, divide the amount of sodium chloride (Step 3) by the sodium chloride equivalent of the other substance.

Example Calculations of the *i* Factor

Zinc sulfate is a 2-ion electrolyte, dissociating 40% in a certain concentration. Calculate its dissociation (i) factor.
On the basis of 40% dissociation, 100 particles of zinc sulfate will yield:

$$
\begin{array}{r}
40 \text{ zinc ions} \\
40 \text{ sulfate ions} \\
\underline{60} \text{ undissociated particles} \\
\text{or } 140 \text{ particles}
\end{array}
$$

Because 140 particles represent 1.4 times as many particles as were present before dissociation, the dissociation (*i*) factor is 1.4, *answer.*

Zinc chloride is a 3-ion electrolyte, dissociating 80% in a certain concentration. Calculate its dissociation (i) factor.
On the basis of 80% dissociation, 100 particles of zinc chloride will yield:

$$
\begin{array}{r}
80 \text{ zinc ions} \\
80 \text{ chloride ions} \\
80 \text{ chloride ions} \\
\underline{20} \text{ undissociated particles} \\
\text{or } 260 \text{ particles}
\end{array}
$$

Because 260 particles represents 2.6 times as many particles as were present before dissociation, the dissociation (*i*) factor is 2.6, *answer.*

Table 11.1 ▼ SODIUM CHLORIDE EQUIVALENTS (*E*-VALUES)

SUBSTANCE	MOLECULAR WEIGHT	IONS	i	SODIUM CHLORIDE EQUIVALENT (E-VALUE)[a]
Antazoline phosphate	363	2	1.8	0.16
Antipyrine	188	1	1.0	0.17
Atropine sulfate·H_2O	695	3	2.6	0.12
Benoxinate hydrochloride	345	2	1.8	0.17
Benzalkonium chloride	360	2	1.8	0.16
Benzyl alcohol	108	1	1.0	0.30
Boric acid	61.8	1	1.0	0.52
Chloramphenicol	323	1	1.0	0.10
Chlorobutanol	177	1	1.0	0.18
Chlortetracycline hydrochloride	515	2	1.8	0.11
Cocaine hydrochloride	340	2	1.8	0.17
Cromolyn sodium	512	2	1.8	0.11
Cyclopentolate hydrochloride	328	2	1.8	0.18
Demecarium bromide	717	3	2.6	0.12
Dextrose (anhydrous)	180	1	1.0	0.18
Dextrose·H_2O	198	1	1.0	0.16
Dipivefrin hydrochloride	388	2	1.8	0.15
Ephedrine hydrochloride	202	2	1.8	0.29
Ephedrine sulfate	429	3	2.6	0.20
Epinephrine bitartrate	333	2	1.8	0.18
Epinephryl borate	209	1	1.0	0.16
Eucatropine hydrochloride	328	2	1.8	0.18
Fluorescein sodium	376	3	2.6	0.31
Glycerin	92	1	1.0	0.35
Homatropine hydrobromide	356	2	1.8	0.17
Hydroxyamphetamine hydrobromide	232	2	1.8	0.25
Idoxuridine	354	1	1.0	0.09
Lidocaine hydrochloride	289	2	1.8	0.22
Mannitol	182	1	1.0	0.18
Morphine sulfate·$5H_2O$	759	3	2.6	0.11
Naphazoline hydrochloride	247	2	1.8	0.27
Oxymetazoline hydrochloride	297	2	1.8	0.20
Oxytetracycline hydrochloride	497	2	1.8	0.12
Phenacaine hydrochloride	353	2	1.8	0.17
Phenobarbital sodium	254	2	1.8	0.24
Phenylephrine hydrochloride	204	2	1.8	0.32
Physostigmine salicylate	413	2	1.8	0.14
Physostigmine sulfate	649	3	2.6	0.13
Pilocarpine hydrochloride	245	2	1.8	0.24
Pilocarpine nitrate	271	2	1.8	0.23
Potassium biphosphate	136	2	1.8	0.43
Potassium chloride	74.5	2	1.8	0.76
Potassium iodide	166	2	1.8	0.34
Potassium nitrate	101	2	1.8	0.58
Potassium penicillin G	372	2	1.8	0.18
Procaine hydrochloride	273	2	1.8	0.21
Proparacaine hydrochloride	331	2	1.8	0.18
Scopolamine hydrobromide·$3H_2O$	438	2	1.8	0.12
Silver nitrate	170	2	1.8	0.33
Sodium bicarbonate	84	2	1.8	0.65
Sodium borate·$10H_2O$	381	5	4.2	0.42
Sodium carbonate	106	3	2.6	0.80

(continued)

Table 11.1 ▼ SODIUM CHLORIDE EQUIVALENTS (E-VALUES) (*continued*)

SUBSTANCE	MOLECULAR WEIGHT	IONS	i	SODIUM CHLORIDE EQUIVALENT (E-VALUE)[a]
Sodium carbonate·H₂O	124	3	2.6	0.68
Sodium chloride	58	2	1.8	1.00
Sodium citrate·2H₂O	294	4	3.4	0.38
Sodium iodide	150	2	1.8	0.39
Sodium lactate	112	2	1.8	0.52
Sodium phosphate, dibasic, anhydrous	142	3	2.6	0.53
Sodium phosphate, dibasic·7H₂O	268	3	2.6	0.29
Sodium phosphate, monobasic, anhydrous	120	2	1.8	0.49
Sodium phosphate, monobasic·H₂O	138	2	1.8	0.42
Tetracaine hydrochloride	301	2	1.8	0.18
Tetracycline hydrochloride	481	2	1.8	0.12
Tetrahydrozoline hydrochloride	237	2	1.8	0.25
Timolol maleate	432	2	1.8	0.14
Tobramycin	468	1	1.0	0.07
Tropicamide	284	1	1.0	0.11
Urea	60	1	1.0	0.59
Zinc chloride	136	3	2.6	0.62
Zinc sulfate·7H₂O	288	2	1.4	0.16

[a]Values rounded off to two decimal places.

Example Calculations of the Sodium Chloride Equivalent (E-values)

The sodium chloride equivalent of a substance may be calculated as follows:

$$\frac{\text{Molecular weight of sodium chloride}}{i \text{ Factor of sodium chloride}} \times \frac{i \text{ factor of the substance}}{\text{Molecular weight of the substance}} = \text{Sodium chloride equivalent}$$

Papaverine hydrochloride (m.w. 376) is a 2-ion electrolyte, dissociating 80% in a given concentration. Calculate its sodium chloride equivalent.

Because papaverine hydrochloride is a 2-ion electrolyte, dissociating 80%, its i factor is 1.8.

$$\frac{58.5}{1.8} \times \frac{1.8}{376} = 0.156, \text{ or } 0.16, \textit{answer}.$$

Calculate the sodium chloride equivalent for glycerin, a nonelectrolyte with a molecular weight of 92.[2]

Glycerin, i factor = 1.0

$$\frac{58.5}{1.8} \times \frac{1.0}{92} = 0.35, \textit{answer}.$$

Calculate the sodium chloride equivalent for timolol maleate, which dissociates into two ions and has a molecular weight of 432.[2]

Timolol maleate, i factor = 1.8

$$\frac{58.5}{1.8} \times \frac{1.8}{432} = 0.14, \textit{answer}.$$

Calculate the sodium chloride equivalent for fluorescein sodium, which dissociates into three ions and has a molecular weight of 376.[2]

Fluorescein sodium, *i* factor = 2.6

$$\frac{58.5}{1.8} \times \frac{2.6}{367} = 0.23, \ answer.$$

The agent brimonidine tartrate has a molecular weight of 442 and dissociates into two ions when in solution. It is used as a 0.1% ophthalmic solution in the treatment of glaucoma. Calculate (a) the sodium chloride equivalent of brimonidine tartrate, and (b) whether, without additional formulation agents, a 0.1% solution would be isotonic, hypotonic, or hypertonic with tears.

(a) $\frac{58.5}{1.8} \times \frac{1.8}{442} = 0.13$ sodium chloride equivalent, *answer.*

(b) Arbitrarily select a volume of solution as a basis for the calculation. The commercial product is available in 10 mL containers, so that volume would be a good choice.

For isotonicity, a 10 mL volume would require the following amount of sodium chloride or its equivalent:

10 mL × 0.9% w/v = 0.09 g sodium chloride or its equivalent

A 10-mL volume of a 0.1% w/v solution of brimonidine tartrate would contain

10 mL × 0.1% w/v = 0.01 g brimonidine tartrate

Applying the sodium chloride equivalent (0.13):

0.01 g brimonidine tartrate × 0.13 = 0.0013 g of sodium chloride equivalence

Thus, this solution would be hypotonic, *answer.*

If 1 g of epinephrine bitartrate, when dissolved in water, prepares 20 mL of an isotonic solution, calculate its sodium chloride equivalent.

20 mL of an isotonic *sodium chloride* solution would be calculated by

20 mL × 0.9% w/v = 0.18 g sodium chloride (in 20 mL of solution).

Therefore, 1 g of epinephrine bitartrate is equal in tonic effect to 0.18 g sodium chloride, and thus its sodium chloride equivalent is 0.18, *answer.*

Example Calculations of Tonicic Agent Required

How many grams of sodium chloride should be used in compounding the following prescription?

R   Pilocarpine Nitrate   0.3 g
        Sodium Chloride   q.s.
        Purified Water ad   30 mL
        Make isoton. sol.
        Sig. For the eye.

Step 1. 0.23 × 0.3 g = 0.069 g of sodium chloride represented by the pilocarpine nitrate
Step 2. 30 × 0.009 = 0.270 g of sodium chloride in 30 mL of an isotonic sodium chloride solution
Step 3. 0.270 g (from Step 2)
      − 0.069 g (from Step 1)
      0.201 g of sodium chloride to be used, *answer.*

How many grams of boric acid should be used in compounding the following prescription?

℞   Phenacaine Hydrochloride   1%
      Pilocarpine Hydrochloride   ½%
      Boric Acid   q.s.
      Purified Water ad   60
      Make isoton. sol.
      Sig. One drop in each eye.

The prescription calls for 0.6 g of phenacaine hydrochloride and 0.3 g of pilocarpine hydrochloride.

Step 1. 0.20×0.6 g = 0.120 g of sodium chloride represented by phenacaine hydrochloride
         0.24×0.3 g = 0.072 g of sodium chloride represented by pilocarpine hydrochloride
         Total: 0.192 g of sodium chloride represented by both ingredients
Step 2. 60×0.009 = 0.540 g of sodium chloride in 60 mL of an isotonic sodium chloride solution
Step 3. 0.540 g (from Step 2)
    − 0.192 g (from Step 1)
     0.348 g of sodium chloride required to make the solution isotonic

But because the prescription calls for boric acid:
Step 4. 0.348 g ÷ 0.52 (sodium chloride equivalent of boric acid) = 0.669 g of boric acid to be used, *answer.*

How many grams of potassium nitrate could be used to make the following prescription isotonic?

℞   Sol. Silver Nitrate   60
      1:500 w/v
      Make isoton. sol.
      Sig. For eye use.

The prescription contains 0.12 g of silver nitrate.

Step 1. 0.33×0.12 g = 0.04 g of sodium chloride represented by silver nitrate
Step 2. 60×0.009 = 0.54 g of sodium chloride in 60 mL of an isotonic sodium chloride solution
Step 3. 0.54 g (from Step 2)
    − 0.04 g (from Step 1)
     0.50 g of sodium chloride required to make solution isotonic

Because, in this solution, sodium chloride is incompatible with silver nitrate, the tonic agent of choice is potassium nitrate. Therefore,
Step 4. 0.50 g ÷ 0.58 (sodium chloride equivalent of potassium nitrate) = 0.86 g of potassium nitrate to be used, *answer.*

How many grams of sodium chloride should be used in compounding the following prescription?

℞   Ingredient X   0.5
      Sodium Chloride   q.s.
      Purified Water ad   50
      Make isoton. sol.
      Sig. Eye drops.

Let us assume that ingredient X is a new substance for which no sodium chloride equivalent is to be found in Table 11.1, and that its molecular weight is 295 and its *i* factor is 2.4. The sodium chloride equivalent of ingredient X may be calculated as follows:

$$\frac{58.5}{1.8} \times \frac{2.4}{295} = 0.26, \text{ the sodium chloride equivalent for ingredient X}$$

Then,

Step 1. 0.26 × 0.5 g = 0.13 g of sodium chloride represented by ingredient X

Step 2. 50 × 0.009 = 0.45 g of sodium chloride in 50 mL of an isotonic sodium chloride solution

Step 3. 0.45 g (from Step 2)
   − 0.13 g (from Step 1)
   0.32 g of sodium chloride to be used, *answer.*

Preparing Isotonic Solutions by Volume Adjustment

As a convenience in compounding, a method of preparing isotonic solutions by volume adjustment may be employed. The method, once described in the *United States Pharmacopeia— National Formulary,*[3] is based on the following:

By adding purified water to a 1-g quantity of a drug with a known E-value, a calculated volume of an isotonic solution may be prepared. Then, by diluting this volume of solution with an isotonic vehicle, the drug strength may be reduced while maintaining the solution's isotonicity.

For example, 1 g of tetracaine hydrochloride ($E = 0.18$) can prepare 20 mL of an isotonic solution, calculated as follows:

$$\frac{0.18 \text{ g [sodium chloride (equiv.)]}}{x \text{ mL (isotonic solution)}} = \frac{0.9 \text{ g (sodium chloride)}}{100 \text{ mL (isotonic solution)}}; x = 20 \text{ mL}.$$

This isotonic solution would contain 5% w/v tetracaine hydrochloride (1 g/20 mL). If a solution of lesser strength is desired, a calculated quantity of an isotonic vehicle, such as 0.9% sodium chloride, may be added. For example, if a 1% w/v solution of tetracaine hydrochloride is desired, a total volume of 100 mL (1 g tetracaine hydrochloride/100 mL) may be prepared by adding 80 mL of isotonic vehicle to the 20 mL of the 5% w/v solution.

If pilocarpine hydrochloride has a sodium chloride equivalent of 0.24 (a) how many milliliters of isotonic solution may be prepared from 1 g of the drug, and (b) how many milliliters of 0.9% w/v sodium chloride solution may be added to the resultant solution to prepare an isotonic solution having a 1.5% w/v concentration of pilocarpine hydrochloride?

(a) $\dfrac{0.24 \text{ g [sodium chloride (equiv.)]}}{x \text{ mL (isotonic solution)}} = \dfrac{0.9 \text{ g (sodium chloride)}}{100 \text{ mL (isotonic solution)}}; x = 26.7 \text{ mL}$

(b) Although there are a number of ways to solve this problem, use of the equation in Chapter 15 is perhaps the most convenient method:

1st quantity (Q1) × 1st concentration (C1) = 2nd quantity (Q2) × 2nd concentration (C2)

First, one must calculate the concentration of pilocarpine hydrochloride in 26.7 mL of solution:

$$\frac{1 \text{ g}}{26.7 \text{ mL}} \times 100\% = 3.75\% \text{ w/v}$$

Table 11.2 ▼ **EXAMPLES OF ISOTONIC SOLUTIONS THAT MAY BE PREPARED FROM 1 GRAM QUANTITIES OF DRUGS**[a]

DRUG, 1 g	VOLUME OF ISOTONIC SOLUTION, mL
Boric acid	57.8
Ephedrine sulfate	22.2
Phenylephrine hydrochloride	35.6
Pilocarpine hydrochloride	26.7
Tetracaine hydrochloride	20.0
Zinc sulfate·7H$_2$O	17.8

[a]Calculated from the E-values in Table 11.1.

Then, applying the above equation:

$$26.7 \text{ mL (Q1)} \times 3.75\% \text{ (C1)} = x \text{ mL (Q2)} \times 1.5\% \text{ (C2)}$$

$$x = \frac{26.7 \text{ mL} \times 3.75\%}{1.5\%} = 66.75 \text{ mL}$$

Thus, 66.75 mL of solution may be prepared, and 40.05 mL (66.75 mL − 26.7 mL) of 0.9% sodium chloride solution should be added, *answer.*

Proof that the concentration of pilocarpine hydrochloride is 1.5%:

$$\frac{1 \text{ g pilocarpine hydrochloride}}{66.75 \text{ mL}} \times 100\% = 1.498 \text{ or } 1.5\% \text{ w/v pilocarpine hydrochloride}$$

Other examples of calculated volumes of isotonic solutions that may be prepared from 1 g of drug are given in Table 11.2 and available from other references.[3,4]

Determine the volume of purified water and 0.9% w/v sodium chloride solution needed to prepare 20 mL of a 1% w/v solution of hydromorphone hydrochloride (E = 0.22).

Step 1. 20 mL × 1% w/v = 0.2 g hydromorphone hydrochloride needed
Step 2. 0.2 g (hydromorphone hydrochloride) × 0.22 (E-value) = 0.044 g (sodium chloride equivalence)

$$\frac{0.044}{x \text{ mL}} = \frac{0.9 \text{ g NaCl}}{100 \text{ mL}}; x = 4.89 \text{ mL of an isotonic solution of hydromorphone hydrochloride}$$

may be prepared by the addition of a sufficient quantity (*qs*) of purified water, *answer.*

Step 3. 20 mL − 4.89 mL = 15.11 mL 0.9% w/v sodium chloride solution required, *answer.*

Proof: 20 mL × 0.9% = 0.18 g sodium chloride or equivalent required
          0.2 × 0.22 = 0.044 g (sodium chloride represented by 0.2 g hydromorphone hydrochloride)
   15.11 mL × 0.9% = 0.136 g sodium chloride present
   0.044 g + 0.136 g = 0.18 g sodium chloride required for isotonicity

Use of Freezing Point Data in Isotonicity Calculations

Freezing point data (ΔT_f) can be used in isotonicity calculations when the agent has a tonicic effect and does not penetrate the biologic membranes in question (e.g., red blood cells). As

Table 11.3 ▼ FREEZING POINT DATA FOR SELECT AGENTS

AGENT	FREEZING POINT DEPRESSION, 1% SOLUTIONS ($\Delta T_f^{1\%}$)
Atropine sulfate	0.07
Boric acid	0.29
Butacaine sulfate	0.12
Chloramphenicol	0.06
Chlorobutanol	0.14
Dextrose	0.09
Dibucaine hydrochloride	0.08
Ephedrine sulfate	0.13
Epinephrine bitartrate	0.10
Ethylmorphine hydrochloride	0.09
Glycerin	0.20
Homatropine hydrobromide	0.11
Lidocaine hydrochloride	0.063
Lincomycin	0.09
Morphine sulfate	0.08
Naphazoline hydrochloride	0.16
Physostigmine salicylate	0.09
Pilocarpine nitrate	0.14
Sodium bisulfite	0.36
Sodium chloride	0.58
Sulfacetamide sodium	0.14
Zinc sulfate	0.09

stated previously, the freezing point of both blood and lacrimal fluid is −0.52°C. Thus, a pharmaceutical solution that has a freezing point of −0.52°C is considered isotonic.

Representative data on freezing point depression by medicinal and pharmaceutical substances are presented in Table 11.3. Although these data are for solution strengths of 1% ($\Delta T_f^{1\%}$), data for other solution strengths and for many additional agents may be found in physical pharmacy textbooks and in the literature.

Freezing point depression data may be used in isotonicity calculations as shown by the following.

Example Calculations Using Freezing Point Data

How many milligrams each of sodium chloride and dibucaine hydrochloride are required to prepare 30 mL of a 1% solution of dibucaine hydrochloride isotonic with tears?

To make this solution isotonic, the freezing point must be lowered to −0.52. From Table 11.3, it is determined that a 1% solution of dibucaine hydrochloride has a freezing point lowering of 0.08°. Thus, sufficient sodium chloride must be added to lower the freezing point an additional 0.44° (0.52° − 0.08°).

Also from Table 11.3, it is determined that a 1% solution of sodium chloride lowers the freezing point by 0.58°. By proportion:

$$\frac{1\% \text{ (NaCl)}}{x\% \text{ (NaCl)}} = \frac{0.58°}{0.44°}$$

$$x = 0.76\% \text{ (the concentration of sodium chloride}$$
$$\text{needed to lower the freezing point by 0.44°,}$$
$$\text{required to make the solution isotonic)}$$

CALCULATIONS CAPSULE

Isotonicity

To calculate the "equivalent tonic effect" to sodium chloride represented by an ingredient in a preparation, multiply its weight by its *E*-value:

$$g \times E\text{-}value = g, \text{ equivalent tonic effect to sodium chloride}$$

To make a solution isotonic, calculate and ensure the quantity of sodium chloride and/or the equivalent tonic effect of all other ingredients to total 0.9% w/v in the preparation:

$$\frac{g \ (NaCl) + g \ (NaCl \ tonic \ equivalents)}{mL \ (preparation)} \times 100 = 0.9\% \ w/v$$

To make an isotonic solution from a drug substance, add sufficient water by the equation:

$$\frac{g \ (drug \ substance) \times E\text{-}value \ (drug \ substance)}{0.009} = mL \ water$$

This solution may then be made to any volume with isotonic sodium chloride solution to maintain its isotonicity.

The *E*-value can be derived from the same equation, given the grams of drug substance and the milliliters of water required to make an isotonic solution.

Thus, to make 30 mL of solution,

30 mL × 1% = 0.3 g = 300 mg dibucaine hydrochloride, and
30 mL × 0.76% = 0.228 g = 228 mg sodium chloride, *answers*.

Note: Should a prescription call for more than one medicinal and/or pharmaceutic ingredient, the sum of the freezing points is subtracted from the required value in determining the additional lowering required by the agent used to provide isotonicity.

CASE IN POINT 11.1[5] A local ophthalmologist is treating one of his patients for a post-LASIK eye infection that is not responding to topical ciprofloxacin. These infections, although rare, can occur after laser in situ keratomileusis (LASIK) surgery for vision correction.

Topical amikacin sulfate has been shown to be effective for the treatment of eye infections due to ciprofloxacin-resistant *Pseudomonas*,[6,7] *Burkholderia ambifaria*,[8] Mycobacterium chelonae, and *Mycobacterium fortuitum*.[9–11]

The ophthalmologist prescribes 60 mL of a 2.5% amikacin sulfate isotonic solution, 2 drops in the affected eye every 2 hours.
Amikacin sulfate USP ($C_{22}H_{43}N_5O_{13} \cdot 2H_2SO_2$), m.w., 781.76, is an aminoglycoside-type antibiotic containing 3 ions.

(a) Determine the weight in grams of amikacin sulfate needed to prepare the solution.
(b) Calculate the sodium chloride equivalent (*E*-value) for amikacin sulfate.
(c) Calculate the amount of sodium chloride needed to make the prepared solution isotonic.
(d) How many milliliters of 23.5% sodium chloride injection should be used to obtain the needed sodium chloride?

Buffers and Buffer Solutions

When a minute trace of hydrochloric acid is added to pure water, a significant increase in *hydrogen-ion* concentration occurs immediately. In a similar manner, when a minute trace of sodium hydroxide is added to pure water, it causes a correspondingly large increase in the *hydroxyl-ion* concentration. These changes take place because water alone cannot neutralize even traces of acid or base, that is, it has no ability to resist changes in hydrogen-ion concentration or pH. A solution of a neutral salt, such as sodium chloride, also lacks this ability. Therefore, it is said to be *unbuffered*.

The presence of certain substances or combinations of substances in aqueous solution imparts to the system the ability to maintain a desired pH at a relatively constant level, even with the addition of materials that may be expected to change the hydrogen–ion concentration. These substances or combinations of substances are called *buffers*; their ability to resist changes in pH is referred to as *buffer action*; their efficiency is measured by the function known as *buffer capacity*; and solutions of them are called *buffer solutions*. By definition, then, a *buffer solution* is a system, usually an aqueous solution, that possesses the property of resisting changes in pH with the addition of small amounts of a strong acid or base.

Buffers are used to establish and maintain an ion activity within rather narrow limits. In pharmacy, the most common buffer systems are used in (i) the preparation of such dosage forms as injections and ophthalmic solutions, which are placed directly into pH-sensitive body fluids; (ii) the manufacture of formulations in which the pH must be maintained at a relatively constant level to ensure maximum product stability; and (iii) pharmaceutical tests and assays requiring adjustment to or maintenance of a specific pH for analytic purposes.

A buffer solution is usually composed of a weak acid and a salt of the acid, such as acetic acid and sodium acetate, or a weak base and a salt of the base, such as ammonium hydroxide and ammonium chloride. Typical buffer systems that may be used in pharmaceutical formulations include the following pairs: acetic acid and sodium acetate, boric acid and sodium borate, and disodium phosphate and sodium acid phosphate. Formulas for standard buffer solutions for pharmaceutical analysis are given in the *United States Pharmacopeia*.[12]

In the selection of a buffer system, due consideration must be given to the dissociation constant of the weak acid or base to ensure maximum buffer capacity. This dissociation constant, in the case of an acid, is a measure of the strength of the acid; the more readily the acid dissociates, the higher its dissociation constant and the stronger the acid. Selected dissociation constants, or K_a values, are given in Table 11.4.

Table 11.4 ▼ DISSOCIATION CONSTANTS OF SOME WEAK ACIDS AT 25°C

ACID	K_a
Acetic	1.75×10^{-5}
Barbituric	1.05×10^{-4}
Benzoic	6.30×10^{-5}
Boric	6.4×10^{-10}
Formic	1.76×10^{-4}
Lactic	1.38×10^{-4}
Mandelic	4.29×10^{-4}
Salicylic	1.06×10^{-3}

The dissociation constant, or K_a value, of a weak acid is given by the equation:

$$K_a = \frac{(H^+)(A^-)}{(HA)} \qquad \text{where } A^- = \text{salt} \\ HA = \text{acid}$$

Because the numeric values of most dissociation constants are small numbers and may vary over many powers of 10, it is more convenient to express them as negative logarithms:

$$pK_a = -\log K_a$$

When equation $K_a = \frac{(H^+)(A^-)}{(HA)}$ is expressed in logarithmic form, it is written:

$$pK_a = -\log (H^+) - \log \frac{\text{salt}}{\text{acid}}$$

and because $pH = -\log (H^+)$:

then

$$pK_a = pH - \log \frac{\text{salt}}{\text{acid}}$$

and

$$pH = pK_a + \log \frac{\text{salt}}{\text{acid}}$$

Buffer Equation

The equation just derived is the Henderson-Hasselbalch equation for weak acids, commonly known as the *buffer equation*.

Similarly, the dissociation constant, or K_b value, of a weak base is given by the equation:

$$K_b = \frac{(B^+)(OH^-)}{(BOH)} \qquad \text{in which } B^+ = \text{salt} \\ \text{and } BOH = \text{base}$$

and the buffer equation for weak bases, which is derived from this relationship, may be expressed as:

$$pH = pK_w - pK_b + \log \frac{\text{base}}{\text{salt}}$$

The buffer equation is useful for calculating (1) the pH of a buffer system if its composition is known and (2) the molar ratio of the components of a buffer system required to give a solution of a desired pH. The equation can also be used to calculate the change in pH of a buffered solution with the addition of a given amount of acid or base.

pK_a Value of a Weak Acid with Known Dissociation Constant

Calculating the pK_a value of a weak acid, given its dissociation constant, K_a:

The dissociation constant of acetic acid is 1.75×10^{-5} at 25°C. Calculate its pK_a value.

$$K_a = 1.75 \times 10^{-5}$$

and
$$\log K_a = \log 1.75 + \log 10^{-5}$$
$$= 0.2430 - 5 = -4.757 \text{ or } -4.76$$

Because
$$pK_a = -\log K_a$$
$$pK_a = -(-4.76) = 4.76, \textit{answer.}$$

pH Value of a Salt/Acid Buffer System

Calculating the pH value:

What is the pH of a buffer solution prepared with 0.05 M sodium borate and 0.005 M boric acid? The pK_a value of boric acid is 9.24 at 25°C.

Note that the ratio of the components of the buffer solution is given in molar concentrations.

Using the buffer equation for weak acids:

$$pH = pK_a + \log\frac{salt}{acid}$$

$$= 9.24 + \log\frac{0.05}{0.005}$$

$$= 9.24 + \log 10$$

$$= 9.24 + 1$$

$$= 10.24, \ answer.$$

pH Value of a Base/Salt Buffer System

Calculating the pH value:

What is the pH of a buffer solution prepared with 0.05 M ammonia and 0.05 M ammonium chloride? The K_b value of ammonia is 1.80×10^{-5} at 25°C.

Using the buffer equation for weak bases:

$$pH = pK_w - pK_b + \log\frac{base}{salt}$$

Because the K_w value for water is 10^{-14} at 25°C, $pK_w = 14$.

$$K_b = 1.80 \times 10^{-5}$$

and
$$\log K_b = \log 1.8 + \log 10^{-5}$$
$$= 0.2553 - 5 = -4.7447 \ or \ -4.74$$
$$pK_b = -\log K_b$$
$$= -(-4.74) = 4.74$$

and
$$pH = 14 - 4.74 + \log\frac{0.05}{0.05}$$

$$= 9.26 + \log 1$$

$$= 9.26, \ answer.$$

Molar Ratio of Salt/Acid for a Buffer System of Desired pH

Calculating the molar ratio of salt/acid required to prepare a buffer system with a desired pH value:

What molar ratio of salt/acid is required to prepare a sodium acetate-acetic acid buffer solution with a pH of 5.76? The pK_a value of acetic acid is 4.76 at 25°C.

Using the buffer equation:

$$pH = pK_a + \log\frac{salt}{acid}$$

$$\log \frac{\text{salt}}{\text{acid}} = \text{pH} - \text{pK}_a$$

$$= 5.76 - 4.76 = 1$$
antilog of $1 = 10$
ratio $\quad = 10/1$ or $10{:}1$, *answer*.

Quantity of Components in a Buffer Solution to Yield a Specific Volume

Calculating the amounts of the components of a buffer solution required to prepare a desired volume, given the molar ratio of the components and the total buffer concentration:

The molar ratio of sodium acetate to acetic acid in a buffer solution with a pH of 5.76 is 10:1. Assuming the total buffer concentration is 2.2×10^{-2} mol/L, how many grams of sodium acetate (m.w. 82) and how many grams of acetic acid (m.w. 60) should be used in preparing a liter of the solution?

Because the molar ratio of sodium acetate to acetic acid is 10:1,

$$\text{the mole fraction of sodium acetate} = \frac{10}{1+10} \text{ or } \frac{10}{11}$$

$$\text{and the mole fraction of acetic acid} = \frac{1}{1+10} \text{ or } \frac{1}{11}$$

If the total buffer concentration $= 2.2 \times 10^{-2}$ mol/L,

$$\text{the concentration of sodium acetate} = \frac{10}{11} \times (2.2 \times 10^{-2})$$

$$= 2.0 \times 10^{-2} \text{ mol/L}$$

$$\text{and the concentration of acetic acid} = \frac{1}{11} \times (2.2 \times 10^{-2})$$

$$= 0.2 \times 10^{-2} \text{ mol/L}$$

then 2.0×10^{-2} or $0.02 \times 82 = 1.64$ g of sodium acetate per liter of solution, *and* 0.2×10^{-2} or $0.002 \times 60 = 0.120$ g of acetic acid per liter of solution, *answers*.

The efficiency of buffer solutions—that is, their specific ability to resist changes in pH—is measured in terms of *buffer capacity*; the *smaller* the pH change with the addition of a given amount of acid or base, the *greater* the buffer capacity of the system. Among other factors, the buffer capacity of a system depends on (1) the relative concentration of the buffer components and (2) the ratio of the components. For example, a 0.5 M-acetate buffer at a pH of 4.76 would have a higher buffer capacity than a 0.05 M-buffer.

If a strong base such as sodium hydroxide is added to a buffer system consisting of equimolar concentrations of sodium acetate and acetic acid, the base is neutralized by the acetic acid forming more sodium acetate, and the resulting *increase* in pH is slight. Actually, the addition of the base increases the concentration of sodium acetate and decreases *by an equal amount* the concentration of acetic acid. In a similar manner, the addition of a strong acid to a buffer system consisting of a weak base and its salt would produce only a small *decrease* in pH.

Change in pH with Addition of an Acid or Base

Calculating the change in pH of a buffer solution with the addition of a given amount of acid or base:

Calculate the change in pH after adding 0.04 mol of sodium hydroxide to a liter of a buffer solution containing 0.2 M concentrations of sodium acetate and acetic acid. The pK$_a$ value of acetic acid is 4.76 at 25°C.

The pH of the buffer solution is calculated by using the buffer equation as follows:

$$pH = pK_a + \log\frac{salt}{acid}$$
$$= 4.76 + \log\frac{0.2}{0.2}$$
$$= 4.76 + \log 1$$
$$= 4.76$$

The addition of 0.04 mol of sodium hydroxide converts 0.04 mol of acetic acid to 0.04 mol of sodium acetate. Consequently, the concentration of acetic acid is *decreased* and the concentration of sodium acetate is *increased* by equal amounts, according to the following equation:

$$pH = pK_a + \log\frac{salt + base}{acid - base}$$
$$\text{and}\quad pH = pK_a + \log\frac{0.2 + 0.04}{0.2 - 0.04}$$
$$= pK_a + \log\frac{0.24}{0.16}$$
$$= 4.76 + 0.1761 = 4.9361 \text{ or } 4.94$$

Because the pH before the addition of the sodium hydroxide was 4.76, the change in pH = 4.94 − 4.76 = 0.18 unit, *answer.*

PRACTICE PROBLEMS

Calculations of Tonicity

1. Isotonic sodium chloride solution contains 0.9% w/v sodium chloride. If the *E*-value of boric acid is 0.52, calculate the percentage strength (w/v) of an isotonic solution of boric acid.

2. Sodium chloride is a 2-ion electrolyte, dissociating 90% in a certain concentration. Calculate (a) its dissociation factor, and (b) the freezing point of a molal solution.

3. A solution of anhydrous dextrose (m.w. 180) contains 25 g in 500 mL of water. Calculate the freezing point of the solution.

4. Procaine hydrochloride (m.w. 273) is a 2-ion electrolyte, dissociating 80% in a certain concentration.
   (a) Calculate its dissociation factor.
   (b) Calculate its sodium chloride equivalent.
   (c) Calculate the freezing point of a molal solution of procaine hydrochloride.

5. The freezing point of a molal solution of a nonelectrolyte is −1.86°C. What is the freezing point of a 0.1% solution of zinc chloride (m.w. 136), dissociating 80%? (For lack of more definite information, assume that the volume of the molal solution is approximately 1 liter.)

6. The freezing point of a 5% solution of boric acid is −1.55°C. How many grams of boric acid should be used in preparing 1000 mL of an isotonic solution?

7. ℞ Ephedrine Sulfate   0.3 g
       Sodium Chloride   q.s.
       Purified Water ad   30 mL
       Make isoton. sol.
       Sig. Use as directed.

   How many milligrams of sodium chloride should be used in compounding the prescription?

8. ℞ Dipivefrin Hydrochloride ½%
       Scopolamine
          Hydrobromide   ⅓%
       Sodium Chloride   q.s.
       Purified Water ad   30
       Make isoton. sol.
       Sig. Use in the eye.

   How many grams of sodium chloride should be used in compounding the prescription?

9. ℞ Zinc Sulfate   0.06
       Boric Acid   q.s.
       Purified Water ad   30
       Make isoton. sol.
       Sig. Drop in eyes.

   How many grams of boric acid should be used in compounding the prescription?

10. ℞ Cromolyn Sodium   4% (w/v)
        Benzalkonium   1:10,000
           Chloride   (w/v)
        Buffer Solution (pH 5.6) q.s.
        Water for Injection ad 10 mL
        Sig. One (1) drop in each eye b.i.d.

    How many milliliters of the buffer solution ($E = 0.30$) should be used to render the solution isotonic?

11. Dextrose, anhydrous 2.5%
    Sodium Chloride q.s.
    Sterile Water for Injection ad 1000 mL
    Label: Isotonic Dextrose and Saline Solution.

    How many grams of sodium chloride should be used in preparing the solution?

12. A sterile ophthalmic preparation contains 0.6% besifloxacin ($E = 0.08$) in each 5-mL. Calculate the quantity of sodium chloride required for isotonicity.

13. Calculate the *effective quantity (g) of sodium chloride* in 100 mL of an intravenous fluid labeled "5% dextrose in 0.45% sodium chloride," and indicate whether the solution is isotonic, hypotonic, or hypertonic.

14. ℞ Cocaine Hydrochloride   0.6
        Eucatropine
           Hydrochloride   0.6
        Chlorobutanol   0.1
        Sodium Chloride   q.s.
        Purified Water ad   30
        Make isoton. sol.
        Sig. For the eye.

    How many grams of sodium chloride should be used in compounding the prescription?

15. ℞ Tetracaine Hydrochloride 0.1
        Zinc Sulfate   0.05
        Boric Acid   q.s.
        Purified Water ad   30
        Make isoton. sol.
        Sig. Drop in eye.

    How many grams of boric acid should be used in compounding the prescription?

16. ℞ Sol. Homatropine
           Hydrobromide 1%   15
        Make isoton. sol. with
           boric acid.
        Sig. For the eye.

    How many grams of boric acid should be used in compounding the prescription?

17. ℞ Procaine Hydrochloride   1%
       Sodium Chloride   q.s.
       Sterile Water for
           Injection ad   100
       Make isoton. sol.
       Sig. For injection.

    How many grams of sodium chloride should be used in compounding the prescription?

18. ℞ Phenylephrine
           Hydrochloride   1%
       Chlorobutanol   0.5%
       Sodium Chloride   q.s.
       Purified Water ad   15
       Make isoton. sol.
       Sig. Use as directed.

    How many milliliters of an 0.9% solution of sodium chloride should be used in compounding the prescription?

19. ℞ Oxymetazoline Hydrochloride ½%
       Boric Acid Solution   q.s.
       Purified Water ad   15
       Make isoton. sol.
       Sig. For the nose, as decongestant.

    How many milliliters of a 5% solution of boric acid should be used in compounding the prescription?

20. ℞ Ephedrine Hydrochloride   0.5
       Chlorobutanol   0.25
       Dextrose, monohydrate   q.s.
       Rose Water ad   50
       Make isoton. sol.
       Sig. Nose drops.

    How many grams of dextrose monohydrate should be used in compounding the prescription?

21. ℞ Naphazoline
           Hydrochloride   1%
       Sodium Chloride   q.s.
       Purified Water ad   30 mL
       Make isoton. sol.
       Sig. Use as directed in the eye.

    How many grams of sodium chloride should be used in compounding the prescription? Use the freezing point depression method.

22. ℞ Oxytetracycline
           Hydrochloride   0.05
       Chlorobutanol   0.1
       Sodium Chloride   q.s.
       Purified Water ad   30
       Make isoton. sol.
       Sig. Eye drops.

    How many milligrams of sodium chloride should be used in compounding the prescription?

23. How many milligrams of sodium chloride may be used in the preparation of 15 mL of an eye drop containing 1% phenacaine hydrochloride and 0.5% chlorobutanol to render the solution isotonic with tears?

    (a) 25.5 mg
    (b) 135 mg
    (c) 13.5 mg
    (d) 96 mg

24. Monobasic Sodium
        Phosphate, anhydrous   5.6 g
    Dibasic Sodium
        Phosphate, anhydrous   2.84 g
    Sodium Chloride   q.s.
    Purified Water ad   1000 mL
    Label: Isotonic Buffer
        Solution, pH 6.5.

    How many grams of sodium chloride should be used in preparing the solution?

25. How many grams of anhydrous dextrose should be used in preparing 1 liter of a ½% isotonic ephedrine sulfate nasal spray?

26. ℞   Ephedrine Sulfate   1%
         Chlorobutanol   ½%
         Purified Water ad   100
         Make isoton. sol. and
             buffer to pH   6.5
         Sig. Nose drops.

    You have on hand an isotonic buffered solution, pH 6.5. How many milliliters of purified water and how many milliliters of the buffered solution should be used in compounding the prescription?

27. ℞   Oxytetracycline
        Hydrochloride   0.5%
        Tetracaine Hydro-
        chloride Sol. 2%   15 mL
        Sodium Chloride   q.s.
        Purified Water ad   30 mL
        Make isoton. sol.
        Sig. For the eye.

   The 2% solution of tetracaine hydrochloride is already isotonic. How many milliliters of an 0.9% solution of sodium chloride should be used in compounding the prescription?

28. Determine if the following commercial products are hypotonic, isotonic, or hypertonic:

   (a) An ophthalmic solution containing 40 mg/mL of cromolyn sodium and 0.01% of benzalkonium chloride in purified water.
   (b) A parenteral infusion containing 20% (w/v) of mannitol.
   (c) A 500-mL large volume parenteral containing D5W (5% w/v of anhydrous dextrose in sterile water for injection).

29. For agents having the following sodium chloride equivalents, calculate the percentage concentration of an isotonic solution:

   (a) 0.20
   (b) 0.32
   (c) 0.61

30. How many milliliters each of purified water and an isotonic sodium chloride solution should be used to prepare 30 mL of a 1% w/v isotonic solution of fentanyl citrate ($E = 0.11$)?

31. Using the E-values in Table 11.1, calculate the number of milliliters of water required to make an isotonic solution from 0.3 g of each of the following:

   (a) antipyrine
   (b) chlorobutanol
   (c) ephedrine sulfate
   (d) silver nitrate
   (e) zinc sulfate

32. Calculate the E-values for each of the following, given that the number of milliliters of water shown will produce an isotonic solution from 0.3 g of drug substance.

   (a) apomorphine hydrochloride, 4.7 mL water
   (b) ethylmorphine hydrochloride, 5.3 mL water
   (c) holocaine hydrochloride, 6.7 mL water
   (d) procainamide hydrochloride, 7.3 mL water
   (e) viomycin sulfate, 2.7 mL water

Calculations of Buffer Solutions

33. The dissociation constant of ethanolamine is 2.77×10^{-5} at 25°C. Calculate its pK_b value.

34. What is the pH of a buffer solution prepared with 0.055 M sodium acetate and 0.01 M acetic acid? The pK_a value of acetic acid is 4.76 at 25°C.

35. What molar ratio of salt to acid would be required to prepare a buffer solution with a pH of 4.5? The pK_a value of the acid is 4.05 at 25°C.

36. What is the change in pH on adding 0.02 mol of sodium hydroxide to a liter of a buffer solution containing 0.5 M of sodium acetate and 0.5 M acetic acid? The pK_a value of acetic acid is 4.76 at 25°C.

37. The molar ratio of salt to acid needed to prepare a sodium acetate-acetic acid buffer solution is 1:1. Assuming that the total buffer concentration is 0.1 mol/L, how many grams of sodium acetate (m.w. 60) should be used in preparing 2 liters of the solution?

38. What is the change in pH with the addition of 0.01 mol hydrochloric acid to a liter of a buffer solution containing 0.05 M of ammonia and 0.05 M of ammonium chloride? The K_b value of ammonia is 1.80×10^{-5} at 25°C.

CALCQUIZ

11.A. A 3-mL container of a 0.5% ophthalmic solution of moxifloxacin hydrochloride (m.w. 401; $i = 1.8$) is prepared in an aqueous solution of 0.45% sodium chloride. Calculate the quantity, in milligrams, of boric acid required to render the solution isotonic.

11.B. How many grams of boric acid should be used to render this prescription isotonic?

Rx:	Tetracaine Hydrochloride	0.5%
	0.1% Epinephrine Bitartrate in NSS	10 mL
	Boric Acid, qs	
	Purified Water, ad	30 mL

11.C. A formulation pharmacist has developed an injection for dental local anesthesia that contains the following agents:

Lidocaine Hydrochloride	1%
Epinephrine Bitartrate	1:50,000
Sodium Chloride	6.5 mg/mL
Potassium Metabisulfite	1.2 mg/mL
Edetate Disodium	0.25 mg/mL
Sterile Purified Water, ad	1.7 mL

Using the following data, determine the *total tonic effect,* expressed in terms of percent strength of "sodium chloride" or its equivalent.

Lidocaine Hydrochloride ($E = 0.22$)
Epinephrine Bitartrate ($E = 0.18$)
Potassium Metabisulfite (m.w. 222; $i - 2.6$)
Edetate Disodium (m.w. 372; $i = 2.6$)

11.D. A FLEET saline enema delivers in each 118 mL, 19 g monobasic sodium phosphate (monohydrate) and 7 g dibasic sodium phosphate (heptahydrate). Calculate the product's percent strength in terms of "sodium chloride or its equivalent," and indicate whether the enema is hypotonic, isotonic, or hypertonic.

11.E. What would be the pH of a buffer solution prepared with 0.5-M disodium phosphate and 1-M sodium acid phosphate? The pK_a of sodium acid phosphate is 7.21 at 25°C.

ANSWERS TO "CASE IN POINT" AND PRACTICE PROBLEMS

Case in Point 11.1

(a) 60 mL × 2.5% w/v = 1.5 g amikacin sulfate, *answer.*

(b) sodium chloride m.w. = 58.5
amikacin m.w. = 781.76

$i = 2.6$

$$\frac{58.5}{1.8} \times \frac{2.6}{781.76} = E$$

$E = 0.108$, *answer.*

(c) 60 mL × 0.9% w/v = 0.54 g sodium chloride, *answer.*

(d) 1.5 g (amikacin sulfate) × 0.108 (NaCl equivalent) = 0.162 g
0.54 g − 0.162 g = 0.378 g sodium chloride required for isotonicity

$$\frac{23.5 \text{ g}}{100 \text{ mL}} = \frac{0.378 \text{ g}}{x \text{ mL}};$$

x = 1.61 mL sodium chloride injection, *answer.*

Practice Problems

1. 1.73% w/v

2. (a) 1.9
   (b) −3.53°C

3. −0.52°C

4. (a) 1.8
   (b) 0.21
   (c) −3.35°C

5. −0.036°C

6. 16.8 g

7. 210 mg sodium chloride

8. 0.236 g sodium chloride

9. 0.501 g boric acid

10. 0.153 mL buffer solution

11. 4.5 g sodium chloride

12. 42.6 mg sodium chloride

13. 1.35 g sodium chloride, hypertonic

14. 0.042 g sodium chloride

15. 0.469 g boric acid

16. 0.211 g boric acid

17. 0.69 g sodium chloride

18. 8.17 mL sodium chloride solution

19. 4.62 mL boric acid solution

20. 1.625 g dextrose monohydrate

21. 0.189 g sodium chloride

22. 236 mg sodium chloride

23. (d) 96 g sodium chloride

24. 4.751 g sodium chloride

25. 43.61 g anhydrous dextrose

26. 32.22 mL purified water
    67.78 mL buffered solution

27. 13 mL sodium chloride solution

28. (a) hypotonic
    (b) hypertonic
    (c) isotonic

29. (a) 4.5%
    (b) 2.81%
    (c) 1.48%

30. 3.67 mL purified water
    26.33 mL sodium chloride solution

31. (a) 5.7 mL water
    (b) 6 mL water
    (c) 6.67 mL water
    (d) 11 mL water
    (e) 5.33 mL water

32. (a) 0.14
    (b) 0.16
    (c) 0.20
    (d) 0.22
    (e) 0.08

33. 4.56

34. 5.5

35. 2.82:1

36. 0.03 unit

37. 8.2 g
    6 g

38. 0.18 unit

References

1. Reich I, Poon CY, Sugita ET. Tonicity, osmoticity, osmolality, and osmolarity. In: Gennaro AR, ed. *Remington: The Science and Practice of Pharmacy*. 20th Ed. Baltimore, MD: Lippincott Williams & Wilkins, 2000:246–250.
2. Ansel HC, Prince SJ. Pharmaceutical calculations. In: *The Pharmacist's Handbook*. Baltimore, MD: Lippincott Williams & Wilkins, 2004:111.
3. *United States Pharmacopeia 21 National Formulary 16*. Rockville, MD: United States Pharmacopeial Convention, 1985:1339.
4. Allen LV, Popovich NG, Ansel HC. *Ansel's Pharmaceutical Dosage Forms and Drug Delivery Systems*. Baltimore, MD: Lippincott Williams & Wilkins, 2005;8:546.
5. Beach W. Athens, GA: College of Pharmacy, University of Georgia, 2004.
6. Titcomb LC. *Pharmaceutical Journal* 2000;264:441–445.
7. Garg P, et al. *Ophthalmology* 1999;106:1319–1323.
8. Matoba AY. *American Journal of Ophthalmology* 2003;136:748–749.
9. Chung MS, et al. *American Journal of Ophthalmology* 2000;129:382–384.
10. Chandra NS, et al. *American Journal of Ophthalmology* 2001;132:819–830.
11. Ford JG, et al. *Ophthalmology* 1998;105:1652–1658.
12. United States Pharmacopeia 32. National Formulary 27. Rockville, MD: United States Pharmacopeial Convention, 2009;1:862.

Electrolyte Solutions: Milliequivalents, Millimoles, and Milliosmoles

12

Objectives

Upon successful completion of this chapter, the student will be able to:

- Calculate the milliequivalent weight from an atomic or formula weight.
- Calculate problems involving milliequivalents.
- Calculate problems involving millimoles and milliosmoles.

As noted in Chapter 11, the molecules of chemical compounds in solution may remain intact, or they may dissociate into particles known as *ions*, which carry an electric charge. Substances that are not dissociated in solution are called *nonelectrolytes*, and those with varying degrees of dissociation are called *electrolytes*. Urea and dextrose are examples of nonelectrolytes in body water; sodium chloride in body fluids is an example of an electrolyte.

Electrolyte ions in the blood plasma include the cations Na^+, K^+, Ca^{++}, and Mg^{++} and the anions Cl^-, HCO_3^-, HPO_4^{--}, SO_4^{--}, organic acids$^-$, and protein$^-$. Electrolytes in body fluids play an important role in maintaining the acid-base balance in the body. They play a part in controlling body water volumes and help to regulate metabolism.

Applicable Dosage Forms

Electrolyte preparations are used in the treatment of disturbances of the electrolyte and fluid balance in the body. They are provided by the pharmacy as oral solutions, syrups, tablets, capsules, and when necessary, as intravenous infusions.

Milliequivalents

A *chemical unit*, the ***milliequivalent (mEq)***, is used almost exclusively in the United States by clinicians, physicians, pharmacists, and manufacturers to express the concentration of electrolytes in solution. This unit of measure is related to the total number of ionic charges in solution, and it takes note of the valence of the ions. In other words, it is a unit of measurement of the amount of *chemical activity* of an electrolyte. In the International System (SI), which is used in European countries and in many others throughout the world, molar concentrations [as millimoles per liter (mmol/L) and micromoles per liter (μmol/L)] are used.

Table 12.1 ▾ BLOOD PLASMA ELECTROLYTES
IN MILLIEQUIVALENTS PER LITER
(mEq/L)

CATIONS	mEq/L	ANIONS	mEq/L
Na$^+$	142	HCO$_3^-$	24
K$^+$	5	Cl$^-$	105
Ca^{++}	5	HPO$_4^{--}$	2
Mg^{++}	2	SO$_4^{--}$	1
		Org. Ac.$^-$	6
		Proteinate$^-$	16
	154		154

Under normal conditions, blood plasma contains 154 mEq of cations and an equal number of anions (Table 12.1). However, it should be understood that normal laboratory values of electrolytes vary, albeit within a rather narrow range, as shown in Table 12.2. The total concentration of cations always equals the total concentration of anions. Any number of milliequivalents of Na$^+$, K$^+$, or any cation$^+$ always reacts with precisely the same number of milliequivalents of Cl$^-$, HCO$_3^-$, or any anion$^-$. *For a given chemical compound, the milliequivalents of cation equals the milliequivalents of anion equals the milliequivalents of the chemical compound.*

In preparing a solution of K$^+$ ions, a potassium salt is dissolved in water. In addition to the K$^+$ ions, the solution will also contain ions of opposite negative charge. These two components will be chemically equal in that the milliequivalents of one are equal to the milliequivalents of the other. The interesting point is that if we dissolve enough potassium chloride in water to give us 40 mEq of K$^+$ per liter, we also have exactly 40 mEq of Cl$^-$, but the solution will *not* contain the *same weight* of each ion.

A milliequivalent represents the amount, in milligrams, of a solute equal to $\frac{1}{1000}$ of its gram equivalent weight, taking into account the valence of the ions. The milliequivalent expresses the chemical activity or combining power of a substance relative to the activity of 1 mg of hydrogen. Thus, based on the atomic weight and valence of the species, 1 mEq is represented by 1 mg of hydrogen, 20 mg of calcium, 23 mg of sodium, 35.5 mg of chlorine, 39 mg of potassium, and so forth. Important values for some ions are presented

Table 12.2 ▾ USUAL REFERENCE RANGE OF
BLOOD SERUM VALUES FOR
SOME ELECTROLYTES^a

CATION/ANION	mEq/L	SI UNITS (mmol/L)
Sodium	135–145	135–145
Potassium	3.5–5.5	3.5–5.5
Calcium	4.6–5.5	2.3–2.75
Magnesium	1.5–2.5	0.75–1.25
Chloride	96–106	96–106
Carbon Dioxide	24–30	24–30
Phosphorus	2.5–4.5	0.8–1.5

^{a}Reference ranges may vary slightly between clinical laboratories based, in part, on the analytical methods and equipment used.

Table 12.3 ▼ VALUES FOR SOME IMPORTANT IONS

ION	FORMULA	VALENCE	ATOMIC OR FORMULA WEIGHT	EQUIVALENT WEIGHT[a]
Aluminum	Al^{+++}	3	27	9
Ammonium	NH_4^+	1	18	18
Calcium	Ca^{++}	2	40	20
Ferric	Fe^{+++}	3	56	18.7
Ferrous	Fe^{++}	2	56	28
Lithium	Li^+	1	7	7
Magnesium	Mg^{++}	2	24	12
Potassium	K^+	1	39	39
Sodium	Na^+	1	23	23
Acetate	$C_2H_3O_2^-$	1	59	59
Bicarbonate	HCO_3^-	1	61	61
Carbonate	CO_3^{--}	2	60	30
Chloride	Cl^-	1	35.5	35.5
Citrate	$C_6H_5O_7^{---}$	3	189	63
Gluconate	$C_6H_{11}O_7^-$	1	195	195
Lactate	$C_6H_5O_3^-$	1	89	89
Phosphate	$H_2PO_4^-$	1	97	97
	HPO_4^{--}	2	96	48
Sulfate	SO_4^{--}	2	96	48

[a]Equivalent weight = $\dfrac{\text{Atomic or formula weight}}{\text{Valence}}$

in Table 12.3, and a complete listing of atomic weights is provided on the back pages of this text.

Example Calculations of Milliequivalents

To convert the concentration of electrolytes in solution expressed as milliequivalents per unit volume to weight per unit volume and vice versa, use the following:

CALCULATIONS CAPSULE

Milliequivalents

To convert milligrams (mg) to milliequivalents (mEq):

$$mEq = \frac{mg \times Valence}{\text{Atomic, formula, or molecular weight}}$$

To convert milliequivalents (mEq) to milligrams (mg):

$$mg = \frac{mEq \times \text{Atomic, formula, or molecular weight}}{Valence}$$

To convert milliequivalents per milliliter (mEq/mL) to milligrams per milliliter (mg/mL):

$$mg/mL = \frac{mEq/mL \times \text{Atomic, formula, or molecular weight}}{Valence}$$

$$mEq = \frac{mg \times Valence}{Atomic,\ formula,\ or\ molecular\ weight}$$

$$mg = \frac{mEq \times Atomic,\ formula,\ or\ molecular\ weight}{Valence}$$

$$mg/mL = \frac{mEq/mL \times Atomic,\ formula,\ or\ molecular\ weight}{Valence}$$

A physician prescribes 10 mEq of potassium chloride for a patient. How many milligrams of KCl would provide the prescribed quantity?

Molecular weight of KCl = 74.5 g
Equivalent weight of KCl = 74.5 g
1 mEq of KCl = 1/1000 × 74.5 g = 0.0745 g = 74.5 mg
10 mEq = 74.5 mg × 10 = 745 mg, *answer.*

If a patient is prescribed 300 mg of potassium chloride, what is the corresponding mEq?

Molecular weight of KCl = 74.5 g
Equivalent weight of KCl = 74.5 g
1 mEq of KCl = 1/1000 × 74.5 g = 0.0745 g = 74.5 mg

$$\frac{1\ mEq}{74.5\ mg} = \frac{x\ mEq}{300\ mg}; \ x = 4.03\ mEq, \ answer.$$

A physician prescribes 3 mEq/kg of NaCl to be administered to a 165-lb patient. How many milliliters of a half-normal saline solution (0.45% NaCl) should be administered?

Molecular weight of NaCl = 58.5 g
Equivalent weight of NaCl = 58.5 g
1 mEq of NaCl = 1/1000 of 58.5 g = 0.0585 g = 58.5 mg
165 lb/2.2 lb/kg = 75 kg (pt. wt.)
3 mEq/kg × 75 kg = 225 mEq (dose)
0.45% NaCl = 0.45 g/100 mL = 450 mg/100 mL
450 mg/58.5 mg/mEq = 7.69 mEq/100 mL = 0.0769 mEq/mL
225 mEq (dose)/0.0769 mEq/mL = 2925.9 mL, *answer.*

What is the concentration, in milligrams per milliliter, of a solution containing 2 mEq of potassium chloride (KCl) per milliliter?

Molecular weight of KCl = 74.5
Equivalent weight of KCl = 74.5
1 mEq of KCl = $\frac{1}{1000}$ × 74.5 g = 0.0745 g = 74.5 mg
2 mEq of KCl = 74.5 mg × 2 = 149 mg/mL, *answer.*

Or, by using the preceding equation:

$$mg/mL = \frac{2\ (mEq/mL) \times 74.5}{1}$$
$$= 149\ mg/mL, \ answer.$$

What is the concentration, in grams per milliliter, of a solution containing 4 mEq of calcium chloride (CaCl$_2 \cdot$ 2H$_2$O) per milliliter?

Recall that the equivalent weight of a binary compound may be found by dividing the formula weight by the *total valence* of the positive or negative radical.

$$\text{Formula weight of } CaCl_2 \cdot 2H_2O = 147$$
$$\text{Equivalent weight of } CaCl_2 \cdot 2H_2O = {}^{147}\!/_2 = 73.5$$
$$1 \text{ mEq of } CaCl_2 \cdot 2H_2O = {}^{1}\!/_{1000} \times 73.5 \text{ g} = 0.0735 \text{ g}$$
$$4 \text{ mEq of } CaCl_2 \cdot 2H_2O = 0.0735 \text{ g} \times 4 = 0.294 \text{ g/mL, } \textit{answer.}$$

Or, solving by dimensional analysis:

$$\frac{1 \text{ g } CaCl_2 \cdot 2H_2O}{1000 \text{ mg } CaCl_2 \cdot 2H_2O} \times \frac{147 \text{ mg}}{1 \text{ mmole}} \times \frac{1 \text{ mmole}}{2 \text{ mEq}} \times \frac{4 \text{ mEq}}{1 \text{ mL}} = 0.294 \text{ g/mL, } \textit{answer.}$$

Note: The water of hydration molecules do not interfere in the calculations as long as the correct molecular weight is used.

What is the percent (w/v) concentration of a solution containing 100 mEq of ammonium chloride per liter?

$$\text{Molecular weight of } NH_4Cl = 53.5$$
$$\text{Equivalent weight of } NH_4Cl = 53.5$$
$$1 \text{ mEq of } NH_4Cl = {}^{1}\!/_{1000} \times 53.5 = 0.0535 \text{ g}$$
$$100 \text{ mEq of } NH_4Cl = 0.0535 \text{ g} \times 100 = 5.35 \text{ g/L or}$$
$$0.535 \text{ g per } 100 \text{ mL, or } 0.535\%, \textit{answer.}$$

A solution contains 10 mg/100 mL of K^+ ions. Express this concentration in terms of milliequivalents per liter.

$$\text{Atomic weight of } K^+ = 39$$
$$\text{Equivalent weight of } K^+ = 39$$
$$1 \text{ mEq of } K^+ = {}^{1}\!/_{1000} \times 39 \text{ g} = 0.039 \text{ g} = 39 \text{ mg}$$
$$10 \text{ mg/100 mL of } K^+ = 100 \text{ mg of } K^+ \text{ per liter}$$
$$100 \text{ mg} \div 39 = 2.56 \text{ mEq/L, } \textit{answer.}$$

Or, by the equation detailed previously:

$$\text{mEq/L} = \frac{100 \, (\text{mg/L}) \times 1}{39}$$
$$= 2.56 \text{ mEq/L, } \textit{answer.}$$

A solution contains 10 mg/100 mL of Ca^{++} ions. Express this concentration in terms of milliequivalents per liter.

$$\text{Atomic weight of } Ca^{++} = 40$$
$$\text{Equivalent weight of } Ca^{++} = {}^{40}\!/_2 = 20$$
$$1 \text{ mEq of } Ca^{++} = {}^{1}\!/_{1000} \times 20 \text{ g} = 0.020 \text{ g} = 20 \text{ mg}$$
$$10 \text{ mg/100 mL of } Ca^{++} = 100 \text{ mg of } Ca^{++} \text{ per liter}$$
$$100 \text{ mg} \div 20 = 5 \text{ mEq/L, } \textit{answer.}$$

A magnesium (Mg^{++}) level in blood plasma is determined to be 2.5 mEq/L. Express this concentration in terms of milligrams.

$$\text{Atomic weight of } Mg^{++} = 24$$
$$\text{Equivalent weight of } Mg^{++} = {}^{24}\!/_2 = 12$$
$$1 \text{ mEq of } Mg^{++} = {}^{1}\!/_{1000} \times 12 \text{ g} = 0.012 \text{ g} = 12 \text{ mg}$$
$$2.5 \text{ mEq of } Mg^{++} = 30 \text{ mg}$$
$$30 \text{ mg/L, } \textit{answer.}$$

How many milliequivalents of potassium chloride are represented in a 15-mL dose of a 10% (w/v) potassium chloride elixir?

$$\text{Molecular weight of KCl} = 74.5$$
$$\text{Equivalent weight of KCl} = 74.5$$
$$1 \text{ mEq of KCl} = \tfrac{1}{1000} \times 74.5 \text{ g} = 0.0745 \text{ g} = 74.5 \text{ mg}$$
$$15\text{-mL dose of } 10\% \text{ (w/v) elixir} = 1.5 \text{ g or } 1500 \text{ mg of KCl}$$
$$\frac{74.5 \text{ (mg)}}{1500 \text{ (mg)}} = \frac{1 \text{ (mEq)}}{x \text{ (mEq)}}$$
$$x = 20.13 \text{ mEq, } answer.$$

How many milliequivalents of magnesium sulfate are represented in 1 g of anhydrous magnesium sulfate (MgSO$_4$)?

$$\text{Molecular weight of MgSO}_4 = 120$$
$$\text{Equivalent weight of MgSO}_4 = 60$$
$$1 \text{ mEq of MgSO}_4 = \tfrac{1}{1000} \times 60 \text{ g} = 0.06 \text{ g} = 60 \text{ mg}$$
$$1.0 \text{ g of MgSO}_4 = 1000 \text{ mg}$$
$$\frac{60 \text{ (mg)}}{1000 \text{ (mg)}} = \frac{1 \text{ (mEq)}}{x \text{ (mEq)}}$$
$$x = 16.67 \text{ mEq, } answer.$$

How many milliequivalents of Na$^+$ would be contained in a 30-mL dose of the following solution?

Disodium hydrogen phosphate	18 g
Sodium biphosphate	48 g
Purified water ad	100 mL

Each salt is considered separately in solving the problem.

Disodium hydrogen phosphate

$$\text{Formula} = \text{Na}_2\text{HPO}_4 \cdot 7\text{H}_2\text{O}$$
$$\text{Molecular weight} = 268 \text{ and the equivalent weight} = 134$$
$$\frac{18 \text{ (g)}}{x \text{ (g)}} = \frac{100 \text{ (mL)}}{30 \text{ (mL)}}$$
$$x = 5.4 \text{ g of disodium hydrogen phosphate per 30 mL}$$
$$1 \text{ mEq} = \tfrac{1}{1000} \times 134 \text{ g} = 0.134 \text{ g} = 134 \text{ mg}$$
$$\frac{134 \text{ (mg)}}{5400 \text{ (mg)}} = \frac{1 \text{ (mEq)}}{x \text{ (mEq)}}$$
$$x = 40.3 \text{ mEq of disodium hydrogen phosphate}$$

Because the milliequivalent value of Na$^+$ ion equals the milliequivalent value of disodium hydrogen phosphate, then

$$x = 40.3 \text{ mEq of Na}^+$$

Sodium biphosphate

$$\text{Formula} = \text{NaH}_2\text{PO}_4 \cdot \text{H}_2\text{O}$$
$$\text{Molecular weight} = 138 \text{ and the equivalent weight} = 138$$
$$\frac{48 \text{ (g)}}{x \text{ (g)}} = \frac{100 \text{ (mL)}}{30 \text{ (mL)}}$$
$$x = 14.4 \text{ g of sodium biphosphate per 30 mL}$$

$$1 \text{ mEq} = \tfrac{1}{1000} \times 138 \text{ g} = 0.138 \text{ g} = 138 \text{ mg}$$

$$\frac{138 \text{ (mg)}}{14,400 \text{ (mg)}} = \frac{1 \text{ (mEq)}}{x \text{ (mEq)}}$$

$$x = 104.3 \text{ mEq of sodium biphosphate}$$
$$\text{and also, } = 104.3 \text{ mEq of Na}^+$$

Adding the two milliequivalent values for Na^+ = 40.3 mEq + 104.3 mEq = 144.6 mEq, *answer*.

A person is to receive 2 mEq of sodium chloride per kilogram of body weight. If the person weighs 132 lb., how many milliliters of a 0.9% sterile solution of sodium chloride should be administered?

$$\text{Molecular weight of NaCl} = 58.5$$
$$\text{Equivalent weight of NaCl} = 58.5$$
$$1 \text{ mEq of NaCl} = \tfrac{1}{1000} \times 58.5 \text{ g} = 0.0585 \text{ g}$$
$$2 \text{ mEq of NaCl} = 0.0585 \text{ g} \times 2 = 0.117 \text{ g}$$

$$1 \text{ kg} = 2.2 \text{ lb.} \qquad \text{Weight of person in kg} = \frac{132 \text{ lb.}}{2.2 \text{ lb.}} = 60 \text{ kg}$$

Because the person is to receive 2 mEq/kg, then 2 mEq or 0.117 g × 60 = 7.02 g of NaCl needed and because 0.9% sterile solution of sodium chloride contains

9 g of NaCl per liter,

then

$$\frac{9 \text{ (g)}}{7.02 \text{ (g)}} = \frac{1000 \text{ (mL)}}{x \text{ (mL)}}$$
$$x = 780 \text{ mL, } \textit{answer}.$$

CASE IN POINT 12.1[a] A hospital pharmacist receives a medication order calling for 10 mEq of calcium to be added to a 500-mL bag of normal saline solution. The intravenous fluid is to be administered at a rate of 0.5 mEq of calcium per hour. The pharmacist has available 10-mL vials of a 10% injection of calcium chloride dihydrate. (a) How many milliliters of this injection should be added to the bag of IV fluid to make the desired product? (b) If the nurse administering the IV fluid uses an intravenous set that delivers 12 drops/mL, how many drops per minute should be delivered to provide the desired dose?

[a]Problem courtesy of Flynn Warren, Bishop, GA.

Millimoles and Micromoles

As noted previously, electrolyte concentrations may be expressed in *millimoles per liter (mmol/L)*. For monovalent species, the numeric values of the milliequivalent and millimole are identical.

A *mole* is the molecular weight of a substance in grams. A *millimole* is one thousandth of a mole and a *micromole* is one millionth of a mole.

Example Calculations of Millimoles and Micromoles

How many millimoles of monobasic sodium phosphate (m.w. 138) are present in 100 g of the substance?

$$\text{m.w.} = 138$$
$$1 \text{ mole} = 138 \text{ g}$$
$$\frac{1 \, (\text{mole})}{x \, (\text{mole})} = \frac{138 \, (g)}{100 \, (g)}$$
$$x = 0.725 \text{ moles} = 725 \text{ mmol, } answer.$$

How many milligrams would 1 mmol of monobasic sodium phosphate weigh?

$$1 \text{ mole} = 138 \text{ g}$$
$$1 \text{ mmol} = 0.138 \text{ g} = 138 \text{ mg, } answer.$$

What is the weight, in milligrams, of 1 mmol of $HPO_4^=$?

$$\text{Atomic weight of } HPO_4^= = 95.98$$
$$1 \text{ mole of } HPO_4^= = 95.98 \text{ g}$$
$$1 \text{ mmol of } HPO_4^= = 95.98 \text{ g} \times \frac{1}{1000} = 0.09598 \text{ g}$$
$$= 95.98 \text{ mg, } answer.$$

Convert blood plasma levels of 0.5 µg/mL and 2 µg/mL of tobramycin (mw = 467.52) to µmol/L.[1]

By dimensional analysis:

$$\frac{0.5 \, \mu g}{1 \text{ mL}} \times \frac{1 \, \mu mol}{467.52 \, \mu g} \times \frac{1000 \text{ mL}}{1 \text{ L}} = 1.07 \, \mu mol/L$$

and,

$$\frac{2 \, \mu g}{1 \text{ mL}} \times \frac{1 \, \mu mol}{467.52 \, \mu g} \times \frac{1000 \text{ mL}}{1 \text{ L}} = 4.28 \, \mu mol/L, \, answers.$$

If Lactated Ringer's Injection contains 20 mg of calcium chloride dihydrate ($CaCl_2 \cdot 2H_2O$) in each 100 mL, calculate the millimoles of calcium present.

$$\text{Molecular weight of } CaCl_2 \cdot 2H_2O = 147 \text{ g}$$
$$1 \text{ mole} = 147 \text{ g}$$
$$1 \text{ mmol} = 0.147 \text{ g or } 147 \text{ mg}$$
$$\frac{1 \text{ mmol}}{147 \, mg} = \frac{x \text{ mmol}}{20 \, mg}; x = 0.136 \text{ mmol, } answer.$$

Calculate the millimoles of calcium present in 1 L of Lactated Ringer's Injection.

$$0.136 \text{ mmol (per 100 mL)} \times 10 = 1.36 \text{ mmol, } answer.$$

How many micromoles of calcium are present in each milliliter of Lactated Ringer's Injection?

$$1.36 \text{ mmol/L} = 1360 \, \mu moles/L = 1.36 \, \mu mol/mL, \, answer.$$

A patient is receiving a slow intravenous infusion containing 40 mEq of potassium chloride in 1000 mL of fluid. If, after 12 hours, 720 mL of infusion had been infused, how many millimoles of potassium chloride were administered?

$$\text{Molecular weight of KCl} = 74.5 \text{ g}$$
$$1 \text{ mEq KCl} = 74.5 \text{ mg}$$

$$40 \text{ mEq KCl} = 74.5 \text{ mg} \times 40 \text{ (mEq)} = 2980 \text{ mg (in 1000 mL)}$$
$$2980 \text{ mg} \times 720 \text{ mL}/1000 \text{ mL} = 2145.6 \text{ mg (in 720 mL)}$$
$$2145.6 \text{ mg}/74.4 \text{ mg per mmol} = 28.8 \text{ mmol, } answer.$$

Or, more simply, since for KCl:

$$1 \text{ mEq} = 1 \text{ mmol, and thus}$$
$$40 \text{ mEq} = 40 \text{ mmol;}$$

and, 72% of fluid (720 mL of 1000 mL) was administered,

$$72\% \text{ of } 40 \text{ mmol} = 28.8 \text{ mmol, } answer.$$

A medication order calls for 1.8 g of potassium chloride in 60 mL of solution. How many millimoles of KCl are contained in each milliliter?

$$\text{Molecular weight of KCl} = 74.5 \text{ g}$$
$$1 \text{ mmol KCl} = 74.5 \text{ mg}$$
$$1.8 \text{ g KCl} = 1800 \text{ mg}$$
$$1800 \text{ mg}/74.5 \text{ mg per mmol} = 24.16 \text{ mmol}$$
$$24.16 \text{ mmol}/60 \text{ mL} = 0.4 \text{ mmol/mL, } answer.$$

Calculate the concentrations in mmol/L for each of the following infusion solutions: (a) 5% NaCl; (b) 3% NaCl; (c) 0.9% NaCl (NSS); (d) 0.45% NaCl (half-NSS); and (e) 0.2% NaCl.

(a) 1 L of a 5% NaCl solution contains 50 g or 50,000 mg NaCl.
    1 mole of NaCl = 23 g + 35.5 g = 58.5 g
    1 mmol of NaCl = 58.5 mg
    50,000 mg/58.5 mg/mmol = 854.7 or 855 mmol/L, *answer.*
(b) 30,000 mg/58.5 mg/mmol = 512.8 or 513 mmol/L, *answer.*
(c) 9000 mg/58.5 mg/mmol = 153.8 or 154 mmol/L, *answer.*
(d) 4500 mg/58.5 mg/mmol − 76.9 or 77 mmol/L, *answer.*
(e) 2000 mg/58.5 mg/mmol = 34.2 or 34 mmol/L, *answer.*

Osmolarity

As indicated in Chapter 11, osmotic pressure is important to biologic processes that involve the diffusion of solutes or the transfer of fluids through semipermeable membranes. The labels of solutions that provide intravenous replenishment of fluid, nutrients, or electrolytes, and the osmotic diuretic mannitol are required to state the osmolar concentration. This information indicates to the practitioner whether the solution is hypoosmotic, iso-osmotic, or hyperosmotic with regard to biologic fluids and membranes.

Osmotic pressure is proportional to the *total number* of particles in solution. The unit used to measure osmotic concentration is the *milliosmole* (mOsmol). For dextrose, a nonelectrolyte, 1 mmol (1 formula weight in milligrams) represents 1 mOsmol. This relationship is not the same with electrolytes, however, because the total number of particles in solution depends on the degree of dissociation of the substance in question. Assuming complete dissociation, 1 mmol of NaCl represents 2 mOsmol ($Na^+ + Cl^-$) of total particles, 1 mmol of $CaCl_2$ represents 3 mOsmol ($Ca^{++} + 2Cl^-$) of total particles, and 1 mmol of sodium citrate ($Na_3C_6H_5O_7$) represents 4 mOsmol ($3Na^+ + C_6H_5O_7^-$) of total particles.

The milliosmolar value of *separate* ions of an electrolyte may be obtained by dividing the concentration, in milligrams per liter, of the ion by its atomic weight. The milliosmolar value of the *whole* electrolyte in solution is equal to the sum of the milliosmolar values of the separate ions. According to the *United States Pharmacopeia*, the ideal osmolar concentration may be calculated according to the equation[2]:

$$\text{mOsmol/L} = \frac{\text{Weight of substance (g/L)}}{\text{Molecular weight (g)}} \times \text{Number of species} \times 1000$$

In practice, as the concentration of the solute increases, physicochemical interaction among solute particles increases, and actual osmolar values decrease when compared to ideal values. Deviation from ideal conditions is usually slight in solution within the physiologic range and for more dilute solutions, but for highly concentrated solutions, the actual osmolarities may be appreciably lower than ideal values. For example, the ideal osmolarity of 0.9% sodium chloride injection is:

$$\text{mOsmol/L} = \frac{9 \text{g/L}}{58.5 \text{ g}} \times 2 \times 1000 = 308 \text{ mOsmol/L}$$

Because of bonding forces, however, n is slightly less than 2 for solutions of sodium chloride at this concentration, and the actual measured osmolarity of the solution is about 286 mOsmol/L.

Some pharmaceutical manufacturers label electrolyte solutions with ideal or stoichiometric osmolarities calculated by the equation just provided, whereas others list experimental or actual osmolarities. The pharmacist should appreciate this distinction.

A distinction also should be made between the terms *osmolarity* and *osmolality*. Whereas **osmolarity** is the *milliosmoles of solute per liter of solution*, **osmolality** is the *milliosmoles of solute per kilogram of solvent*. For dilute aqueous solutions, osmolarity and osmolality are nearly identical. For more concentrated solutions, however, the two values may be quite dissimilar. The pharmacist should pay particular attention to a product's label statement regarding molarity versus molality.

Normal serum osmolality is considered to be within the range of 275 to 300 mOsmol/kg. The contribution of various constituents to the osmolality of normal serum is shown in Table 12.4. *Osmometers* are commercially available for use in the laboratory to measure osmolality.[3] Abnormal blood osmolality that deviates from the normal range can occur in association with shock, trauma, burns, water intoxication (overload), electrolyte imbalance, hyperglycemia, or renal failure.[3]

Example Calculations of Milliosmoles

A solution contains 5% of anhydrous dextrose in water for injection. How many milliosmoles per liter are represented by this concentration?

Formula weight of anhydrous dextrose = 180
1 mmol of anhydrous dextrose (180 mg) = 1 mOsmol
5% solution contains 50 g or 50,000 mg/L
50,000 mg ÷ 180 = 278 mOsmol/L, *answer.*

Or, solving by dimensional analysis:

$$\frac{50,000 \text{ mg}}{1 \text{ L}} \times \frac{1 \text{ mOsmol}}{180 \text{ mg}} = 278 \text{ mOsmol/L, } answer.$$

Table 12.4 ▼ **THE CONTRIBUTION OF VARIOUS CONSTITUENTS OF NORMAL HUMAN SERUM TO THE TOTAL SERUM OSMOTIC PRESSURE**[a]

CONSTITUENT	MEAN CONCENTRATION (mEq/L)	OSMOTIC PRESSURE (mOsmol/kg of water)[b]	PERCENTAGE OF TOTAL OSMOTIC PRESSURE
Sodium	142.0	139.0	48.3%
Potassium	5.0	4.9	1.7
Calcium	2.5	1.2	0.4
Magnesium	2.0	1.0	0.3
Chloride	102.0	99.8	34.7
Bicarbonate	27.0	26.4	9.2
Proteinate	16.0	1.0	0.3
Phosphate	2.0	1.1	0.4
Sulfate	1.0	0.5	0.2
Organic Anions	3.5	3.4	1.2
Urea	30 (mg/100 mL)	5.3	1.8
Glucose	70 (mg/100 mL)	4.1	1.4
TOTALS		287.7 mOsmol/kg	99.9%
OBSERVED NORMAL MEAN		289.0 mOsmol/kg	

[a]From Chughtai MA, Hendry EB. Serum electrolytes, urea, and osmolality in cases of chloride depletion. *Clinical Biochemistry* 1967;1:91. Adapted from Fluid and Electrolytes. Chicago: Abbott Laboratories, 1970.
[b]Water content of normal serum taken as 94 g/100 mL.

A solution contains 156 mg of K^+ ions per 100 mL. How many milliosmoles are represented in a liter of the solution?

$$\text{Atomic weight of } K^+ = 39$$
$$1 \text{ mmol of } K^+ (39 \text{ mg}) = 1 \text{ mOsmol}$$
$$156 \text{ mg of } K^+ \text{ per } 100 \text{ mL} = 1560 \text{ mg of } K^+ \text{ per liter}$$
$$1560 \text{ mg} \div 39 = 40 \text{ mOsmol}, \textit{answer}.$$

A solution contains 10 mg% of Ca^{++} ions. How many milliosmoles are represented in 1 liter of the solution?

$$\text{Atomic weight of } Ca^{++} = 40$$
$$1 \text{ mmol of } Ca^{++} (40 \text{ mg}) = 1 \text{ mOsmol}$$
$$10 \text{ mg\% of } Ca^{++} = 10 \text{ mg of } Ca^{++} \text{ per } 100 \text{ mL or}$$
$$100 \text{ mg of } Ca^{++} \text{ per liter}$$
$$100 \text{ mg} \div 40 = 2.5 \text{ mOsmol}, \textit{answer}.$$

How many milliosmoles are represented in a liter of a 0.9% sodium chloride solution?

Osmotic concentration (in terms of milliosmoles) is a function of the total number of particles present. Assuming complete dissociation, 1 mmol of sodium chloride (NaCl) represents 2 mOsmol of total particles (Na^+ + Cl^-).

$$\text{Formula weight of NaCl} = 58.5$$
$$1 \text{ mmol of NaCl } (58.5 \text{ mg}) = 2 \text{ mOsmol}$$
$$1000 \times 0.009 = 9 \text{ g or } 9000 \text{ mg of NaCl per liter}$$
$$\frac{58.5 \text{ (mg)}}{9000 \text{ (mg)}} = \frac{2 \text{ (mOsmol)}}{x \text{ (mOsmol)}}$$
$$x = 307.7, \text{ or } 308 \text{ mOsmol}, \textit{answer}.$$

Calculate the milliosmoles of sodium chloride in 100 mL of a 3% hypertonic solution of sodium chloride injection.

$$\text{Formula weight of NaCl} = 58.5 \text{ g}$$
$$1 \text{ mmol of NaCl } (58.5 \text{ mg}) = 2 \text{ mOsmol}$$
$$100 \text{ mL} \times 3\% = 3 \text{ g or } 3000 \text{ mg NaCl}$$
$$2 \text{ (mOsmol)} \times 3000 \text{ mg (NaCl)}/58.5 \text{ mg (NaCl)} = 102.6 \text{ mOsmol, } \textit{answer.}$$

Calcium chloride dihydrate injection is a 10% solution of $CaCl_2 \cdot 2H_2O$. *How many milliosmoles are present in a 10-mL vial?*

$$\text{Formula weight of } CaCl_2 \cdot H_2O = 147 \text{ g}$$
1 mmol $CaCl_2 \cdot H_2O$ (147 mg) = 3 mOsmol (*Note:* water of hydration provides no "parti-cles" to contribute to the number of osmols in solution)
$$10 \text{ mL} \times 10\% = 1 \text{ g or } 1000 \text{ mg } CaCl_2 \cdot 2H_2O$$
$$3 \text{ (mOsmol)} \times 1000 \text{ mg } (CaCl_2 \cdot 2H_2O)/147 \text{ mg } (CaCl_2 \cdot 2H_2O) = 20.4 \text{ mOsmol, } \textit{answer.}$$

If a pharmacist wished to prepare 100 mL of a solution containing 50 mOsmol of calcium chloride, how many grams of calcium chloride would be needed?

$$\text{Formula weight of } CaCl_2 = 111 \text{ g}$$
$$1 \text{ mmol } CaCl_2 \text{ (111 mg)} = 3 \text{ mOsmol}$$
$$111 \text{ mg} \times 50 \text{ mOsmol}/3 \text{ mOsmol} = 1850 \text{ mg} = 1.85 \text{ g, } \textit{answer.}$$

The molecular weight of Dextrose, USP is 198.17. How many grams are required to prepare a solution providing 120 mOsmol?

$$\text{Formula weight, } C_6H_{12}O_6 \cdot H_2O = 198.17 \text{ g}$$
$$1 \text{ mmol } C_6H_{12}O_6 \cdot H_2O \text{ (198.17 mg)} = 1 \text{ mOsmol}$$
$$198.17 \text{ mg}/1 \text{ mOsmol} \times 120 \text{ mOsmol} = 23,780.4 \text{ mg} = 23.78 \text{ g, } \textit{answer.}$$

Calculate the milliequivalents of sodium, potassium and chloride, the millimoles of anhydrous dextrose, and the osmolarity of the following parenteral fluid.

Dextrose, anhydrous	50	g
Sodium Chloride	4.5	g
Potassium Chloride	1.49	g
Water for Injection, ad	1000	mL

$$\text{Molecular weight of NaCl} = 58.5$$
$$\text{Equivalent weight of NaCl} = 58.5$$
$$1 \text{ mEq of NaCl} = \tfrac{1}{1000} \times 58.5 = 0.0585 \text{ g} = 58.5 \text{ mg}$$
$$4.5 \text{ g of NaCl} = 4500 \text{ mg}$$
$$\frac{58.5 \text{ mg}}{4500 \text{ mg}} = \frac{1 \text{ mEq}}{x \text{ mEq}}$$
$$x = 76.9 \text{ or } 77 \text{ mEq of Na}^+ \text{ and}$$
$$76.9 \text{ or } 77 \text{ mEq of Cl}^-$$

$$\text{Molecular weight of KCl} = 74.5$$
$$\text{Equivalent weight of KCl} = 74.5$$
$$1 \text{ mEq of KCl} = \tfrac{1}{1000} \times 74.5 = 0.0745 \text{ g} = 74.5 \text{ mg}$$
$$1.49 \text{ g of KCl} = 1490 \text{ mg}$$
$$\frac{74.5 \text{ mg}}{1490} = \frac{1 \text{ mEq}}{x \text{ mEq}}$$
$$x = 20 \text{ mEq of K}^+ \text{ and}$$
$$20 \text{ mEq of Cl}^-$$

$$\text{Total: } Na^+ = 77 \text{ mEq}$$
$$K^+ = 20 \text{ mEq}$$
$$Cl^- = 77 \text{ mEq} + 20 \text{ mEq} = 97 \text{ mEq, } answers.$$

$$\text{Molecular weight of anhydrous dextrose} = 180$$
$$1 \text{ mmol of anhydrous dextrose} = 180 \text{ mg}$$
$$50 \text{ g of anhydrous dextrose} = 50,000 \text{ mg}$$
$$\frac{180 \text{ mg}}{50,000 \text{ mg}} = \frac{1 \text{ mmol}}{x \text{ mmol}}$$
$$x = 277.7 \text{ or } 278 \text{ mmol, } answer.$$

Osmolarity:

$$\text{Dextrose, anhyd.: } 278 \text{ mmol} \times 1 \text{ particle per mmol} = 278 \text{ mOsmol}$$
$$\text{NaCl: } 77 \text{ mEq} \times 2 \text{ particles per mEq (or mmol)} = 154 \text{ mOsmol}$$
$$\text{KCl: } 20 \text{ mEq} \times 2 \text{ particles per mEq (or mmol)} = \;\;40 \text{ mOsmol}$$
$$\text{Total} = 472 \text{ mOsmol, } answer.$$

Clinical Considerations of Water and Electrolyte Balance

Maintaining body water and electrolyte balance is an essential component of good health. Water provides the environment in which cells live and is the primary medium for the ingestion of nutrients and the excretion of metabolic waste products. Normally, the osmolality of body fluid is maintained within narrow limits through dietary input, the regulatory endocrine processes, and balanced output via the kidneys, lungs, skin, and the gastrointestinal system.

In clinical practice, fluid and electrolyte therapy is undertaken either to provide maintenance requirements or to replace serious losses or deficits. Body losses of water and/or electrolytes can result from a number of causes, including vomiting, diarrhea, profuse sweating, fever, chronic renal failure, diuretic therapy, surgery, and others. The type of therapy undertaken (i.e., oral or parenteral) and the content of the fluid administered depend on a patient's specific requirements.

For example, a patient taking diuretics may simply require a daily oral potassium supplement along with adequate intake of water. An athlete may require rehydration with or without added electrolytes. Hospitalized patients commonly receive parenteral maintenance therapy of fluids and electrolytes to support ordinary metabolic function. In severe cases of deficit, a patient may require the prompt and substantial intravenous replacement of fluids and electrolytes to restore acute volume losses resulting from surgery, trauma, burns, or shock.

Total body water in adult males normally ranges between 55% and 65% of body weight depending on the proportion of body fat. The greater the proportion of fat, the lesser the proportion of water. Values for adult women are about 10% less than those for men. Newborn infants have approximately 75% body water, which decreases with growth and increases in body fat. Of the adult body's water content, up to two thirds is intracellular and one third is extracellular. The proportion of extracellular body water, as a fraction of total body weight, decreases in infants in the first year from approximately 45% to 30% while the intracellular portion increases.[4] For an adult, approximately 2500 mL of daily water intake (from ingested liquids and foods and from oxidative metabolism) are needed to balance the daily water output.

In general terms, 1500 mL of water per square meter of body surface area may be used to calculate the daily requirement for adults. On a weight basis, estimates of 32 mL/kg for adults and 100 to 150 mL/kg for infants have been cited as average daily requirements of water intake for healthy individuals.[5] These estimated requirements differ greatly in persons with clinical disorders affecting water and electrolyte homeostasis and in conditions of acute deficit.

The composition of body fluids generally is described with regard to body compartments: *intracellular* (within cells), *intravascular* (blood plasma), or *interstitial* (between cells in the tissue). Intravascular and interstitial fluids commonly are grouped together and termed *extracellular* fluid.

The usual reference ranges of electrolytes in blood plasma are shown in Table 12.2. Although all electrolytes and nonelectrolytes in body fluids contribute to osmotic activity, sodium and chloride exert the principal effect in *extra*cellular fluid, and potassium and phosphate predominate in *intra*cellular fluid.

Since cell membranes generally are freely permeable to water, the osmolality of the extracellular fluid (about 290 mOsm/kg water) is about equal to that of the intracellular fluid. Therefore, the plasma osmolality is a convenient and accurate guide to intracellular osmolality and may be approximated by the formula[4]:

$$\text{Plasma osmolality (mOsm/kg)} = 2\,([\text{Na}]+[\text{K}])\text{ plasma} + \frac{[\text{BUN}]}{2.8} + \frac{[\text{Glucose}]}{18}$$

where: sodium (Na) and potassium (K) are in mEq/L, and blood urea nitrogen (BUN) and glucose concentrations are in mg/100 mL (mg/dL).

Example Calculations of Water Requirements and Plasma Osmolality

Calculate the estimated daily water requirement for a healthy adult with a body surface area of 1.8 m².

$$\text{Water Requirement} = 1500 \text{ mL/m}^2$$
$$\frac{1 \text{ m}^2}{1.8 \text{ m}^2} = \frac{1500 \text{ mL}}{\text{x mL}}$$
$$\text{x} = 2700 \text{ mL, } answer.$$

Estimate the plasma osmolality from the following data: sodium, 135 mEq/L; potassium, 4.5 mEq/L; blood urea nitrogen, 14 mg/dL; and glucose, 90 mg/dL.

Equation from text:

$$\text{mOsm/kg} = 2\,([\text{Na}]+[\text{K}]) + \frac{[\text{BUN}]}{2.8} + \frac{[\text{Glucose}]}{18}$$
$$\text{mOsm/kg} = 2\,(135 \text{ mEq/L} + 4.5 \text{ mEq/L}) + \frac{14 \text{ mg/dL}}{2.8} + \frac{90 \text{ mg/dL}}{18}$$
$$= 2\,(139.5) + 5 + 5$$
$$= 289, answer.$$

CALCULATIONS CAPSULE

Millimoles and Milliosmoles

To calculate millimoles (mmol):
   A *millimole* is $\frac{1}{1000}$ of the gram molecular weight of a substance.

$$1\ millimole = \frac{Molecular\ weight,\ grams}{1000}$$

To calculate milliosmoles (mOsmol):

   A *milliosmole* is $\frac{1}{1000}$ of an osmol. When substances do not dissociate, the numbers of millimoles and milliosmoles are the same. There are 2 milliosmoles per millimole for substances that dissociate into two particles and 3 milliosmoles per millimole for substances that dissociate into three particles.

$$mOsmol = mg\ of\ drug \times \frac{1\ mmol\ of\ drug}{Molecular\ weight\ (mg)}$$

CASE IN POINT 12.2[a] A hospital pharmacist fills a medication order calling for an intravenous fluid of dextrose 5% in a 0.9% sodium chloride injection and 40 mEq of potassium chloride in a total volume of 1000 mL. The intravenous infusion is administered through an IV set that delivers 15 drops per milliliter. The infusion has been running at a rate of 12 drops per minute for 15 hours.

   During the 15-hour period:
(a) How many mEq of KCl have been administered?
(b) How many grams of KCl have been administered?
(c) How many millimoles of KCl have been administered?
(d) What is the total osmolarity of the intravenous fluid?
   Express the answer in millimoles (rounded to the nearest whole number) per 1000 mL.

   [a]Problem courtesy of Flynn Warren, Bishop GA.

PRACTICE PROBLEMS

Calculations Based on Millimoles, Micromoles, and Milliequivalents

1. Convert a blood plasma level range of 5 to 20 µg/mL of tobramycin (m.w. = 467.52) to µmol/L.[1]

2. A preparation contains in each milliliter, 236 mg of dibasic potassium phosphate (m.w. = 174.18) and 224 mg of monobasic potassium phosphate (m.w. = 136.09). Calculate the total concentration of phosphate, in mmol/mL, in the preparation.[7]

3. A 10-mL ampul contains 2.98 g of potassium chloride. What is the concentration of the solution in milliequivalents per milliliter?

4. A 154-lb patient is to receive 36 mg/kg of ammonium chloride. How many milliliters of an ammonium chloride (NH_4Cl—m.w. 53.5) injection containing 5 mEq/mL should be added to the patient's intravenous infusion?

5. A sterile solution of potassium chloride contains 2 mEq/mL. If a 20-mL ampul of the solution is diluted to 1 liter, what is the percentage strength of the resulting solution?

6. A certain electrolyte solution contains, as one of the ingredients, the equivalent of 4.6 mEq of calcium per liter. How many grams of calcium chloride ($CaCl_2 \cdot 2H_2O$—m.w. 147) should be used in preparing 20 liters of the solution?

7. Ammonium chloride injection contains 267.5 mg of NH_2Cl (m.w. 53.5) per milliliter. How many mEq of ammonium chloride are present in a 20-mL vial?

8. A solution contains, in each 5 mL, 0.5 g of potassium acetate ($C_2H_3KO_2$—m.w. 98), 0.5 g of potassium bicarbonate ($KHCO_3$—m.w. 100), and 0.5 g of potassium citrate ($C_6H_5K_3O_7 \cdot H_2O$—m.w. 324). How many milliequivalents of potassium (K^+) are represented in each 5 mL of the solution?

9. How many grams of sodium chloride should be used in preparing 20 liters of a solution containing 154 mEq/L?

10. Sterile solutions of potassium chloride containing 5 mEq/mL are available in 20-mL containers. Calculate the amount, in grams, of potassium chloride in the container.

11. How many milliliters of a solution containing 2 mEq of potassium chloride per milliliter should be used to obtain 2.98 g of potassium chloride?

12. A patient is given 125 mg of phenytoin sodium ($C_{15}H_{11}N_2NaO_2$—m.w. 274) three times a day. How many milliequivalents of sodium are represented in the daily dose?

13. If a 40-mL vial of sodium chloride is added to a 1 L container of water for injection, calculate the concentration of sodium chloride, in mEq/mL in the original vial, if the resultant dilution is 0.56% in strength.

14. How many grams of sodium bicarbonate ($NaHCO_3$—m.w. 84) should be used in preparing a liter of a solution to contain 44.6 mEq per 50 mL?

15. A liter of an electrolyte solution contains the following: 131 mEq Na^+, 111 mEq Cl^-, 5 mEq K^+, 29 mEq $C_3H_5O_3^-$ (lactate), and 4 mEq Ca^{2+}. Convert each of these values to mmol/L.

16. Sterile sodium lactate solution is available commercially as a $\frac{1}{6}$-molar solution of sodium lactate in water for injection. How many milliequivalents of sodium lactate ($C_3H_5NaO_3$—m.w. 112) would be provided by a liter of the solution?

17. A certain electrolyte solution contains 0.9% of sodium chloride in 10% dextrose solution. Express the concentration of sodium chloride (NaCl) in terms of milliequivalents per liter.

18. ℞ Potassium Chloride   10%
       Cherry Syrup q.s. ad   480 mL
       Sig. Tablespoonful b.i.d.

    How many milliequivalents of potassium chloride are represented in each prescribed dose?

19. How many milliequivalents of potassium are in 5 million units of Penicillin V Potassium ($C_{16}H_{17}KN_2O_6S$—m.w. 388)? One milligram of penicillin V potassium represents 1380 Penicillin V Units.

20. The normal potassium level in the blood plasma is 17 mg% (17 mg/100 mL). Express this concentration in terms of milliequivalents per liter.

21. How many grams of potassium citrate ($C_6H_5K_3O_7 \cdot H_2O$—m.w. 324) should be used in preparing 500 mL of a potassium ion elixir so as to supply 15 mEq of K^+ in each 5-mL dose?

22. A potassium supplement tablet contains 2.5 g of potassium bicarbonate ($KHCO_3$—m.w. 100). How many milliequivalents of potassium (K^+) are supplied by the tablet?

23. Ringer's injection contains 0.86% of sodium chloride, 0.03% of potassium chloride, and 0.033% of calcium chloride dihydrate. Calculate the sodium, potassium, calcium, and chloride content in mEq/L.

24. Calculate the mEq of Na^+ in each gram of ampicillin sodium ($C_{16}H_{18}N_3NaO_4S$—m.w. 371).

25. A 20-mL vial of concentrated ammonium chloride solution containing 5 mEq/mL is diluted to 1 liter with sterile distilled water. Calculate (a) the total milliequivalent value of the ammonium ion in the dilution and (b) the percentage strength of the dilution.

26. If a liter of an intravenous fluid contains 5% dextrose and 34 mEq sodium (as NaCl), calculate the percent strength of sodium chloride in the solution.

27. How many milliequivalents of potassium would be supplied daily by the usual dose (0.3 mL three times a day) of saturated potassium iodide solution? Saturated potassium iodide solution contains 100 g of potassium iodide per 100 mL.

28. An intravenous solution calls for the addition of 25 mEq of sodium bicarbonate. How many milliliters of 8.4% w/v sodium bicarbonate injection should be added to the formula?

29. Calcium gluconate ($C_{12}H_{22}CaO_{14}$—m.w. 430) injection 10% is available in a 10-mL ampul. How many milliequivalents of Ca^{++} does the ampul contain?

30. A flavored potassium chloride packet contains 1.5 g of potassium chloride. How many milliequivalents of potassium chloride are represented in each packet?

31. How many milliequivalents of Li^+ are provided by a daily dose of four 300-mg tablets of lithium carbonate (Li_2CO_3—m.w. 74)?

32. How many milliequivalents of ammonium (NH_4^+) ion are contained in 1 liter of a 4.2% w/v solution of ammonium chloride?

33. A patient is to receive 10 mEq of potassium gluconate ($C_6H_{11}KO_7$—m.w. 234) four times a day for 3 days. If the dose is to be 1 teaspoonful in a cherry syrup vehicle, (a) how many grams of potassium gluconate should be used, and (b) what volume, in milliliters, should be dispensed to provide the prescribed dosage regimen?

34. A physician wishes to administer 1,200,000 units of penicillin G potassium every 4 hours. If 1 unit of penicillin G potassium ($C_{16}H_{17}KN_2O_4S$—m.w. 372) equals 0.6 μg, how many milli-equivalents of K^+ will the patient receive in a 24-hour period?

35. Five milliliters of lithium citrate syrup contain the equivalent of 8 mEq of Li^+. Calculate the equivalent, in milligrams, of lithium carbonate (Li_2CO_3—m.w. 74) in each 5-mL dose of the syrup.

36. How many milligrams of magnesium sulfate ($MgSO_4$—m.w. 120) should be added to an intravenous solution to provide 5 mEq of Mg^{++} per liter?

37. K-TAB, a slow-release potassium chloride tablet, contains 750 mg of potassium chloride in a wax/polymer matrix. How many milliequivalents of potassium chloride are supplied by a dosage of one tablet three times a day?

38. An electrolyte solution contains 222 mg of sodium acetate ($C_2H_3NaO_2$—m.w. 82) and 15 mg of magnesium chloride ($MgCl_2$—m.w. 95) in each 100 mL. Express these concentrations in milliequivalents of Na^+ and Mg^{++} per liter.

39. Ammonium chloride (NH_4Cl—m.w. 53.5) is to be used as a urinary acidifier with a dose of 150 mEq. How many 500-mg tablets should be administered?

40. A patient has a sodium deficit of 168 mEq. How many milliliters of isotonic sodium chloride solution (0.9% w/v) should be administered to replace the deficit?

41. A normal 70 kg (154 lb) adult has 80 to 100 g of sodium. It is primarily distributed in the extracellular fluid. Body retention of 1 g additional of sodium results in excess body water accumulation of approximately 310 mL. If a person retains 100 mEq of extra sodium, how many milliliters of additional water could be expected to be retained?

42. A patient receives 3 liters of an electrolyte fluid containing 234 mg of sodium chloride (NaCl—m.w. 58.5), 125 mg of potassium acetate ($C_2H_3KO_2$—m.w. 98), and 21 mg of magnesium acetate ($C_4H_6MgO_4$—m.w. 142) per 100 mL. How many milliequivalents each of Na^+, K^+, and Mg^{++} does the patient receive?

43. How many milliliters of a 2% w/v solution of ammonium chloride (NH_4Cl—m.w. 53.5) should be administered intravenously to a patient to provide 75 mEq?

44. The usual adult dose of calcium for elevating serum calcium is 7 to 14 mEq. How many milliliters of a calcium gluceptate injection, each milliliter of which provides 18 mg of elemental calcium, would provide the recommended dosage range?

45. The oral pediatric maintenance solution PEDIALYTE liquid has the following electrolyte content per liter: sodium, 45 mEq; potassium, 20 mEq; chloride, 35 mEq; and citrate, 30 mEq. Calculate the equivalent quantities of each in terms of milligrams.

46. Calculate the milliequivalents of chloride per liter of the following parenteral fluid:

Sodium Chloride	516 mg
Potassium Chloride	89.4 mg
Calcium Chloride, anhyd.	27.8 mg
Magnesium Chloride, anhyd.	14.2 mg
Sodium Lactate, anhyd.	560 mg
Water for Injection ad	100 mL

47. The pediatric infusion rate for potassium is 5 mEq/hour. If 9 mL of a 39.2% solution of potassium acetate ($KC_2H_3O_2$) is diluted to 1 L of infusion solution, calculate the proper infusion rate in mL/hr.

48. HALFLYTELY, a colon lavage preparation contains the following mixture of dry powder to prepare 2 liters of solution:

Sodium Chloride	5.6 g
Potassium Chloride	0.74 g
Sodium Bicarbonate	2.86 g
Polyethylene Glycol (3350)	210 g

Calculate the milliequivalents each of sodium and chloride present in the prepared solution.

Calculations Including Milliosmoles

49. At 3:00 P.M., a pharmacist received an order to add 30 mEq/L of potassium chloride to the already running intravenous fluid for a patient. After checking the medication order, the pharmacist found that the patient is receiving a 5% dextrose/0.9% sodium chloride infusion at a rate of 85 mL/hour, and that the patient's liter of fluid was started at 1:30 PM.[6]

(a) Assuming that it took 30 minutes to provide the needed potassium chloride to the floor nurse, how many milliequivalents of potassium chloride should have been added to the patient's running IV fluid to achieve the ordered concentration?

(b) How many milliliters of an injection containing 2 mEq of potassium chloride/mL should have been used to supply the amount of potassium chloride needed?

(c) What was the osmolality of the infusion with the potassium chloride added? Assume complete dissociation of the sodium chloride and potassium chloride.

50. A solution contains 322 mg of Na^+ ions per liter. How many milliosmoles are represented in the solution?

51. How many milliosmoles of sodium are represented in 1 liter of 3% hypertonic sodium chloride solution? Assume complete dissociation.

52. A solution of sodium chloride contains 77 mEq/L. Calculate its osmolar strength in terms of milliosmoles per liter. Assume complete dissociation.

53. Calculate the osmolar concentration, in terms of milliosmoles, represented by 1 liter of a 10% w/v solution of anhydrous dextrose (m.w. 180) in water.

54. Calculate the osmolarity, in milliosmoles per milliliter, of a parenteral solution containing 2 mEq/mL of potassium acetate ($KC_2H_3O_2$—m.w. 98).

55. Calculate (a) the milliequivalents per milliliter, (b) the total milliequivalents, and (c) the osmolarity of a 500-mL parenteral fluid containing 5% w/v of sodium bicarbonate.

56. What is the osmolarity of an 8.4% w/v solution of sodium bicarbonate?

57. A hospital medication order calls for the administration of 100 g of mannitol to a patient as an osmotic diuretic over a 24-hour period. Calculate (a) how many milliliters of a 15% w/v mannitol injection should be administered per hour, and (b) how many milliosmoles of mannitol (m.w. 182) would be represented in the prescribed dosage.

58. How many (a) millimoles, (b) milliequivalents, and (c) milliosmoles of calcium chloride ($CaCl_2 \cdot 2H_2O$—m.w. 147) are represented in 147 mL of a 10% w/v calcium chloride solution?

59. From the information in this chapter, calculate the daily water requirement for a healthy adult weighing 165 lb.

60. Estimate the plasma osmolality, in milliosmoles per kilogram, from the following data: sodium, 136 mEq/L; potassium, 5 mEq/L; blood urea nitrogen, 26 mg/100 mL; and glucose, 90 mg/dL.

CALCQUIZ

Note: In solving the following problems, refer to Table 12.2 as needed.

12.A. A veterinarian ordered a liter of *Hartmann's Irrigation* (Lactated Ringer's Irrigation) with the following formula:

Sodium Chloride	600 mg
Sodium Lactate	310 mg
Potassium Chloride	30 mg
Calcium Chloride, dihydrate	20 mg
Water for Injection, ad	100 mL

Calculate the mEq/L of Na^+, K^+, Ca^{2+}, Cl^-, and $C_3H_5O_3^-$.

12.B. Calculate the content of *Hartmann's Irrigation* in mOsmol/L.

12.C. A multiple electrolytes injection (PLASMA–LYTE) contains the following electrolytes in each 100 mL;

Sodium Chloride	526 mg
Sodium Gluconate	502 mg
Sodium Acetate trihydrate	368 mg
Potassium Chloride	37 mg
Magnesium Chloride	30 mg

The formula for sodium gluconate is $C_6H_{11}NaO_7$; for sodium acetate trihydrate, $C_2H_3NaO_2 \cdot 3H_2O$; and for magnesium chloride, $MgCl_2 \cdot 6H_2O$.
Calculate the mEq/L of Na^+ in the injection.

12.D.[a] A patient has been receiving lithium carbonate (Li_2CO_3) capsules but, due to difficulty in swallowing, needs to change to a liquid form. If the patient's dose of lithium carbonate is 300 mg three times a day, how many millimoles of lithium is the patient receiving per day? If lithium citrate syrup contains 300 mg of lithium citrate ($C_6H_5Li_3O_7$) per 5 mL, how many milliliters of syrup per day would be equivalent to the lithium in the capsules?

12.E.[a] A patient is receiving an intravenous infusion containing 40 mEq of potassium chloride in 1000 mL of Dextrose 5% in Half Normal Saline. The infusion has been running at a rate of 80 mL/h for the past 6.5 hours. Following a lab report showing the patient's serum potassium level to be 3.5 mEq/L, the physician decides to increase the potassium dose while slowing the infusion flow rate to 40 mL/h. The physician prescribes potassium chloride injection (14.9% KCl) to be added to the IV such that the patient will receive a total of 80 mEq of potassium over the remaining time for completion of the infusion. How many milliliters of the potassium chloride injection should be added by the pharmacist?

[a]Problem courtesy of Flynn Warren, Bishop, GA.

ANSWERS TO "CASE IN POINT" AND PRACTICE PROBLEMS

Case in Point 12.1

(a) $CaCl_2 \cdot 2H_2O$: m.w. = 147 g
Equivalent weight = 147/2 = 73.5 g
1 mEq = 0.735 g = 73.5 mg
10 mEq = 735 mg

Calcium chloride dihydrate in 10-mL vial
= 10 mL × 10% (w/v) = 1 g = 1000 mg

By proportion: $\dfrac{1000 \text{ mg}}{10 \text{ mL}} = \dfrac{735 \text{ mg}}{x \text{ mL}}$;

$x = 7.35$ mL, *answer*.

Thus, 7.35 mL of the injection contains 10 mEq of calcium and should be added to the 500-mL bag of normal saline solution.

(b) Since 0.5 mEq of calcium is to be administered per hour and there are 10 mEq of calcium in 507.35 mL of fluid (500 mL of NSS + 7.35 mL of calcium chloride dihydrate injection), the volume of fluid to be administered per hour may be calculated by proportion:

$\dfrac{10 \text{ mEq}}{507.35 \text{ mL}} = \dfrac{0.5 \text{ mEq}}{x \text{ mL}}$; $x = 25.37$ mL/h

Then, the milliliters to be delivered per minute may be calculated:

25.37 mL (per hour)/60 min
= 0.43 mL/min

Finally, the drops per minute may be calculated:

0.43 mL/min × 12 drops/mL
= 5.07 = 5 drops/min, *answer*.

Case in Point 12.2

(a) $\dfrac{15 \text{ drops}}{1 \text{ mL}} = \dfrac{12 \text{ drops}}{x \text{ mL}}$

= 0.8 mL administered per minute

0.8 mL/min × 60 min/hr × 15 hr
= 720 mL infused in 15 hr

$\dfrac{40 \text{ mEq KCl}}{1000 \text{ mL}} = \dfrac{x \text{ mEq}}{720 \text{ mL}} = 28.8$ mEq

KCl, *answer*.

(b) 39 (K) + 35.5 (Cl) = 74.5 molecular weight of KCl; monovalent salt, so 74.5 mg = 1 mEq

74.5 mg/mEq × 28.8 mEq = 2145.6 mg
÷ 1000 mg/g = 2.1456 g, *answer*.

(c) 74.5 mg KCl = 1 mmol KCl = 1 mEq KCl

74.5 mg KCl/mEq × 40 mEq KCl/1000 mL = 2980 mg KCl in 1000 mL

720 mL infused in 15 hr [from (a)]

$\dfrac{2980 \text{ mg KCl}}{1000 \text{ mL}} = \dfrac{x \text{ mg KCl}}{720 \text{ mL}}$;

$x = 2145.6$ mg KCl

$\dfrac{1 \text{ mmol KCl}}{74.5 \text{ mg}} = \dfrac{x \text{ mmol KCl}}{2145.6 \text{ mg}}$;

$x = 28.8$ mmol KCl, *answer*.

(d) *For the NaCl*

23 (Na) + 35.5 (Cl) = 58.5 mg, millimolecular weight of NaCl

$NaCl \rightarrow Na^+$ and Cl^- or 2 mOsmol/mmol of 58.8 mg

0.9% sodium chloride = 9 mg NaCl/mL × 1000 mL = 9000 mg NaCl in the IV fluid

$\dfrac{2 \text{ mOsmol}}{58.5 \text{ mg}} = \dfrac{x \text{ mOsmol}}{9000 \text{ mg}}$;

$x = 307.6923 \approx 308$ mOsmol NaCl per 1000 mL

For the KCl

39 (K) + 35.5 (Cl) = 74.5 mg = millimolecular weight of KCl

$KCl \rightarrow K^+$ and Cl^- or 2 mOsmol/mmol of 74.5 mg

2980 mg KCl in 1000 mL of infusion [from (c)]

$\dfrac{2 \text{ mOsmol}}{74.5 \text{ mg}} = \dfrac{x \text{ mOsmol}}{2980 \text{ mg}}$;

$x = 80$ mOsmol KCl per 1000 mL

For the dextrose

dextrose = 180 mg/mmol and does not hydrolyze, so 180 mg = 1 mOsmol

Dextrose 5% = 50 mg/mL × 1000 mL = 50,000 mg per 1000 mL of IV fluid

$$\frac{1\ \text{mOsmol}}{180\ \text{mg}} = \frac{x\ \text{mOsmol}}{50,000\ \text{mg}};$$

$$x = 277.7778 \approx 278\ \text{mOsmol}$$
$$\text{dextrose per 1000 mL}$$

Total osmolarity

mOsmol NaCl =   308
mOsmol KCl =   80
mOsmol dextrose = 278
total =   666 mOsmol/1000 mL
  of IV fluid, *answer.*

Note: The osmolarity of serum is about 300 mOsmol/L, so this solution is *hyperosmotic.*

Practice Problems

1. 10.69 to 42.78 μmol/L tobramycin
2. 3.001 mmol/mL phosphate
3. 4 mEq/mL potassium chloride
4. 9.4 mL ammonium chloride injection
5. 0.298% potassium chloride
6. 6.762 g calcium chloride
7. 100 mEq ammonium chloride
8. 14.73 mEq potassium
9. 180.18 g sodium chloride
10. 7.45 g potassium chloride
11. 20 mL potassium chloride solution
12. 1.37 mEq sodium
13. 2.5 mEq/mL sodium chloride
14. 74.928 g sodium bicarbonate
15. 131 mmol/L Na^+
    111 mmol/L Cl^-
    29 mmol/L $C_3H_5O_3^-$
    5 mmol/L K^+
    2 mmol/L Ca^{2+}
16. 166.67 mEq sodium lactate
17. 153.85 mEq/mL sodium chloride
18. 20.13 mEq potassium chloride
19. 9.34 mEq potassium
20. 4.36 mEq/L potassium
21. 162 g potassium citrate
22. 25 mEq potassium
23. 147 mEq sodium
    4.03 mEq potassium
    4.49 mEq calcium
    155.5 mEq chloride
24. 2.7 mEq sodium
25. (a) 100 mEq ammonium
    (b) 0.54% ammonium chloride
26. 0.2% sodium chloride
27. 5.42 mEq potassium
28. 25 mL sodium bicarbonate injection
29. 4.65 mEq calcium
30. 20.13 mEq potassium chloride
31. 32.43 mEq lithium
32. 785.05 mEq ammonium
33. (a) 28.08 g potassium gluconate
    (b) 60 mL syrup
34. 11.61 mEq potassium
35. 296 mg lithium carbonate
36. 300 mg magnesium sulfate
37. 30.2 or 30 mEq potassium chloride
38. 27.07 mEq/L sodium
    3.16 mEq/L magnesium
39. 16 ammonium chloride tablets
40. 1092 mL isotonic sodium chloride solution
41. 713 mL water
42. 120 mEq sodium
    38.27 mEq potassium
    8.87 mEq magnesium
43. 200.63 mL ammonium chloride solution
44. 7.78 to 15.56 mL calcium gluceptate injection
45. 1035 mg/L sodium
    1242.5 mg/L chloride
    780 mg/L potassium
    1890 mg/L citrate
46. 108.2 mEq/L sodium

47. 138.89 mL/h potassium acetate infusate

48. 129.8 mEq sodium
    105.6 mEq chloride

49. (a) 24.9 mEq potassium chloride
    (b) 12.45 mL potassium chloride injection
    (c) 645.47 mOsmol

50. 14 mOsmol

51. 512.82 mOsmol

52. 154 mOsmol/L

53. 555.56 mOsmol

54. 4000 mOsmol/mL

55. (a) 0.595 mEq/mL sodium bicarbonate
    (b) 297.6 mEq sodium bicarbonate
    (c) 1190.48 mOsmol/L

56. 2000 mOsmol/L

57. (a) 27.78 mL/h mannitol injection
    (b) 549.49 mOsmol mannitol

58. (a) 100 mmol calcium chloride
    (b) 200 mEq calcium chloride
    (c) 300 mOsmol calcium chloride

59. 2400 mL water

60. 296.29 mOsmol/kg

References

1. Prince SJ. Calculations. *International Journal of Pharmaceutical Compounding* 2001;5:485.
2. *United States Pharmacopeia 32 National Formulary 27*. Rockville, MD: United States Pharmacopeial Convention, 2009;(785)1:305–306.
3. VAPRO Vapor Pressure Osmometer [product literature]. Logan, UT: Wescor, Inc., 1997.
4. Berkow R, ed. *The Merck Manual*. 14th Ed. Rahway, NJ: Merck Sharpe & Dohme Research Laboratories, 1982: 922–952, 1833–1850.
5. The Fundamentals of Body Water and Electrolytes. Deerfield, IL: Travenol Laboratories, 1967.
6. Prince SJ. Calculations. *International Journal of Pharmaceutical Compounding* 1999;3:311.

Intravenous Infusions, Parenteral Admixtures, and Rate-of-Flow Calculations

13

Objectives

Upon successful completion of this chapter, the student will be able to:

- Perform calculations for standard adult and pediatric intravenous infusions.
- Perform calculations for additives to intravenous infusions.
- Perform rate-of-flow calculations for intravenous infusions utilizing medication orders, standard tables, and nomograms.

Injections

Injections are sterile pharmaceutical solutions or suspensions of a drug substance in an aqueous or nonaqueous vehicle. They are administered by needle into almost any part of the body, including the joints (*intra-articular*), joint fluid (*intrasynovial*), spinal column (*intraspinal*), spinal fluid (*intrathecal*), arteries (*intra-arterial*), and in an emergency, even the heart (*intracardiac*). However, most injections are administered into a vein (*intravenous, I.V., IV*), muscle (*intramuscular, I.M., IM*), skin (*intradermal, I.D., ID, intracutaneous*), or under the skin (*subcutaneous, sub-Q, SQ, hypodermic*).

Depending upon their use, injections are packaged in small volumes in *ampuls*[a] or in prefilled disposable syringes for single-dose use; in *vials* and pen-injectors for single- or multiple-dose use; or in large volume plastic bags or glass containers for administration by slow intravenous *infusion*.

Some injections are available as *prepared* solutions or suspensions with their drug content labeled as, for example, "10 mg/mL." Others contain dry powder for reconstitution *to form* a solution or suspension by adding a specified volume of diluent prior to use and are labeled as, for example, "10 mg/vial." In the latter case, the calculations required to determine the correct volume of diluent needed to prepare an injection of a certain concentration are provided in Chapter 17.

Small-volume injections may be administered as such or they may be used as *additives* to large-volume parenteral fluids for intravenous infusion. The term *parenteral* is defined as *any medication route other than the alimentary canal* and thus includes all routes of injection.

---

[a]An *ampul* (also *ampule* or *ampoule*) is a small hermetically sealed glass container.

Intravenous Infusions

Intravenous (IV) infusions are sterile, aqueous preparations administered intravenously in relatively large volumes. They are used to extend blood volume and/or provide electrolytes, nutrients, or medications. Most intravenous infusions are administered to critical care, infirm, dehydrated, or malnourished patients, or to patients prior to, during, and/or following surgery. Intravenous infusions are widely employed in emergency care units, in hospitals and other patient care institutions, and in home care. Pharmacists participate in the preparation and administration of institutional as well as home intravenous infusion therapy. The *United States Pharmacopeia* has established requirements for the compounding of sterile preparations.[1]

Most intravenous infusions are solutions; however, some are very fine dispersions of nutrients or therapeutic agents, or blood and blood products. Although some intravenous solutions are isotonic or nearly isotonic with blood, isotonicity is not absolutely necessary because the volumes of fluid usually administered are rapidly diluted by the circulating blood.[2]

Commercially prepared infusions are available in glass or plastic bottles or collapsible plastic "bags" in volumes of 50 mL (a *minibag*), 100 mL, 250 mL, 500 mL, and 1000 mL. The smaller volumes find particular application in treating pediatric patients and adults who require relatively small volumes of infusate. When a smaller IV bag is attached to the tubing of a larger IV being administered, it is referred to as an IV piggyback (IVPB). The abbreviation LVP is commonly used to indicate a *large-volume parenteral*, and SVP indicates a *small-volume parenteral*.

Some common solutions for intravenous infusion are listed in Table 13.1. Additional components or *additives* frequently are added to these basic solutions.

An *administration set* is attached to an intravenous bottle or bag to deliver the fluid into a patient's vein. The sets may be standard (macrodrip) or pediatric (microdrip). Depending on the particular set used, the drip rate can vary from 10 to 15 drops/mL for standard sets to 60 drops/mL for microdrip sets.[a]

Table 13.1 ▼ **SOME COMMON INTRAVENOUS INFUSION SOLUTIONS**

SOLUTION[a]	ABBREVIATION
0.9% Sodium Chloride	NS (Normal Saline)
0.45% Sodium Chloride	½NS
5% Dextrose in Water	D5W or D_5W
10% Dextrose in Water	D10W or $D_{10}W$
5% Dextrose in 0.9% Sodium Chloride	D5NS or D_5NS
5% Dextrose in 0.45% Sodium Chloride	D5½NS or $D_5$1/2NS
Lactated Ringer's (0.86% Sodium Chloride, 0.03% Potassium Chloride, 0.033% Calcium Chloride)	LR
5% Dextrose in Lactated Ringer's	D5LR or D_5LR

[a]All solutions are prepared in Water for Injection, USP. In addition to the solutions listed, other concentrations of dextrose and sodium chloride are commercially available. These solutions may be administered as such or used as vehicles for therapeutic agents, nutrients, or other additives.

---

[a]In some literature, particularly that of nursing, the abbreviations *gtt* for drop and *mcgtt* for microdrop are used.

The passage of an infusion solution into a patient's vein of entry may be assisted by gravity (the solution is hung on a stand well above the portal of entry) or by electronic volumetric infusion pumps. Some infusion pumps can be calibrated to deliver microinfusion volumes, such as 0.1 mL per hour, to as much as 2000 mL per hour, depending on the drug being administered and the requirements of the patient. Electronic controllers can be used to maintain the desired flow rate. The use of latest technology "smart" pumps can reduce intravenous administration errors by virtue of software that requires fewer human programming entries at the patient's bedside. Errors may also be reduced through the use of bar codes to ensure correct medication delivery, and through wireless technology that allows a nurse to monitor the rate of flow and the remaining volume of an infusion when not physically present in a patient's room.

In the administration of infusions, special needles or catheters provide intravenous entry for the intravenous fluid. Large-, intermediate-, and small-gauge (bore) needles or catheters are used, with the portal of entry selected based on the patient's age (i.e., adult, child, infant, or neonate) and the clinical circumstances. The narrower the gauge, the slower the flow rate and thus the longer period required to infuse a specified volume. Veins of the back of the hand, forearm, subclavian, jugular, and scalp (e.g., in premature neonates) may be used. Figure 13.1 depicts an intravenous fluid and attached administration set (see also Fig. 14.1). Figure 13.2 shows a typical intravenous set-up with a piggyback attachment.

Intravenous infusions may be continuous or intermittent. In ***continuous infusions***, large volumes of fluid (i.e., 250 to 1000 mL), with or without added drug, are run into a vein uninterrupted, whereas ***intermittent infusions*** are administered during scheduled periods.[2] The rapid infusion of a medication into a vein is termed ***IV push*** and is usually conducted in 1 to 5 minutes depending upon the medication.

Common Intravenous Infusion Solutions

Aqueous solutions of dextrose, sodium chloride, and lactated Ringer's solution are the most commonly used intravenous fluids. Table 13.1 describes the content of these solutions, which may be administered as such, or with additional drug or nutritional components.

Example Calculations of Basic Intravenous Infusions

How many grams each of dextrose and sodium chloride are used to prepare a 250-mL bag of D5½NS *for intravenous infusion?*

$$250 \text{ mL} \times 0.05 \ (5\% \text{ w/v}) = 12.5 \text{ g dextrose, and}$$
$$250 \text{ mL} \times 0.0045 \ (0.45\% \text{ w/v}) = 1.125 \text{ g sodium chloride, } answers.$$

Calculate the milliequivalents of sodium and millimoles of dextrose in the above solution.

Molecular weight of NaCl = 58.5 g
Equivalent weight of NaCl = 58.5 g
1 mEq NaCl = 58.5 mg
mEq in 1.125 g NaCl = 1125 mg/58.5 mg per 1 mEq = 19.2 mEq Na^+, and
Molecular weight of dextrose ($C_6H_{12}O_6$) = 180.16 g
1 mmol dextrose = 180.16 mg
mmol in 12.5 g dextrose = 12,500 mg/180.16 mg per 1 mmol
= 69.38 or 69.4 mmol, *answers.*

Medication port

Solution port and cover

Piercing device

Airway valve

Drip chamber

Back check valve

Injection or y site

Slide clamp

Roller clamp

Injection or y site

Threaded lock

Cap

▼ FIGURE 13.1 A depiction of an intravenous fluid with an administration set.

▼ FIGURE 13.2 A typical intravenous infusion set-up with a piggybacked antibiotic. (*Courtesy of Lacher B. Pharmaceutical Calculations for the Pharmacy Technician. Baltimore: Lippincott Williams & Wilkins, 2008.*)

A pharmacist prepared a liter of a 15% dextrose solution in sterile water for injection using a dextrose injection, 700 mg/mL. How many milliliters of the injection were required?

$$\text{Dextrose needed: } 1000 \text{ mL} \times 15\% = 150 \text{ g}$$
$$700 \text{ mg/mL} = 0.7 \text{ g/mL}$$
$$150 \text{ g} \times \frac{1 \text{ mL}}{0.7 \text{ g}} = 214.28 \text{ or } 214.3 \text{ mL}, \textit{ answer.}$$

Example Calculations of Infusion Administration Sets

Calculate the total drops in the delivery of 250 mL of an infusion when using the following administration sets: (a) 15 drops/mL, (b) 20 drops/mL, and (c) 60 mcgtts/mL.

(a) 15 drops/mL × 250 mL = 3750 drops, and
(b) 20 drops/mL × 250 mL = 5000 drops, and
(c) 60 microdrops/mL × 250 mL = 15,000 microdrops, *answers.*

For each of the above, calculate the number of drops delivered each minute if the infusion is to last 2 hours.

$$2 \text{ hours} = 120 \text{ minutes}$$
$$250 \text{ mL}/120 \text{ min} = 2.08 \text{ mL/min}$$

(a) 15 drops/mL × 2.08 mL (per minute) = 31.2 or 31 drops/min, and
(b) 20 drops/mL × 2.08 mL = 41.6 or 42 drops/min, and
(c) 60 microdrops/mL × 2.08 mL = 124.8 or 125 microdrops/min, *answers.*

$$\text{Or,}\quad \frac{250 \text{ mL}}{2 \text{ h}} \times \frac{1 \text{ h}}{60 \text{ min}} \times \frac{60 \text{ mcgtt}}{1 \text{ mL}} = \frac{15{,}000 \text{ mcgtt}}{120 \text{ min}} = 125 \text{ microdrops/minute}$$

Alternatively, the answers may be derived by dividing the total drops delivered by each administration set by the delivery time of 120 minutes:

(a) 3750 drops/120 min = 31.2 or 31 drops/min, and
(b) 5000 drops/120 min = 41.6 or 42 drops/min, and
(c) 15,000 microdrops/120 min = 125 microdrops/min, *answers.*

A rural patient is being transported by ambulance to a hospital 3 hours away. During transport, the patient is to be infused with 750 mL of normal saline injection. For each delivery set, calculate the rate of flow in drops/min: (a) 15 gtts/mL, (b) 20 gtts/mL, and (c) 60 mcgtts/mL.

$$3 \text{ hours} = 180 \text{ minutes}$$
$$750 \text{ mL}/180 \text{ min} = 4.17 \text{ mL/min}$$

(a) 15 drops/mL × 4.17 mL/min = 62.55 or 63 drops/min, and
(b) 20 drops/mL × 4.17 mL/min = 83.4 or 83 drops/min, and
(c) 60 microdrops/mL × 4.17 mL/min = 250.2 or 250 microdrops/min, *answers.*

$$\text{Or,}\quad \frac{750 \text{ mL}}{3 \text{ h}} \times \frac{1 \text{ h}}{60 \text{ min}} \times \frac{60 \text{ mcgtt}}{1 \text{ mL}} = \frac{45{,}000 \text{ mcgtt}}{180 \text{ min}} = 250 \text{ microdrops/minute}$$

Or,

(a) 750 mL × 15 gtts/mL = 11,250 drops
    11,250/180 min = 62.5 or 63 drops/min, and
(b) 750 mL × 20 gtts/mL = 15,000 drops
    15,000 drops/180 min = 83.3 or 83 drops/min, and
(c) 750 mL × 60 mcgtts/mL = 45,000 microdrops
    45,000 mcgtts/180 min = 250 microdrops/min, *answers.*

Compare (a) the number of drops and (b) the length of time, in minutes, required to deliver 50-mL of intravenous solutions when using a microdrip set, at 60 drops/mL, and a standard administration set, at 15 drops/mL, if in each case one drop is to be administered per second.

Microdrip set:
(a) 60 drops/mL × 50 mL = 3000 drops
(b) 3000 drops ÷ 60 drops/minute = 50 minutes, *answers.*

Standard set:
(a) 15 drops/mL × 50 mL = 750 drops
(b) 750 drops ÷ 60 drops/minute = 12.5 minutes, *answers.*

Or, by dimensional analysis:

$$50 \text{ mL} \times \frac{60 \text{ drops}}{1 \text{ mL}} \times \frac{1 \text{ min}}{60 \text{ drops}} = 50 \text{ minutes, } answer.$$

$$50 \text{ mL} \times \frac{15 \text{ drops}}{1 \text{ mL}} \times \frac{1 \text{min}}{60 \text{ drops}} = 12.5 \text{ minutes, } answer.$$

Intravenous Push (IVP) Drug Administration

The rapid injection of intravenous medications, as in emergency or critical care situations, is termed *IV push, IVP, IV Stat*, or sometimes a **bolus** dose. For the most part, drugs administered by IV push are intended to quickly control heart rate, blood pressure, cardiac output, respiration, or other life-threatening conditions. Intravenous push medications frequently are administered in a short time frame (from less than 1 to 5 minutes), but slowly enough so as to not cause a too-rapid effect. The safe administration of a drug by IV push depends on precise calculations of dose and rate of administration. When feasible, a diluted injection rather than a highly concentrated one (e.g., 1 mg/mL versus 5 mg/mL) may be administered as an added safety precaution.[3]

The IV push may be injected directly into a vein or into a portal of an intravenous set. If the medication is administered via an administration set, a second injection of saline may be used to "flush" or help to push the medication into the bloodstream. A *flush* also may be used to clean an infusion line before and/or after use. An example of an intravenous *flush syringe* is shown in Figure 13.3.

Example Calculations of IV Push Drug Administration

A physician orders enalaprilat (VASOTEC IV) 2 mg IVP for a hypertensive patient. A pharmacist delivers several 1-mL injections, each containing 1.25 mg of enalaprilat. How many milliliters of the injection should be administered?

▼ FIGURE 13.3 An intravenous flush syringe. *(Courtesy of Becton Dickinson.)*

$$\frac{1.25 \text{ mg}}{1 \text{ mL}} = \frac{2 \text{ mg}}{x \text{ mL}}; x = 1.6 \text{ mL (1 mL from one syringe and 0.6 mL from another)}, \textit{answer}.$$

Or, by dimensional analysis:

$$2 \text{ mg} \times \frac{1 \text{ mL}}{1.25 \text{ mg}} = 1.6 \text{ mL}, \textit{ answer}.$$

A physician orders midazolam hydrochloride (VERSED) 2 mg IV Stat. A pharmacist delivers a vial containing midazolam hydrochloride 5 mg/mL. How many milliliters should be administered?

$$\frac{5 \text{ mg}}{1 \text{ mL}} = \frac{2 \text{ mg}}{x \text{ mL}}; x = 0.4 \text{ mL}, \textit{ answer}.$$

Or, by dimensional analysis:

$$2 \text{ mg} \times \frac{1 \text{ mL}}{5 \text{ mg}} = 0.4 \text{ mL}, \textit{ answer}.$$

General guidelines in the treatment of severe diabetic ketoacidosis include an initial bolus dose of 0.1 to 0.4 unit of insulin/kg IVP, followed by an insulin drip. Calculate the bolus dosage range for a 200-lb patient.

$$200 \text{ lb} \div 2.2 \text{ lb/kg} = 90.9 \text{ kg},$$
$$90.9 \text{ kg} \times 0.1 \text{ unit/kg} = 9.09 \text{ units, and}$$
$$90.9 \text{ kg} \times 0.4 \text{ unit/kg} = 36.36 \text{ units}, \textit{answers}.$$

Special Considerations in Pediatric IV Infusion Delivery

Medication errors in pediatric patients is a special concern in institutional practice.[4] There is the ever-present need for weight-based dosing and highly individualized dose calculations that must be diligently performed. A reduction in errors has been achieved by the use of web-based calculators to perform infusion calculations, use of a limited number of standardized drug concentrations to prepare infusions (as noted below), and the utilization of smart-pump technology that reduces the number of human calculations required in dose and rate-of-flow determinations.

Depending on the institutional protocol, a medication order for an intravenous infusion for a 10-kg child may be stated as, for example, "dopamine 60 mg/100 mL, IV to run at 5 mL/hr to give 5 mcg/kg/min." At some institutions in which *standardized drug products and established protocols* have been developed, the same medication order may be written simply as "dopamine 5 mcg/kg/min IV" to provide equivalently accurate drug dosing of the patient.[5] This is because the standard solution of dopamine used in the institution, containing 60 mg of dopamine in each 100 mL and run at 5 mL/hr, *would deliver the same dose of 5 mcg/kg/min* to the 10-kg patient. Calculate it:

$$\frac{60 \text{ mg}}{100 \text{ mL}} = \frac{x \text{ mg}}{5 \text{ mL}}; x = 3 \text{ mg or 3000 mcg dopamine administered per hour}$$

$$3000 \text{ mcg} \div 60 \text{ min/hr} = 50 \text{ mcg dopamine administered per minute}$$

Since the 50 mcg/min are administered to a 10-kg child, the dose, per kg per minute, is:

$$\frac{50 \text{ mcg}}{10 \text{ kg}} = \frac{x \text{ mcg}}{1 \text{ kg}}; \ x = 5 \text{ mcg dopamine/kg/min, } answer.$$

Or, by dimensional analysis:

$$\frac{60 \text{ mg}}{100 \text{ mL}} \times \frac{1000 \text{ mcg}}{1 \text{ mg}} \times \frac{5 \text{ mL}}{1 \text{ hr}} \times \frac{1 \text{ hr}}{60 \text{ min}} =$$

$$50 \text{ mcg/min (dose for 10-kg child)} = 5 \text{ mcg/kg/min}$$

All medication doses for pediatric patients, including those administered intravenously, must be carefully determined from available literature and reference sources.

In addition to medications administered by intravenous infusion to pediatric patients, fluid and electrolyte therapy is especially important in the clinical management of preterm and term neonates, particularly those with extremely low birth weights who tend to have greater loss of water through the skin, especially when they are maintained in a warm incubator.[6]

Example Calculations of Pediatric Infusions

Calculate the daily infusion volume of D10W to be administered to a neonate weighing 3 lb. 8 oz. on the basis of 60 mL/kg/day.

$$3 \text{ lb. 8 oz.} = 3.5 \text{ lb.} \div 2.2 \text{ lb./kg} = 1.59 \text{ kg or } 1.6 \text{ kg}$$
$$1.6 \text{ kg} \times 60 \text{ mL} = 96 \text{ mL, } answer.$$

Using an administration set that delivers 60 drops/mL at 20 drops per minute, calculate the total time for the above infusion.

$$96 \text{ mL} \times \frac{60 \text{ drops}}{1 \text{ mL}} \times \frac{1 \text{ minute}}{20 \text{ drops}} = 288 \text{ minutes, or 4 hours 48 minutes, } answer.$$

Gentamicin sulfate, 2.5 mg/kg, is prescribed for a 1.5-kg neonate. Calculate (a) the dose of the drug, and (b) when the drug is placed in a 50-mL IV bag, the flow rate, in mL/minute, if the infusion is to run for 30 minutes.

(a) $2.5 \text{ mg/kg} \times 1.5 \text{ kg} = 3.75 \text{ mg gentamicin sulfate}$
(b) $50 \text{ mL} \div 30 \text{ minutes} = 1.67 \text{ mL/minute, } answers.$

A neonate born at 32 weeks' gestation weighs 2005 g and is transferred to the hospital's neonate intensive care unit with a diagnosis of sepsis. Among the physician's orders are aminophylline 5 mg/ kg IV q6h, cefotaxime 50 mg/kg q12h, and vancomycin 10 mg/kg q12h.[7]

(a) *Calculate the initial dose of each drug, in milligrams.*

$$\text{Neonate's weight} = 2005 \text{ g} \times \frac{1 \text{ kg}}{1000 \text{ g}} = 2.005 \text{ kg}$$

$$\text{Aminophylline initial dose} = 5 \text{ mg/kg} \times 2.005 \text{ kg} = 10.025 \text{ or } 10 \text{ mg, and}$$
$$\text{Cefotaxime initial dose} = 50 \text{ mg/kg} \times 2.005 \text{ kg} = 100.25 \text{ or } 100 \text{ mg, and}$$
$$\text{Vancomycin initial dose} = 10 \text{ mg/kg} \times 2.005 \text{ kg} = 20.05 \text{ or } 20 \text{ mg, } answers.$$

(b) *If aminophylline injection, 25 mg/mL, is available, how many milliliters of injection should be added to a 100-mL container of D10W for IV infusion?*

$$10 \text{ mg} \times \frac{1 \text{ mL}}{25 \text{ g}} = 0.4 \text{ mL, } answer.$$

A 4-day-old neonate born at 35 weeks' gestation and weighing 2210 g is prescribed gentamicin, 4 mg/kg, in 60 mL/kg of D10W for intravenous infusion.[7] If a pediatric injection contains gentamicin, 10 mg/mL, how many milliliters each of injection and D10W should be administered?

$$\text{Neonate's weight} = 2210 \text{ g} \times \frac{1 \text{ kg}}{1000 \text{ g}} = 2.21 \text{ kg}$$

$$\text{Gentamicin dose} = 4 \text{ mg/kg} \times 2.21 \text{ kg} = 8.84 \text{ mg}$$

$$\text{Gentamicin injection to administer} = 8.84 \text{ mg} \times \frac{1 \text{ mL}}{10 \text{ mg}} = 0.884 \text{ or } 0.9 \text{ mL, and}$$

$$\text{D10W to administer} = 60 \text{ mL/kg} \times 2.21 \text{ kg} = 132.6 \text{ mL, } \textit{answers.}$$

A 2-year-old child weighing 30 lb is hospitalized with severe respiratory distress. Physicians' orders include aminophylline 5 mg/kg in 50-mL D5W½NS to infuse over 60 minutes. If aminophylline injection, 25 mg/mL, is available, how many milliliters should be used in the infusion?

$$\text{Child's weight} = 30 \text{ lb} \times \frac{1 \text{ kg}}{2.2 \text{ lb}} = 13.6 \text{ kg}$$

$$\text{Aminophylline dose} = 5 \text{ mg/kg} \times 13.6 \text{ kg} = 68 \text{ mg}$$

$$\text{Aminophylline injection to use} = 68 \text{ mg} \times \frac{1 \text{ mL}}{22 \text{ mg}} = 2.72 \text{ or } 2.7 \text{ mL, } \textit{answer.}$$

Intravenous Admixtures

The preparation of an intravenous admixture involves the transfer of one or more additives to a large-volume parenteral fluid. The additive may be incorporated into the fluid in the pharmacy, or at the patient's bedside by injecting the additive into a port of the intravenous line or by administering by piggyback. Additives may include therapy-specific medications, antibiotics, electrolytes, vitamins, trace minerals, and other agents. Figure 13.4 shows the transfer of an additive to a large volume fluid prior to administration.

Examples of calculations involving additives for *pediatric patients* are provided above and further examples are provided as follows.

Example Calculations of Additives to Intravenous Infusion Solutions

A medication order for a patient weighing 154 lb. calls for 0.25 mg of amphotericin B per kilogram of body weight to be added to 500 mL of 5% dextrose injection. If the amphotericin B is to be obtained from a constituted injection that contains 50 mg/10 mL, how many milliliters should be added to the dextrose injection?

$$1 \text{ kg} = 2.2 \text{ lb.}$$

$$\frac{154 \text{ (lb.)}}{2.2 \text{ (lb.)}} = 70 \text{ kg}$$

$$0.25 \text{ mg} \times 70 = 17.5 \text{ mg}$$

Constituted solution contains 50 mg/10 mL:

$$\frac{50 \text{ (mg)}}{17.5 \text{ (mg)}} = \frac{10 \text{ (mL)}}{x \text{ (mL)}}$$

$$x = 3.5 \text{ mL, } \textit{answer.}$$

▼ FIGURE 13.4 The transfer of an additive to a large-volume parenteral solution. *(Courtesy of Millipore Corporation.)*

Or, solving by dimensional analysis:

$$154 \text{ lb.} \times \frac{1 \text{ kg}}{2.2 \text{ lb.}} \times \frac{0.25 \text{ mg}}{1 \text{ kg}} \times \frac{10 \text{ mL}}{50 \text{ mg}} = 3.5 \text{ mL}, \textit{ answer.}$$

An intravenous infusion is to contain 15 mEq of potassium ion and 20 mEq of sodium ion in 500 mL of 5% dextrose injection. Using potassium chloride injection containing 6 g/30 mL and 0.9% sodium chloride injection, how many milliliters of each should be used to supply the required ions?

15 mEq of K⁺ ion will be supplied by 15 mEq of KCl, and 20 mEq of Na⁺ ion will be supplied by 20 mEq of NaCl

$$1 \text{ mEq of KCl} = 74.5 \text{ mg}$$
$$15 \text{ mEq of KCl} = 1117.5 \text{ mg or } 1.118 \text{ g}$$
$$\frac{6 \text{ (g)}}{1.118 \text{ (g)}} = \frac{30 \text{ (mL)}}{\text{x (mL)}}$$
$$\text{x} = 5.59 \text{ or } 5.6 \text{ mL}, \textit{ and}$$

$$1 \text{ mEq of NaCl} = 58.5 \text{ mg}$$
$$20 \text{ mEq of NaCl} = 1170 \text{ mg or } 1.170 \text{ g}$$
$$\frac{0.9 \text{ (g)}}{1.17 \text{ (g)}} = \frac{100 \text{ (mL)}}{\text{x (mL)}}$$
$$\text{x} = 130 \text{ mL}, \textit{ answers.}$$

Or, solving by dimensional analysis:

$$15 \text{ mEq} \times \frac{74.5 \text{ mg}}{1 \text{ mEq}} \times \frac{1 \text{ g}}{1000 \text{ mg}} \times \frac{30 \text{ mL}}{6 \text{ g}} = 5.59 \text{ or } 5.6 \text{ mL, and}$$

$$20 \text{ mEq} \times \frac{58.5 \text{ mg}}{1 \text{ mEq}} \times \frac{1 \text{ g}}{1000 \text{ mg}} \times \frac{100 \text{ mL}}{0.9 \text{ g}} = 130 \text{ mL}, \text{ } answers.$$

A medication order for a child weighing 44 lb. calls for polymyxin B sulfate to be administered by the intravenous drip method in a dosage of 7500 units/kg of body weight in 500 mL of 5% dextrose injection. Using a vial containing 500,000 units of polymyxin B sulfate and sodium chloride injection as the solvent, explain how you would obtain the polymyxin B sulfate needed in preparing the infusion.

$$1 \text{ kg} = 2.2 \text{ lb.}$$

$$\frac{44}{2.2} = 20 \text{ kg}$$

$$7500 \text{ units} \times 20 = 150,000 \text{ units}$$

Step 1. Dissolve contents of vial (500,000 units) in 10 mL of sodium chloride injection.
Step 2. Add 3 mL of constituted solution to 500 mL of 5% dextrose injection, *answer.*

Rate of Flow of Intravenous Fluids

On medication orders, the physician specifies the rate of flow of intravenous fluids in milliliters per minute, drops per minute, amount of drug (as milligrams per hour), or, more frequently, as the approximate duration of time of administration of the total volume of the infusion. Pharmacists may be called on to perform or check rate-of-flow calculations as those described in some previous problem examples as well as those in this section.

Oftentimes, the following equation finds use in rate-of-flow calculations:

$$\text{Rate of flow (drops/minute)} = \frac{\text{Volume infusion (mL)} \times \text{Drip set (drops/mL)}}{\text{Time (minutes)}}$$

In common usage are *macro sets* that deliver 10, 15, or 20 drops per milliliter and *microdrip* or *minidrip sets* that deliver 60 drops per milliliter.

Examples of Rate-of-Flow Calculations

A medication order calls for 1000 mL of D5W to be administered over an 8-hour period. Using an IV administration set that delivers 10 drops/mL, how many drops per minute should be delivered to the patient?

$$\text{Volume of fluid} = 1000 \text{ mL}$$

$$8 \text{ hours} = 480 \text{ minutes}$$

$$\frac{1000 \text{ (mL)}}{480 \text{ (minutes)}} = 2.08 \text{ mL per minute}$$

$$2.08 \text{ mL/min} \times 10 \text{ (drops/mL)} = 20.8 \text{ or } 21 \text{ drops per minute, } answer.$$

Or, solving by dimensional analysis:

$$\frac{10 \text{ drops}}{1 \text{ mL}} \times \frac{1000 \text{ mL}}{8 \text{ hr}} \times \frac{1 \text{ hr}}{60 \text{ min}} = 20.8, \text{ or } 21 \text{ drops per minute, } answer.$$

Or, solving by the equation:

$$\text{Rate of flow (drops/minute)} = \frac{\text{Volume infused (mL)} \times \text{Drip set (drops/mL)}}{\text{Time (minutes)}}$$

$$= \frac{1000 \text{ mL} \times 10 \text{ drops/mL}}{480 \text{ minutes}}$$

$$= 20.8 \text{ or } 21 \text{ drops per minute, } \textit{answer.}$$

Ten (10) milliliters of 10% calcium gluconate injection and 10 mL of multivitamin infusion are mixed with 500 mL of a 5% dextrose injection. The infusion is to be administered over 5 hours. If the dropper in the venoclysis set calibrates 15 drops/mL, at what rate, in drops per minute, should the flow be adjusted to administer the infusion over the desired time interval?

Total volume of infusion =
10 mL + 10 mL + 500 mL = 520 mL
Dropper calibrates 15 drops/mL
520×15 drops = 7800 drops

$$\frac{7800 \text{ (drops)}}{300 \text{ (minutes)}} = 26 \text{ drops per minute, } \textit{answer.}$$

Or, solving by dimensional analysis:

$$\frac{15 \text{ drops}}{1 \text{ mL}} \times \frac{520 \text{ mL}}{5 \text{ hours}} \times \frac{1 \text{ hr}}{60 \text{ min}} = 26 \text{ drops per minute, } \textit{answer.}$$

Or, solving by the equation:

$$\text{Rate of flow (drops/minute)} = \frac{\text{Volume infused (mL)} \times \text{Drip set (drops/mL)}}{\text{Time (minutes)}}$$

$$= \frac{520 \text{ mL} \times 15 \text{ drops/mL}}{300 \text{ minutes}}$$

$$= 26 \text{ drops per minute, } \textit{answer.}$$

An intravenous infusion contains 10 mL of a 1:5000 solution of isoproterenol hydrochloride and 500 mL of a 5% dextrose injection. At what flow rate should the infusion be administered to provide 5 μg of isoproterenol hydrochloride per minute, and what time interval will be necessary for the administration of the entire infusion?

10 mL of a 1:5000 solution contain 2 mg
2 mg or 2000 μg are contained in a volume of 510 mL

$$\frac{2000 \text{ (μg)}}{5 \text{ (μg)}} = \frac{510 \text{ (mL)}}{x \text{ (mL)}}$$

$$x = 1.275 \text{ or } 1.28 \text{ mL per minute, } \textit{and}$$

$$\frac{1.28 \text{ (mL)}}{510 \text{ (mL)}} = \frac{1 \text{ (minute)}}{x \text{ (minutes)}}$$

$$x = 398 \text{ minutes or approx. } 6\tfrac{1}{2} \text{ hours, } \textit{answers.}$$

Or, solving by dimensional analysis:

$$\frac{1 \text{ min}}{5 \text{ μg}} \times \frac{0.002 \text{ g}}{510 \text{ mL}} \times \frac{1,000,000 \text{ μg}}{1 \text{ g}} \times 510 \text{ mL} = 400 \text{ minutes} \approx 6 \tfrac{1}{2} \text{ hours, } \textit{answer.}$$

If 10 mg of a drug are added to a 500-mL large-volume parenteral fluid:

(a) what should be the rate of flow, in milliliters per hour, to deliver 1 mg of drug per hour?

$$\frac{10 \ (mg)}{1 \ (mg)} = \frac{500 \ (mL)}{x \ (mL)}$$
$$x = 50 \ mL \text{ per hour, } answer.$$

(b) If the infusion set delivers 15 drops/mL, what should be the rate of flow in drops per minute?

$$15 \text{ drops/mL} \times 50 \text{ mL/hr} = 750 \text{ drops per hour}$$
$$\frac{750 \ (drops)}{x \ (drops)} = \frac{60 \ (minutes)}{1 \ (minute)}$$
$$x = 12.5 \text{ drops/minute, } answer.$$

Or, solving by dimensional analysis:

$$\frac{15 \text{ drops}}{1 \text{ mL}} \times \frac{50 \text{ mL}}{1 \text{ hr}} \times \frac{1 \text{ hr}}{60 \text{ min}} = 12.5 \text{ drops per minute, } answer.$$

(c) How many hours should the total infusion last?

$$\frac{50 \ (mL)}{500 \ (mL)} = \frac{1 \ (hour)}{x \ (hour)}$$
$$x = 10 \text{ hours, } answer.$$

A physician's medication order calls for 800 mg of erythromycin to be added to 100 mL of D5W for intravenous infusion over 60 minutes. The source of erythromycin is a 1-g vial requiring dilution to 20 mL with sterile water for injection before being added to the D5W. Calculate (a) the milliliters of the erythromycin dilution that should be added to the D5W and (b) the rate of flow of the infusion, in milliliters per minute.

(a) $\dfrac{1 \text{ g}}{20 \text{ mL}} = \dfrac{0.8 \text{ g}}{x}$; x = 16 mL, *answer.*

(b) 100 mL (D5W) + 16 mL (erythromycin dilution) = 116 mL
116 mL/60 min = 1.93 mL/min, *answer.*

A physician's medication order calls for 400 mg of clindamycin to be added to 600 mL of D5W for intravenous infusion over 90 minutes. Clindamycin is available as an injection containing 600 mg/4 mL. (a) How many milliliters of the clindamycin injection should be used, (b) how many mg/mL of clindamycin will the infusion contain, and (c) how many milliliters per minute of the infusion should be delivered?

(a) $\dfrac{600 \text{ mg}}{4 \text{ mL}} = \dfrac{400 \text{ mg}}{x}$; x = 2.67 mL, *answer.*

(b) infusion = 600 mL (D5W) + 2.67 mL (clindamycin injection) = 602.67 mL
400 mg clindamycin/602.67 mL infusion = clindamycin 0.66 mg/mL, *answer.*

(c) 602.67 mL/90 min = 6.69 or 6.7 mL/min, *answer.*

An intravenous fluid that contains 25 mg nitroglycerin in 250 mL is to be administered at 20 μg/min. Calculate the correct drip rates, in drops/min, from administration sets which deliver (a) 15 drops/mL, (b) 20 drops/mL, and (c) 60 drops/mL.

25 mg in 250 mL = 0.1 mg/mL = 100 μg/mL
Therefore, *20 μg/min* = 0.2 mL/min

Thus,

(a) 15 drops/mL × 0.2 mL/min = 3 drops/min, and
(b) 20 drops/mL × 0.2 mL/min = 4 drops/min, and
(c) 60 drops/mL × 0.2 mL/min = 12 drops/min, *answers.*

IV Infusion Rate Calculations for the Critical Care Patient

Many patients, including those in critical care, require both a maintenance fluid, as D5W, and a therapeutic drug additive, as an antibiotic (see Fig. 13.2). However, many critical care patients have fluid restrictions and must be maintained and treated within a stated maximum volume of fluid intake per day. Thus, consideration must be given to the *rate* and *volumes* of any infusions administered including intravenous piggybacked (IVPB) additives.

Example:

An order for a patient, with a 3-liter daily IV fluid limit, calls for 3 L of D5W with a 100-mL IVPB antibiotic to be run-in alone over a 1-hour period and administered every 6 hours. The administration set is calibrated to deliver 10 drops per milliliter. Calculate:

(a) *The flow rate of the IVPB antibiotic;*
(b) *The total flow time for the IV antibiotic;*
(c) *The total volume for the IV antibiotic;*
(d) *The total flow time for the D5W;*
(e) *The total volume for the D5W;*
(f) *The flow rate for the D5W.*

(a) $\dfrac{10 \text{ mL} \times 10 \text{ drops/mL}}{60 \text{ min}}$ = 16.6 or 17 drops per minute;

(b) 1 hour × 4 times a day = 4 hours or 240 minutes;
(c) 100 mL × 4 times a day = 400 mL;
(d) 24 hours − 4 hours (run time for the antibiotic) = 20 hours or 1200 minutes;
(e) 3000 mL − 400 mL (the IVPB antibiotic) = 2600 mL;

(f) $\dfrac{2600 \text{ mL} \times 10 \text{ drops/mL}}{1200 \text{ min}}$ = 21.6 or 22 drops per minute, *answers.*

Using a Nomogram

A nomogram, as that shown in Figure 13.5, may be used in determining the rate of flow of a parenteral fluid. Given the volume to be administered, the infusion time (duration), and the drops per milliliter delivered by the infusion set, the rate of flow, in drops per minute, may be determined directly.

Example:

If 1 liter of a parenteral fluid is to be infused over a 12-hour period using an infusion set that delivers 20 drops/mL, what should be the rate of flow in drops per minute?

First, locate the intercept of the diagonal line representing an infusion time of 12 hours with the horizontal line representing 1 liter of fluid. Next, follow the point of the intercept down to the drop counter scale representing "20 drops/mL" to determine the answer. In the example, the horizontal line would be crossed between 20 and 30 drops per minute—closer to the 30, or approximately 28 drops per minute, *answer.*

Nomogram for number of drops per minute

The number of drops per minute required to administer a particular quantity of infusion solution in a certain time can be read off directly from this nomogram. The nomogram allows for the increase in drop size as the dropping rate increases and is based on the normal drop defined by the relationship: 20 drops distilled water at 15° C = 1 g (±0.05 g) when falling at the rate of 60/min. The dependence of drop size on dropping rate is allowed for by the increasing width of the scale units of the three abscissae as the dropping rate. increases.

▼ FIGURE 13.5 Rate of flow versus quantity of infusion solution versus time nomogram. *(From Documenta Geigy Scientific Tables, 7th Ed., 1970. With permission of Ciba-Geigy Limited, Basel, Switzerland.)*

As a check to the proper use of the nomogram, the preceding example may be calculated as follows:

$$\text{Infusion time} = 12 \text{ hours} = 720 \text{ minutes}$$
$$\text{Infusion fluid} = 1 \text{ liter} = 1000 \text{ mL}$$
$$\text{Drops per milliliter} = 20$$
$$\text{Total drops in infusion liquid} = 20 \text{ drops/mL} \times 1000 \text{ mL} = 20,000$$
$$\frac{20,000 \text{ (drops)}}{720 \text{ (minutes)}} = 27.7 \text{ or } 28 \text{ drops per minute, } \textit{answer.}$$

Or, solving by dimensional analysis:

$$\frac{20 \text{ drops}}{1 \text{ mL}} \times \frac{1000 \text{ mL}}{12 \text{ hrs}} \times \frac{1 \text{ hr}}{60 \text{ min}} = 27.7 \text{ or } 28 \text{ drops per minute, } \textit{answer.}$$

Or, solving by the equation:

$$\text{Rate of flow (drops/minute)} = \frac{\text{Volume infused (mL)} \times \text{Drip set (drops/mL)}}{\text{Time (minutes)}}$$

$$= \frac{1000 \text{ mL} \times 20 \text{ drops/mL}}{720 \text{ minutes}}$$

$$= 27.7 \text{ or } 28 \text{ drops per minute, } \textit{answer.}$$

Table 13.2 ▼ **INFUSION RATE OF A HYPOTHETICAL DRUG FOR A CONCENTRATION OF 0.2 mg/mL**

PATIENT WEIGHT (kg)	DRUG DELIVERY RATE (mcg/kg per minute)								
	5	6	7	8	9	10	11	12	13
	INFUSION DELIVERY RATE (mL/hr)								
30	45	54	63	72	81	90	99	108	117
35	53	63	74	84	95	105	116	126	137
40	60	72	84	96	108	120	132	144	156
45	68	81	95	108	122	135	149	162	176
50	75	90	105	120	135	150	165	180	195
55	83	99	116	132	149	165	182	198	215
60	90	108	126	144	162	180	198	216	234
65	98	117	137	156	176	195	215	234	254
70	105	126	147	168	189	210	231	252	273
75	113	135	158	180	203	225	248	270	293
80	120	144	168	192	216	240	264	288	312
90	135	162	189	216	243	270	297	324	351
100	150	180	210	240	270	300	330	360	390

Using an Infusion Rate Table

An infusion rate table, as exemplified by Table 13.2, may accompany a commercial product to facilitate dosing. The composition of the example table is based on the concentration of the infusion solution to be used, the desired dose of the drug, and the patient's weight. Other tables may be designed differently; for example, rather than the patient's weight, the

---

CALCULATIONS CAPSULE

Intravenous Infusions

In certain calculations, the following equations find application.

To calculate infusion time:

$$\text{Infusion time} = \frac{\text{Volume of infusion in mL}}{\text{Flow rate in mL/hr or mL/min}}$$

To calculate flow rate in drops/minute:

$$\text{Rate of flow (drops/minute)} = \frac{\text{Volume infused (mL)} \times \text{Drip set (drops/mL)}}{\text{Time (minutes)}}$$

To calculate flow rate in mL/hour when based on dose[4]:

$$\text{Infusion rate (mL/hr)} = \frac{\text{Patient's weight (kg)} \times \text{Dose (mcg, mg, or units/kg/min)} \times 60}{\text{Drug concentration, infusion (mcg, mg, or units/mL)}}$$

In using this equation, the denominations for the dose and drug concentration must be the same (e.g., mcg, mg, or units). Also, if the dosage rate is stated in hours (e.g., mcg/kg/hr), the 60 is not needed in the equation to arrive at flow rate per hour.

CASE IN POINT 13.1 A physician prescribes amiodarone HCl IV (CORDARONE) for a patient with ventricular fibrillation. The prescribing information is:

Loading infusions:

Rapid infusion over first 10 minutes:	15 mg/min
Slow infusion over the next 6 hours:	1 mg/min

Maintenance infusion:

Slow infusion over the remaining 18 hours:	0.5 mg/min

Amiodarone HCl IV is available in 3-mL ampuls containing 50 mg/mL.
The pharmacist uses a 100-mL bag of D5W for the rapid infusion and 250-mL bottles of D5W for the slow infusions.

(a) How many milliliters from an amiodarone HCl IV ampul should be placed in the 100-mL bag for the rapid infusion?
(b) What is the drug concentration in the rapid infusion, in mg/mL?
(c) If the pharmacist added the contents of 3 ampuls to each 250-mL bottle of D5W needed for the slow infusions, calculate the drug concentration in mg/mL.
(d) What rate of administration, in mL/hr, should the pharmacist have recommend during the 6-hour infusion segment?
(e) Calculate the rate of administration in (d) in drops/minute with an administration set that delivers 15 drops/mL.
(f) Calculate the milligrams of drug administered by slow infusion over the 6-hour segment.
(g) Make the same calculation as that in (f) but over the 18-hour segment.

patient's body surface area, in square meters, may be used. In each case, however, the table provides guidelines for the delivery rate of an infusion. Table 13.2 is used by matching the column of the desired drug delivery rate against the patient's weight to yield the infusion delivery rate in mL/hr.

Examples:

Using Table 13.2, determine the delivery rate, in mL/hr, for a drug to be administered at 10 mcg/kg/minute to a patient weighing 65 kg.

$$\text{Drug delivery rate} = 10 \text{ mcg/kg/minute}$$
$$\text{Patient weight} = 65 \text{ kg}$$
$$\text{Table intercept} = 195 \text{ mL/hr, } answer.$$

If the infusion pump used in the previous example delivers 60 microdrops per milliliter, how many microdrops would be administered to the patient per minute?

$$195 \text{ (mL/hr)} \times 60 \text{ (microdrops/mL)} = 11,700 \text{ (microdrops/hr)}$$
$$11,700 \text{ (microdrops/hr)} \div 60 \text{ (minutes/hr)} = 195 \text{ microdrops per minute, } answer.$$

Calculate the entry shown in Table 13.2 for the infusion delivery rate as determined in the first example problem (i.e., 195 mL/hr).

Drug concentration: 0.2 mg/mL = 200 mcg/mL
Desired delivery rate: 10 mcg/kg/min
Patient weight: 65 kg

Drug to be delivered = 10 (mcg/kg/min) × 65 (kg) = 650 mcg/min
650 (mcg/min) × 60 (min) = 3900 mcg/hr
Infusion delivery rate = 3900 (mcg/hr) ÷ 200 (mcg/mL) = 195 mL/hr, *answer.*

Note: For data such as these, when the patient's weight, the dose of the drug, and the drug concentration in the infusion are given or may be calculated, the infusion rate may be calculated by the following equation[5]:

$$\text{Infusion rate (mL/hr)} = \frac{\text{Patient's weight (kg)} \times \text{Dose (mcg, mg, or units/kg/min)} \times 60}{\text{Drug concentration, infusion (mcg, mg, or units/mL)}}$$

$$= \frac{65\,(\text{kg}) \times 10\,(\text{mcg/kg/min}) \times 60}{200\,(\text{mcg/mL})}$$

$$= 195\ \text{mL/hr,}\ \ answer.$$

In using this equation, the denominations for the dose and drug concentration must be the same (e.g., mcg, mg, or units). Also, if the dosage rate is stated in hours (e.g., mcg/kg/hr), the 60 is not needed in the equation to arrive at flow rate per hour.

A different type of flow rate table is shown in Table 13.3. This type of table is used for determining flow rates for different doses when using a specific drug concentration. The data in the table are calculated as by the following illustration:

Drug concentration: 200 μg/mL
Dose selected: 5 μg/min
Calculation of mL of infusion providing 5 μg dose:

$$\frac{200\ \mu g}{1\ \text{mL}} = \frac{5\ \mu g}{x\ \text{mL}}; \ x = 0.025\ \text{mL} = \text{dose/min}$$

Calculation, dose in mL/h:
0.025 mL (dose/min) × 60 (min/h) = 1.5 mL/h, *answer.*

Table 13.3 ▼ EXAMPLE OF A FLOW RATE TABLE FOR AN INFUSION CONTAINING DRUG IN A CONCENTRATION OF 200 μg/mL[a]

DOSE, μg/min:	1	2	3	4	5	6	7	8	9	10	15	20	30	40	50
RATE, mL/h:	0.3	0.6	0.9	1.2	1.5	1.8	2.1	2.4	2.7	3	4.5	6	9	12	15

[a]After finding the desired dose in μg/min in the top column, the rate of flow in mL/h is found by the number below. The table may be extrapolated; for example, a dose of 80 μg/min would translate into a rate of 24 mL/h. Also, the table may be changed for a different drug concentration; for example, a drug concentration of 100 μg/mL and a dose of 5 μg/min would necessitate a flow rate of 3 mL/h.

Examples:

Use Table 13.3 to determine the infusion administration rate, in mL/h, to deliver drug at 16 µg/min.

For 8 µg/min, the rate is 2.4 mL/h
Thus, for 16 µg/min the rate would be double, or 4.8 mL/h, *answer.*
Proof: the infusion contains 200 µg/mL

$$16 \text{ µg (per minute)}/200 \text{ µg/mL} = 0.08 \text{ mL (per minute)}$$
$$0.08 \text{ mL/min} \times 60 \text{ minutes (per hour)} = 4.8 \text{ mL/h}$$

Or, note from the table that the rate in mL/h for each dose may be determined by multiplying by the factor 0.3. Thus, 16 µg/min × 0.3 = 4.8 mL/h.

Monoclonal Antibodies (mAbs) Infusion Calculations

Monoclonal antibodies (mAbs) are used in the diagnosis and treatment of various diseases. In general, mAbs are dosed on the basis of body weight or body surface area and are administered by injection or infusion. Table 13.4 presents some examples of mAb infusions.

Example:

In preparing an infusion of the drug trastuzumab, a pharmacist adds 20 mL of bacteriostatic water for injection to a vial containing 440 mg of the mAb. The resulting solution contains trastuzumab, 21 mg/mL. Using the information from Table 13.4, (a) calculate the milliliters of solution required for the loading dose for a 165-lb patient. The pharmacist then transfers the calculated volume into an infusion bag containing 250 mL of sodium chloride injection. Calculate (b) the quantity of trastuzumab administered in mg/min and (c) the drip rate, in drops/min, using an administration set that delivers 20 drops/mL.

(a) weight of patient: 165 lb/2.2 lb per kg = 75 kg
     loading dose in mg: 75 kg × 4 mg/kg = 300 mg

     volume of injection (dose): $\dfrac{21 \text{ mg}}{1 \text{ mL}} = \dfrac{300 \text{ mg}}{\text{x mL}}$; x = 14.29 or 14.3 mL, *answer.*

(b) 300 mg/90 min = 3.33 mg/min, *answer.*
(c) volume of infusion: 250 mL + 14.3 mL = 264.3 mL
     drops in infusion: 264.3 mL × 20 drops/mL = 5286 drops
     drops per minute: 5286 drops/90 min = 58.7 or 59 drops/min, *answer.*

Table 13.4 ▼ EXAMPLES OF MONOCLONAL ANTIBODIES (mAbs) ADMINISTERED BY INTRAVENOUS INFUSION

mAb	PRIMARY USE	USUAL ADULT DOSE AND INFUSION RATE[a]
Cetuximab	Agent or coagent in the treatment of colorectal and head and neck cancer	400 mg/m² (120-min infusion); then 250 mg/m² (60-min infusion) weekly
Natalizumab	Monotherapy in treatment of relapsing forms of multiple sclerosis and in Crohn's disease	300 mg (60-min infusion)
Tocilizumab	Rheumatoid arthritis	4 mg/kg once every 4 wk (60-min infusion)
Trastuzumab	Sole or coagent in treatment of breast cancer	4 mg/kg loading dose (90-min infusion) 2 mg/kg/wk maintenance dose (30-min infusion)

[a]Stated usual doses/rates are for illustration; actual clinical doses/rates are determined based on individual patient parameters.

Calculations of Basic Intravenous Infusion Solutions

1. How many grams each of sodium chloride and dextrose are present in a 1000-mL IV bag of 0.18% sodium chloride and 4% dextrose?

2. A medication calls for 1000 mL of D5W½NSS to be administered over 8 hours. Calculate the quantity, in grams, each of dextrose and sodium chloride administered in a 20-minute period.

Calculations of Infusion Time

3. If a standard *microdrop* infusion set is used to administer 100 mL of an infusion over a 2-hour period, calculate the rate of delivery, in drops/min.

4. A patient was administered 150 mL of D_5W at a rate of 25 mL/hr. If the infusion was begun at 8 AM, at what time was it completed?

5. A patient received 500 mL of D_5W½NS at a rate of 15 drops/minute. If the administration set used delivered 15 drops/mL, calculate the infusion time in hours, minutes.

6. A pediatric patient received 50 mL of an infusion at 10 drops/minute with an administration set that delivered 60 drops/mL. Calculate the duration of the infusion in minutes.

7. An intravenous drip contains 2 g of Xylocaine and is administered at a rate of 4 mg/min. Calculate the total time, in minutes, for the complete infusion.

Calculations of Intravenous Infusions with Additives

8. Daptomycin (CUBICIN), 4 mg/kg, is recommended for administration over a 30-minute period by intravenous infusion in 0.9% sodium chloride. How many milliliters of a vial containing 500 mg of daptomycin in 10 mL should be added to a 100-mL bag of normal saline in treating a 165-lb. patient?

9. An emergency syringe contains lidocaine, 1 g/5 mL. How many milliliters should be used in preparing 250 mL of an infusion to contain 4 mg/mL of lidocaine in D5W?

10. A fluconazole injection contains 400 mg of fluconazole in 200 mL of normal saline injection for infusion. Calculate the concentration of fluconazole in mg/mL.

11. Intravenous immunoglobulin (IVIG) has been administered in the pretransplantation of organs at a rate of 0.08 mL/kg/min. Calculate the number of milliliters administered to a 154-lb patient over a period of 4 hours.

12. A pharmacist prepared a "standard concentration" of a dopamine HCl solution to contain 400 mg/250 mL D5W. Calculate (a) the concentration of dopamine HCl in the infusion, in mg/mL, and (b) the infusion flow rate, in mL/hr, for a 150-lb. patient, based on a dose of 5 mcg/kg/minute.

13. A pharmacist receives a medication order for 300,000 units of penicillin G potassium to be added to 500 mL of D5W. The directions on the 1,000,000-unit vial state that if 1.6 mL of solvent are added, the solution will measure 2 mL. How many milliliters of the solution must be withdrawn and added to the D5W?

14. A physician orders 2 g of an antibiotic to be placed in 1000 mL of D5W. Using an injection that contains 300 mg of the antibiotic per 2 mL, how many milliliters should be added to the dextrose injection in preparing the medication order?

15. An intravenous infusion for a patient weighing 132 lb. calls for 7.5 mg of amikacin sulfate per kilogram of body weight to be added to 250 mL of 5% dextrose injection. How many milliliters of an amikacin sulfate injection containing 500 mg per 2 mL should be used in preparing the infusion?

16. Lidocaine injection may be administered by continuous intravenous infusion to treat cardiac arrhythmias at a dose of 2 mg/min. Solutions for intravenous infusion may be prepared by the addition of 1 g of lidocaine hydrochloride to 1 L of 5% dextrose in water. Calculate the maximum duration of this infusion in minutes.

17. A medication order calls for acyclovir, 355 mg, to be administered by intravenous infusion over 60 minutes. A 500-mg vial of acyclovir is available that must be mixed with sterile water for injection to prepare 10 mL of injection. The proper amount is then admixed with 100 mL of normal saline solution. Calculate (a) the volume to be taken from the vial of mixed acyclovir, (b) the rate of infusion in mL/min, and (c) the drops/min if using an intravenous set that delivers 20 drops/mL.

18. A medication order for a 20-lb pediatric patient calls for vancomycin, 10 mg/kg, to be administered by intravenous infusion. The pharmacy has a 10-mL injection containing 500 mg of vancomycin. The pharmacist adds the correct amount to a 100-mL bag of normal saline solution. (a) How many milliliters of the injection were added and (b) what is the content of vancomycin in the infusion, in mg/mL?

Various Calculations of Infusions Including Drip Rates

19. A medication order calls for a dopamine drip at 5 μg/kg/min for a 185-lb patient. The pharmacy adds 400 mg dopamine in 250 mL of D5W. Calculate the drip rates per minute when using administration sets delivering (a) 15 drops/mL, (b) 20 drops/mL, and (c) 60 drops/mL.

20. A physician orders 4 L of intravenous fluids for a dehydrated patient to be administered over a period of 24 hours using an intravenous set that delivers 15 drops/mL. Calculate the drip rate in (a) drops per minute and in (b) milliliters per hour.

21. How many milliliters of an injection containing 1 g of drug in 4 mL should be used in filling a medication order requiring 275 mg of the drug to be added to 500 mL of D5W solution? If the solution is administered at the rate of 1.6 mL per minute, how many milligrams of the drug will the patient receive in 1 hour?

22. A physician orders a 2-g vial of a drug to be added to 500 mL of D5W. If the administration rate is 125 mL per hour, how many milligrams of the drug will a patient receive per minute?

23. The drug labetalol has a dose of 300 mg and is administered in 300 mL of an intravenous infusion at a rate of 2 mg/min. Using an infusion set that delivers 20 drops/mL, calculate the required drip rate in drops/min.

24. A physician orders 35 mg of amphotericin B and 25 units of heparin to be administered intravenously in 1000 mL of D5W over an 8-hour period. In filling the medication order, the available sources of the additives are a vial containing 50 mg of amphotericin B in 10 mL and a syringe containing 10 units of heparin per milliliter.

    (a) How many milliliters of each additive should be used in filling the medication order?

    (b) How many milliliters of the intravenous fluid per minute should the patient receive?

25. A solution containing 500,000 units of polymyxin B sulfate in 10 mL of sterile water for injection is added to 250 mL of 5% dextrose injection. The infusion is to be administered over 2 hours. If the administration set delivers 15 drops/mL, at what rate, in drops per minute, should the flow be adjusted to administer the infusion over the designated time interval?

26. Five hundred (500) milliliters of a 2% sterile solution of a drug are to be administered by intravenous infusion over a period of 4 hours. If the administration set delivers 20 drops/mL, at what rate, in drops per minute, should the infusion flow? Solve the problem by calculation *and* by using the nomogram in this chapter.

27. An 8-kg infant requires a continuous infusion of a drug to run at 1 mL/hour to deliver 4 mcg of drug/kg per minute. Calculate the milligrams of drug that must be added to a 100-mL intravenous infusion solution.

28. Five hundred milliliters of an intravenous solution contain 0.2% of succinylcholine chloride. At what flow rate should the infusion be administered to provide 2.5 mg of succinylcholine chloride per minute?

29. A hospital pharmacist prepared thirty 100-mL epidural bags containing 0.125% of bupivacaine hydrochloride and 1 μg/mL of fentanyl citrate in 0.9% sodium chloride injection. How many (a) 30-mL vials of 0.5% bupivacaine hydrochloride, (b) 20-mL vials of 50 μg/mL of fentanyl citrate, and (c) 1-L bags of 0.9% sodium chloride were required?

30. An intravenous fluid of 1000 mL of lactated Ringer's injection was started in a patient at 8 AM and was scheduled to run for 12 hours. At 3 PM, 800 mL of the fluid remained in the bottle. At what rate of flow should the remaining fluid be regulated using an IV set that delivers 15 drops/mL to complete the administration of the fluid in the scheduled time?

31. If a physician orders 5 units of insulin to be added to a 1-liter intravenous solution of D5W to be administered over 8 hours, (a) how many drops per minute should be administered using an IV set that delivers 15 drops/mL, and (b) how many units of insulin would be administered in each 30-minute period?

32. A patient is to receive 3 μg/kg/min of nitroglycerin from a solution containing 100 mg of the drug in 500 mL of D5W. If the patient weighs 176 lb. and the infusion set delivers 60 drops/mL, (a) how many milligrams of nitroglycerin would be delivered per hour, and (b) how many drops per minute would be delivered?

33. Using the nomogram in Figure 13.5, determine the approximate rate of infusion delivery, in drops per minute, based on 1.5 liters of fluid to be used over a period of 8 hours with an infusion set calibrated to deliver 16 drops/mL.

34. The drug alfentanil hydrochloride is administered by infusion at the rate of 2 μg/ kg/min for anesthesia induction. If a total of 0.35 mg of the drug is to be administered to a 110-lb. patient, how long should be the duration of the infusion?

35. The recommended maintenance dose of aminophylline for children is 1 mg/kg/hr by injection. If 10 mL of a 25 mg/mL solution of aminophylline is added to a 100-mL bottle of dextrose injection, what should be the rate of delivery, in milliliters per hour, for a 40-lb. child?

36. A patient is to receive an infusion of a drug at the rate of 5 mg/hr for 8 hours. The drug is available in

10-mL vials containing 8 mg of drug per milliliter. If a 250-mL bottle of D5W is used as the vehicle, (a) how many milliliters of the drug solution should be added, and (b) what should be the flow rate in milliliters per minute?

37. A patient is receiving 500 mL of an intravenous drip containing 25,000 units of sodium heparin in sodium chloride injection. Calculate (a) the administration rate, in mL/h, to deliver 1200 units of sodium heparin per hour and (b) the administration rate, in drops/min, with an IV set that delivers 15 drops/mL.

38. A 50-mL vial containing 1 mg/mL of the drug alteplase is added to 100 mL of D5W and administered intravenously with an infusion set that delivers 15 drops/mL. How many drops per minute should be given to administer 25 mg of the drug per hour?

39. If the loading dose of phenytoin in children is 20 mg/kg of body weight to be infused at a rate of 0.5 mg/kg/min, over how many minutes should the dose be administered to a 32-lb. child?

40.[8] The following was ordered for a critical care patient: 2 L of D5/0.45% NS to run over 24 hours with a 2000 mL IV fluid daily limit. An IVPB antibiotic is ordered to run every 6 hours separately in 50 mL of D5W over 30 minutes. The drop factor is 60 drops per milliliter. Calculate the flow rate of the IVPB and the D5W/0.45% NS.

41. If a medication order calls for a dobutamine drip, 5 μg/kg/min, for a patient weighing 232 lb. what should be the drip rate, in drops per minute, if the 125-mL infusion bag contains 250 mg of dobutamine and a micro-drip chamber is used that delivers 60 drops/mL?

42. At what rate, in drops per minute, should a dose of 20 μg/kg/min of dopamine be administered to a 65-kg patient using a solution containing dopamine, 1200 μg/mL, and a drip set that delivers 60 drops/mL?

43. A pharmacist places 5 mg/mL of acyclovir sodium in 250 mL of D5W for parenteral infusion into a pediatric patient. If the infusion is to run for 1 hour and the patient is to receive 500 mg/m^2 BSA, what would be the rate of flow in milliliters per minute for a patient measuring 55 cm in height and weighing 10 kg?

44. Aminophylline is not to be administered in pediatric patients at a rate greater than 25 mg per minute to avoid excessive peak serum concentrations and possible circulatory failure. What should be the maximum infusion rate, in milliliters per minute, for a solution containing 10 mg/mL of aminophylline in 100 mL of D5W?

45. An intravenous infusion contains 5 mg of RECLAST (zoledronic acid) in 100 mL. If the infusion is to be administered in 15 minutes, how many (a) milligrams of zoledronic acid, and (b) milliliters of infusion must be administered per minute? And (c), using a drip-set that delivers 20 drops/milliliter, how many drops per minute must be infused?

46. ORENCIA (abatacept), used to treat rheumatoid arthritis, is available in vials, each containing 250 mg of powdered drug, intended to be reconstituted to 10 mL with sterile water for injection. The dose of abatacept depends on a patient's

body weight: <60 kg, 500 mg; 60 to 100 kg, 750 mg; and >100 kg, 1 g. The contents of the appropriate number of vials are aseptically added to a 100-mL infusion bag or bottle of sodium chloride injection *after* the corresponding volume of sodium chloride injection has been removed. The concentration of abatacept in an infusion for a 200-lb. patient would be:

(a) 5.8 mg/mL
(b) 6.25 mg/mL
(c) 6.8 mg/mL
(d) 7.5 mg/mL

47. TORISEL (temsirolimus), for use in advanced renal cell carcinoma, is prepared for infusion by adding 1.8 mL of special diluent to the drug vial resulting in 3 mL of injection containing 10 mg/mL of temsirolimus. The required quantity is then added to a 250-mL container of sodium chloride injection for infusion. The recommended dose of temsirolimus is 25 mg infused over 30 to 60 minutes. The quantity of drug delivered, in mg/mL, and the rate of infusion, in mL/min, for a 30-minute infusion are:

(a) 0.099 mg/mL and 8.42 mL/min
(b) 0.099 mg/mL and 8.33 mL/min
(c) 1 mg/mL and 8.42 mL/min
(d) 1 mg/mL and 8.33 mL/min

48. CARDENE IV (nicardipine hydrochloride) is administered in the short-term treatment of hypertension by slow intravenous infusion at a concentration of 0.1 mg/mL. A 10-mL ampule containing 25 mg of nicardipine hydrochloride should be added to what volume of D5W to achieve the desired concentration of infusion?

(a) 80 mL
(b) 100 mL
(c) 240 mL
(d) 250 mL

Calculations of Monoclonal Antibody (mAb) Infusions

49. The mAb eculizumab is available in 30-mL vials containing 300 mg of drug. Prior to administration by intravenous infusion, the solution is diluted with sodium chloride injection to a concentration of 5 mg/mL. The dose of eculizumab is 600 mg infused over a 35-minute period. Calculate the rate of infusion in drops/min using an administration set that delivers 15 drops/mL.

50. Using Table 13.4 and Figure 8.2 as references, (a) calculate the initial dose of cetuximab for a 140-lb patient measuring 65 in. in height. If cetuximab is available in vials containing 200 mg/100 mL, (b) calculate the volume to be used in an infusion. If the infusion is delivered over 120 minutes and the package insert states that rate of delivery of cetuximab should not exceed 10 mg/min, calculate whether or not that standard is being met.

51. The mAb natalizumab is available in vials containing 300 mg/15 mL. Prior to infusion, the contents are added to 100 mL of normal saline injection. Refer to Table 13.4 as needed, and calculate (a) the concentration of natalizumab in the infusion, in mg/mL, and (b) the rate of infusion, in mL/min.

CALCQUIZ

13.A.[a] A hospital pharmacy receives a medication order for 500 mg aminophylline in 250 mL normal saline solution for a 132-lb patient. The aminophylline is to be administered at a dose of 300 μg/kg/h using an IV set that delivers 60 drops/mL. The pharmacy has 20-mL vials of injection containing aminophylline, 25 mg/mL. Calculate the following:

(a) The milliliters of aminophylline injection that should be added to the normal saline solution.
(b) The total volume of the intravenous infusion.
(c) The milligrams of aminophylline administered per hour.
(d) The duration, in hours, for the complete infusion.
(e) The number of milliliters of infusion delivered per hour (flow rate, mL/h).
(f) The number of drops administered per minute (flow rate, drops/min).

13.B.[a] A hospitalized patient is receiving an intravenous infusion containing 40 mEq of potassium chloride in a liter of fluid. The IV set being used is calibrated to deliver 15 drops/mL with a flow rate of 12 drops/min. How many (a) milligrams, (b) milliequivalents, and (c) millimoles of potassium chloride are delivered each hour?

13.C. A physician submits a medication order for a 110-lb patient calling for an intravenous drip containing 400 mg of dopamine in a 250-mL bag of normal saline solution. The drip is to be run at 5 μg/kg/min with an IV set that delivers 15 drops/mL. Calculate the following:

(a) The milliliters of a dopamine injection, 40 mg/mL, to use in the infusion.
(b) The concentration of dopamine in the infusion in mg/mL.
(c) The drip rate in drops/min.
(d) The infusion rate in mL/h.

13.D. A medication order for a patient in the critical care unit of a hospital calls for a continuous intravenous infusion of isoproterenol, 5 μg/min. The standard protocol is to add the contents of a 5-mL ampule of a 1:5000 isoproterenol injection to 250 mL of dextrose 5% in water. The critical care nurse uses an IV set programmed to deliver 12 drops/mL. Calculate the following:

(a) The quantity of isoproterenol, in μg/mL, in the 5-mL ampule of isoproterenol injection.
(b) The concentration of isoproterenol, in μg/mL, in the infusion.
(c) The flow rate of the intravenous infusion in drops/min.
(d) The duration of the completed infusion in minutes.

13.E. A hospital pharmacy received an order for 250 mL of a premixed injection containing 50 mg of nitroglycerin in D5W. The initial infusion rate was prescribed at 5 μg/min to be increased by 5 μg/min every 5 minutes as needed up to a maximum of 20 μg/min. An infusion set delivering 60 microdrops/mL was used. Calculate the following:

(a) The concentration of nitroglycerin in the infusion in μg/mL.
(b) The initial rate of infusion in mL/h.
(c) The maximum rate of infusion (20 μg/min) in microdrops/min *and* in mL/h.

[a]Problem courtesy of Flynn Warren, Bishop, GA.

ANSWERS TO "CASE IN POINT" AND PRACTICE PROBLEMS

Case in Point 13.1

(a) 15 mg/min × 10 min = 150 mg amiodarone HCl needed for the rapid infusion. Ampul contains 50 mg/mL, so 3 mL are needed = one 3-mL ampul, *answer*.

(b) 150 mg amiodarone in 103 mL; 150 mg ÷ 103 mL = 1.46 mg/mL, *answer*.

(c) 3 (ampuls) × 3 mL = 9 mL × 50 mg/mL = 450 mg amiodarone HCl
450 mg ÷ 259 mL = 1.74 mg/mL amiodarone HCl, *answer*.

(d) 60 minutes × 1 mg/min = 60 mg amiodarone HCl
60 mg ÷ 1.74 mg/mL = 34.5 mL/hr, *answer*.

(e) 34.5 mL × 15 drops/mL = 517.5 drops in 1 hour
517.5 drops ÷ 60 = 8.625 or about 9 drops per minute, *answer*.

(f) 1 mg/min × 60 min/hr × 6 hr = 360 mg, *answer*.

(g) 0.5 mg/min × 60 min/hr × 18 hr = 540 mg, *answer*.

Practice Problems

1. 1.8 g sodium chloride
   40 g dextrose

2. 2.083 g dextrose
   0.187 g sodium chloride

3. 50 drops/minute

4. 2:00 PM

5. 8 hours, 20 minutes

6. 300 minutes

7. 500 minutes

8. 6 mL daptomycin injection

9. 5 mL lidocaine injection

10. 2 mg/mL fluconazole

11. 1344 mL IVIG

12. (a) 1.6 mg/mL dopamine
    (b) 12.78 mL/hour

13. 0.6 mL

14. 13.33 mL

15. 1.8 mL amikacin sulfate injection

16. 500 minutes

17. (a) 7.1 mL
    (b) 1.785 or 1.8 mL/minute
    (c) 35.7 or 36 drops/minute

18. (a) 1.8 mL
    (b) 0.89 mg/mL vancomycin

19. (a) 3.9 or 4 drops/minute
    (b) 5.25 or 5 drops/minute
    (c) 15.7 or 16 drops/minute

20. (a) 41.7 or 42 drops/minute
    (b) 166.7 mL/hour

21. 1.1 mL
    52.8 mg

22. 8.33 mg

23. 40 drops/minute

24. (a) 7 mL amphotericin B
        2.5 mL heparin
    (b) 2.08 mL/minute

25. 32.6 or 33 drops/minute

26. 41.7 or 42 drops/minute

27. 192 mg

28. 1.25 mL/minute

29. (a) 25
    (b) 3
    (c) 3

30. 40 drops/minute

31. (a) 31.25 or 31 drops/minute
    (b) 0.3 unit

32. (a) 14.4 mg/hour
    (b) 72 drops/minute

33. approximately 50 drops/minute

34. 3.5 minutes

35. 8 mL/hour

36. (a) 5 mL
    (b) 0.53 mL/minute

37. (a) 24 mL/hour
    (b) 6 drops/minute

38. 18.75 or 19 drops/minute

39. 40 minutes

40. IVPB, 100 drops/minute
    D5/0.45NS, 82 drops/minute
41. 15.82 or 16 drops/minute
42. 66 drops/minute
43. 0.58 mL/minute
44. 2.5 mL/minute
45. (a) 0.33 mg zoledronic acid
    (b) 6.67 mL
    (c) 133 drops/minute

46. (d) 7.5 mg/mL
47. (a) 0.099 mg/mL and 8.42 mL/minute
48. (c) 240 mL
49. 51.4 or 51 drops/minute
50. (a) 680 mg cetuximab
    (b) 340 mL
    (c) 5.7 mg/minute, yes
51. (a) 2.6 mg/mL natalizumab
    (b) 1.9 mL/minute

References

1. <797> Pharmaceutical Compounding—Sterile Preparations. *United States Pharmacopeia 32 National Formulary 27*. Rockville, MD. The United States Pharmacopeial Convention, 2009;1:318–354.
2. Boh L. *Pharmacy Practice Manual: A Guide to the Clinical Experience*. Baltimore, MD: Lippincott Williams & Wilkins, 2001:418.
3. Institute for Safe Medication Practices. ISMP medication safety alert: how fast is too fast for IV push medications? May 15, 2003. Available at: https://www.ismp.org/Newsletters/acutecare/articles/20030515.asp. Accessed June 15, 2011.
4. Larsen GY, Howard PB, Cash J, et al. Standard drug concentrations and smart-pump technology reduce continuous-medication-infusion errors in pediatric patients. *Pediatrics* 2005;116:e21–e25. Available at: http://pediatrics.aappublications.org/content/116/1/e21.full. Accessed June 6, 2011.
5. Mitchell A, Sommo P, Mocerine T, et al. A standardized approach to pediatric parenteral medication delivery. *Hospital Pharmacy* 2004;39:433–459.
6. Gomella TL, Cunningham MD, Eyal FG, et al. *Neonatology: Management Procedures, On-Call Problems, Diseases, and Drugs*. New York: Lange Medical Books, 2004:69–73.
7. Craig GP. *Clinical Calculations Made Easy*. 2nd Ed. Philadelphia, PA: Lippincott Williams & Wilkins, 2001:225–228.
8. Lacher B. *Pharmaceutical Calculations for the Pharmacy Technician*. Baltimore, MD: Lippincott Williams & Wilkins, 2008:287.

Enteral and Parenteral Nutrition, Body Mass Index, and the Food Nutrition Label

14

Objectives

Upon successful completion of this chapter, the student will be able to:

- Perform basic calculations for enteral and parenteral nutrition.
- Calculate body mass index (BMI) from a standard formula.
- Apply the food nutrition label in related calculations.

Pharmacists are increasingly involved in providing enteral and parenteral nutrition services in the institutional as well as in the home care setting. In this role, pharmacists may take part in the selection of the nutritional formula, prepare the product for use, and/or participate in its administration.

In community pharmacies, pharmacists routinely counsel patients on matters of nutrition. It is well recognized that poor dietary choices contribute to obesity and many chronic conditions, including hypertension, coronary heart disease, sleep apnea, and type 2 diabetes mellitus (the term *diabesity* has been coined to describe the relationship between type 2 diabetes and obesity).[1-4] Community pharmacists frequently advise patients on general dietary requirements for the maintenance of good health, provide counseling with regard to weight control, help patients understand the nutritional labeling on food products, and explain the use and composition of various dietary supplements.

Figure 14.1 depicts the three routes of nutrition: oral, enteral, and parenteral.

Enteral Nutrition

Enteral nutrition is a method of providing nutritional support via tubes inserted into the stomach or small intestine. It finds application in patients who have an inability or decreased ability to ingest nutrients by mouth. As shown in Figure 14.1, nasogastric tubes may be used, or tubes may be inserted through surgical openings into the stomach, duodenum, or jejunum.[5] Surgical insertions generally are reserved for the relatively long-term feeding requirements of patients (e.g., more than 4 weeks). Enteral nutrition may be used for total nutrition, for supplemental nutrition, or as a transitional phase for patients coming off parenteral nutrition. Tube feedings may be intermittent or continuous, and in addition to nutritional requirements, they address the need to replace water lost daily through urination, bowel function, respiration, and perspiration.

Enteral nutrition takes into account a patient's caloric requirements and his or her need for protein, carbohydrate and fat, vitamins and minerals, dietary fiber, electrolytes, and fluids. Commercial formulas for enteral feeding are multiple and varied. Some are designed

▼ FIGURE 14.1 Routes of nutrition: oral, enteral, and parenteral.

specifically for pediatric or adult patients. Some provide a balanced or general requirement; others are high in calories, protein, amino acids, fat, and/or fiber; and still others are low in carbohydrate, sodium, or cholesterol. Some commercial formulas are designed to meet the disease-specific requirements of certain patients, such as those with renal or hepatic disease or those who are diabetic, lactose intolerant, or allergic to specific foods. As required, additions may be made to commercial formulas to meet the needs of a specific patient.

The osmolality of an enteral formula is an important consideration. Some patients exhibit intolerance to a hyperosmolar formula, resulting in vomiting, osmotic diarrhea, abdominal distention, and other symptoms.[6] Most infant formulas have osmolalities between 150 and

380 mOsmol/kg, and adult formulas from about 270 to 700 mOsmol/kg. It should be recalled that the osmolality of extracellular fluid is considered to be 285 to 295 mOsmol/kg.

When necessary, medications can be administered through the enteral feeding tubes, preferably with liquid dosage forms. As required, well-diluted slurries can be prepared and administered from the solid contents of tablets or capsules. Liquid medications with high osmolalities (some are greater than 1000 mOsmol/kg) can be diluted with 10 to 30 mL of sterile water prior to administration.[5,7]

Medications generally are administered separately from the nutrient formulas, with care taken not to conflict with the feeding schedule, to avoid drug incompatibilities with other medications and nutritional components, to consider a medication's possible gastrointestinal effects (e.g., diarrhea or constipation), and to make certain that no residual medication remains in the feeding tubes after medication delivery.[5,7]

Parenteral Nutrition

Parenteral nutrition (PN) or *intravenous hyperalimentation (IVH or HAL)* is the feeding of a patient by the intravenous infusion of fluids and basic nutrients. *Partial parenteral nutrition (PPN)* is nutritional support that *supplements* oral intake and provides only part of daily nutritional requirements. *Total parenteral nutrition (TPN)* provides *all* the patient's daily nutritional requirements.

Parenteral nutrition is used for patients who cannot obtain adequate nutrition by oral means. This includes patients who are severely malnourished, those whose critical illness temporarily precludes their receiving oral or enteral nutrition and there is need to *prevent* starvation-induced complications, those whose gastrointestinal tracts are unavailable or malfunctioning, those with a demonstrated or assessed probability of ineffective nourishment by enteral feeding, and patients in renal or hepatic failure, among others.[8,9]

Figure 14.2 is an example of a hospital adult parenteral nutrition form. Note that the prescribing physician may select the standard formulas or modifications for central or peripheral administration. In the example, the quantities of the basic components, amino acids (protein), dextrose (carbohydrate), and fat (lipid), are expressed in percent strength; however, other such forms may express these quantities in grams per stated volume. Added electrolytes are expressed in milliequivalents and phosphorous in millimoles. The patient's *dosing weight* (the actual, ideal, or adjusted body weight) is used to determine the component doses. Central administration lines are inserted into the superior vena cava, whereas peripheral lines are inserted into veins of the arm or hand (see Fig. 14.1). Because concentrated dextrose solutions are hypertonic and may be damaging to veins, central lines are preferred over peripheral lines for higher concentrations of dextrose (e.g., 25%). Nutritional formulas for peripheral parenteral nutrition generally are isotonic or near isotonic.

Typically, parenteral nutrition formulas contain the following:

- *Macronutrients:*
  Carbohydrate (e.g., dextrose)
  Protein (e.g., amino acids)
  Fat (e.g., lipid emulsions)
- *Micronutrients:*
  Electrolytes
  Vitamins
  Trace elements
- *Sterile water for injection*

STANDARD CENTRAL LINE FORMULA	STANDARD PERIPHERAL LINE FORMULA	STANDARD RENAL CENTRAL LINE FORMULA
Standard ☐ Modified ☐	Standard ☐ Modified ☐	Standard ☐ Modified ☐
Amino Acid 4.25% _____%	Amino Acid 2.75% _____%	Amino Acid 1.95% _____%
Dextrose 25% _____%	Dextrose 10% _____%	Dextrose 44% _____%
Rate _____mL/hr	Rate _____mL/hr	Rate _____mL/hr

Electrolytes (per liter)

Standard ☐   Modified ☐

Na	35 mEq	_____mEq	
K	30 mEq	_____mEq	
Mg	5 mEq	_____mEq	
Ca	3 mEq	_____mEq	
P	15 mM	_____mM	

Acetate: Cl = 1:1 _____

Each bag contains the standard amount of multi-vitamins and trace elements.

Additional Ingredients (per liter)

Standard ☐   Modified ☐

___Cimetidine
900 mg/24 hr OR:_____ mg/24 hr

___Ranitidine
150 mg/24 hr OR:_____ mg/24 hr

___Reg Insulin _____units/L
Other:

_____
_____
_____

STANDARD PERIPHERAL LINE FORMULA — Electrolytes (per liter)

Standard ☐   Modified ☐

Na	35 mEq	_____mEq	
K	30 mEq	_____mEq	
Mg	5 mEq	_____mEq	
Ca	3 mEq	_____mEq	
P	15 mM	_____mM	

Acetate: Cl = 1:1 _____

Each bag contains the standard amount of multi-vitamins and trace elements.

Additional Ingredients (per liter)

_____
_____
_____
_____

STANDARD RENAL CENTRAL LINE FORMULA — Electrolytes (per liter)

Standard ☐   Modified ☐

Na	0 mEq	_____mEq	
K	0 mEq	_____mEq	
Mg	0 mEq	_____mEq	
Ca	0 mEq	_____mEq	
P	0 mM	_____mM	

Check if you wish to add the standard amount of trace elements and multivitamins.

Trace Elements _____

Multivitamins _____

Additional Ingredients (per liter)

_____
_____
_____
_____

Intravenous Fat 10% 500 mL (1.1 kcal/mL):_____(rate)

Intravenous Fat 20% 500 mL (2 kcal/mL):_____(rate)

Date:_____ MD _____

NOTE:
Standing physician's orders for line management and patient monitoring of parenteral hyperalimentation will be followed unless initialed here:_____

▼ FIGURE 14.2 Example of part of an order form for adult parenteral nutrition. *(Published with the permission of Wake Medical Center, Raleigh, NC.)*

Parenteral nutrition formulas can be obtained commercially or they may be prepared in the pharmacy, often through the use of automated compounding devices that mix the basic as well as additive ingredients according to input managed by computer software. Nutritional requirements and thus formulations differ based on age groups (e.g., neonates, general pediatrics, adults) as well as patient-specific diseases (e.g., renal, liver, pulmonary). In preparing formulas for parenteral nutrition, pharmacists use calculated quantities of small-volume parenterals (ampuls and vials) as the source of electrolytes, vitamins, and minerals, and large-volume parenterals (LVPs) as the source of amino acids, dextrose, and sterile water for injection.

Typically, infusion rates are begun at about 25 to 50 mL per hour and adjusted every 8 to 12 hours as dictated by the patient's condition and fluid and nutritional status.[9] TPN solutions may be administered continuously over a 24-hour period or cyclically, depending on a patient's requirements. Infusions may be administered by gravity flow or through the use of automated, high-speed multichannel pumping devices. The duration of an infusion is referred to as its *hang time*.

In many instances, parenteral nutrition begun in a hospital is continued in a long-term care or rehabilitation facility or in home care.

Nutritional Requirements

Nutritional requirements are the quantities of macronutrients and micronutrients needed for a patient to obtain or maintain the desired nutritional status. The quantitative amounts of fluid and specific nutrients required vary with an individual's age, gender, physical parameters, disease state, and current nutritional status. The purpose of this section is to provide only *general* considerations. More detailed and patient-specific considerations are presented in other resources, including those referenced.[7-14]

Fluid Requirements

A factor of 30–35 mL/kg of body weight, 1500 mL per square meter of body surface area, or 1 mL/kcal of nutrition required are among the methods used to estimate a patient's daily fluid or water requirement. On a case-by-case basis, these values may be increased (e.g., for patients who are dehydrated) or decreased (e.g., for patients with renal failure or congestive heart failure). A daily requirement of between 2 and 3 liters per day is usual for adults. For neonates, infants, children, and adolescents without abnormal water losses, the approximate daily water requirement may be calculated by:

Parameter	*Estimated Water Requirement*
Based on age:	
Neonates	120 to 180 mL/kg/day
1 to 12 months	150 mL/kg/day (maximum, 200 mL)
Based on Weight:	
<10 kg	100 mL/kg/day
10 to 20 kg	1000 mL + 50 mL/kg/day over 10 kg
>20 kg	1500 mL + 20 mL/kg/day over 20 kg
Based on Body Surface Area:	
1500 mL/day/m^2	__mL/day
Based on Caloric Requirement:	
1.2 mL/kcal × kcal/day	__mL/day

Example:

Compare the estimated daily fluid requirement for a 35-lb child with a BSA of 0.65 m^2 based on (a) weight and (b) body surface area.

Weight of child, kg = 35-lb/2.2 lb per kg = 15.9 kg

(a) Requirement, based on weight = 1000 mL + 50 mL/kg/day over 10 kg
= 1000 mL + 50 mL × 5.9 (kg) = 295 mL
= 1000 mL + 295 mL = 1295 mL, and

(b) Requirement, based on BSA = 1500 mL/day/m^2
= 1500 mL × 0.65 (m^2) = 975 mL, *answers.*

Caloric Requirements

The **kilocalorie** (*kcal*) is the unit used in metabolism studies. By definition, the kilocalorie (or large Calorie, C, or Cal.) is the amount of heat required to raise the temperature of 1 kg of water 1°C. The caloric requirements for patients vary, depending on their physical state and medical condition. The Harris-Benedict equations,[15] which follow, are commonly used to estimate the *daily basal energy expenditure* (*BEE*) requirements for nonprotein calories. The BEE is also referred to as the *resting metabolic energy* (*RME*) or the *resting energy expenditure* (*REE*).

For males:

BEE = 66.65 + [13.75 × Weight (kg)] + [5 × Height (cm)] − [6.78 × Age (yr)]

For females:

BEE = 655.1 + [9.56 × Weight (kg)] + [1.85 × Height (cm)] − [4.68 × Age (yr)]

The *total daily expenditure* (*TDE*) of energy, as calculated, may be adjusted for activity and stress factors[8,14]:

BEE × activity factors × stress factors = TDE

Activity factors: Confined to bed: 1.2
                       Ambulatory: 1.3

Stress factors: Surgery: 1.2
                       Infection: 1.4 to 1.6
                       Trauma: 1.3 to 1.5
                       Burns: 1.5 to 2.1
                       Nonstressed: 1.0

(Note: unless otherwise indicated, for calculations in this chapter the lowest appropriate stress factor should be used.)

As an alternative to the use of the Harris-Benedict equations, clinicians can estimate the BEE for adults as 25 kcal/kg/day for mildly stressed hospitalized patients, up to 35 kcal/kg/day for moderately stressed patients, up to 45 kcal/kg/day for postoperative patients, and up to 60 kcal/kg/day for hypercatabolic patients. Energy requirements for infants, children, and teenagers are different than those for adults and vary according to age, growth rate, and clinical/metabolic status. The caloric requirements are about 100 kcal/kg/day for infants, 80 to 100 kcal/kg/day for children, and 35 to 60 kcal/kg/day for teenagers.

Examples:

Using the Harris-Benedict equation, calculate the BEE for a 78-year-old male patient, measuring 5 ft 8 in. in height and weighing 160 lb (without using activity or stress factors).

$$5 \text{ ft 8 in.} = 68 \text{ in.}; 68 \text{ in.} \times 2.54 \text{ cm/in.} = 172.72 \text{ cm}$$
$$160 \text{ lb} \div 2.2 \text{ lb/kg} = 72.72 \text{ kg}$$

$$\begin{aligned} \text{BEE} &= 66.5 + (13.75 \times \text{weight, kg}) + (5 \times \text{height, cm}) - (6.78 \times \text{age, y}) \\ &= 66.5 + (13.75 \times 72.72 \text{ [kg]}) + (5 \times 172.72 \text{ [cm]}) - (6.78 \times 78 \text{ y}) \\ &= 66.5 + 999.9 + 863.6 - 528.84 \\ &= 1401.16 \text{ kcal, } \textit{answer.} \end{aligned}$$

Calculate the TDE for the above patient factoring in an activity factor of 1.2 (confined to bed) and a stress factor of 1.2 (surgery).

$$\text{TDE} = \text{BEE} \times \text{activity factor} \times \text{stress factor}$$
$$= 1401.16 \text{ kcal} \times 1.2 \times 1.2 = 2017.67 \text{ kcal}, \textit{answer.}$$

Calculate the BEE for the above patient using the alternative method of 25 kcal/kg/day.

$$25 \text{ kcal/kg} \times 72.72 \text{ kg} = 1818 \text{ kcal}, \textit{answer.}$$

Carbohydrate Requirements

Carbohydrates are the primary source of cellular energy. In formulas for parenteral nutrition, dextrose provides 3.4 kcal of energy per gram; for example, each 100 mL of a 25% dextrose injection provides 85 kcal of energy. For enteral nutrition, the factor used is 4 kcal/g.

Protein Requirements

In TPN, protein is provided as protein hydrolysate or amino acids. The purpose of the protein support is not to produce energy, although energy is produced by proteins by a factor of 4 kcal/g, but rather to build tissues and body strength.[14] A patient's caloric needs should be provided by *nonprotein calories*. The daily quantity of protein required in adults is generally estimated to be about:

- 0.8 g/kg/day in an unstressed patient;
- 0.8 to 1 g/kg of body weight for a mildly stressed patient;
- 1.2 g/kg for a renal dialysis patient;
- 1.1 to 1.5 g/kg for a moderately stressed patient;
- 1.5 to 2 g/kg for a severely stressed patient and those with a critical illness or trauma; and
- 3 g/kg for a severely burned patient.

Infants may require 2 to 3 g/kg/day, children 1.5 to 2 g/kg/day, and teenagers 1 to 1.5 g/kg/day of protein.[8,14]

Lipid (Fat) Requirements

Lipids may be used to provide energy when the body cannot obtain all the necessary energy requirement from carbohydrates. The proportion of calories provided by lipids is usually restricted to 20% to 40% of the total daily calories. Lipids provide 9 kcal of energy per gram. Lipids are generally administered in the form of an emulsion containing carbohydrate-based emulsifying agents, which also contribute to the caloric content. The abbreviation *IVFE*, for *intravenous fat emulsion*, is often used to indicate the lipid component of a parenteral nutritional formula. It has been determined that a 10% lipid emulsion provides 11 kcal/g of total energy, and a 20% to 30% lipid emulsion provides 10 kcal/g of total energy.[12]

Fiber Requirements

Dietary guidelines generally recommend a daily intake of 14 g of fiber for each 1000 calories consumed. This translates to approximately 21 to 25 grams of daily fiber for women and between 30 to 38 g for men. *Insoluble* fiber reaches the large intestine after ingestion and is associated with good bowel function whereas *soluble* fiber partially dissolves in the upper gastrointestinal tract and is associated with reduced absorption of dietary fat and cholesterol.[16]

Electrolytes

As shown in Figure 14.2, the standard quantities of electrolytes may be used or modified by the following parameter, or other.[11]

Sodium, 1 to 2 mEq/kg/day
Potassium, 1 to 2 mEq/kg/day
Calcium, 10 to 15 mEq/kg/day
Magnesium, 8 to 20 mEq/kg/day
Phosphorus, 20 to 40 mmol/day

Special Considerations in Parenteral and Enteral Nutrition

The content provided in this chapter is introductory. Pharmacists' actual participation in providing parenteral and enteral nutrition services requires a comprehensive understanding of all aspects of this specialized field. Practice guidelines and critical reports are provided by the *American Society for Parenteral and Enteral Nutrition (ASPEN)*, its publication, *Journal of Parenteral and Enteral Nutrition*, and its Web site, *http://www.nutritioncare.org*

The following points are emphasized within the context of the limited scope of this chapter:

- The order form for PN presented by Figure 14.2 is an *example*. Such forms and their content vary between institutions.
- Nutritional orders are individualized for each patient based on age, metabolic condition, organ function, disease state, and medication usage.
- Calculations are often performed to provide the "targets" for nutritional components, which then may be rounded or modified based on individual patient requirements.
- The most common errors associated with PN involve dosage formulation, dosage calculations, and infusion rates.[11]
- Standard units of measure used are *grams* for the base components (i.e., dextrose, amino acids, and lipids), *milliequivalents* for electrolytes, and *millimoles* for phosphate, all in a specified volume, as per *liter*, or volume for a 24-hour infusion. The rate of flow is stated in *milliliters per hour* for a designated period of time (*hang time*), usually 24 hours.
- Parenteral and enteral nutrition orders should be clearly labeled with all *identifiers* of the patient, formula and quantity, route and rate of administration, hang time, expiration date, and for enteral preparations, the statement "Not for I.V. Use."[11]

Enteral and Parenteral Nutrition Calculations

Example Calculations of Enteral Nutrition

The nutritional requirements for a 76-year-old male who is 6 ft. 2 in. tall and weighs 201 lb. have been determined to be as follows:

Protein: 73.09 g/day
Lipids: 81.23 g/day
Carbohydrates: 266.34 g/day
Water: 2088.82 to 2740.91 mL/day
Total calories: 2088.82 kcal/day

A ready-to-drink nutritional liquid product is selected for this patient. A quart container provides 37 g protein, 143 g carbohydrates, 37 g lipids, and 1.06 kcal/mL.

(a) *How many milliliters of the product should this patient receive daily to meet his caloric requirements?*

$$\frac{2088.82\,\text{kcal}}{1\,\text{day}} \times \frac{1\,\text{mL}}{1.06\,\text{kcal}} = 1970.58\,\text{mL/day},\ \textit{answer}.$$

(b) *How many grams each of protein, carbohydrates, and lipids would this volume provide?*

$$\text{Protein}: \frac{1970.58\,\text{mL}}{1\,\text{day}} \times \frac{1\,\text{qt}}{946\,\text{mL}} \times \frac{37\,\text{g}}{1\,\text{qt}} = 77.07\,\text{g/day};$$

$$\text{Carbohydrates}: \frac{1970.58\,\text{mL}}{1\,\text{day}} \times \frac{1\,\text{qt}}{946\,\text{mL}} \times \frac{143\,\text{g}}{1\,\text{qt}} = 297.88\,\text{g/day};\ \textit{and}$$

$$\text{Lipids}: \frac{1970.58\,\text{mL}}{1\,\text{day}} \times \frac{1\,\text{qt}}{946\,\text{mL}} \times \frac{37\,\text{g}}{1\,\text{qt}} = 77.07\,\text{g/day},\ \textit{answers}.$$

(c) *If the product contains 85% free water, does it meet the patient's daily water requirement?*

$$1970.58\,\text{mL/day} \times 85\% = 1675\,\text{mL/day}$$

Therefore, the amount of water provided by 1970.58 mL of the formula would *not* fully meet the patient's daily water requirement, *answer*.

(d) *If the formula is to be delivered continuously over a 24-hour period, what would be the flow rate in mL/hr?*

$$\frac{1970.58\,\text{mL}}{1\,\text{day}} \times \frac{1\,\text{day}}{24\,\text{hrs}} = 82.11\,\text{mL/hr} \approx 82\,\text{mL/hr},\ \textit{answer}.$$

(e) *If the patient is to continue receiving this formula at home by intermittent feedings over 40 minutes every 4 hours, what volume would be administered with each feeding, and what would be the flow rate in mL/hr?*

$$\frac{1970.58\,\text{mL}}{1\,\text{day}} \times \frac{1\,\text{day}}{24\,\text{hrs}} \times \frac{4\,\text{hrs}}{1\,\text{dose}} = 328.43\,\text{mL/dose},\ \textit{and}$$

$$\frac{328.43\,\text{mL}}{40\,\text{min}} \times \frac{60\,\text{min}}{1\,\text{hr}} = 492.65\,\text{mL/hr} \approx 493\,\text{mL/hr},\ \textit{answers}.$$

Example Calculations of Parenteral Nutrition

The following basic steps may be used as a guide in TPN calculations.

Step 1. Calculate the total daily calories required using the Harris-Benedict equations, and apply the appropriate stress or activity factors.

Step 2. Calculate the daily quantity (g) of amino acids (protein) required based on 0.8 g/kg of body weight, and adjust as needed for stress factors and certain disease states.

Step 3. Calculate the number of calories supplied by the amino acids (from Step 2) at 4 kcal/g.

Step 4. Calculate the kcal of lipids required at 20% to 40% of the total daily calories.

Step 5. Calculate the grams of lipids required (from Step 4) based on 9 kcal/g or based on the lipid emulsion used [as discussed in the section titled "Lipid (Fat) Requirements" earlier in the text].

Step 6. Calculate the quantity of carbohydrate required based on 3.4 kcal/g after accounting for the contribution of the lipids.

Step 7. Calculate the daily fluid requirement using 30 mL/kg/day or one of the other methods described earlier in the text.

Notes: In some clinical practices (a) a patient's actual body weight, the ideal body weight, or some middle ground may be used in the calculations (in Step 1), and (b) in Step 6, the energy provided by the protein, in addition to that from lipids, may or may not be taken into account. In addition to Steps 1 through 7, TPN calculations also can include:

- determination of the quantities of the pharmaceutical sources of the macronutrients (e.g., vials) and micronutrients (e.g., LVPs) to use to obtain the required components; and
- determination of the total TPN volume, the number of TPN bags to be prepared, and the rate of flow.

Calculate the parenteral nutrition and fluid requirements for a 58-year-old woman who is 5 ft. 3 in. tall and weighs 140 lb., assuming that she has no disease states that would alter her nutritional requirements.

Step 1. Total daily kcal required by Harris-Benedict equation:

$$655.1 + (9.56 \times 63.63 \text{ kg}) + (1.85 \times 160 \text{ cm}) - (4.68 \times 58 \text{ yr}) = 1287.96 \text{ kcal}$$

Step 2. Protein required (grams):

$$140 \text{ lb.} \times \frac{1 \text{ kg}}{2.2 \text{ lb.}} \times \frac{0.8 \text{ g}}{1 \text{ kg/day}} = 50.91 \text{ g/day}$$

Step 3. Protein (kcal):

$$\frac{50.91 \text{ g}}{1 \text{ day}} \times \frac{4 \text{ kcal}}{1 \text{ g}} = 203.64 \text{ kcal/day}$$

Step 4. Lipids required (kcal), using 35% of total daily calories:

$$1287.96 \text{ kcal/day (total)} \times 35\% = 450.79 \text{ kcal/day}$$

Step 5. Lipids required (grams), using a 10% lipid emulsion:

$$\frac{450.79 \text{ kcal}}{1 \text{ day}} \times \frac{1 \text{ g}}{11 \text{ kcal}} = 40.98 \text{ g/day}$$

Step 6. Carbohydrates (dextrose) required (grams), accounting for kcal from both protein and lipids:

$$1287.96 \text{ kcal/day} - 203.64 \text{ kcal/day (protein)} - 450.79 \text{ kcal/day (lipids)} = 633.53 \text{ kcal/day}$$

$$\frac{633.53 \text{ kcal}}{1 \text{ day}} \times \frac{1 \text{ g}}{3.4 \text{ kcal}} = 186.33 \text{ g/day}$$

Step 7. Fluid required (milliliters):

Based on 30 mL/kg/day:

$$140 \text{ lb.} \times \frac{1 \text{ kg}}{2.2 \text{ lb.}} \times \frac{30 \text{ mL}}{1 \text{ kg/day}} = 1909.09 \text{ mL/day}$$

Based on 1 mL/kcal required/day:

$$\frac{1287.96 \text{ kcal}}{1 \text{ day}} \times \frac{1 \text{ mL}}{1 \text{ kcal}} = 1287.96 \text{ mL/day}$$

The patient should receive 50.91 g of protein, 41.03 g of lipids, 186.33 g of dextrose, and between 1287.96 and 1909.09 mL of fluid per day, *answer.*

Using the Harris-Benedict equation, calculate the caloric requirement for an ambulatory 56-year-old hospitalized female patient weighing 121 lb. and measuring 5 ft 3 in. in height.

$$121 \text{ lb.} = 55 \text{ kg}$$
$$5 \text{ ft. } 3 \text{ in.} = 63 \text{ in.} = 160 \text{ cm}$$
$$\text{BEE} = 655.1 + (9.56 \times 55) + (1.85 \times 160) - (4.68 \times 56)$$
$$= 655.1 + (525.8) + (296) - (262)$$
$$= 1217.9 \text{ kcal}$$

Using the activity factor of 1.3 for a mildly stressed patient:

$$1217.9 \times 1.3 = 1583.27 \text{ kcal, } answer.$$

Calculate the daily quantity of protein required for the 55-kg-patient based on 0.8 g/kg and the caloric value based on 4 kcal/g for proteins.

$$55 \text{ kg} \times 0.8 \text{ g/kg} = 44 \text{ g protein, } and$$
$$44 \text{ g} \times 4 \text{ kcal/g} = 176 \text{ kcal, } answers.$$

From the previous two example problems, calculate the number of milliliters of 50% dextrose solution (170 kcal/dL) that may be used to provide the additional kilocalories required.

$$\text{Total kcal required} = 1583.27$$
$$\text{kcal provided by proteins} = 176$$
$$\text{Additional kcal required} = 1407.27 \ (1583.27 - 176)$$

Thus,

$$\frac{1407.27 \text{ kcal}}{170 \text{ kcal}} = \frac{x \text{ mL}}{100 \text{ mL}}$$
$$x = 827.8 \text{ mL, } answer.$$

The following is a formula for a desired parenteral nutrition solution. Using the source of each drug as indicated, calculate the amount of each component required in preparing the solution.

Formula	Component Source
(*a*) Sodium Chloride 35 mEq	Vial, 5 mEq per 2 mL
(*b*) Potassium Acetate 35 mEq	Vial, 10 mEq per 5 mL
(*c*) Magnesium Sulfate 8 mEq	Vial, 4 mEq per mL
(*d*) Calcium Gluconate 9.6 mEq	Vial, 4.7 mEq per 10 mL
(*e*) Potassium Chloride 5 mEq	Vial, 40 mEq per 20 mL
(*f*) Folic Acid 1.7 mg	Ampul, 5 mg per mL
(*g*) Multiple Vitamin Infusion 10 mL	Ampul, 10 mL

To be added to:

Amino Acids Infusion (8.5%) 500 mL
Dextrose Injection (50%) 500 mL

(a)
$$\frac{5\,(\text{mEq})}{35\,(\text{mEq})} = \frac{2\,(\text{mL})}{x\,(\text{mL})}$$
$$x = 14\;\text{mL};$$

(b)
$$\frac{10\,(\text{mEq})}{35\,(\text{mEq})} = \frac{5\,(\text{mL})}{x\,(\text{mL})}$$
$$x = 17.5\;\text{mL};$$

(c)
$$\frac{4\,(\text{mEq})}{8\,(\text{mEq})} = \frac{1\,(\text{mL})}{x\,(\text{mL})}$$
$$x = 2\;\text{mL};$$

(d)
$$\frac{4.7\,(\text{mEq})}{9.6\,(\text{mEq})} = \frac{10\,(\text{mL})}{x\,(\text{mL})}$$
$$x = 20.4\;\text{mL};$$

(e)
$$\frac{40\,(\text{mEq})}{5\,(\text{mEq})} = \frac{20\,(\text{mL})}{x\,(\text{mL})}$$
$$x = 2.5\;\text{mL};$$

(f)
$$\frac{5\,(\text{mg})}{1.7\,(\text{mg})} = \frac{1\,(\text{mL})}{x\,(\text{mL})}$$
$$x = 0.34\;\text{mL; and}$$

(g)   10 mL, *answers.*

The formula for a TPN solution calls for the addition of 2.7 mEq of Ca^{++} and 20 mEq of K$^+$ per liter. How many milliliters of an injection containing 20 mg of calcium chloride per milliliter and how many milliliters of a 15% (w/v) potassium chloride injection should be used to provide the desired additives?

$$\text{Formula weight of } CaCl_2 \cdot 2\,H_2O = 147$$
$$\text{Formula weight of KCl} = 74.5$$
$$1\;\text{mEq of Ca}^{++} = 20\;\text{mg}$$
$$2.7\;\text{mEq of Ca}^{++} = 20\;\text{mg} \times 2.7 = 54\;\text{mg}$$

54 mg of Ca^{++} are furnished by 198.45 or 198 mg of calcium chloride

Because the injection contains 20 mg of calcium chloride per mL, then $198 \div 20 = 9.9\;\text{mL}$, and

$$1\;\text{mEq of K}^+ = 39\;\text{mg}$$
$$20\;\text{mEq of K}^+ = 39\;\text{mg} \times 20 = 780\;\text{mg}$$

780 mg of K$^+$ are furnished by 1.49 g of potassium chloride
15% (w/v) solution contains 15 g of potassium chloride per 100 mL, then

$$\frac{15\,(\text{g})}{1.49\,(\text{g})} = \frac{100\,(\text{mL})}{x\,(\text{mL})}$$
$$x = 9.9\;\text{mL, } answers.$$

A potassium phosphate injection contains a mixture of 224 mg of monobasic potassium phosphate *(KH₂PO₄) and 236 mg of dibasic potassium phosphate (K₂HPO₄) per milliliter. If 10 mL of the injection are added to 500 mL of D5W (5% dextrose in water for injection), (a) how many milliequivalents of K⁺ and (b) how many millimoles of total phosphate are represented in the prepared solution?*

$$\text{Formula weight of } KH_2PO_4 = 136$$
$$1 \text{ mmol of } KH_2PO_4 = 136 \text{ mg}$$

10 mL of injection contains 2240 mg of KH_2PO_4

and thus provide $2240 \div 136 = 16.4$ or 16 mmol of KH_2PO_4
or 16 mmol of K^+ and 16 mmol of $H_2PO_4 =$

$$\text{Formula weight of } K_2HPO_4 = 174$$
$$1 \text{ mmol of } K_2HPO_4 = 174 \text{ mg}$$

10 mL of injection contain 2360 mg of K_2HPO_4
and thus provide $2360 \div 174 = 13.6$ or 14 mmol of K_2HPO_4
or 14 (mmol) $\times 2$ (K^+) = 28 mmol of K^+, and 14 mmol of $HPO_4 =$
thus 10 mL of injection provide a total of:
44 mmol of K^+ or (because the valence of K^+ is 1) 44 mEq of K^+, *and*
30 mmol of total phosphate, *answers.*

CASE IN POINT 14.1 A hospital pharmacist is asked to provide TPN for a 75-year-old female patient who is 5 ft 2 in. in height and weighs 120 lb. The patient is confined to bed but has no stress factors. The pharmacist reviews the patient's laboratory records and based on experience decides to prepare a 2000 mL TPN, utilizing a 10% amino acid injection as the protein source, D50W as the source of dextrose, and a 20% lipid emulsion as the fat source, with a standard mixture of electrolytes, minerals, and vitamins. The pharmacist asks a student on a pharmacy practice experience program to perform these basic calculations:

(a) target amount of the patient's daily fluid requirement,
(b) target amount of daily protein requirements (g/day)
(c) volume of amino acid injection that may be required
(d) target amount of non-protein calories (kcal)
(e) the volume of D50W that could supply the non-protein calories

---

Body Mass Index (BMI)

As previously stated, being overweight carries an increased risk for a number of health consequences. However, being *grossly* overweight, or *obese*, predisposes one to an even greater risk of disease, disease complications, and mortality.[3] In addition to diet, other factors that can result in obesity include behavioral, cultural, metabolic, and genetic disposition.

The initial phase in managing the overweight or obese patient is an assessment of the degree of excessive weight. Today, **body mass index (BMI)** is accepted as the clinical standard for judging excessive weight and obesity. BMI is defined as body weight in kilograms divided by the square of height measured in meters. According to the National Institutes of Health (NIH),[3] individuals with a BMI (kg/m²):

- ≤18.5 (kg/m²) are considered underweight;
- 18.5 to 24.9 (kg/m²) are considered normal;
- 25.0 to 29.9 (kg/m²) are considered overweight;
- 30.0 to 39.9 (kg/m²) are considered obese; and
- ≥40 (kg/m²) are considered extremely obese.

For an elderly person, a BMI of less than 21 can be a sign of malnutrition.[17] BMI in *most people* is an indicator of high body fat (this may not be the case for persons who are especially muscular).

Calculations Involving Body Mass Index

Determining BMI from a Standardized Table

BMI may be determined by using a standardized table like that shown in Table 14.1, in which the intercept of a person's height and weight indicates the body mass index. Many of the standardized tables available are in units of the common systems of measurement (i.e., feet/inches and pounds) to facilitate ease of use by the general public. Others are available in metric or dual scale.

> *Using Table 14.1, determine the BMI for a person measuring 5 ft. 8 in. and weighing 160 lb.*
> The intercept of 5 ft. 8 in. and 160 lb. shows a BMI of 24, *answer.*

> *Using Table 14.1, determine the BMI for a person 183 cm in height and weighing 82 kg.*

Table 14.1 ▼ DETERMINING BODY MASS INDEX (BMI, kg/m²)

HEIGHT	\<WEIGHT\> 100	110	120	130	140	150	160	170	180	190	200	210	220	230	240	250
5'0"	20	21	23	25	27	29	31	33	35	37	39	41	43	45	47	49
5'1"	19	21	23	25	26	28	30	32	34	36	38	40	42	43	45	47
5'2"	18	20	22	24	26	27	29	31	33	35	37	38	40	42	44	46
5'3"	18	19	21	23	25	27	28	30	32	34	35	37	39	41	43	44
5'4"	17	19	21	22	24	26	27	29	31	33	34	36	38	39	41	43
5'5"	17	18	20	22	23	25	27	28	30	32	33	35	37	38	40	42
5'6"	16	18	19	21	23	24	26	27	29	31	32	34	36	37	39	40
5'7"	16	17	19	20	22	23	25	27	28	30	31	33	34	36	38	39
5'8"	15	17	18	20	21	23	24	26	27	29	30	32	33	35	36	38
5'9"	15	16	18	19	21	22	24	25	27	28	30	31	32	34	35	37
5'10"	14	16	17	19	20	22	23	24	26	27	29	30	32	33	34	36
5'11"	14	15	17	18	20	21	22	24	25	26	27	28	30	32	33	35
6'0"	14	15	16	18	19	20	22	23	24	26	27	28	30	31	33	34
6'1"	13	15	16	17	18	20	21	22	24	25	26	28	29	30	32	33
6'2"	13	14	15	17	18	19	21	22	23	24	26	27	28	30	31	32
6'3"	12	14	15	16	17	19	20	21	22	24	25	26	27	29	30	31
6'4"	12	13	15	16	17	18	19	21	22	23	24	26	27	28	29	30

BMI interpretation

Underweight: under 18.5

Normal: 18.5–24.9

Overweight: 25–29.9

Obese: 30–39.9

Extremely obese ≥ 40

$$\frac{2.54 \text{ cm}}{183 \text{ cm}} = \frac{1 \text{ in.}}{x \text{ in.}}; x = 72 \text{ in.}$$

$$\frac{1 \text{ kg}}{82 \text{ kg}} = \frac{2.2 \text{ lb.}}{x \text{ lb.}}; x = 180 \text{ lb.}$$

Then, in Table 14.1, the intercept of 72 in, or 6 ft. 0 in. in height and 180 lb., shows a BMI of 24, *answer.*

Determining BMI by Calculation

If a person's height and weight are outside the range of a BMI table, or if a BMI table is unavailable, BMI may be determined by the formula:

$$BMI = \frac{\text{Weight (kg)}}{\text{Height (m}^2)}$$

Calculate the BMI of a person 4 ft. 11 in. in height and weighing 98 lb.

$$\frac{2.2 \text{ lb.}}{98 \text{ lb.}} = \frac{1 \text{ kg}}{x \text{ kg}}; x = 44.5 \text{ kg}$$

$$\frac{39.37 \text{ in.}}{59 \text{ in.}} = \frac{1 \text{ meter}}{x \text{ meter}}; x = 1.5 \text{ meters}$$

$$\frac{44.5 \text{ kg}}{1.5 \text{ m} \times 1.5 \text{ m}} = \frac{44.5 \text{ kg}}{2.25 \text{ m}^2} = 19.8 \text{ BMI}, \textit{answer.}$$

Calculate the BMI of a person 6 ft. 0 in. in height weighing 182 lb.

$$\frac{2.2 \text{ lb.}}{182 \text{ lb.}} = \frac{1 \text{ kg}}{x \text{ kg}} \quad x = 82.7 \text{ kg, and}$$

$$\frac{39.37 \text{ in.}}{72 \text{ in.}} = \frac{1 \text{ meter}}{x \text{ meter}}; x = 1.83 \text{ meters, thus}$$

$$\frac{82.7 \text{ kg}}{1.83 \text{ m} \times 1.83 \text{ m}} = \frac{82.7 \text{ kg}}{3.35 \text{ m}^2} = 24.7 \text{ BMI}, \textit{answer.}$$

Note: In these calculations, pounds may be multiplied by 0.454 to get kilograms, and inches may be multiplied by 0.0254 to get meters.

An Alternative Formula for the Calculation of BMI

BMI may be calculated by the formula:

$$\frac{\text{Weight (lb.)}}{\text{Height (in.)}^2} \times 704.5 = BMI$$

Note: The factor 704.5, used by the National Institutes of Health, is derived by dividing the square of 39.37 (in./m) by 2.2 (lb./kg).

Calculate the BMI for a person weighing 182 lb. and standing 72 in. in height.

$$\frac{182 \text{ lb.}}{(72 \text{ in.})^2} = \frac{182 \text{ lb.}}{5184 \text{ in.}} \times 704.5 = 24.7 \text{ BMI}, \textit{answer.}$$

The Nutrition Label

The *2010 Dietary Guidelines for Americans*,[18] issued by the United States Departments of Agriculture (USDA) and Health and Human Services (HHS), provide guidance aimed at improving health and reversing obesity and related diseases. The document includes basic nutritional information and dietary recommendations while the Web site offers interactive tools to assist consumers in meeting dietary objectives. The familiar "Nutrition Facts" (Fig. 14.3) that accompanies packaged foods is a labeling requirement of the FDA and provides direct guidance to the consumer.[18–20] Through knowledge of dietary requirements and the nutrition label, pharmacists have a unique opportunity to counsel patients.

Percent Daily Value (% DV)

As is depicted in Figure 14.3, nutrition labeling includes a listing of Daily Reference Values (DRVs) based on a 2000 calorie diet (most labels also include values based on a 2500 calorie diet). These values allow consumers to ascertain the amount of a particular nutrient in a food product and to compare the nutritional content between products.

Nutrition Facts

Serving Size 1 cup (228g)
Servings Per Container 2

Amount Per Serving

Calories 260	Calories from Fat 120

	% Daily Value*
Total Fat 13g	**20%**
Saturated Fat 5g	**25%**
Trans Fat 2g	
Cholesterol 30mg	**10%**
Sodium 660mg	**28%**
Total Carbohydrate 31g	**10%**
Dietary Fiber 0g	**0%**
Sugars 5g	
Protein 5g	

Vitamin A	4%
Vitamin C	2%
Calcium	15%
Iron	4%

* Percent Daily Values are based on a 2,000 calorie diet. Your Daily Values may be higher or lower depending on your calorie needs:

	Calories:	2,000	2,500
Total Fat	Less than	65g	80g
Sat Fat	Less than	20g	25g
Cholesterol	Less than	300mg	300mg
Sodium	Less than	2,400mg	2,400mg
Total Carbohydrate		300g	375g
Dietary Fiber		25g	30g

Calories per gram:
  Fat 9 • Carbohydrate 4 • Protein 4

▼ FIGURE 14.3 Example of a nutrition label.

Required labeling includes the *percent daily value* (%DV) for certain nutritional components. In order to calculate the %DV, the quantity of a nutrient in a serving is compared to its daily value and expressed as a percent. For example, in Figure 14.3, the total fat per serving is 13 g and the total DV for total fat (on the bottom of label, based on a 2000 calorie diet) is 65 g. Thus, 13 g/65 g × 100% = 20%, the labeled %DV for total fat.

Serving Size and Servings per Container

The labeled *serving size* reflects the amount that people generally eat at one time and is indicated in common household units (e.g., 1 cup) and approximate corresponding metric measure (e.g., 240 g). Items of discrete size, such as cookies, are listed in both units and metric equivalent, e.g., "2 cookies (26 g)." The *servings per container* indicates the number of servings in the package.

Calories

On the nutrition label, *calories per serving* and the number of *calories derived from fat* are of special importance to many consumers. High-calorie and high-fat diets are linked to overweight and obesity and the consequent illnesses.

A *calorie* (spelled with a small *c*) is the amount of energy needed to raise the temperature of 1 g of water 1°C. A *kilocalorie (kcal)* equals 1000 calories. The kilocalorie, or Calorie (spelled with a capital *C*), is the unit used in metabolism studies and in nutrition to describe the energy provided by various foods. In common usage, the "small-C" *calorie* is often used interchangeably (albeit incorrectly).

According to the *2010 Dietary Guidelines for Americans*,[18] the caloric requirements as stated in Table 14.2 generally are suitable for most persons.

For the calculations in this section, it is important to note that:

> **carbohydrates yield 4 kcal/g;**
> **protein, 4 kcal/g; and**
> **fat, 9 kcal/g.**

Table 14.2 ▼ ESTIMATED DAILY CALORIE REQUIREMENTS[a]

AGE (YEARS)	SEDENTARY[b]		MODERATELY ACTIVE[c]		ACTIVE[d]	
	FEMALE	MALE	FEMALE	MALE	FEMALE	MALE
2	1000	1000	1000	1000	1000	1000
5	1200	1200	1400	1400	1600	1600
10	1400	1600	1800	1800	2000	2200
15	1800	2200	2000	2600	2400	3000
20–29	2000	2600	2200	2800	2400	3000
30–39	1800	2400	2000	2600	2200	2800
40–50	1800	2200	2000	2400	2200	2800
60	1600	2000	1800	2400	2000	2600
70+	1600	2000	1800	2200	2000	2600

[a]Adapted with modification from *2010 Dietary Guidelines for Americans*.[18]
[b]*Sedentary* includes only light physical activity associated with daily life.
[c]*Moderately active* includes walking 1.5 to 3 miles/day at 3 to 4 miles/h or equivalent other activity.
[d]*Active* includes walking more than 3 miles/day at 3 to 4 miles/h or equivalent other activity.

Macronutrients—Carbohydrates, Protein, and Fats

The recommended *relative proportions* of daily dietary calories between carbohydrate, protein, and fat for age groups are shown in Table 14.3.[18]

Carbohydrates are important components of a healthy diet providing the fuel for energy and organ function. Dietary fiber (a carbohydrate) is a food component providing valuable "roughage" to the digestive tract. The generally recommended daily amount of carbohydrate intake for adults is about 300 g based on a 2000-calorie diet. Daily fiber requirements were stated previously in this chapter.

Protein intake is not considered a general health concern for adults and children over 4 years of age.[18] Consequently, a labeled percent of the daily value *is not* required unless a protein claim is made for the product or if the product is intended for use by infants or children under 4 years of age. Guidelines suggest a daily protein requirement of 0.8 g/kg or 50 g for adults and children 4 or more years of age; 16 g for children less than 4 years of age; 14 g for infants; 60 g for pregnant women; and 65 g for lactating women.

In addition to the listing requirement for *total fat*, the nutrition label also is required to contain the content of *saturated fat* and *trans fat*. Intake of these components increases the body's low density lipoprotein (LDL) cholesterol and the risk of developing coronary heart disease. Guidelines suggest total dietary fat of less than 65 g/day with less than 20 g being saturated fat. It is recommended that the intake of cholesterol be less than 300 mg daily.

Sodium and Potassium

The labeling of sodium and potassium content is required. Guidelines suggest that sodium intake should be less than 2300 mg daily and reduced to 1500 mg for persons who are 51 years of age and older, and for persons of any age who are African American or have hypertension, diabetes, or chronic kidney disease.[18] Presently, the daily 1500 mg recommendation applies to about half of the United States population, including children, and the majority of adults.

The adult requirement of potassium is considered to be about 4 g/day.

Micronutrients—Vitamins and Minerals

The nutrition label must specify the content of vitamins A and C and the minerals, calcium and iron. Any additional content of vitamins and minerals must appear in a food's general ingredient list.

Use of Special Terms on the Nutrition Label

Descriptive terms as "*lite, free, low, reduced,*" as used with reference to calories, fat, saturated fat, cholesterol, sodium and sugars, are defined and regulated by the FDA. The qualifying definitions are found in the reference.[21]

Table 14.3 ▼ **RECOMMENDED MACRONUTRIENT PROPORTIONS OF DAILY DIETARY CALORIES BY AGE**[18]

	CARBOHYDRATE (%)	PROTEIN (%)	TOTAL FAT (%)[a]
Young Children (1–3 years)	45–65	5–20	30–40
Older Children and Adolescents (4–18 years)	45–65	10–30	25–35
Adults (19 years and older)	45–65	10–35	20–35

[a]Saturated fat, less than 10% of daily calories.

Example Calculations Involving the Nutrition Label

Note: In calculations of the labeled "% Daily Values," the FDA allows latitude in rounding.

Based on the "Nutrition Facts" depicted in Figure 14.3, for a 2500 calorie intake and with the consumption of one serving size, calculate the percent daily value (% DV) for (a) total fat, (b) cholesterol, and (c) sodium.

(a) 13 g/80 g × 100% = 16% total fat (rounded), and
(b) 30 mg/300 mg × 100% = 10% cholesterol, and
(c) 660 mg/2400 mg × 100% = 28% sodium (rounded), *answers.*

For a person on a sodium-reduced diet (i.e., 1500 mg/day), recalculate the % DV in the above-problem.

$$660 \text{ mg}/1500 \text{ mg} \times 100\% = 40\% \text{ sodium, } answer.$$

Using the data from Tables 14.2 and 14.3, calculate the caloric intake of each macronutrient by a moderately active 20-year-old female who consumes 45% carbohydrate, 35% protein, and 20% fat.

Total daily intake = 2200 calories (Table 14.2).
Carbohydrate: 2200 calories × 45% = 990 calories, and
protein: 2200 calories × 35% = 770 calories, and
fat: 2200 calories × 20% = 440 calories, *answers.*

For the previous problem, calculate the intake in grams for each macronutrient.

Carbohydrate: 990 calories/4 calories per gram = 247.5 g, and
protein: 770 calories/4 calories per gram = 192.5 g, and
fat: 440 calories/9 calories per gram = 48.9 g, *answers.*

For a diet of 3000 calories, calculate the dietary grams of fat based on the daily reference values (DRVs) for this substance. Is the calculated amount of fat "acceptable" according to the standards of upper limits for a healthy diet?

DRV for fat = 30% of calories
Thus, for fat, 30% of 3000 calories = 900 calories

Since fat provides 9 calories/g:

$$\frac{9 \text{ calories}}{900 \text{ calories}} = \frac{1 \text{ g fat}}{x \text{ g fat}}; \ x = 100 \text{ g fat}$$

Since the "upper limit" of fat for a healthy diet is "less than 65 g," 100 g of fat is not acceptable, *answers.*

How many calories from fat and how many grams of fat should be the limit per day for a person on a 2000-calorie diet?

$$2000 \times 35\% = 700 \text{ calories from fat, and}$$

$$\frac{9 \text{ calories}}{700 \text{ calories}} = \frac{1 \text{ g}}{x \text{ g}}; \ x = 78 \text{ grams of fat, } answers$$

How many food calories would be provided by a diet of 65 grams of fat, 500 grams of carbohydrate, and 180 grams of protein?

65 g fat × 9 calories/g	= 585 calories
500 g carbohydrate × 4 calories/g	= 2000 calories
180 g protein × 4 calories/g	= 720 calories
	3305 calories, *answer.*

If a food item contains 100 calories per serving with 10 calories coming from fat, is it considered both "low calorie" and "low fat"?

By definition, *low calorie* is less than 40 calories per serving. Thus, the food item is not "low calorie," and on the basis of 9 calories per gram of fat:

$$\frac{9\,\text{calories}}{10\,\text{calories}} = \frac{1\,\text{g}}{\text{x}\,\text{g}}; x = 1.1\,\text{g fat}$$

Low fat is defined as less than 3 g per serving, and thus the food item *is* low fat, *answers*.

A multiple vitamin tablet contains 7500 international units of vitamin A. If this amount represents a %DV of 150%, what is the 100% daily requirement of vitamin A?

$$\frac{150\%\,\text{DV}}{100\%\,\text{DV}} = \frac{7500\,\text{I.U.}}{\text{x}\,\text{I.U.}}; x = 5000 \text{ international units}, \textit{answer}.$$

A multiple vitamin and mineral tablet contains 162 mg of calcium. If the minimum daily value for calcium is 1000 mg, what percentage of the minimum daily value of calcium is contained in each tablet?

$$\frac{162\,\text{mg}}{1000\,\text{mg}} \times 100 = 16.2\%, \textit{answer}.$$

CALCULATIONS CAPSULE

Adult Nutrition

Basal energy expenditure (BEE):

The Harris-Benedict equations may be used to approximate the BEE, in kcal:

$BEE_{males} = 66.65 + [13.75 \times Weight\ (kg)] + [5 \times Height\ (cm)] - [6.78 \times Age\ (yr)]$
$BEE_{females} = 655.1 + [9.56 \times Weight\ (kg)] + [1.85 \times Height\ (cm)] - [4.68 \times Age\ (yr)]$

The BEE is adjusted by activity and stress factors to yield the estimated total daily energy expenditure (TDE).

kcal/g values:
   Carbohydrates @ 4 kcal/g (enteral), 3.4 kcal/g (parenteral)
   Proteins @ 4 kcal/g
   Fats (lipids) @ 9 kcal/g

Fluid requirement:
   30 mL/kg patient weight, or
   1 mL/kcal, nutrition provided, or
   1500 mL/m² BSA

CASE IN POINT 14.2 A parent asks a pharmacist to explain the nutritional content of PEDIASURE Enteral Formula, which has been recommended for her 12-year-old child. The label indicates that 1500 mL of the product, taken daily, provides complete nutrition for children 9 to 13 years of age. The product is packaged in 237-mL cans containing 7.1 g protein, 9.4 g fat, 31.4 g carbohydrate, 202 g water, and over 30 vitamins and minerals. Calculate:

(a) The kilocalories per milliliter of product.
(b) The grams each of protein, fat, and carbohydrate, consumed from a daily intake of 1500 mL of product.
(c) The proportion, expressed in percentage, of daily kilocalories derived from each of protein, fat, and carbohydrate.
(d) Whether or not the answers in (c) compare favorably with the recommended parameters as stated in Table 14.3.

PRACTICE PROBLEMS

Calculations of Nutritional Requirements

1. From the information in this chapter, calculate the estimated daily protein requirement, in g/day, for a 141-lb. renal dialysis patient.

2. A nutritional formula calls for 500 g of dextrose. How many milliliters of a 70% w/v dextrose injection are needed to provide the required amount of dextrose?

3. A patient requires 1800 kcal/day, including 60 g of protein. How many kilocalories would be provided by the protein?

4. If the source of the protein in problem 3 is a 5% amino acid solution, how many milliliters of the solution would be needed to provide the requirement?

5. Calculate the following for enteral nutrition:
   (a) Grams of dextrose needed to supply 1400 kcal
   (b) grams of protein needed to supply 800 kcal
   (c) grams of lipid needed to supply 1000 kcal (111.1 g lipid)

6. Calculate the approximate daily water requirement for a/an:
   (a) 165-lb. patient
   (b) adult patient with a BSA of 1.6 m²
   (c) patient receiving 1500 kcal by TPN
   (d) 2.2-kg neonate
   (e) 19-kg child
   (f) child with a BSA of 0.65

7. The daily caloric requirement for a 201-lb. 76-year-old male has been determined to be 2088.82 kcal/day. Calculate the protein, carbohydrate, lipid (35% TDC), and fluid requirements for enteral nutrition, assuming no stress factors.

8. A TPN order calls for a liter of solution to contain 2.125% of amino acids and 20% of dextrose. How many milliliters each of 8.5% amino acid injection, 50% dextrose injection, and sterile water for injection should be used to prepare the solution?

9. If a 50% dextrose injection provides 170 kcal in each 100 mL, how many milliliters of a 70% dextrose injection would provide the same caloric value?

10. Using the Harris-Benedict equation and assuming no stress factor, calculate (a) the daily calories required, and (b) the daily protein needed for a 58-year-old woman who is 5 ft. 3 in. tall and weighs 152 lb.

11. Using the Harris-Benedict equation, calculate the TPN caloric requirement for a hospitalized, bedridden, 60-year-old male surgical patient, weighing 160 lb, and measuring 5 ft 8 in. in height.

12. If amino acids have a caloric value of 4 kcal/g and the daily protein requirement is 0.8g/kg, calculate the kilocalories administered to a patient weighing 180 lb.

13. A medication order for a TPN solution calls for additives as indicated in the following formula. Using the sources designated below, calculate the amount of each component required in filling the medication order.

TPN Solution Formula	Component Source
Sodium Chloride 40 mEq	10-mL vial of 30% solution
Potassium Acetate 15 mEq	20-mL vial containing 40 mEq
Vitamin B_{12} 10 μg	Vial containing 1 mg in 10 mL
Insulin 8 units	Vial of Insulin U-100

To be added to:
500 mL of 50% dextrose injection
500 mL of 7% protein hydrolysate injection

14. A solution of potassium phosphate contains a mixture of 164 mg of monobasic potassium phosphate and 158 mg of dibasic potassium phosphate per milliliter.

    (a) If a TPN fluid calls for the addition of 45 mEq of K^+, how many milliliters of the solution should be used to provide this level of potassium?

    (b) How many millimoles of total phosphate will be represented in the calculated volume of potassium phosphate solution?

15. Using the component sources as indicated, calculate the amount of each component required in preparing 1000 mL of the following parenteral nutrition solution:

Parenteral Nutrition Solution Formula	Component Source
(a) Amino Acids 2.125%	500 mL of 8.5% amino acids injection
(b) Dextrose 20%	500 mL of 50% dextrose injection
(c) Sodium Chloride 30 mEq	20-mL vial of 15% solution
(d) Calcium Gluconate 2.5 mEq	10-mL vial containing 4.6 mEq
(e) Insulin 15 units	Vial of U-100 insulin
(f) Heparin 2500 units	5-mL vial containing 1000 units/mL
(g) Sterile Water for Injection to make 1000 mL	500 mL of sterile water for injection

Calculations of Body Mass Index

16. Using Table 14.1, determine the body mass index for a person measuring 62 in. in height and weighing 150 lb.

17. Calculate the body mass index for a person measuring 1.7 meters in height and weighing 87 kilograms (round answer).

18. An investigational drug for obesity is being dosed at either of two protocols: (a) 7.6 mg/0.5 BMI for persons with a BMI over 25 but less than 30, or (b) 9.6 mg/0.5 BMI for persons with a BMI greater than 30. In each protocol, the dose is equally divided and administered "t.i.d.a.c." What would be the divided dose for a male standing 5 ft. 8 in. and weighing 230 pounds?

Calculations of Nutrition Label Information

19. If a person consumes 3000 calories per day, calculate the intake of fat, in grams, based on dietary fat being 30 percent of caloric intake.

20. A high-fiber cereal contains 13 g of dietary fiber in each 30 g of cereal. Calculate the %DV of dietary fiber, based on a 2000-calorie diet and the general requirement of 14 g fiber per 1000 calorie intake.

21. A sweetened cereal contains 14 g of sugar (carbohydrate) per 30 g serving size of cereal. Calculate the %DV based on a 2000-calorie diet.

22. How many grams of fat are contained in a 2500-calorie diet if 450 of those calories are derived from fat?

23. If an 8-oz. container of yogurt contains 300 mg of calcium, calculate the percent daily requirement for a young adult met by consuming half the contents of the container. The daily requirement of calcium is listed as 1000 mg.

24. If a food serving contains 240 mg of potassium, listed as 6 percent of the daily value, calculate 100% of the daily value of potassium in milligrams.

25. Using the information in Figure 14.3, calculate the %DV for sodium if a different product contained 140 mg of sodium.

CALCQUIZ

14.A. A pharmacist is providing TPN for hospitalized patients. One patient is a 75-year-old female weighing 115 lb and measuring 5 ft 1 in. in height. She is confined to her bed and is somewhat stressed following a surgical procedure. Another patient is an 80-year-old male weighing 162 lb and measuring 5 ft 10 in. in height. He is ambulatory but stressed due to a severe infection. The pharmacist uses the Harris-Benedict equations adjusted for activity and stress factors to determine patients' daily energy requirements. Perform the same calculations.

14.B.[a] A TPN formula is as follows:

Dextrose injection, 50%	1000 mL
Amino acids, 10%	400 mL
Electrolyte/Vitamin mix	200 mL
Sterile water for injection	800 mL

If the TPN fluid is to be administered over 24 hours, (a) how many calories will be administered per hour, and (b) what would be the flow rate, in drops/min, when using an IV set that delivers 10 drops/mL?

(continued)

CALCQUIZ (continued)

14.C.[a] A TPN formula is as follows:

Dextrose	15%
Amino acids	4%
Sodium chloride	0.75%
Potassium chloride	0.2%
Multivitamin injection	10 mL
Sterile water for injection, ad	1000 mL

(a) How many milliliters of each of the following will be needed to prepare the formula?

Dextrose injection, 700 mg/mL
Amino acid injection, 10%
Sodium chloride injection, 4 mEq/mL
Potassium chloride injection, 2 mEq/mL

(b) If the flow rate for the TPN is prescribed at 1 mL/kg/h, how many total calories will a 187-lb patient receive in 24 hours?

14.D. Compare a 152-lb 5 ft 8 in. patient's target daily fluid requirement based on (a) weight, (b) body surface area, and (c) a daily nutritional requirement of 2000 kcal.

14.E. A high-protein oral nutritional drink has the following label content based on a 2000-calorie diet. For each item with a question mark (?), fill in the missing number.

NUTRITION FACTS		CALORIES 210	
Serving size: 1 bottle (14 fl. oz.)		Calories from fat: (?)	
Amount per serving	% DV	Amount per serving	% DV
Total fat 2.5 g	(?)	Potassium 440 mg	(?)
Saturated fat 0.5 g	(?)	Total carbohydrates (?) g	8%
Trans fat 0 g		Dietary fiber 3 g	12%
Cholesterol (?) mg	7%	Sugars 5 g	
Sodium 280 mg	(?)	Protein 25 g	(?)

[a]Problem courtesy of Flynn Warren, Bishop, GA.

ANSWERS TO "CASE IN POINT" AND PRACTICE PROBLEMS

Case in Point 14.1

(a) The patient weighs 120 lb equivalent to 54.5 kg (120 lb/2.2 lb per kg).

Daily fluid requirement:
based on 1500 mL + 20 mL/kg over 20 kg:
    1500 mL + 690 mL (20 mL × 34.5 kg)
    = 2190 mL

based on 30 to 35 mL/kg/day:
    54.5 kg × 30 mL/kg/day = 1635 mL
    54.5 kg × 35 mL/kg/day = 1908 mL

Thus, the target is between 1635 and 2190 mL/day and the predetermined TPN volume of 2000 mL would suffice.

(b) A hospitalized patient may be considered mildly to moderately stressed, and thus, a target protein requirement may be based on 1 to 1.2 g/kg/day:

54.5 kg × 1 g/kg/day = 54.5 g/day
54.5 kg × 1.2 g/kg/day = 65.4 g/day

Thus, the acceptable target for protein would be between 54.5 g and 65.4 g/day

(c) The 10% amino acid injection that would be required:

100 mL/10 g × 54.5 g = 545 mL, and
100 mL/10 g × 65.4 g = 654 mL.

Thus, the target for protein would be met by between 545 and 654 mL of the 10% amino acid injection.

(d) The target of the patient's nonprotein caloric requirements (BEE) is determined by the Harris-Benedict equation:

655.1 + (9.56 × weight, kg) + (1.85 × height, cm) − (4.68 × age, y) =

655.1 + (9.56 × 54.5 kg) + (1.85 × 157.5 cm) − (4.68 × 75) =

655.1 + 521 + 291.4 − 351 = 1116.5 kcal/day × 1.2 (activity factor) − 1339.8 or 1340 kcal/day

(e) 1340 kcal/day @ 3.4 kcal/g = 394 g/day dextrose required.

D50W = 50 g dextrose/100 mL;
100 mL/50 g × 394 g dextrose provided by 788 mL D50W

(Note: in practice the quantities, as calculated, may be rounded and individualized based on clinical factors.)

Case in Point 14.2

(a) Protein: 7.1 g × 4 kcal/g = 28.4 kcal;
Fat: 9.4 g × 9 kcal/g = 84.6 kcal;
Carbohydrate: 31.4 g × 4 kcal/g = 125.6 kcal.
Total kcal = 28.4 + 84.6 + 125.6 = 238.6 kcal.
kcal/mL = 238.6 kcal/237 mL = 1.007 kcal/mL, *answer*.

(b) Protein: 7.1 g/237 mL × 1500 mL = 44.94 g protein, and
Fat: 9.4 g/237 mL × 1500 mL = 59.49 g fat, and
Carbohydrate: 31.4 g/237 mL × 500 mL = 198.7 g carbohydrate, *answers*.

(c) Daily kcal: Protein, 44.94 g × 4 kcal/g = 179.76 kcal,
Fat, 59.49 g × 9 kcal/g = 535.41 kcal,
Carbohydrate, 198.7 g × 4 kcal/g = 794.8 kcal.
Total daily kcal = 179.76 + 535.41 + 794.8 = 1509.97 kcal
% kcal from protein = 179.76 kcal/1509.97 kcal × 100% = 11.9%, and
% kcal from fat = 535.41 kcal/1509.97 kcal × 100% = 35.46%, and
% kcal from carbohydrate = 794.8 kcal/1509.97 kcal × 100% = 52.64%, *answers*.

(d) Yes, they compare favorably.

Practice Problems

1. 76.9 g

2. 714.29 mL

3. 240 kcal

4. 1200 mL

5. (a) 350 g dextrose
   (b) 200 g protein
   (c) 111.1 g lipid

6. (a) 2250 mL
   (b) 2400 mL
   (c) 1500 mL
   (d) 264 mL to 396 mL
   (e) 1450 mL
   (f) 975 mL

7. 73.09 g protein
   266.34 g carbohydrate
   81.23 g lipid
   2088.82 to 2740.91 mL fluid

8. 250 mL amino acids injection
   400 mL dextrose injection
   350 mL sterile water for injection

9. 71.43 mL dextrose injection

10. (a) 1340.2 kcal
    (b) 55.27 g protein

11. 2193.4 kcal

12. 261.8 kcal

13. 7.8 mL sodium chloride solution
    7.5 mL potassium acetate solution
    0.1 mL vitamin B_{12}
    0.08 mL insulin

14. (a) 14.89 mL
    (b) 31.48 mmol

15. (a) 250 mL amino acids injection
    (b) 400 mL dextrose injection
    (c) 11.7 mL sodium chloride solution
    (d) 5.43 mL calcium gluconate solution
    (e) 0.15 mL insulin

(f) 2.5 mL heparin
(g) sterile water for injection to make 1 L

16. 27 BMI

17. 30 BMI

18. 224 mg

19. 100 g fat

20. 46% DV

21. 4.7% DV

22. 50 g fat

23. 15%

24. 4000 mg potassium

25. 5.8% DV

References

1. Dombrowski SR. Pharmacist counseling on nutrition and physical activity—part 1 of 2: understanding current guidelines. *Journal of the American Pharmacists Association* 1999;39:479–491.
2. Diabesity®. Available at: http://www.carbs-information.com/diabesity-obesity-diabetes.htm. Accessed June 21, 2011.
3. National Heart Lung and Blood Institute, National Institutes of Health. Clinical guidelines on the identification, evaluation, and treatment of overweight and obesity in adults. Available at: http://www.nhlbi.nih.gov/guidelines/obesity/ob__gdlns.pdf. Accessed June 21, 2011.
4. Continuing Education Monograph: Managing Obesity as a Chronic Disease. Washington, DC: American Pharmacists Association, 2001.
5. Beckwith MC, Feddema SS, Barton RG, et al. A guide to drug therapy in patients with enteral feeding tubes: dosage form selection and administration methods. *Hospital Pharmacy* 2004;39:225–237.
6. Davis A. Indications and techniques for enteral feeds. In: Baker SB, Baker RD Jr, Davis A, eds. *Pediatric Enteral Nutrition*. New York: Chapman Hall, 1994:67–94.
7. Wolf TD. Enteral nutrition. In: Boh LE, ed. *Pharmacy Practice Manual: A Guide to the Clinical Experience*. Baltimore, MD: Lippincott Williams & Wilkins, 2001:431–459.
8. Whitney J. Parenteral nutrition. In: Boh LE, ed. *Pharmacy Practice Manual: A Guide to the Clinical Experience*. Baltimore, MD: Lippincott Williams & Wilkins, 2001:460–506.
9. Wallace JI. Malnutrition and enteral/parenteral alimentation. In: Hazzard WR, Blass JP, Halter JB, et al., eds. *Principles of Geriatric Medicine and Gerontology*. New York: McGraw-Hill, 2003:1179–1192.
10. DiPiro JT, Talbert RL, Yee GC, et al. *Pharmacotherapy: A Pathophysiologic Approach*. 5th Ed. New York: McGraw-Hill, 2002:2456–2457, 2523.
11. Mirtallo J, Canada T, Johnson D, et al. Safe practices for parenteral nutrition. *Journal of Parenteral and Enteral Nutrition* 2004;28:S39–S70. Available at: http://www.nutritioncare.org/lcontent.aspx?id=660. Accessed June 28, 2011.
12. DiPiro JT, Talbert RL, Yee GC, et al. *Pharmacotherapy: A Pathophysiologic Approach*. 5th Ed. New York: McGraw-Hill, 2002:2480.
13. Craig SB, Dietz WH. Nutritional requirements. In: Baker SB, Baker RD Jr, Davis A, eds. *Pediatric Enteral Nutrition*. New York: Chapman Hall, 1994:67–94.
14. O'Sullivan TA. Parenteral nutrition calculations. In: *Understanding Pharmacy Calculations*. Washington, DC: American Pharmacists' Association, 2002:143–237.
15. Basal Energy Expenditure: Harris Benedict Equation. Available at: http://www-users.med.cornell.edu/~spon/picu/calc/beecalc.htm Accessed June 21, 2011.
16. Dlugosz C. Pharmacist's guide to fiber and digestive health. *Pharmacy Today* 2008;14.
17. Zagaria MAE. Nutrition in the elderly. *U.S. Pharmacist* 2000;25:42–44.

18. 2010 Dietary Guidelines for Americans, Available at: http://www.cnpp.usda.gov/Publications/ DietaryGuidelines/2010/PolicyDoc/PolicyDoc.pdf. Accessed June 29, 2011.
19. How to Understand and Use the Nutrition Facts Label. Available at: http://www.fda.gov/Food/ LabelingNutrition/ConsumerInformation/ucm078889.htm. Accessed June 30, 2011.
20. Food Labeling Guide. Department of Health and Human Services, Food and Drug Administration, Center for Food Safety and Applied Nutrition Office of Nutrition. Available at: http://www.fda.gov/ Food/GuidanceComplianceRegulatoryInformation/GuidanceDocuments/FoodLabelingNutrition/ FoodLabelingGuide/default.htm. Accessed June 30, 2011.
21. Definitions of Nutrient Content Claims. Guidance for Industry: A Food Labeling Guide. Food and Drug Administration, Department of Health and Human Services. Available at: http://www.fda.gov/ Food/GuidanceComplianceRegulatoryInformation/GuidanceDocuments/FoodLabelingNutrition/ FoodLabelingGuide/ucm064911.htm. Accessed June 30, 2011.

Altering Product Strength, Use of Stock Solutions, and Problem-Solving by Alligation

15

Objectives

Upon successful completion of this chapter, the student will be able to:

- Perform calculations for altering product strength by dilution, concentration, or fortification.
- Perform calculations for the preparation and use of stock solutions.
- Apply *alligation medial* and *alligation alternate* in problem-solving.

The strength of a pharmaceutical preparation may be increased or decreased by changing the proportion of active ingredient to the whole. A preparation may be *strengthened* or made more *concentrated* by the addition of active ingredient, by admixture with a like preparation of greater strength, or through the evaporation of its vehicle, if liquid. The strength of a preparation may be decreased or *diluted* by the addition of diluent or by admixture with a like preparation of lesser strength.

Alternative methods of calculation for the alteration of the strength of pharmaceutical preparations are presented in this chapter.

Special Considerations of Altering Product Strength in Pharmaceutical Compounding

In the course of pharmacy practice, there are occasions in which the alteration of the strength of a pharmaceutical preparation is either desirable or required.

CALCULATIONS CAPSULE

Concentration/Quantity Relationship

The percentage or ratio strength (concentration) of a component in a pharmaceutical preparation is based on its quantity relative to the total quantity of the preparation. If the quantity of the component remains constant, any change in the total quantity of the preparation, through dilution or concentration, changes the concentration of the component in the preparation inversely.

An equation useful in these calculations is:

(1st quantity) × *(1st concentration)* = *(2nd quantity)* × *(2nd concentration)*

The *dilution* of a liquid dosage form, as a solution or suspension, may be desired to provide a product strength more suitable for use by a particular patient (e.g., pediatric, elderly, those in disease states). The diluent is selected based on its compatibility with the vehicle of the original product; that is, aqueous, alcoholic, hydroalcoholic, or other. The dilution of a solid dosage form (as a powder or the contents of a capsule) or a semisolid dosage form (as an ointment or cream) also may be performed to alter the dose or strength of a product. Again, the diluent is selected based on its compatibility with the original formulation. Pharmacists also may find occasion to dilute concentrated acids, alcohol preparations, or very potent therapeutic agents, as discussed in this chapter, to meet special compounding requirements.

The *concentration* of a liquid preparation, as through the evaporation of a portion of its solvent or vehicle, rarely is performed nowadays. However, the *fortification* of a liquid, solid, or semisolid dosage form, by the addition of a calculated quantity of additional therapeutic agent, remains a viable practice in pharmacy compounding.

Relationship Between Strength and Total Quantity

If a mixture of a given percentage or ratio strength is diluted to twice its original quantity, its active ingredient will be contained in twice as many parts of the whole, and its strength therefore will be reduced by one half. By contrast, if a mixture is concentrated by evaporation to one-half its original quantity, the active ingredient (assuming that none was lost by evaporation) will be contained in one half as many parts of the whole, and the strength will be doubled. So, if 50 mL of a solution containing 10 g of active ingredient with a strength of 20% or 1:5 w/v are diluted to 100 mL, the original volume is doubled, but the original strength is now reduced by one half to 10% or 1:10 w/v. If, by evaporation of the solvent, the volume of the solution is reduced to 25 mL or one half the original quantity, the 10 g of the active ingredient will indicate a strength of 40% or 1:2.5 w/v.

If, then, *the amount of active ingredient remains constant, any change in the quantity of a solution or mixture of solids is inversely proportional to the percentage or ratio strength;* that is, the percentage or ratio strength decreases as the quantity increases, and conversely.

This relationship is generally true for all mixtures except solutions containing components that contract when mixed together.

Problems in this section generally may be solved by any of the following methods:

1. Inverse proportion.
2. The equation: **(1st quantity)** × **(1st concentration)** = **(2nd quantity)** × **(2nd concentration)**, or **Q1 × C1 = Q2 × C2.**
3. By determining the quantity of active ingredient (solute) present or required and relating that quantity to the known or desired quantity of the preparation.
   Note: This will become clear as the chapter proceeds.

Dilution and Concentration of Liquids

Example Calculations of the Dilution and Concentration of Liquids

If 500 mL of a 15% v/v solution are diluted to 1500 mL, what will be the percentage strength (v/v)?

$$\frac{1500 \ (\text{mL})}{500 \ (\text{mL})} = \frac{15 \ (\%)}{x \ (\%)}$$

$$x = 5\%, \ answer.$$

Or,

$$\text{Q1 (quantity)} \times \text{C1 (concentration)} = \text{Q2 (quantity)} \times \text{C2 (concentration)}$$
$$500 \text{ (mL)} \times 15 \text{ (\%)} = 1500 \text{ (mL)} \times \text{x (\%)}$$
$$\text{x} = 5\%, \textit{ answer.}$$

Or,

500 mL of 15% v/v solution contains 75 mL of solute

$$\frac{1500 \text{ (mL)}}{75 \text{ (mL)}} = \frac{100 \text{ (\%)}}{\text{x (\%)}}$$

$$\text{x} = 5\%, \textit{ answer.}$$

If 50 mL of a 1:20 w/v solution are diluted to 1000 mL, what is the ratio strength (w/v)?
Note: A student may find it simpler in solving certain problems to convert a given ratio strength to its equivalent percentage strength.

$$1:20 = 5\%$$
$$\frac{1000 \text{ (mL)}}{50 \text{ (mL)}} = \frac{5 \text{ (\%)}}{\text{x (\%)}}$$
$$\text{x} = 0.25\% = 1{:}400, \textit{ answer.}$$

Or,

$$\frac{1000 \text{ (mL)}}{50 \text{ (mL)}} = \frac{\frac{1}{20}}{\text{x}}$$

$$\text{x} = \frac{1}{400} = 1{:}400, \textit{ answer.}$$

Or,

$$\text{Q1 (quantity)} \times \text{C1 (concentration)} = \text{Q2 (quantity)} \times \text{C2 (concentration)}$$
$$50 \text{ (mL)} \times 5 \text{ (\%)} = 1000 \text{ (mL)} \times \text{(\%)}$$
$$\text{x} = 0.25\% = 1{:}400, \textit{ answer.}$$

Or,

50 mL of a 1:20 solution contains 2.5 g of solute

$$\frac{2.5 \text{ (g)}}{1 \text{ (g)}} = \frac{1000 \text{ (mL)}}{\text{x (mL)}}$$
$$\text{x} = 400 \text{ mL}$$
$$\text{Ratio strength} = 1{:}400, \textit{ answer.}$$

If a syrup containing 65% w/v of sucrose is evaporated to 85% of its volume, what percentage (w/v) of sucrose will it contain?

Any convenient amount of the syrup, for example, 100 mL, may be used in the calculation. If we evaporate 100 mL of the syrup to 85% of its volume, we will have 85 mL.

$$\frac{85 \text{ (mL)}}{100 \text{ (mL)}} = \frac{65 \text{ (\%)}}{\text{x (\%)}}$$
$$\text{x} = 76.47\% \text{ or } 76\%, \textit{ answer.}$$

How many grams of 10% w/w ammonia solution can be made from 1800 g of 28% w/w strong ammonia solution?

$$\frac{10\ (\%)}{28\ (\%)} = \frac{1800\ (g)}{x\ (g)}$$
$$x = 5040\ g,\ answer.$$

Or,

$$Q1 \times C1 = Q2 \times C2$$
$$1800\ (g) \times 28\ (\%) = x\ (g) \times 10\ (\%)$$
$$x = 5040\ g,\ answer.$$

Or,

1800 g of 28% ammonia water contains 504 g of ammonia (100%)

$$\frac{10\ (\%)}{100\ (\%)} = \frac{504\ (g)}{x\ (g)}$$
$$x = 5040\ g,\ answer.$$

How many milliliters of a 1:5000 w/v solution of the preservative lauralkonium chloride can be made from 125 mL of a 0.2% solution?

$$1{:}5000 = 0.02\%$$
$$\frac{0.02\ (\%)}{0.2\ (\%)} = \frac{125\ (mL)}{x\ (mL)}$$
$$x = 1250\ mL,\ answer.$$

Or,

$$0.2\% = 1{:}500$$
$$\frac{\frac{1}{5000}}{\frac{1}{500}} = \frac{125\ (mL)}{x\ (mL)}$$
$$x = 1250\ mL,\ answer.$$

Or,

125 mL of a 0.2% solution contains 0.25 g of lauralkonium chloride

$$\frac{1\ (g)}{0.25\ (g)} = \frac{5000\ (mL)}{x\ (mL)}$$
$$x = 1250\ mL,\ answer.$$

Or,

$$125\ (mL) \times 0.2\ (\%) = x\ (mL) \times 0.02\ (\%)$$
$$x = 1250\ mL,\ answer.$$

How many milliliters of water should be added to 80 mL of a 20% w/v aqueous solution to prepare a 3% solution?

$$80\ (mL) \times 20\%\ w/v = 16\ g\ solute\ present$$

$$\frac{3\ g}{100\ mL} = \frac{16\ g}{x};\ x = 533.3\ mL\ (quantity\ of\ a\ 3\%\ solution\ that\ 16\ g\ solute\ can\ prepare)$$

$$533.3\ mL - 80\ mL = 453.3\ mL\ of\ water\ to\ add,\ answer.$$

Or,

$$Q1 \times C1 = Q2 \times C2$$
$$80 \text{ (mL)} \times 20 \text{ (\%)} = x \text{ (mL)} \times 3 \text{ (\%)}$$
$$x = 533.3 \text{ mL} - 80 \text{ mL} = 453.3 \text{ mL, } answer.$$

If a solution containing drug, 50 mg/10 mL, is diluted to 1 L, calculate the ratio strength of the resultant product.

$$50 \text{ mg} = 0.05 \text{ g}$$
$$\frac{0.05 \text{ g}}{1000 \text{ mL}} = \frac{1 \text{ g}}{x \text{ mL}}; \ x = 20,000 \text{ mL};$$

Ratio strength (1 g/20,000 mL) = 1:20,000 w/v, *answer.*

If 1 gallon of a 30% w/v solution is to be evaporated so that the solution will have a strength of 50% w/v, what will be its volume in milliliters?

$$1 \text{ gallon} = 3785 \text{ mL}$$
$$\frac{50 \text{ (\%)}}{30 \text{ (\%)}} = \frac{3785 \text{ (mL)}}{x \text{ (mL)}}$$
$$x = 2271 \text{ mL, } answer.$$

Strengthening of a Pharmaceutical Product

As noted previously, there is occasion in which a pharmacist may be called upon to strengthen an existing pharmaceutical product. This may be accomplished by the addition of active ingredient or by the admixture with a calculated quantity of a like-product of greater concentration. The latter type of calculation is presented later in this chapter under the discussion of *alligation alternate*.

The following problem and Case in Point 15.1 offer example calculations of product strengthening.

Example:

If a cough syrup contains in each teaspoonful, 1 mg of chlorpheniramine maleate and if a pharmacist desired to double the strength, how many milligrams of that ingredient would need to be added to a 60-mL container of the syrup. Assume no increase in volume.

$$\frac{1 \text{ mg}}{5 \text{ mL}} \times 60 \text{ mL} = 12 \text{ mg chlorpheniramine maleate in original syrup}$$

To double the strength, 12 mg of additional chlorpheniramine maleate would be required, *answer.*

CASE IN POINT 15.1 A pharmacist received a prescription for 100 mL of a cefuroxime axetil suspension to contain 300 mg of drug in each 5 mL. The pharmacist has 100 mL of a suspension containing 250 mg/5 mL and also has 250-mg scored tablets of the drug. How many tablets should be pulverized and added to the suspension to achieve the desired strength? Assume no increase in the volume of the suspension.

<u>A Second Look</u>

The pharmacist observed that after adding the pulverized tablets, the suspension measured 102 mL in volume. Calculations revealed that rather than the prescribed drug strength of 300 mg/5 mL, there were 294.1 mg/5 mL. What could the pharmacist do to bring the suspension to the desired strength?

Stock Solutions
. . . .

Stock solutions are concentrated solutions of active (e.g., drug) or inactive (e.g., colorant) substances and are used by pharmacists as a convenience to prepare solutions of lesser concentration.

Example Calculations of Stock Solutions

How many milliliters of a 1:400 w/v stock solution should be used to make 4 liters of a 1:2000 w/v solution?

$$4 \text{ liters} = 4000 \text{ mL}$$
$$1:400 = 0.25\%$$
$$1:2000 = 0.05\%$$
$$\frac{0.25\,(\%)}{0.05\,(\%)} = \frac{4000\,(\text{mL})}{x\,(\text{mL})}$$
$$x = 800 \text{ mL}, \textit{answer}.$$

Or,

4000 mL of a 1:2000 w/v solution requires 2 g of active constituent (solute); thus:

$$\frac{1\,(\text{g})}{2\,(\text{g})} = \frac{400\,(\text{mL})}{x\,(\text{mL})}$$
$$x = 800 \text{ mL}, \textit{answer}.$$

Or,

$$Q1 \times C1 = Q2 \times C2$$
$$4000\,(\text{mL}) \times 0.25\,(\%) = x \times 0.05\,(\%)$$
$$x = 800 \text{ mL}, \textit{answer}.$$

How many milliliters of a 1:400 w/v stock solution should be used in preparing 1 gallon of a 1:2000 w/v solution?

$$1 \text{ gallon} = 3785 \text{ mL}$$
$$1:400 = 0.25\%$$
$$1:2000 = 0.05\%$$
$$\frac{0.25\,(\%)}{0.05\,(\%)} = \frac{3785\,(\text{mL})}{x\,(\text{mL})}$$
$$x = 757 \text{ mL}, \textit{answer}.$$

Or,

1 gallon of a 1:2000 w/v solution requires 1.89 g of active constituent; thus:

$$\frac{1.89\,(\text{g})}{1\,(\text{g})} = \frac{x\,(\text{mL})}{400\,(\text{mL})}$$
$$x = 756 \text{ mL}, \textit{answer}.$$

How many milliliters of a 1% stock solution of a certified red dye should be used in preparing 4000 mL of a mouthwash that is to contain 1:20,000 w/v of the certified red dye as a coloring agent?

$$1:20,000 = 0.005\%$$
$$Q1 \times C1 = Q2 \times C2$$
$$4000 \text{ (mL)} \times 0.005 \text{ (\%)} = x \text{ (mL)} \times (1\%)$$
$$x = 20 \text{ mL, } answer.$$

A pharmacist has a 5% stock solution of potassium permanganate from which to prepare 1 L of a 1:5000 solution to dispense as a foot soak. How many milliliters of the stock solution are needed?

$$1:5000 \text{ w/v} = 0.02\%$$
$$Q1 \times C1 = Q2 \times C2$$
$$1000 \text{ (mL)} \times 0.02 \text{ (\%)} = x \text{ (mL)} \times 5 \text{ (\%)}$$
$$x = 4 \text{ mL, } answer.$$

How many milliliters of a 10% stock solution are needed to prepare 120 mL of a 0.1 % solution?

$$Q1 \times C1 = Q2 \times C2$$
$$120 \text{ (mL)} \times 0.1 \text{ (\%)} = x \text{ (mL)} \times 10 \text{ (\%)}$$
$$x = 1.2 \text{ mL, } answer.$$

Some interesting calculations are used in pharmacy practice in *which the strength of a diluted portion of a solution is defined, but the strength of the concentrated stock solution used to prepare it must be determined.* The relevance to pharmacy practice may be explained, for example, by the need of a pharmacist to prepare and dispense a concentrated solution of a drug and direct the patient to use a specific household measure of a solution (e.g., 1 teaspoonful) in a specified volume of water (e.g., a pint) to make of solution of the desired concentration (e.g., for irrigation or soaking). This permits the dispensing of a relatively small volume of liquid, enabling a patient to prepare relatively large volumes as needed, rather than carrying home gallons of a diluted solution from a pharmacy.

How much drug should be used in preparing 50 mL of a solution such that 5 mL diluted to 500 mL will yield a 1:1000 solution?

1:1000 means 1 g of drug in 1000 mL of solution

$$\frac{1000 \text{ (mL)}}{500 \text{ (mL)}} = \frac{1 \text{ (g)}}{x \text{ (g)}}$$

$$x = 0.5 \text{ g of drug in 500 mL of}$$
diluted solution (1:1000), which
is *also* the amount in 5 mL of the
stronger (stock) solution

And,

$$\frac{5 \text{ (mL)}}{50 \text{ (mL)}} = \frac{0.5 \text{ (g)}}{y \text{ (g)}}$$
$$y = 5 \text{ g, } answer.$$

The accompanying diagrammatic sketch should prove helpful in solving the problem.

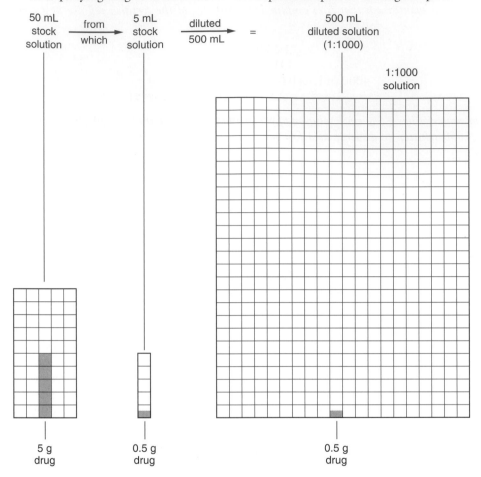

How many grams of sodium chloride should be used in preparing 500 mL of a stock solution such that 50 mL diluted to 1000 mL will yield a "⅓ normal saline" (0.3% w/v) for irrigation?

1000 (mL) × 0.003 = 3 g of sodium chloride in 1000 mL of " ⅓ normal saline" (0.3% w/v), which is *also* the amount in 50 mL of the *stronger* (stock) solution to be prepared.

And,

$$\frac{50 \ (mL)}{500 \ (mL)} = \frac{3 \ (g)}{x \ (g)}$$
$$x = 30 \ g, \textit{answer.}$$

How many milliliters of a 17% w/v concentrate of benzalkonium chloride should be used in preparing 300 mL of a stock solution such that 15 mL diluted to 1 liter will yield a 1:5000 solution?

1 liter = 1000 mL
1:5000 means 1 g of benzalkonium chloride in 5000 mL of solution

$$\frac{5000 \ (mL)}{1000 \ (mL)} = \frac{1 \ (g)}{x \ (g)}$$

x = 0.2 g of benzalkonium chloride in 1000 mL of *diluted* solution (1:5000), which is *also* the amount in 15 mL of the *stronger* (stock) solution to be prepared, and:

$$\frac{15\,(\text{mL})}{300\,(\text{mL})} = \frac{0.2\,(\text{g})}{y\,(\text{g})}$$

y = 4 g of benzalkonium chloride needed,

because a 17% w/v concentrate contains 17 g per 100 mL, then:

$$\frac{17\,(\text{g})}{4\,(\text{g})} = \frac{100\,(\text{mL})}{z\,(\text{mL})}$$

z = 23.5 mL, *answer.*

A solution of known volume and strength may be diluted with water to prepare a solution of lesser strength. In such calculations, first calculate the quantity of diluted solution that may be prepared from the concentrated solution. Then, subtract the volume of the concentrated solution from the total quantity that may be prepared to determine the volume of water needed.

How many milliliters of water should be added to 300 mL of a 1:750 w/v solution of benzalkonium chloride to make a 1:2500 w/v solution?

$$1:2500 = 0.04\%$$
$$1:750 = 0.133\%$$
$$\frac{0.04\,(\%)}{0.133\,(\%)} = \frac{300\,(\text{mL})}{x\,(\text{mL})}$$

x = 997.5 or 1000 mL of 0.04%
w/v solution to be prepared

The difference between the volume of *diluted* (weaker) solution prepared and the volume of *stronger* solution used represents the volume of water (diluent) to be used.

1000 mL – 300 mL = 700 mL, *answer.*

Or,

300 mL of a 1:750 (w/v) solution contains 0.4 g of benzalkonium chloride

$$\frac{1\,(\text{g})}{0.4\,(\text{g})} = \frac{2500\,(\text{mL})}{x\,(\text{mL})}$$

x = 1000 mL
1000 mL – 300 mL = 700 mL, *answer.*

How many milliliters of water should be added to a pint of a 5% w/v solution to make a 2% w/v solution?

$$1\ \text{pint} = 473\ \text{mL}$$
$$\frac{2\,(\%)}{5\,(\%)} = \frac{473\,(\text{mL})}{x\,(\text{mL})}$$

x = 1182.5 mL

And,

1182.5 mL – 473 mL = 709.5 mL, *answer.*

If the *quantity of a component* is given rather than the *strength of a solution*, the solution may be diluted to a desired strength as shown by the following example.

How many milliliters of water should be added to 375 mL of a solution containing 0.5 g of benzalkonium chloride to make a 1:5000 solution?

1:5000 means 1 g in 5000 mL of solution

$$\frac{1\,(g)}{0.5\,(g)} = \frac{5000\,(mL)}{x\,(mL)}$$

$$x = 2500 \text{ mL of 1:5000 (w/v) solution containing}$$
$$0.5 \text{ g of benzalkonium chloride}$$

And,

$$2500 \text{ mL} - 375 \text{ mL} = 2125 \text{ mL}, \textit{answer.}$$

If 15 mL of a 0.06% ATROVENT (ipratropium bromide) nasal spray were diluted with 6 mL of normal saline solution, what would be the final drug concentration?

$$15 \text{ mL} \times 0.06\% = 0.009 \text{ g of ipratropium bromide}$$
$$15 \text{ mL} + 6 \text{ mL} = 21 \text{ mL, new total volume}$$
$$\frac{0.009\,g}{21\,mL} \times 100 = 0.043\ \%, \textit{ answer.}$$

Or,

$$15\,(mL) \times 0.06\,(\%) = 21\,(mL) \times x\,(\%)$$
$$x = 0.043\ \%, \textit{answer.}$$

Dilution of Alcohol

Example Calculations of Alcohol Dilutions

When water and alcohol are mixed, there is a physical contraction such that the resultant volume is less than the total of the individual volumes of the two liquids. Thus, to prepare a *volume-in-volume* strength of an alcohol dilution, the alcohol "solute" may be determined and water used to "q.s." to the appropriate volume.

How much water should be mixed with 5000 mL of 85% v/v alcohol to make 50% v/v alcohol?

$$Q1 \times C1 = Q2 \times C2$$
$$5000\,(mL) \times 85\,(\%) = x\,(mL) \times 50\,(\%)$$
$$x = 8500 \text{ mL}$$

Therefore, use 5000 mL of 85% v/v alcohol and enough water to make 8500 mL, *answer.*

How many milliliters of 95% v/v alcohol and how much water should be used in compounding the following prescription?

> ℞ Xcaine   1 g
>   Alcohol 70%   30 mL
>   Sig. Ear drops.

$$Q1 \times C1 = Q2 \times C2$$
$$30\,(mL) \times 70\,(\%) = x\,(mL) \times 95\,(\%)$$
$$x = 22.1 \text{ mL}$$

Therefore, use 22.1 mL of 95% v/v alcohol and enough water to make 30 mL, *answer.*

Dilution of Acids

The strength of an official undiluted (*concentrated*) acid is expressed as percentage weight-in-weight. For example, Hydrochloric Acid, NF, contains not less than 36.5% and not more than 38.0%, by weight, of HCl. However, the strength of an official *diluted* acid is expressed as percentage weight-in-volume. For example, Diluted Hydrochloric Acid, NF, contains, in each 100 mL, not less than 9.5 g and not more than 10.5 g of HCl.[1]

It is necessary, therefore, to consider the specific gravity of concentrated acids in calculating the volume to be used in preparing a desired quantity of a diluted acid.

Example Calculations of Acid Dilutions

How many milliliters of 37% w/w hydrochloric acid having a specific gravity of 1.20 are required to make 1000 mL of diluted hydrochloric acid 10% w/v?

1000 g × 0.10 = 100 g of HCl (100%) in 1000 mL of 10% w/v acid

$$\frac{37\,(\%)}{100\,(\%)} = \frac{100\,(g)}{x\,(g)}$$
$$x = 270 \text{ g of } 37\% \text{ acid}$$

270 g of water measure 270 mL

$$270\,(mL) \div 1.20 = 225 \text{ mL, } answer.$$

How many milliliters of 85% w/w phosphoric acid having a specific gravity of 1.71 should be used in preparing 1 gallon of ¼% w/v phosphoric acid solution to be used for bladder irrigation?

1 gallon = 3785 mL
3785 (g) × 0.0025 = 9.46 g of H_3PO_4 (100%) in 3785 mL (1 gallon) of ¼% w/v solution

$$\frac{85\,(\%)}{100\,(\%)} = \frac{9.46\,(g)}{x\,(g)}$$
$$x = 11.13 \text{ g of } 85\% \text{ phosphoric acid}$$

11.13 g of water measures 11.13 mL

$$11.13\,(mL) \div 1.71 = 6.5 \text{ mL, } answer.$$

Dilution and Fortification of Solids and Semisolids

The dilution of solids in pharmacy occurs when there is need to achieve a lower concentration of an active component in a more concentrated preparation. There also is a type of diluted pharmaceutical preparation, termed a *trituration* (as discussed in the next section) that represents a useful means of preparing and administering very potent therapeutic substances.

Example Calculations of Solid and Semisolid Dilutions

If 30 g of a 1% hydrocortisone ointment were diluted with 12 g of Vaseline, what would be the concentration of hydrocortisone in the mixture?

$$30 \text{ g} \times 1\% = 0.3 \text{ g hydrocortisone}$$
$$30 \text{ g} + 12 \text{ g} = 42 \text{ g, weight of mixture}$$
$$\frac{0.3 \text{ g}}{42 \text{ g}} \times 100 = 0.71\% \text{ (w/w), } answer.$$

Or,

$$30 \text{ (g)} \times 1 \text{ (\%)} = 42 \text{ (g)} \times x \text{ (\%)}$$
$$x = 0.71\% \text{ (w/w), } answer.$$

How many grams of 20% benzocaine ointment and how many grams of ointment base (diluent) should be used in preparing 5 lb. of 2.5% benzocaine ointment?

$$5 \text{ lb.} = 454 \text{ g} \times 5 = 2270 \text{ g}$$

$$\frac{20 \text{ (\%)}}{2.5 \text{ (\%)}} = \frac{2270 \text{ (g)}}{x \text{ (g)}}$$
$$x = 283.75 \text{ or } 284 \text{ g of } 20\% \text{ ointment, } and$$
$$2270 \text{ g} - 284 \text{ g} = 1986 \text{ g of ointment base, } answers.$$

Or,

$$5 \text{ lb.} = 454 \text{ g} \times 5 = 2270 \text{ g}$$
$$2270 \text{ g} \times 2.5\% = 56.75 \text{ g of benzocaine needed}$$
$$\frac{20 \text{ (g)}}{56.75 \text{ (g)}} = \frac{100 \text{ (g)}}{x \text{ (g)}}$$
$$x = 283.75 \text{ or } 284 \text{ g of } 20\% \text{ ointment, } and$$
$$2270 \text{ g} - 284 \text{ g} = 1986 \text{ g of ointment base, } answers.$$

How many grams of zinc oxide should be added to 3200 g of 5% zinc oxide ointment to prepare an ointment containing 20% of zinc oxide?

$$3200 \text{ g} \times 0.05 = 160 \text{ g of zinc oxide in } 3200 \text{ g of } 5\% \text{ ointment}$$
$$3200 \text{ g} - 160 \text{ g} = 3040 \text{ g of base (diluent) in } 3200 \text{ g of } 5\% \text{ ointment}$$

In the 20% ointment, the diluent will represent 80% of the total weight

$$\frac{80 \text{ (\%)}}{20 \text{ (\%)}} = \frac{3040 \text{ (g)}}{x \text{ (g)}}$$
$$x = 760 \text{ g of zinc oxide in the } 20\% \text{ ointment}$$

Because the 5% ointment already contains 160 g of zinc oxide,

$$760 \text{ g} - 160 \text{ g} = 600 \text{ g, } answer.$$

A simpler method of solving this problem can be used if we mentally translate it to read: *How many grams of zinc oxide should be added to 3200 g of zinc oxide ointment containing 95% diluent to prepare an ointment containing 80% diluent?*

$$\frac{80 \text{ (\%)}}{95 \text{ (\%)}} = \frac{3200 \text{ (g)}}{x \text{ (g)}}$$

$$x = 3800 \text{ g of ointment containing } 80\% \text{ diluent and } 20\% \text{ zinc oxide}$$
$$3800 \text{ g} - 3200 \text{ g} = 600 \text{ g, } answer.$$

Note: For another simple method, using alligation alternate (see subsequent section in this chapter).

Triturations

Triturations are dilutions of potent medicinal substances. They were at one time official and were prepared by *diluting one part by weight of the drug with nine parts of finely powdered lactose.* They are, therefore, *10%* or *1:10 w/w* mixtures.

These dilutions offer a means of obtaining conveniently and accurately small quantities of potent drugs for compounding purposes. Although no longer official as such, triturations exemplify a method for the calculation and use of dilutions of solid medicinal substances in compounding and manufacturing procedures.

A modern-day example of a trituration is the product Trituration of MUSTARGEN (mechlorethamine hydrochloride for injection), in which 10 mg of the highly toxic drug is triturated with 90 mg of sodium chloride. When dissolved with 10 mL Sterile Water for Injection or 0.9% sodium chloride injection, the solution that results has a concentration of 1 mg mechlorethamine hydrochloride per milliliter.

Note: The term *trituration* as used in this context should not be confused with the like term *trituration*, which is the pharmaceutical *process* of reducing substances to fine particles through grinding in a mortar and pestle.

Example Calculations of Triturations

How many grams of a 1:10 trituration are required to obtain 25 mg of drug?

$$10 \text{ g of trituration contain 1 g of drug}$$
$$25 \text{ mg} = 0.025 \text{ g}$$
$$\frac{1\,(g)}{0.025\,(g)} = \frac{10\,(g)}{x\,(g)}$$
$$x = 0.25 \text{ g, } answer.$$

How many milliliters of an injection prepared by dissolving 100 mg of a 1:10 trituration of mechlorethamine hydrochloride in sufficient water for injection to prepare 10 mL of injection is required to obtain 5 mg of drug?

$$100 \text{ mg of trituration} = 10 \text{ mg of drug}$$
$$10 \text{ mg of drug in 10 mL of injection}$$
$$\frac{10\,(mg)}{5\,(mg)} = \frac{10\,(mL)}{x\,(mL)}$$
$$x = 5 \text{ mL, } answer.$$

How many milligrams of a 1:10 dilution of colchicine should be used by a manufacturing pharmacist in preparing 100 capsules for a clinical drug study if each capsule is to contain 0.5 mg of colchicine?

$$0.5 \text{ mg} \times 100 = 50 \text{ mg of colchicine needed}$$
$$10 \text{ mg of dilution contain 1 mg of colchicine}$$
$$\frac{1\,(mg)}{50\,(mg)} = \frac{10\,(mg)}{x\,(mg)}$$
$$x = 500 \text{ mg, } answer.$$

Alligation

Alligation is an arithmetical method of solving problems that involves the mixing of solutions or mixtures of solids possessing different percentage strengths.

Alligation Medial. *Alligation medial* is a method by which the "weighted average" percentage strength of a mixture of two or more substances of known quantity and concentration may be easily calculated. The example calculations that follow demonstrate the process.

Example Calculations Using Alligation Medial

What is the percentage of zinc oxide in an ointment prepared by mixing 200 g of 10% ointment, 50 g of 20% ointment, and 100 g of 5% ointment?

$$0.10 \times 200 \text{ g} = 20 \text{ g}$$
$$0.20 \times 50 \text{ g} = 10 \text{ g}$$
$$0.05 \times \underline{100 \text{ g}} = \underline{5 \text{ g}}$$
$$\text{Totals:} \quad 350 \text{ g} \quad\quad 35 \text{ g}$$
$$35 \text{ (g)} \div 350 \text{ (g)} = 0.10 \times 100 = 10\%, answer.$$

In some problems, the addition of a solvent or vehicle must be considered. It is generally best to consider the diluent as of zero percentage strength, as in the following problem.

What is the percentage strength of alcohol in a mixture of 500 mL of a solution containing 40% v/v alcohol, 400 mL of a second solution containing 21% v/v alcohol, and a sufficient quantity of a nonalcoholic third solution to make a total of 1000 mL?

$$0.40 \times 500 \text{ mL} = 200 \text{ mL}$$
$$0.21 \times 400 \text{ mL} = 84 \text{ mL}$$
$$0 \times \underline{100 \text{ mL}} = \underline{0 \text{ mL}}$$
$$\text{Totals:} \quad 1000 \text{ mL} \quad 284 \text{ mL}$$
$$284 \text{ (mL)} \div 1000 \text{ (mL)} = 0.284 \times 100 = 28.4\%, answer.$$

Alligation Alternate. *Alligation alternate* is a method used to determine the quantities of ingredients of differing strengths needed to make a mixture of a desired strength. *It involves matching pairs of ingredients, one higher in strength and one lower in strength than the desired strength, which lies somewhere in between.* As shown in the example below, the desired strength is placed in the center of the working diagram.

Example Calculations Using Alligation Alternate

In what proportion should alcohols of 95% and 50% strengths be mixed to make 70% alcohol?

Note that the difference between the *strength of the stronger component* (95%) and the *desired strength* (70%) indicates the *number of parts of the weaker* to be used (25 parts), and the difference between the *desired strength* (70%) and the *strength of the weaker component* (50%) indicates the *number of parts of the stronger* to be used (20 parts).

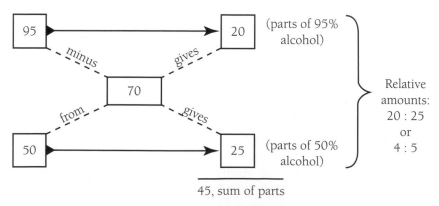

45, sum of parts

The mathematical validity of this relationship can be demonstrated.

Percent given	Percent desired	Proportional parts required
a		x
	c	
b		y

Given these data, the ratio of x to y may be derived algebraically as follows:

$$ax + by = c(x + y)$$
$$ax + by = cx + cy$$
$$ax - cx = cy - by$$
$$x(a - c) = y(c - b)$$
$$\frac{x}{y} = \frac{c - b}{a - c}$$

Given a = 95%, b = 50%, and c = 70%, we may therefore solve the problems as follows:

$$0.95x + 0.50y = 0.70(x + y)$$

Or,

$$95x + 50y = 70x + 70y$$
$$95x - 70x = 70y - 50y$$
$$x(95 - 70) = y(70 - 50)$$

$$\frac{x}{y} = \frac{70 - 50}{95 - 70} = \frac{20}{25} = \frac{4 \text{ (parts)}}{5 \text{ (parts)}}, \ answer.$$

The result can be shown to be correct by *alligation medial:*

$$95 \times 4 = 380$$
$$50 \times 5 = \underline{250}$$
$$\text{Totals: } 9 \quad 630$$

$$630 \div 9 = 70\%$$

The customary layout of *alligation alternate*, used in the subsequent examples, is a convenient simplification of the preceding diagram.

In what proportion should 20% benzocaine ointment be mixed with an ointment base to produce a 2.5% benzocaine ointment?

Note that an "ointment base" has no drug content, and thus is represented by a zero in the scheme.

20%		2.5 parts of 20% ointment
	2.5%	
0%		17.5 parts of ointment base

Relative amounts: 2.5:17.5, or 1:7, *answer.*

$$\text{Check: } 20 \times 1 = 20$$
$$0 \times 7 = \underline{\ 0}$$
$$\text{Totals: } 8 \quad 20$$
$$20 \div 8 = 2.5\%$$

A hospital pharmacist wants to use three lots of zinc oxide ointment containing, respectively, 50%, 20%, and 5% of zinc oxide. In what proportion should they be mixed to prepare a 10% zinc oxide ointment?

Note that *pairs* must be used in each determination, one lower and one greater in strength than the desired strength.

$$
\begin{array}{lll}
\quad 50\% & & 5 \text{ parts of } 50\% \text{ ointment} \\[4pt]
\quad 20\% & & 5 \text{ parts of } 20\% \text{ ointment} \\[4pt]
& 10\% & \\[4pt]
\quad\ 5\% & & 10 + 40 = 50 \text{ parts of } 5\% \text{ ointment}
\end{array}
$$

Relative amounts: 5:5:50, or 1:1:10, *answer.*

$$
\begin{array}{rcl}
\textit{Check: } 50 \times\ 1 & = & 50 \\
20 \times\ 1 & = & 20 \\
5 \times \underline{10} & = & \underline{50} \\
\text{Totals: } 12 & & 120 \\
120 \div 12 & = & 10\%
\end{array}
$$

Other answers are possible, of course, because the two stronger lots may be mixed first in any proportions desired, yielding a mixture that may then be mixed with the weakest lot in a proportion giving the desired strength.

In what proportions may a manufacturing pharmacist mix 20%, 15%, 5%, and 3% zinc oxide ointments to produce a 10% ointment?

Each of the weaker lots is paired with one of the stronger to give the desired strength, and because we may pair them in two ways, we may get two sets of correct answers.

$$
\begin{array}{lll}
\quad 20\% & & 7 \text{ parts of } 20\% \text{ ointment} \\[6pt]
\quad 15\% & & 5 \text{ parts of } 15\% \text{ ointment} \\[6pt]
& 10\% & \\[6pt]
\quad\ 5\% & & 5 \text{ parts of }\ 5\% \text{ ointment} \\[6pt]
\quad\ 3\% & & 10 \text{ parts of }\ 3\% \text{ ointment}
\end{array}
$$

Relative amounts: 7:5:5:10, *answer.*

The relative amounts, *in parts*, of the ointments to be combined to prepare a 10% ointment are thus determined. To prove the correctness of the process, let's substitute "grams" for each of the "parts" and calculate the resulting percent strength of zinc oxide in the ointment:

$$
\begin{array}{ll}
7 \text{ g of the } 20\% \text{ ointment} = & 7 \text{ g} \times 20\% = 1.4 \ \text{ g zinc oxide} \\
5 \text{ g of the } 15\% \text{ ointment} = & 5 \text{ g} \times 15\% = 0.75 \text{ g zinc oxide} \\
5 \text{ g of the }\ \ 5\% \text{ ointment} = & 5 \text{ g} \times\ \ 5\% = 0.25 \text{ g zinc oxide} \\
\underline{10 \text{ g}} \text{ of the }\ \ 3\% \text{ ointment} = & 10 \text{ g} \times\ \ 3\% = \underline{0.3}\ \text{ g zinc oxide} \\
\text{Total } \quad 27 \text{ g} & 2.7\ \text{ g zinc oxide}
\end{array}
$$

2.7 g zinc oxide/27 g ointment × 100% = 10% zinc oxide in the ointment, *answer.*

Or,

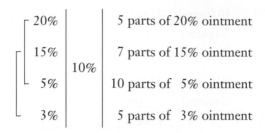

Relative amounts: 5:7:10:5, *answer.*

Proof: again, by substituting "grams" for "parts:"

$$5 \text{ g of the } 20\% \text{ ointment} = 5 \text{ g} \times 20\% = 1 \text{ g zinc oxide}$$
$$7 \text{ g of the } 15\% \text{ ointment} = 7 \text{ g} \times 15\% = 1.05 \text{ g zinc oxide}$$
$$10 \text{ g of the } 5\% \text{ ointment} = 10 \text{ g} \times 5\% = 0.5 \text{ g zinc oxide}$$
$$\underline{5 \text{ g of the } 3\% \text{ ointment} = 5 \text{ g} \times 3\% = 0.15 \text{ g zinc oxide}}$$

Total   27 g   2.7 g zinc oxide

2.7 g zinc oxide/27 g ointment × 100% = 10% zinc oxide in the ointment, *answer.*

How many milliliters of 50% w/v dextrose solution and how many milliliters of 5% w/v dextrose solution are required to prepare 4500 mL of a 10% w/v solution?

$$
\begin{array}{c|c|c}
50\% & & \text{5 parts of 50\% solution} \\
& 10\% & \\
5\% & & \text{40 parts of 5\% solution}
\end{array}
$$

Relative amounts 5:40, or 1:8, with a total of 9 parts

The total of 9 parts equates to the 4500 mL. The milliliters that equate each to the *1 part* and the *8 parts* are then determined:

$$\frac{9 \text{ (parts)}}{1 \text{ (part)}} = \frac{4500 \text{ (mL)}}{x \text{ (mL)}}$$

$$x = 500 \text{ mL of 50\% solution, } and$$

$$\frac{9 \text{ (parts)}}{8 \text{ (parts)}} = \frac{4500 \text{ (mL)}}{y \text{ (mL)}}$$

$$y = 4000 \text{ mL of 5\% solution, } answers.$$

How many milliliters each of a 2% w/v solution and a 7% w/v solution should be used in preparing 1 gallon of a 3.5% w/v solution?

1 gallon = 3785 mL

The total of 10 parts equates to the 3785 mL. The milliliters that equate each to the 7 *parts* and the *3 parts* are then determined.

$$
\begin{array}{c|c|c}
2\% & & \text{3.5 parts of 2\% solution} \\
& 3.5\% & \\
7\% & & \text{1.5 parts of 7\% solution}
\end{array}
$$

Relative amounts: 3.5:1.5, or 7:3, with a total of 10 parts

$$\frac{10 \,(\text{parts})}{7 \,(\text{parts})} = \frac{3785 \,(\text{mL})}{x \,(\text{mL})}$$

$$x = 2650 \text{ mL of 2\% solution, } \textit{and}$$

$$\frac{10 \,(\text{parts})}{3 \,(\text{parts})} = \frac{3785 \,(\text{mL})}{y \,(\text{mL})}$$

$$y = 1135 \text{ mL of 7\% solution, } \textit{answers.}$$

How many grams of 2.5% hydrocortisone cream should be mixed with 360 g of 0.25% cream to make a 1% hydrocortisone cream?

2.5%		0.75 part of 2.5% cream
	1%	
0.25%		1.5 parts of 0.25% cream

Relative amounts: 0.75:1.5, or 1:2

$$\frac{2 \,(\text{parts})}{1 \,(\text{part})} = \frac{360 \,(\text{g})}{x \,(\text{g})}$$

$$x = 180 \text{ g, } \textit{answer.}$$

Alternate (algebraic) solution of the same problem:

$$2.5(x) + 0.25(360) = 1(360 + x)$$
$$2.5x + 90 = 360 + x$$
$$1.5x = 270$$
$$x = 180 \text{ g, } \textit{answer.}$$

How many grams of white petrolatum should be mixed with 250 g of 5% and 750 g of 15% zinc oxide ointments to prepare a 10% ointment?

$$
\begin{array}{rrcr}
5 \times & 250 & = & 1250 \\
15 \times & 750 & = & \underline{11{,}250} \\
\text{Totals:} & \overline{1000} & & 12{,}500
\end{array}
$$

12,500 ÷ 1000 = 12.5% of zinc oxide in 1000 g of a mixture of 5% and 15% ointments

12.5%		10 parts of 12.5% mixture
	10%	
0%		2.5 parts of white petrolatum

Relative amounts: 10:2.5, or 4:1

$$\frac{4 \,(\text{parts})}{1 \,(\text{part})} = \frac{1000 \,(\text{g})}{x \,(\text{g})}$$

$$x = 250 \text{ g, } \textit{answer.}$$

Check:
$$
\begin{array}{rrcr}
12.5 \times & 1000 & = & 12{,}500 \\
0 \times & \underline{250} & = & \underline{0} \\
\text{Totals:} & 1250 & & 12{,}500 \\
\end{array}
$$
$$12500 \div 1250 = 10\%$$

How many grams of zinc oxide should be added to 3200 g of 5% zinc oxide ointment to prepare an ointment containing 20% of zinc oxide?

Zinc oxide (active ingredient) = 100%

$$
\begin{array}{c|c|l}
100\% & & \text{15 parts of 100\% zinc oxide} \\
& 20\% & \\
5\% & & \text{80 parts of \quad 5\% ointment}
\end{array}
$$

Relative amounts: 15:80, or 3:16

$$\frac{16\,(\text{parts})}{3\,(\text{parts})} = \frac{3200\,(\text{g})}{\text{x}\,(\text{g})}$$

$$x = 600 \text{ g, } answer.$$

$$
\begin{aligned}
Check: \quad 100 \times \ \ 600 &= 60,000 \\
5 \times 3200 &= \underline{16,000} \\
\text{Totals:} \quad 3800 \quad &\ \ 76,000 \\
76,000 \div 3800 &= 20\%
\end{aligned}
$$

Compare the solution of this problem by use of alligation alternate with other methods shown for the identical problem earlier in this chapter.

Specific Gravity of Mixtures

The methods of alligation medial and alligation alternate may be used in solving problems involving the specific gravities of liquids as demonstrated below.

CASE IN POINT 15.2[a] A pharmacist received the following prescription:

℞

Clindamycin Phosphate	1.5%
Alcohol (52% v/v) q.s. ad	120 mL
Sig: Apply daily for acne	

The pharmacist has no clindamycin phosphate powder but does have clindamycin phosphate sterile solution, 150 mg/mL, in vials. From the label, the pharmacist learns that the solution is aqueous.

(a) How many milliliters of the clindamycin phosphate sterile solution should the pharmacist use in filling the prescription?

(b) How many milliliters of 95% v/v of alcohol are required?

(c) How many milliliters of water should be added to make 120 mL?

[a]Problem courtesy of Warren Beach, Athens, GA. College of Pharmacy, The University of Georgia.

Example Calculations of Specific Gravity Using Alligation

What is the specific gravity of a mixture of 1000 mL of syrup with a specific gravity of 1.300, 400 mL of glycerin with a specific gravity of 1.250, and 1000 mL of an elixir with a specific gravity of 0.950?

$$1.300 \times 1000 = 1300$$
$$1.250 \times 400 = 500$$
$$0.950 \times \underline{1000} = \underline{950}$$

Totals: 2400 $\quad$ 2750

$$2750 \div 2400 = 1.146, answer.$$

In what proportion must glycerin with a specific gravity of 1.25 and water be mixed to prepare a liquid having a specific gravity of 1.10?

$$
\begin{array}{c|c|l}
1.25 & & 0.10 \text{ parts of glycerin} \\
& 1.10 & \\
1.00 & & 0.15 \text{ parts of water}
\end{array}
$$

Relative amounts: 0.10:0.15, or 2:3, *answer.*

How many milliliters of each of two liquids with specific gravities of 0.950 and 0.875 should be used to prepare 1500 mL of a liquid having a specific gravity of 0.925?

$$
\begin{array}{c|c|l}
0.950 & & 0.050, \text{ or 50 parts of liquid with} \\
& & \quad \text{specific gravity of } 0.950 \\
& 0.925 & \\
0.875 & & 0.025, \text{ or 25 parts of liquid with} \\
& & \quad \text{specific gravity of } 0.875
\end{array}
$$

Relative amounts: 50:25, or 2:1, with a total of 3 parts

$$\frac{3\,(\text{parts})}{2\,(\text{parts})} = \frac{1500\,(\text{mL})}{x\,(\text{mL})}$$

$$x = 1000 \text{ mL of liquid with specific gravity of } 0.950, and$$

$$\frac{3\,(\text{parts})}{1\,(\text{part})} = \frac{1500\,(\text{mL})}{y\,(\text{mL})}$$

$$y = 500 \text{ mL of liquid with specific gravity of } 0.875, answers.$$

CASE IN POINT 15.3 A pharmacist received the following prescription:

℞

Hydrocortisone	0.6%
AQUAPHOR q.s. ad	15 g

Sig. Apply to child's affected area t.i.d.

The pharmacist has no hydrocortisone powder but does have a hydrocortisone cream, 1%. How many grams each of hydrocortisone cream and Aquaphor should be used in filling the prescription?

PRACTICE PROBLEMS

Altering Strength, Stock Solutions, and Alligation Calculations

1. If 250 mL of a 1:800 (v/v) solution were diluted to 1000 mL, what would be the ratio strength?

2. If a pharmacist added 12 g of azelaic acid to 50 g of an ointment containing 15% azelaic acid, what would be the final concentration of azelaic acid in the ointment?

3. If 400 mL of a 20% w/v solution were diluted to 2 liters, what would be the percentage strength?

4. BACTROBAN ointment contains 2% mupirocin. How many grams of a polyethylene glycol ointment base must be mixed with the contents of a 22-g tube of the BACTROBAN ointment to prepare one having a concentration of 5 mg/g?

5. How many grams of an 8% w/w progesterone gel must be mixed with 1.45 g of a single-use 4% w/w progesterone gel to achieve a gel of 5.5% w/w strength?

6. If 150 mL of a 17% (w/v) concentrate of benzalkonium chloride are diluted to 5 gallons, what will be the ratio strength of the dilution?

7. A pharmacist fills a prescription for 30 g of a 0.1% w/w hydrocortisone cream by combining a 1% w/w hydrocortisone cream and a cream base. How many grams of each were used?

8. ℞² Tetracaine
       Hydrochloride   0.75% w/v
    Epinephrine
       Hydrochloride   1:4000 w/v
    Cocaine
       Hydrochloride   3% w/v
    Sodium
       Chloride
       Solution ad   30 mL
    Sig. Use in eye as directed.

How many milliliters each of a 2% w/v solution of tetracaine hydrochloride and a 1:1000 w/v solution of epinephrine hydrochloride should be used in preparing the prescription?

9. If two tablespoonfuls of a 10% w/v povidone iodine solution were diluted to 1 quart with purified water, what would be the ratio strength of the dilution?

10. How many milliliters of a 1:50 w/v boric acid solution can be prepared from 500 mL of a 5% w/v boric acid solution?

11. How many milliliters of water must be added to 250 mL of a 25% w/v stock solution of sodium chloride to prepare a 0.9% w/v sodium chloride solution?

12. How many milliliters of undecylenic acid would need to be added to 30 mL of a 20% undecylenic acid topical solution to change its concentration to 25%?

13. A certain product contains benzalkonium chloride in a concentration of 1:5000 w/v. How many milliliters of a 17% stock solution of benzalkonium chloride should be used in preparing 4 liters of the product?

14. How many milliliters of a 10% stock solution of a chemical are needed to prepare 120 mL of a solution containing 10 mg of the chemical per milliliter?

15. How many milliliters of a 1% w/v epinephrine injection must be used to prepare 20 mL of an injection containing 1:200,000 w/v epinephrine?

16. NEORAL oral solution contains 100 mg/mL of cyclosporine. If, on prescription, a pharmacist desired to prepare 30 mL of an oral solution containing 10% cyclosporine, how many milliliters of diluent should be used?

17. The formula for a buffer solution contains 1.24% w/v of boric acid. How many milliliters of a 5% w/v boric acid solution should be used to obtain the boric acid needed in preparing 1 liter of the buffer solution?

18. In filling a hospital order, a pharmacist diluted 1 mL of an amphotericin B injection (containing 50 mg/10 mL) with a 5% dextrose injection to prepare an intravenous infusion containing amphotericin B, 0.1 mg/mL. How many milliliters of infusion did the pharmacist prepare?

19. ℞ Gentian Violet Solution 500 mL
         1:100,000
     Sig. Mouthwash

    How many milliliters of ½% stock solution of gentian violet should be used in preparing the prescription?

20. A pharmacist combines the contents of a 30-g tube of a 0.5% ointment and a 90-g tube of a 1.5% ointment of the same active ingredient. What is the concentration of the mixture?

21. ℞³ Rhus Toxicodendron
         Extract   10 μg/mL
     Sterile Water for
         Injection qs   100 mL
     Sig. As directed.

    How many milliliters of a 100 mg/mL concentrate of Rhus toxicodendron extract should be used in preparing the prescription?

22. If a pharmacist fortified 10 g of a 0.1% w/w tacrolimus (PROTOPIC) ointment by adding 12.5 g of an ointment containing 0.03% w/w of the same drug, what would be the percentage strength of the mixture?

23. A physician prescribes an ophthalmic suspension to contain 100 mg of cortisone acetate in 8 mL of normal saline solution. The pharmacist has on hand a 2.5% suspension of cortisone acetate in normal saline solution. How many milliliters of this and how many milliliters of normal saline solution should be used in preparing the prescribed suspension?

24. ℞ Benzalkonium Chloride
        Solution   240 mL
    Make a solution such
        that 10 mL diluted
        to a liter equals a
        1:5000 solution.
    Sig. 10 mL diluted to
        a liter for external
        use.

    How many milliliters of a 17% stock solution of benzalkonium chloride should be used in preparing the prescription?

25. How many milliliters of water should be added to 100 mL of a 1:125 w/v solution to make a solution such that 25 mL diluted to 100 mL will yield a 1:4000 dilution?

26. How many milliliters of a lotion base must be added to 30 mL of oxiconazole nitrate (OXISTAT) lotion 1% w/v, to reduce its concentration to 6 mg/mL?

27. ℞⁴ Lactic Acid   10% w/v
     Salicylic Acid   10% w/v
     Flexible Collodion q.s. 15   mL
     Sig. For wart removal. Use externally as directed.

    How many milliliters of an 85% w/w solution of lactic acid with a specific gravity of 1.21 should be used in preparing the prescription?

28. A pharmacist receives a prescription for 60 g of a 0.75% w/w bexarotene gel. How many grams each of a 1% w/w bexarotene gel and gel base must be used?

29. How many milliliters of a syrup containing 85% w/v of sucrose should be mixed with 150 mL of a syrup containing 60% w/v of sucrose to make a syrup containing 80% w/v of sucrose?

30. A pharmacist receives an order for 60 mL of an oral solution containing memantine hydrochloride (NAMENDA) 1.5 mg/mL. She has on hand a 360-mL bottle of oral solution containing memantine hydrochloride, 10 mg/5 mL, and a diluent of sorbitol solution. How many milliliters each of the available oral solution and sorbitol solution may be used to fill the order?

31. How many milliliters of 95% w/w sulfuric acid having a specific gravity of 1.820 should be used in preparing 2 liters of 10% w/v acid?

32. A pharmacist mixes 100 mL of 38% w/w hydrochloric acid with enough purified water to make 360 mL. If the specific gravity of hydrochloric acid is 1.20, calculate the percentage strength (w/v) of the resulting dilution.

33. In using isoproterenol hydrochloride solution (1:5000 w/v), 1 mL of the solution is diluted to 10 mL with sodium chloride injection before intravenous administration. What is the percentage concentration of the diluted solution?

34. A 1:750 w/v solution of benzalkonium chloride diluted with purified water in a ratio of 3 parts of the benzalkonium solution and 77 parts of purified water is recommended for bladder and urethral irrigation. What is the ratio strength of benzalkonium chloride in the final dilution?

35. How many milliliters of a suspension base must be mixed with 250 mL of a paroxetine (PAXIL) oral suspension, 10 mg/5 mL, to change its concentration to 0.1% w/v?

36. An insect venom concentrate for immunotherapy contains 100 μg/mL. How many milliliters of water should be added to 1.2 mL of the venom concentrate to yield a 1:100,000 dilution?

37. How many grams of a 2.5% w/w benzocaine ointment can be prepared by diluting 1 lb. of a 20% w/w benzocaine ointment with white petrolatum?

38. How many grams of salicylic acid should be added to 75 g of a polyethylene glycol ointment to prepare an ointment containing 6% w/w of salicylic acid?

39. How many grams of an ointment base must be added to 45 g of clobestasol (TEMOVATE) ointment, 0.05% w/w, to change its strength to 0.03% w/w?

40. ℞ Hydrocortisone Acetate
    Ointment 0.25%   10 g
    Sig. Apply to the eye.

    How many grams of 2.5% ophthalmic hydrocortisone acetate ointment and how many grams of ophthalmic base (diluent) should be used in preparing the prescription?

41. How many milliliters of a nonmedicated, flavored syrup base must be added to 1 pint of ranitidine (ZANTAC) syrup, 15 mg/mL, to change its concentration to 5 mg/mL?

42. ℞ Zinc Oxide   1.5
    Hydrophilic Petrolatum   2.5
    Purified Water   5
    Hydrophilic Ointment ad   30
    Sig. Apply to affected areas.

    How much zinc oxide should be added to the product to make an ointment containing 10% of zinc oxide?

43. If equal portions of tretinoin gel (RETINA MICRO), 0.1% w/w and 0.04% w/w, are combined, what would be the resultant percentage strength?

44. A vaginal douche powder concentrate contains 2% w/w of active ingredient. What would be the percentage concentration (w/v) of the resultant solution after a 5-g packet of powder is dissolved in enough water to make 1 quart of solution?

45.[5] How many milliliters of a 0.2% solution of a skin-test antigen must be used to prepare 4 mL of a solution containing 0.04 mg/mL of the antigen?

46. How many milligrams of sodium fluoride are needed to prepare 100 mL of a sodium fluoride stock solution such that a solution containing 2 ppm of sodium fluoride results when 0.5 mL is diluted to 250 mL with water?

47. ℞[6] Cyclosporine   2%
        Corn Oil   qs
        Sig. Use as directed.

    (a) How many milliliters each of corn oil and a 10% solution of cyclosporine would be needed to prepare 30 mL of the prescription? (b) If you then wished to dilute the prescription to a concentration of 1.5% cyclosporine, how many additional milliliters of corn oil would be required?

48. If 100 mg of a 1:10 trituration of mechlorethamine hydrochloride (MUSTARGEN) are diluted to 10 mL with water for injection, how many milliliters of the injection should be administered to a 132-lb. patient if the dose of mechlorethamine hydrochloride is 0.1 mg/kg?

49. A hospital worker combined 2 fluidounces of a povidone-iodine cleaner, 7.5% w/v, with 4 fluidounces of a povidone-iodine topical solution, 10 % w/v. Calculate the resulting strength of the povidone-iodine mixture.

50. If 60 mL of a combination gel of hydrocortisone acetate, 1% w/w, and pramoxine, 1% w/w, are mixed with 12.5 mL of a gel containing hydrocortisone acetate, 2.5% w/w, and pramoxine, 1% w/w, calculate the percentage strength of each of the two drugs in the mixture.

51. A drug is commercially available in capsules each containing 12.5 mg of drug and 37.5 mg of diluent. How many milligrams of additional diluent must be added to the contents of one capsule to make a dilution containing 0.5 mg of drug in each 100 mg of powder?

52. In what proportion should 5% and 1% hydrocortisone ointments be mixed to prepare a 2.5% ointment?

53. In what proportion should a 20% zinc oxide ointment be mixed with white petrolatum (diluent) to produce a 3% zinc oxide ointment?

54. A parent diluted 1 mL ibuprofen oral drops (Infant's MOTRIN Concentrated Drops) with 15 mL of water prior to administering the medication. The concentrated drops contain ibuprofen, 50 mg/1.25 mL. Calculate the concentration of ibuprofen in the dilution in (a) mg/mL, and (b) as a percentage strength.

55. How many milliliters of a 2.5% w/v chlorpromazine hydrochloride injection and how many milliliters of 0.9% w/v sodium chloride injection should be used to prepare 500 mL of a 0.3% w/v chlorpromazine hydrochloride injection?

56. How many milliliters of a 2% w/v solution of lidocaine hydrochloride should be used in preparing 500 mL of a solution containing 4 mg of lidocaine hydrochloride per milliliter of solution?

57. Dopamine hydrochloride injection is available in 5-mL ampuls containing 40 mg of dopamine hydrochloride per milliliter. The injection must be diluted before administration. If a physician wishes to use sodium chloride injection as the diluent and wants a dilution containing 0.04% w/v of dopamine hydrochloride, how many milliliters of sodium chloride injection should be added to 5 mL of the injection?

58. A solution of benzalkonium chloride is available in a concentration of 1:750 w/v. How many milliliters of purified water should be added to 30 mL of the solution to prepare a 1:5000 benzalkonium chloride solution for use as a wet dressing to the skin?

59.[7] How many milliliters of sterile water for injection should be added to a vial containing 5 μg/mL of a drug to prepare a solution containing 1.5 μg/mL of the drug?

60. ℞ Zephiran Chloride
          Solution (17% w/v)   q.s.
       Purified Water, to
          make   480 mL
       Sig. One tbsp. diluted to
          1 gallon with water
          to make a 1:10,000
          dilution.

    How many milliliters of zephiran chloride solution should be used in preparing the prescription?

Specific Gravity Calculations of Mixtures

61. What is the specific gravity of a mixture containing 1000 mL of water, 500 mL of glycerin having a specific gravity of 1.25, and 1500 mL of alcohol having a specific gravity of 0.81? (Assume no contraction occurs when the liquids are mixed.)

62. If a pharmacist mixed 1 pint of propylene glycol having a specific gravity of 1.20 with 500 mL of water, how many milliliters additional of propylene glycol should be added to change the specific gravity to 1.15?

63. How many milliliters of a syrup having a specific gravity of 1.350 should be mixed with 3000 mL of a syrup having a specific gravity of 1.250 to obtain a product having a specific gravity of 1.310?

64. How many grams of sorbitol solution having a specific gravity of 1.285 and how many grams (milliliters) of water should be used in preparing 500 g of a sorbitol solution having a specific gravity of 1.225?

CALCQUIZ

15.A.[a] A pharmacist receives a special request from an ophthalmologist to prepare a fortified tobramycin ophthalmic solution. The available solution contains tobramycin, 3 mg/mL. How many milliliters of a tobramycin injection containing 40 mg/mL must be aseptically added to a 5-mL container of the ophthalmic solution to prepare one 0.5% in concentration?

15.B. How many milliliters of water must be added to 15 mL of a 23.4% solution of sodium chloride to dilute the concentration to 0.06 mEq/mL?

15.C.[a] A pharmacy receives a medication order for 1 L of a 3% sodium chloride injection. The pharmacy stocks 0.9% sodium chloride injection in 1-L bags and sodium chloride injection, 23.4% in 50-mL vials. How many milliliters of the latter should be added to the 1-L bag of normal saline solution to fill the order?

15.D. A 60-mL bottle of an oral solution contains a drug in a concentration of 15 mg/mL. A medication order requests that the drug concentration be reduced to 5 mg/mL by using three parts water to one part polyethylene glycol 400. How many milliliters of each of these two agents should be used?

15.E. How many milliliters of a 17% solution of benzalkonium chloride should a pharmacist use in preparing 120 mL of a prescription such that when a patient adds 15 mL of the dispensed medication to a gallon of water, as a foot soak, the resulting benzalkonium chloride concentration will be 1:5000?

[a]Problem courtesy of Flynn Warren, Bishop, GA.

ANSWERS TO "CASE IN POINT" AND PRACTICE PROBLEMS

Case in Point 15.1

Cefuroxime axetil present in original suspension:

$$100 \text{ mL} \times \frac{250 \text{ mg}}{5 \text{ mL}} = 5000 \text{ mg}$$

Cefuroxime axetil required in strengthened suspension:

$$100 \text{ mL} \times \frac{300 \text{ mg}}{5 \text{ mL}} = 6000 \text{ mg}$$

Cefuroxime axetil to add:

6000 mg − 5000 mg = 1000 mg

Tablets required:

$$1000 \text{ mg} \times \frac{1 \text{ tablet}}{250 \text{ mg}} = 4 \text{ tablets, } answer.$$

A Second Look

There are a number of ways in which this problem could be addressed. One way would be to add another 250-mg pulverized tablet, calculate the volume of suspension that could be prepared at a concentration of 300 mg/5 mL, dispense 100 mL of that and discard the remaining volume.

Cefuroxime axetil in strengthened suspension plus another tablet:

6000 mg + 250 mg = 6250 mg cefuroxime axetil

Volume of suspension that could be prepared at a concentration of 300 mg/ 5 mL:

$$\frac{5 \text{ mL}}{300 \text{ mg}} \times 6250 \text{ mg} = 104.17 \text{ mL}$$

Volume to dispense:

100 mL, and

Volume to discard:

4.17 mL, *answers*.

Proof: "If there are 6250 mg of cefuroxime axetil in 104.17 mL, how many milligrams would be present in each 5 mL?"

$$6250 \text{ mg} \times \frac{5 \text{ mL}}{104.17 \text{ mL}} = 299.99 \text{ or}$$

300 mg, *answer*.

Case in Point 15.2

(a) 120 mL × 0.15 (1.5%) = 1.8 g
1.8 g = 1800 mg

$$1800 \text{ mg} \times \frac{1 \text{ mL}}{150 \text{ mg}} = 12 \text{ mL},$$

clindamycin phosphate sterile solution, *answer*.

(b) *If* the pharmacist had had clindamycin phosphate powder with which to fill the prescription, 1.8 g would have been used, and that quantity would have taken up a negligible volume on solution in the 52% v/v alcohol. Thus, the interpretation of the prescription is that the 120 mL (not 120 mL − 12 mL) of 52% v/v alcohol should be used.

120 mL × 0.52 (52% v/v) = 62.4 mL of solute (100% v/v alcohol)

$$\frac{62.4 \text{ mL}}{\text{x mL}} = \frac{95 \text{ mL}}{100 \text{ mL}}; \text{ x} = 65.68 \text{ mL of}$$
95% v/v alcohol, *answer*.

(c) Due to contraction when alcohol and water are mixed, the volume of water cannot be determined by subtracting 65.68 mL from 120 mL; thus, a sufficient volume of water is used (q.s.) to make 120 mL, *answer*.

Case in Point 15.3

15 g × 0.006 (0.6% w/w) = 0.09 g hydrocortisone

1% hydrocortisone cream = 1 g hydrocortisone/100 g

Thus, $\dfrac{0.09 \text{ g}}{\text{x g}} = \dfrac{1 \text{ g}}{100 \text{ g}};$

x = 9 g hydrocortisone cream, *and*
15 g − 9 g = 6 g AQUAPHOR, *answers*.

Note: The problem also may be solved by alligation alternate.

Practice Problems

1. 1:3200 v/v

2. 31.5% w/w

3. 4% w/v

4. 66 g polyethylene glycol ointment base

5. 0.87 g progesterone gel, 8%

6. 1:742 w/v

7. 3 g hydrocortisone cream (1%)
   27 g cream base

8. 11.25 mL tetracaine hydrochloride solution
   7.5 mL epinephrine hydrochloride solution

9. 1:315 w/v

10. 1250 mL boric acid solution

11. 6694.4 mL water

12. 2 mL undecylenic acid

13. 4.7 mL stock solution

14. 12 mL stock solution

15. 0.1 mL epinephrine injection

16. 0 mL diluent

17. 248 mL boric acid solution

18. 50 mL infusion

19. 1 mL stock solution

20. 1.25%

21. 0.01 mL concentrate

22. 0.06% w/w

23. 4 mL cortisone acetate suspension
    4 mL normal saline solution

24. 28.2 mL stock solution

25. 700 mL water

26. 20 mL lotion base

27. 1.46 mL lactic acid solution

28. 45 g bexarotene gel
    15 g gel base

29. 600 mL syrup

30. 45 mL memantine oral solution
    15 mL sorbitol solution

31. 115.67 mL sulfuric acid, 95%

32. 12.67% w/v

33. 0.002% w/v

34. 1:20,000 w/v

35. 250 mL suspension base

36. 10.8 mL water

37. 3632 g benzocaine ointment, 2.5%

38. 4.787 g salicylic acid

39. 30 g ointment base

40. 1 g hydrocortisone acetate ointment, 2.5%
    9 g ophthalmic base

41. 946 mL syrup base

42. 1.667 g zinc oxide

43. 0.07% w/w

44. 0.011% w/v

45. 0.08 mL antigen, 0.2%

46. 100 mg sodium fluoride

47. (a) 24 mL corn oil
         6 mL cyclosporin solution
    (b) 10 mL corn oil

48. 6 mL MUSTARGEN injection

49. 9.17% w/v

50. 1% pramoxine
    1.26% hydrocortisone

51. 2450 mg diluent

52. 3:5

53. 3:17

54. (a) 2.5 mg/mL ibuprofen
    (b) 2.5% ibuprofen

55. 60 mL chlorpromazine hydrochloride injection
    440 mL sodium chloride injection

56. 100 mL lidocaine hydrochloride injection

57. 495 mL sodium chloride injection

58. 170 mL purified water

59. 2.33 mL sterile water for injection

60. 71.2 mL zephiran chloride solution

61. 0.947

62. 1031.38 mL propylene glycol

63. 4500 mL syrup

64. 394.737 g sorbitol solution
    105.263 mL water

References

1. United States Pharmacopeia 32. National Formulary 27. Rockville, MD: United States Pharmacopeial Convention, 2009;1:1249.
2. Prince SJ. Calculations. *International Journal of Pharmaceutical Compounding* 2000;4:221.
3. Karolchyk S. Treating patients allergic to poison ivy. *International Journal of Pharmaceutical Compounding* 1998;2:421.
4. Prince SJ. Calculations. *International Journal of Pharmaceutical Compounding* 1998;2:310.
5. Prince SJ. Calculations. *International Journal of Pharmaceutical Compounding* 1998;2:453.
6. Prince SJ. Calculations. *International Journal of Pharmaceutical Compounding* 2000;4:393.
7. Prince SJ. Calculations. *International Journal of Pharmaceutical Compounding* 1999;3:145.

Reducing and Enlarging Formulas 16

Objectives

Upon successful completion of this chapter, the student will be able to:

• Perform calculations to reduce or enlarge formulas for pharmaceutical preparations.

Pharmacists may have to reduce or enlarge formulas for pharmaceutical preparations in the course of their professional practice or manufacturing activities. Formulas in the United States Pharmacopeia-National Formulary generally are based on the preparation of 1000 mL or 1000 g of product. However, other formulas may be based on different quantities.

The need to prepare different quantities of a formula varies greatly. Whereas only small quantities may be required in a community pharmacy, and modest quantities in a hospital pharmacy, very large quantities are prepared in the pharmaceutical industry. In the latter case, hundreds of thousands of dosage units may be prepared in a single production batch. The key point is that *irrespective of the quantity prepared, it is essential that the correct proportion of one ingredient to the other in a given formula be maintained.*

Methods to Reduce or Enlarge Formulas

As is demonstrated in the following section, *ratio and proportion*, *dimensional analysis*, and a *factor method* each may be used to calculate a reduced or enlarged formula.

The *factor method* is the simplest method to use. It is based on the *relative* quantity of formula to be prepared. For instance, if 240 mL of a 1000-mL standard formula is to be prepared, the factor is derived as follows:

$$\frac{240 \text{ mL (to be prepared)}}{1000 \text{ mL (standard formula)}} = 0.24 \text{ (factor)}$$

Then, by multiplying the quantity of each ingredient in the standard formula by the factor, the correct quantity of that ingredient to use is determined.

Example Calculations of Reducing and Enlarging Formulas

From the following formula for Calamine Topical Suspension, USP,[1] calculate the quantity of each ingredient required to prepare 240 mL of product.

Calamine	80 g
Zinc oxide	80 g
Glycerin	20 mL
Bentonite magma	250 mL
Calcium hydroxide	
Topical solution, qs ad	1000 mL

Solving by *Ratio and Proportion:*

$$\frac{80 \text{ g}}{1000 \text{ mL}} = \frac{\text{x g}}{240 \text{ mL}}; \ \text{x} = 19.2 \text{ g, calamine,}$$

$$\frac{80 \text{ g}}{1000 \text{ mL}} = \frac{\text{x g}}{240 \text{ mL}}; \ \text{x} = 19.2 \text{ g, zinc oxide,}$$

$$\frac{20 \text{ mL}}{1000 \text{ mL}} = \frac{\text{x mL}}{240 \text{ mL}}; \ \text{x} = 4.8 \text{ mL, glycerin,}$$

$$\frac{250 \text{ mL}}{1000 \text{ mL}} = \frac{\text{x mL}}{240 \text{ mL}}; \ \text{x} = 60 \text{ mL, bentonite magma,}$$

and calcium hydroxide topical solution, to make 240 mL, *answers.*

Solving by *Dimensional Analysis:*

$$240 \text{ mL} \times \frac{80 \text{ g}}{1000 \text{ mL}} = 19.2 \text{ g} \ \ \text{calamine, and so forth, for each ingredient, arriving at the}$$

same answers as shown above.

Solving by the *Factor Method:*

$$\frac{240 \text{ mL (to be prepared)}}{1000 \text{ mL (standard formula)}} = 0.24 \text{ (factor)}$$

The quantity of each ingredient in the standard formula is multiplied by the factor:

$$80 \text{ g} \times 0.24 = 19.2 \text{ g calamine,}$$

and so forth, for each ingredient, arriving at the same answers as shown above.

From the following formula for artificial tears,[2] calculate the quantity of each ingredient required to prepare a dozen 30-mL containers.

Polyvinyl Alcohol	1.4 g
Povidone	0.6 g
Chlorobutanol	0.5 g
Sterile Sodium Chloride Solution, 9% ad	100 mL

$$30 \text{ mL} \times 12 = 360 \text{ mL}$$

$$\frac{360 \text{ mL}}{100 \text{ mL}} = 3.6 \text{ (factor)}$$

Using the factor 3.6, the quantity of each ingredient is calculated as follows:

Polyvinyl Alcohol	= 1.4 g × 3.6 = 5.04 g
Povidone	= 0.6 g × 3.6 = 2.16 g
Chlorobutanol	= 0.5 g × 3.6 = 1.8 g

Sterile Sodium Chloride Solution, 9% ad 360 mL, answers.

From the following formula for an estradiol vaginal gel,[3] calculate the quantity of each ingredient required to prepare 1 lb. of gel.

Estradiol	200 g
Polysorbate 80	1 g
Methylcellulose Gel, 2%	95 g

$$1 \text{ lb.} = 454 \text{ g}$$

$$\text{Formula weight} = 200 \text{ g} + 1 \text{ g} + 95 \text{ g} = 296 \text{ g}$$

$$\frac{454 \text{ g}}{296 \text{ g}} = 1.534 \text{ (factor)}$$

Using the factor 1.534, the quantity of each ingredient is calculated as follows:

Estradiol	$= 200 \text{ g} \times 1.534 = 306.8 \text{ g}$
Polysorbate 80	$= 1 \text{ g} \times 1.534 = 1.534 \text{ g}$
Methylcellulose Gel, 2%	$= 95 \text{ g} \times 1.534 = 145.73 \text{ g}$, *answers.*

From the following formula for a dexamethasone ophthalmic ointment,[4] *calculate the quantity of each ingredient needed to prepare 7.5 g of ointment.*

Dexamethasone Sodium Phosphate	55 mg
Lanolin, Anhydrous	5 g
Mineral Oil	10 g
White Petrolatum ad	100 g

$$\frac{7.5 \text{ g}}{100 \text{ g}} = 0.075 \text{ (factor)}$$

Using the factor 0.075, the quantity of each ingredient is calculated as follows:

Dexamethasone Sodium Phosphate	$= 55 \text{ mg} \times 0.075 = 4.125 \text{ mg}$
Lanolin, Anhydrous	$= 5 \text{ g} \times 0.075 = 0.375 \text{ g}$
Mineral Oil	$= 10 \text{ g} \times 0.075 = 0.75 \text{ g}$
White Petrolatum ad	$= 7.5 \text{ g}$, *answers.*

Formulas That Specify Proportional Parts

On a rare occasion, a pharmacist may encounter an old formula that indicates the ingredients in "parts" rather than in measures of weight or volume. The parts indicate the relative proportion of each of the ingredients in the formula by *either* weight or volume, but not both. A formula for solid or semisolid ingredients, therefore, may be considered in terms of *grams*, whereas a formula of liquids may be considered in terms of *milliliters*.

Example Calculation of a Formula Expressed in Parts

From the following formula, calculate the quantity of each ingredient required to make 1000 g of the ointment.

Coal Tar	5 parts
Zinc Oxide	10 parts
Hydrophilic Ointment	50 parts

Total number of parts (by weight) = 65
1000 g will contain 65 parts

$$\frac{65 \text{ (parts)}}{5 \text{ (parts)}} = \frac{1000 \text{ (g)}}{x \text{ (g)}}$$

$$x = 76.92 \text{ g of Coal Tar,}$$

and

$$\frac{65 \ (\text{parts})}{10 \ (\text{parts})} = \frac{1000 \ (\text{g})}{y \ (\text{g})}$$

$$y = 153.85 \text{ g of Zinc Oxide,}$$

and

$$\frac{65 \ (\text{parts})}{50 \ (\text{parts})} = \frac{1000 \ (\text{g})}{z \ (\text{g})}$$

$$z = 769.23 \text{ g of Hydrophilic Ointment, } \textit{answers.}$$
(Check total: 1000 g)

An alternative method at solution would be to determine that there are 15.385 g per part (1000 g/65 parts) and thus

Coal Tar: 5 parts × 15.385   = 76.92 g
Zinc Oxide: 10 parts × 15.385 g/part   = 153.85 g
Hydrophilic Ointment: 50 parts × 15.385 = 769.25 g, *answers.*

PRACTICE PROBLEMS

1. From the following formula for 40 sertraline hydrochloride capsules,[5] calculate the quantity of each ingredient needed to prepare 250 such capsules.

Sertraline Hydrochloride	300 mg
Silica Gel	6 g
Calcium Citrate	4 g

2. From the following formula for a progesterone nasal spray,[6] calculate the quantity of each ingredient needed to prepare twenty-four 15-mL containers of the spray.

Progesterone	20 mg
Dimethyl-β-cyclodextrin	62 mg
Purified Water ad	1 mL

3. From the following formula, calculate the quantities required to make 5 lb. of hydrophilic ointment.

Methylparaben	0.25 g
Propylparaben	0.15 g
Sodium Lauryl Sulfate	10 g
Propylene Glycol	120 g
Stearyl Alcohol	250 g
White Petrolatum	250 g
Purified Water, to make	1000 g

4. The formula for an ophthalmic ointment is as follows:

Sulfacetamide Sodium	10% w/w
Prednisolone Acetate	0.2% w/w
Phenylmercuric Acetate	0.0008% w/w
Mineral Oil	1% w/w
White Petrolatum, qs ad	3.5 g

   How much of each ingredient would be needed to manufacture 2000 such tubes of ointment?

5. Calculate the quantity of each ingredient needed to prepare 15-mL of the following ophthalmic solution.[7]

Erythromycin Lactobionate	500 mg
Dexamethasone Sodium Phosphate	100 mg
Glycerin	2.5 mL
Sterile Water for Injection ad	100 mL

6. According to the literature, the bio-technology product NEULASTA (pegfilgrastim) contains the following in 0.6 mL pre-filled syringes[8]:

Pegfilgrastim	6	mg
Sorbitol	30	mg
Polysorbate 20	0.02	mg
Water for Injection, ad	0.6	mL

How much of the first three ingredients would be needed to manufacture 100,000 such syringes?

7. From the following formula, calculate the quantity of each ingredient required to make 1500 g of the powder.

Calcium Carbonate	5 parts
Magnesium Oxide	1 part
Sodium Bicarbonate	4 parts
Bismuth Subcarbonate	3 parts

8. The following is a formula for 100 triple estrogen capsules.[9] Calculate the quantities of the first three ingredients, in grams, and the last two ingredients, in kilograms, required to prepare 5000 such capsules.

Estriol	200 mg
Estrone	25 mg
Estradiol	25 mg
Polyethylene Glycol 1450	20 g
Polyethylene Glycol 3350	20 g

9. The formula for a ciprofloxacin otic drop is given in the literature as follows[10]:

Ciprofloxacin	1 g
Propylene Glycol	50 mL
Glycerin qs ad	100 mL

How many grams of ciprofloxacin would be required to prepare 200 15-mL bottles of the ear drop?

10. The formula for a sports rub cream is given in the literature as follows[11]:

Methyl Salicylate	15 mL
Menthol	10 g
Eucalyptus Oil	1 g
Hydrophilic Ointment, qs ad	100 g

If the specific gravity of methyl salicylate is 1.18, how many grams of each ingredient would be needed to prepare a dozen 30-g tubes of ointment?

11. From the following formula for gastric lavage prior to colonoscopy, calculate the quantity of sodium bicarbonate needed to prepare 100 liters of the formula.

Polyethylene Glycol 3350	60	mL
Sodium Chloride	1.46	g
Potassium Chloride	0.745	g
Sodium Bicarbonate	1.68	g
Sodium Sulfate	5.68	g
Water q.s. ad	4	L

12. The following is a formula for the preparation of a suppository for the treatment of migraine headaches.[12] Calculate the quantities of each ingredient needed to prepare 250 suppositories.

Ergotamine Tartrate	2	mg
Caffeine	100	mg
Hyoscyamine Sulfate	0.25	mg
Pentobarbital Sodium	60	mg
FATTIBASE ad	2	g

CALCQUIZ

16.A. An ophthalmic solution has the following formula[13]:

Tobramycin sulfate	300 mg
Diclofenac sodium	100 mg
Sodium chloride	806 mg
Sterile water for injection, ad	100 mL

Calculate the quantities of each ingredient required to prepare twenty-four 7.5-mL containers of the ophthalmic solution.

16.B. The formula for "Lubow's Solution" is as follows[14]:

Progesterone	1 g
Hydrocortisone	500 mg
Propylene glycol	2 g
Ethanol (95%) ad	100 mL

(a) Calculate the quantities of each ingredient required to prepare 2.5 mL of solution.
(b) How many milliliters of propylene glycol (sp. gr. 1.04) are needed to prepare a liter of the formula?

16.C. An ophthalmic solution for veterinary use has the following formula[15]:

Miconazole	1 g
PEG 40 castor oil	11.5 mL
Lactic acid 88% solution	0.4 mL
Sterile water for injection qs ad	100 mL

(a) Calculate the quantities of each ingredient required to prepare twelve 1.5-mL drop-containers of the medication.
(b) If the PEG 40 castor oil has a specific gravity of 1.1, calculate the grams present in (a).
(c) Calculate the quantity, in milliliters, of pure (100%) lactic acid in the formula.

16.D. A vial for injection contains 0.6 mL of solution. The dose is 0.5 mL, which contains 7.5 mg of drug. How many grams of drug are needed to manufacture 5000 vials of the product?

ANSWERS TO PRACTICE PROBLEMS

1. 1.875 g sertraline hydrochloride
   37.5 g silica gel
   25 g calcium citrate
2. 7.2 g progesterone
   22.32 g dimethyl-β-cyclodextrin
   ad 360 mL, purified water
3. 0.568 g methylparaben
   0.341 g propylparaben
   22.7 g sodium lauryl sulfate

272.4 g propylene glycol
567.5 g stearyl alcohol
567.5 g white petrolatum
ad 2270 g or 5 lb. purified water
4. 700 g sulfacetamide sodium
   14 g prednisolone acetate
   56 mg phenyl mercuric acetate
   70 g mineral oil
   6215.944 g white petrolatum

5. 75 mg erythromycin lactobionate
   15 mg dexamethasone sodium phosphate
   0.375 mL glycerin
   q.s. ad 15 mL sterile water for injection

6. 600 g pegfilgrastim
   3000 g sorbitol
   2 g polysorbate 20

7. 576.923 g calcium carbonate
   115.385 g magnesium oxide
   461.539 g sodium bicarbonate
   346.154 g bismuth subcarbonate

8. 10 g estriol
   1.25 g estrone
   1.25 g estradiol
   1 kg polyethylene glycol 1450
   1 kg polyethylene glycol 3350

9. 30 g ciprofloxacin

10. 63.72 g methyl salicylate
    36 g menthol
    3.6 g eucalyptus oil
    256.68 g hydrophilic ointment

11. 42 g sodium bicarbonate

12. 500 mg ergotamine tartrate
    25 g caffeine
    62.5 mg hyoscyamine sulfate
    15 g pentobarbital sodium
    459.44 g FATTIBASE

References

1. *United States Pharmacopeia 32 National Formulary 27*. Rockville, MD: United States Pharmacopeial Convention, 2009;2:1745.
2. Allen LV Jr, Editor-In-Chief. *International Journal of Pharmaceutical Compounding* 2000;4:376.
3. Allen LV Jr, Editor-In-Chief. *International Journal of Pharmaceutical Compounding* 1998;2:51.
4. Allen LV Jr, Editor-In-Chief. *International Journal of Pharmaceutical Compounding* 2003;7:215.
5. Allen LV Jr, Editor-In-Chief. *International Journal of Pharmaceutical Compounding* 1998;2:443.
6. Allen LV Jr, Editor-In-Chief. *International Journal of Pharmaceutical Compounding* 1998;2:56.
7. Allen LV Jr, Editor-In-Chief. *International Journal of Pharmaceutical Compounding* 2002;6:452.
8. NEULASTA (pegfilgrastim). *Product Literature*. Thousand Oaks, CA. Amgen, Inc., 2011.
9. Allen LV Jr, Editor-In-Chief. *International Journal of Pharmaceutical Compounding* 1997;1:187.
10. Allen LV Jr. Secundum Artem 2006;13:4. Available at: http://paddocklabs.com/html/resource/pdf/Sec%20Artem%2013.1.pdf. Accessed August 1, 2011.
11. Allen LV Jr. Secundum Artem 2005;12:4. Available at: http://paddocklabs.com/html/resource/pdf/Sec%20Artem%2012.4.pdf. Accessed August 1, 2011.
12. Allen LV Jr, Editor-In-Chief. *International Journal of Pharmaceutical Compounding* 1998;2:151.
13. Allen LV Jr, Editor-In-Chief. *International Journal of Pharmaceutical Compounding* 2010;14:74.
14. Allen LV Jr, Editor-In-Chief. *International Journal of Pharmaceutical Compounding* 2009;13:558.
15. Allen LV Jr, Editor-In-Chief. *International Journal of Pharmaceutical Compounding* 2009;13:559.

Selected Calculations in Contemporary Compounding 17

Objectives

Upon successful completion of this chapter, the student will be able to:

- Perform calculations for the constitution of dry powders for oral solution or suspension.
- Perform calculations for the constitution of dry powders for parenteral use.
- Perform calculations for the use of prefabricated dosage forms in compounding procedures.
- Perform calculations applied to the filling of capsules.
- Perform calculation applied to the preparation of suppositories by molding.
- Perform calculations applicable to specialized formulas and their methods of preparation.

Pharmaceutical compounding is the process by which pharmacists combine therapeutically active ingredients with pharmaceutical materials in the preparation of *customized* prescriptions and medication orders to meet the specific needs of *individual patients*. This is in contrast to the *large-scale* production of pharmaceutical products to meet the needs of the general population that is termed *pharmaceutical manufacturing*.

Compounding is an activity for which pharmacists are uniquely qualified by virtue of their education, training, and experience. Many pharmacists have developed *specialized practices* in compounding that have contributed greatly to the medication needs of their patients.

This chapter presents calculations that apply to the preparation of oral and parenteral fluids by the *constitution* of dry powders; the use of tablets, capsules, and injections as the source of active therapeutic ingredients (ATI) in compounding; calculations specifically applicable to the extemporaneous preparation of suppositories and capsules; and calculations relevant to specialized prescriptions, medication orders, and formulas.

General Considerations in Compounding Practice

Compounded prescriptions may be desired for a number of reasons, including[1,2]:

- the need to adjust the strength or dose of a commercially available product to meet the specific requirements of a patient (e.g., a pediatric patient);
- the need to provide a product more organoleptically acceptable (e.g., taste) to a pediatric or veterinary patient;
- the need to prepare a different dosage form (e.g., a liquid) than the commercially available product (e.g., a tablet) to meet the requirements of a patient unable to swallow the existing dosage form (e.g., a pediatric or elderly patient);
- the need to prepare a dosage form free of an agent (e.g., sugar, preservatives) in the commercially available product that cannot be tolerated by a patient; and
- the need to provide a patient with a specifically designed formulation of an approved drug or drug combination, which is unavailable as a commercial product.

The *United States Pharmacopeia—National Formulary* (USP/NF) devotes several chapters to the compounding of both sterile and non-sterile preparations.[3] These chapters, along with other pharmaceutical references, should be referred to as required to ensure that standards of good pharmaceutical practice in compounding are understood and met. Pharmacists may participate in a comprehensive program of voluntary accreditation conducted by a consortium of national pharmacy organizations.[1]

Constitution of Dry Powders

Constitution of Dry Powders for Oral Solution or Suspension

Some drugs, most notably antibiotics, lose their potency in a relatively short period when prepared in a liquid dosage form. To enhance the shelf-life of these drugs, manufacturers provide products to the pharmacy in dry powder form for *constitution* (or *reconstitution*) with purified water or special diluent at the time a prescription or medication order is received. Depending on the product, the dry powder may be stable for about 24 months. After constitution, the resultant solution or suspension is stable in the quantities usually dispensed, for the treatment period.

Dry powders for constitution are packaged in self-contained bottles of sufficient size to accommodate the addition of the required volume of diluent (Figure 17.1). In addition to the quantitative amount of therapeutic agent, the powder contains such pharmaceutical ingredients as solubilizing or suspending agents, stabilizers, colorants, sweeteners, and flavorants.

▼ FIGURE 17.1 Example of a dry powder for reconstitution to prepare an oral solution. The label calls for the addition of 127 mL of water to prepare 200 mL of solution having a concentration of 125 mg or 200,000 units of penicillin V per 5 mL of solution.

On receipt of a prescription order, the pharmacist follows the label instructions for constitution, adding the proper amount of purified water or other diluent to prepare the liquid form. Depending on the product's formulation, constitution results in the preparation of a clear *solution* (often called a *syrup*) or a *suspension*. The final volume of product is the sum of the volume of solvent or diluent added and the volume occupied by the dissolved or suspended powder mixture. These products generally are intended for infants and children but also can be used by adults who have difficulty swallowing counterpart solid dosage form products.

Manufacturer's products generally are formulated to provide the usual dose by teaspoon or calibrated dropper. Pharmacists may customize products for individual patients, as demonstrated by the calculations that follow.

Example Calculations for the Constitution of Dry Powders for Oral Use

The label for a dry powder package of cefprozil (CEFZIL) for oral suspension directs the pharmacist to add 72 mL of purified water to prepare 100 mL of suspension. If the package contains 2.5 g of cefprozil, how many milligrams of the drug would be contained in each teaspoonful dose of the constituted suspension?

$$2.5 \text{ g} = 2500 \text{ mg}$$

$$\frac{2500 \text{ mg}}{100 \text{ mL}} = \frac{x \text{ mg}}{5 \text{ mL}}$$

$$x = 125 \text{ mg cefprozil, } answer.$$

Or, solving by dimensional analysis:

$$\frac{1000 \text{ mg}}{1 \text{ g}} \times \frac{5 \text{ mL}}{1 \text{ tsp}} \times \frac{2.5 \text{ g}}{100 \text{ mL}} = 125 \text{ mg cefprozil, } answer.$$

Label instructions for an ampicillin product call for the addition of 78 mL of water to make 100 mL of constituted suspension such that each 5 mL contains 125 mg of ampicillin. Calculate the volume represented by the suspended powder in the product and the total content of ampicillin.

Volume of powder: Because the addition of 78 mL of water results in the preparation of 100 mL of product, the volume occupied by the powder is:

$$100 \text{ mL} - 78 \text{ mL} = 22 \text{ mL, } answer.$$

Total drug (ampicillin) present: If, in the constituted product, each 5 mL contains 125 mg of ampicillin, the total amount of ampicillin in the 100-mL product is:

$$\frac{5 \text{ mL}}{125 \text{ mg}} = \frac{100 \text{ mL}}{x}$$

$$x = 2500 \text{ mg, } answer.$$

Using the product in the previous example, if a physician desires an ampicillin concentration of 100 mg/5 mL (rather than 125 mg/5 mL), how many milliliters of water should be added to the dry powder?

Because it was determined that 2500 mg of ampicillin are in the dry product, the volume of product that can be made with a concentration of 100 mg/5 mL may be calculated by:

$$\frac{2500 \text{ mg}}{x \text{ mL}} = \frac{100 \text{ mg}}{5 \text{ mL}}$$

$$x = 125 \text{ mL, } answer.$$

Then, because it had been determined that the dry powder occupies 22 mL of volume, it is possible to determine the amount of water to add:

$$125 \text{ mL} - 22 \text{ mL} = 103 \text{ mL}, answer.$$

The label of a dry powder for oral suspension states that when 111 mL of water are added to the powder, 150 mL of a suspension containing 250 mg of ampicillin per 5 mL are prepared. How many milliliters of purified water should be used to prepare, in each 5 mL of product, the correct dose of ampicillin for a 60-lb. child based on the dose of 8 mg/kg of body weight?

The dose of ampicillin may be determined by:

$$\frac{8 \text{ mg}}{2.2 \text{ lb.}} = \frac{x \text{ mg}}{60 \text{ lb.}}$$
$$x = 218 \text{ mg}$$

Then, the amount of ampicillin in the container is determined by:

$$\frac{250 \text{ mg}}{5 \text{ mL}} = \frac{x \text{ mg}}{150 \text{ mL}}$$
$$x = 7500 \text{ mg}$$

Thus, the amount of product that can be made from 7500 mg of drug such that each 5 mL contains 218 mg of drug may be found by:

$$\frac{218 \text{ mg}}{5 \text{ mL}} = \frac{7500 \text{ mg}}{x \text{ mL}}$$
$$x = 172 \text{ mL}$$

Finally, because the volume of powder occupies 39 mL (150 mL – 111 mL), the amount of water to add is determined by:

$$172 \text{ mL} - 39 \text{ mL} = 133 \text{ mL}, answer.$$

The label of a dry powder for constitution into pediatric drops states that when 12 mL of purified water are added to the powder, 15 mL of a pediatric suspension containing 50 mg of amoxicillin per milliliter results. How many milliliters of water should be added to prepare the dose of amoxicillin in each 10 drops if the dropper delivers 20 drops/mL, the child has a body surface area (BSA) of 0.4 m^2, and the dose of the drug is based on 50 mg/m^2 of BSA?

The dose of amoxicillin may be determined by:

$$\frac{50 \text{ mg}}{1 \text{ m}^2 \text{ BSA}} = \frac{x \text{ mg}}{0.4 \text{ m}^2 \text{ BSA}}$$
$$x = 20 \text{ mg}$$

The volume of product to contain the 20-mg dose is determined by:

$$\frac{10 \text{ drops}}{x \text{ mL}} = \frac{20 \text{ drops}}{1 \text{ mL}}$$
$$x = 0.5 \text{ mL}$$

The amount of amoxicillin in the package is determined by:

$$\frac{50 \text{ mg}}{1 \text{ mL}} = \frac{x \text{ mg}}{15 \text{ mL}}$$
$$x = 750 \text{ mg}$$

The amount of product of the desired dose that may be prepared is determined by:

$$\frac{750 \text{ mg}}{x \text{ mL}} = \frac{20 \text{ mg}}{0.5 \text{ mL}}$$
$$x = 18.75 \text{ mL}$$

Subtracting the volume accounted for by the dry powder (15 mL − 12 mL = 3 mL), the volume of water to add is determined by:

$$18.75 \text{ mL} - 3 \text{ mL} = 15.75 \text{ mL}, \textit{answer}.$$

CASE IN POINT 17.1[a] A pediatrician telephones a pharmacist asking that the concentration of an antibiotic suspension be changed. The pediatrician wants the child-patient to take 200 mg of amoxicillin per teaspoonful dose. The label for amoxicillin powder for oral suspension indicates that the addition of 68 mL of purified water will result in a final volume of 100 mL with a concentration of 250 mg amoxicillin per 5 mL of suspension.

How many milliliters of water should the pharmacist add to the amoxicillin powder to produce a concentration of 200 mg/teaspoonful?

---

[a]Problem courtesy of Flynn Warren, Bishop, GA.

Constitution of Dry Powders for Parenteral Solution

Some medications intended for injection are provided as dry powder in vials to be constituted with sterile water for injection or other designated solvent or diluent immediately before use. Generally, these medications are small-volume products intended for use by injection or as additives to large-volume parenterals.

In contrast to the dry powders intended for oral use after constitution, injectable products may contain only limited amounts of specified added ingredients to increase the stability and effectiveness of the drug (obviously, no colorants, flavorants, or sweeteners are added). So, in effect, the bulk volume of the dry contents of a vial is largely or entirely the medication.

If the quantity of the dry drug powder is small and does not contribute significantly to the final volume of the constituted solution, the volume of solvent used will approximate the final volume of solution. For example, if 1000 units of a certain antibiotic in dry form are to be dissolved, and if the powder does not account for any significant portion of the final volume, the addition of 5 mL of solvent will produce a solution containing 200 units/mL. If the dry powder, however, because of its bulk, contributes to the final volume of the constituted solution, the increase in volume produced by the drug must be considered, and this factor must then be used in calculating the amount of solvent needed to prepare a solution of a desired concentration. For example, the package directions for making injectable solutions of piperacillin sodium specify that 4 mL of sterile solvent should be added to 2 g of the dry powder to produce 5 mL of a solution that is to contain 400 mg/mL. The drug, in this case, accounts for 1 mL of the final volume.

Example Calculations for the Constitution of Dry Powders for Parenteral Use

When a vial containing 3.5 mg of a sterile powder of the monoclonal antibody bortezomib (VELCADE) is reconstituted with 3.5 mL of 0.9% sodium chloride injection, a drug concentration of 1 mg/mL results. Calculate the volume of injection occupied by the bortezomib powder.

1 mg/mL is equivalent to 3.5 mg/3.5 mL; thus, the volume occupied by bortezomib may be considered negligible, *answer.*

When a vial is reconstituted to a volume of 1.2 mL with sterile water for injection, the resulting solution contains 20 mg/mL of drug. Calculate the drug content of the vial.

$$\frac{20 \text{ mL}}{1 \text{ mL}} = \frac{x \text{ mL}}{1.2 \text{ mL}}; \ x = 24 \text{ mg, } answer.$$

Label instructions for the reconstitution of a 500-mg vial of ceftazidime for intramuscular injection (FORTAZ) call for the addition of 1.5 mL of diluent to prepare 1.8 mL of injection. Calculate (a) the volume occupied by the dry drug, (b) the concentration of ceftazidime in the injection, in mg/mL, and (c) the volume of injection to provide a dose of 250 mg of ceftazidime.

(a) 1.8 mL − 1.5 mL = 0.3 mL, volume of ceftazidime,
(b) 500 mg/1.8 mL = 277.8 mg/mL, and
(c) 250 mg × 1.8 mL/500 mg = 0.9 mL, *answers.*

Using a vial containing 200,000 units of penicillin G potassium, how many milliliters of solvent should be added to the dry powder in preparing a solution having a concentration of 25,000 units/mL?

$$\frac{25,000 \text{ (units)}}{200,000 \text{ (units)}} = \frac{1 \text{ (mL)}}{x \text{ (mL)}}$$
$$x = 8 \text{ mL, } answer.$$

Using a vial containing 200,000 units of penicillin G sodium and sodium chloride injection as the solvent, explain how you would obtain the penicillin G sodium needed in preparing the following prescription.

℞	Penicillin G Sodium	15,000 units per mL
	Sodium Chloride Injection ad	10 mL
	Sig. For IM Injection.	

15,000 units × 10 = 150,000 units of penicillin G sodium needed

Because the dry powder represents 200,000 units of penicillin G sodium or $\frac{4}{3}$ *times* the number of units desired, ¾ of the powder will contain the required number of units.

Step 1. Dissolve the dry powder in 4 mL of sodium chloride injection.
Step 2. Use 3 mL of the constituted solution, *answer.*

Or, solving by dimensional analysis:

$$10 \text{ mL} \times \frac{15,000 \text{ units}}{1 \text{ mL}} \times \frac{4 \text{ mL}}{200,000 \text{ units}} = 3 \text{ mL, } answer.$$

The package information enclosed with a vial containing 5,000,000 units of penicillin G potassium (buffered) specifies that when 23 mL of a sterile solvent are added to the dry powder, the resulting concentration is 200,000 units/mL. On the basis of this information, how many milliliters of sterile water for injection should be used in preparing the following solution?

℞   Penicillin G Potassium (buffered)   5,000,000 units
         Sterile Water for Injection   q.s.
         Make solution containing 500,000 units per mL
         Sig. One mL = 500,000 units of Penicillin G Potassium

The package information states that the constituted solution prepared by dissolving 5,000,000 units of the dry powder in 23 mL of sterile solvent has a final volume of 25 mL. The dry powder, then, accounts for 2 mL of this volume.

Step 1. The final volume of the prescription is determined as follows:

$$\frac{500,000 \text{ (units)}}{5,000,000 \text{ (units)}} = \frac{1 \text{ (mL)}}{x \text{ (mL)}}$$
$$x = 10 \text{ mL}$$

Step 2. 10 mL – 2 mL (dry powder accounts for this volume) = 8 mL, *answer*.

Piperacillin sodium is available in 2-g vials, and the dry powder accounts for 1 mL of the volume of the constituted solution. Using a 2-g vial of piperacillin sodium and sodium chloride injection as the solvent, explain how you could fill the following medication order.

Piperacillin Sodium   250 mg
Sodium Chloride Injection   ad   15 mL

Step 1. Dissolve the 2 g of dry powder in 9 mL of sodium chloride injection to prepare 10 mL of solution. Each milliliter will contain 200 mg of piperacillin sodium.
Step 2. Use 1.25 mL of the constituted solution and 13.75 mL of sodium chloride injection, *answer*.

CASE IN POINT 17.2 A hospital pharmacist received the following order for a patient[4]:

Medication Order: Staphcillin, 750 mg IV every 4 hours

The following product and procedures were followed:
   Product: 6-g vial Staphcillin
   Pharmacy Operations: Reconstitute vial with sterile water for injection to yield Staphcillin 500 mg/mL and further dilute in 100 mL of sodium chloride injection.
   Administer: 30-minute IV infusion.

(a) How many milliliters of solution from the reconstituted vial should be used per infusion?
(b) What should be the infusion rate in milliliters per hour?
(c) With a drop factor of 10 drops per milliliter, calculate the infusion rate in drops per minute.

Use of Prefabricated Dosage Forms in Compounding

Pharmacists frequently find that bulk supplies of certain proprietary drug substances are not available for extemporaneous compounding and that prefabricated tablets, capsules, injections, and other dosage forms provide the only available source of the medicinal agents needed.

When using commercially prepared dosage forms as the source of a medicinal agent, the pharmacist selects products that are of the most simple, economic, and convenient form. For example, uncoated tablets or capsules are preferred over coated tablets or sustained-release dosage forms. For both convenience and economy, use of the fewest dosage units is preferred; for example, five 100-mg tablets rather than one hundred 5-mg tablets. An injection often provides a convenient source of medicinal agent when the volume of injection required is small and it is compatible with the physical characteristics of the dosage form being prepared (e.g., an oral liquid rather than dry-filled capsules).

Occasionally, when of the prescribed strength, small whole tablets or broken *scored* (grooved) tablets, may be placed within capsule shells when capsules are prescribed. In most instances, however, tablets are crushed in a mortar and reduced to a powder. When capsules are used as the drug source, the capsule shells are opened and their powdered contents are expelled. The correct quantity of powder is then used to fill the prescription or medication order.

It is important to understand that in addition to the medicinal agent, most solid dosage forms contain additional materials, such as fillers, binders, and disintegrants. These ingredients may need to be considered in the required calculations. For example, a tablet labeled to contain 10 mg of a drug may actually weigh 200 mg or more because of the added ingredients. Calculations involved in the use of injections generally are simplified because injections are labeled according to quantity of drug per unit volume; for example, milligrams per milliliter (mg/mL).

A factor to consider when using manufacturer's dosage forms in compounding is the uncertainty of the *precise* content of active therapeutic agent.[5] This is because there are legally allowable variances which in some cases, may be 90% to 110% of labeled drug content. Thus, whenever possible, use of the bulk chemical in compounding procedure provides better assurance of drug content.

Example Calculations for the Use of Prefabricated Dosage Forms in Compounding

Only capsules, each containing 25 mg of indomethacin, are available. How many capsules should be used to obtain the amount of indomethacin needed in preparing the following prescription?

> ℞   Indomethacin   2 mg/mL
>   Cherry Syrup   ad   150 mL
>   Sig. 5 mL b.i.d.

Because 2 mg/mL of indomethacin are prescribed, 300 mg are needed in preparing the prescription. Given that each capsule contains 25 mg of indomethacin, then 300 (mg) ÷ 25 (mg) = 12 capsules are needed, *answer*.

The drug metoprolol tartrate (LOPRESSOR) is available as 50-mg tablets. Before preparing the following prescription, a pharmacist determined that each tablet weighed 120 mg. Explain how to obtain the proper quantity of LOPRESSOR.

> ℞   LOPRESSOR   15 mg
>   Lactose, qs   ad   300 mg
>   Prepare 24 such capsules.
>   Sig. One cap. 2× a day.

15 (mg) × 24 = 360 mg of LOPRESSOR needed
Crush 8 tablets, which contain:

400 mg (8 × 50 mg) of LOPRESSOR and
960 mg (8 × 120 mg) of total powder

$$\frac{400 \text{ mg LOPRESSOR}}{360 \text{ mg LOPRESSOR}} = \frac{960 \text{ mg total}}{x \text{ mg total}}$$

x = 864 mg quantity of powder to use, *answer.*

How many milliliters of an injection containing 40 mg of triamcinolone per milliliter may be used in preparing the following prescription?

> ℞   Triamcinolone   0.05%
>   Ointment Base   ad   120 g
>   Sig. Apply to affected area.

120 g × 0.0005 = 0.06 g = 60 mg triamcinolone needed

$$\frac{40 \text{ mg}}{60 \text{ mg}} = \frac{1 \text{ mL}}{x \text{ mL}}$$

x = 1.5 mL, *answer.*

A pharmacist receives the following prescription[a]:

> ℞   Diazepam   0.75 mg
>   Ft. charts #30

In filling the prescription, the pharmacist chooses to use 10-mg unscored diazepam tablets.

(a) How many tablets must be used?
(b) If the tablets in answer (a) are powdered and weigh a total of 345 mg, how many milligrams of the powder would provide the diazepam required?
(c) If the desired total weight for the contents of each divided powder is 250 mg, how much lactose should be used as diluent?

(a) 0.75 mg × 30 = 22.5 mg diazepam required.
   22.5 mg/10 mg per tablet = 2.25 tablets, so 3 tablets must be used,

(b) 345 mg × $\dfrac{2.25 \text{ tablets}}{3 \text{ tablets}}$ = 258.75 mg, and

(c) 250 mg × 30 mg = 7500 mg (total weight) − 258. 75 (tablet powder weight) = 7241.25 mg lactose, *answers.*

A pharmacist receives the following prescription[b]:

> ℞   Baby Stephanie Jones (22 lb)
>   Reserpine liquid: 0.1 mg/mL
>   Dispense: 60   mL
>   Sig: 0.01 mg/kg/b.i.d.

---

[a]Problem courtesy of Deborah Elder, Pharmaceutical and Biomedical Sciences, College of Pharmacy, The University of Georgia, Athens, GA.
[b]Problem courtesy of Flynn Warren, Bishop, GA.

In filling the prescription, the pharmacist chooses to use 0.25 mg reserpine tablets.

(a) How many reserpine tablets are required to compound the prescription?
(b) What volume of reserpine liquid will be required per dose?
(c) Using a calibrated dropper that delivers 12 drops/0.5 mL, how many drops would constitute a single dose?
(d) If the medication is taken as directed, how many days will the medication last?

(a) 0.1 mg/mL × 60 mL = 6 mg of reserpine required.
    6 mg/0.25 mg per tablet = 24 tablets,
(b) 22 1b/2.2 lb per kg = 10 kg
    0.01 mg/kg × 10 kg = 0.1 mg reserpine required

$$\frac{6 \text{ mg}}{60 \text{ mL}} = \frac{0.1 \text{ mg}}{\text{x mL}}; \text{ x} = 1 \text{ mL,}$$

(c) $\dfrac{12 \text{ drops}}{0.5 \text{ mL}} = \dfrac{\text{x drops}}{1 \text{ mL}}; \text{ x} = 24 \text{ drops, and}$

(d) 60 mL/2 mL per day = 30 days, *answers.*

CASE IN POINT 17.3 Following FDA-approved directions for the emergency compounding of an oral suspension from TAMIFLU (oseltamivir phosphate) capsules,[6] a pharmacist determined that

- the suspension should have a drug concentration of 15 mg/mL
- the volume to compound is based on the patient's weight, that is

  ≤33 lb = 30 mL
  33 to 51 lb = 40 mL
  51 to 88 lb = 50 mL
  >88 lb = 60 mL

- 75-mg TAMIFLU capsules are to be used.
- Cherry Syrup or Ora-Sweet SF may be used as the vehicle.
- Specific compounding procedures as outlined in the reference should be employed.[6]

(a) How many 75-mg TAMIFLU capsules should be used in compounding a suspension for a 30-kg patient?
(b) If the prophylactic dose for a 30-kg patient is listed as 60 mg once daily, how many milliliters of the compounded oral suspension would constitute a dose?

Special Calculations: Capsule Filling and Suppository Molding

Capsule Filling[7]

The extemporaneous filling of capsules enables the pharmacist to prepare patient-specific doses of drugs in a conveniently administrated form. Empty capsule shells, made of gelatin, are readily available in a variety of sizes, as shown in Figure 17.2, with size 000 being the largest and size 5 the smallest.

▼ FIGURE 17.2 Hard gelatin capsule sizes, from left to right: 000, 00, 0, 1, 2, 3, 4, and 5.

Filled capsules should be neither underfilled nor overfilled but should hold the ingredients snugly. Different drug powders have different densities, and thus different weights can be packed into a given size capsule (see Table 17.1). In filling a prescription or medication order, a pharmacist should select a capsule size that accommodates the fill and will be easy for the patient to swallow.

Most oral drugs have relatively small doses; thus, a diluent, like lactose, commonly is added to provide the necessary bulk to completely fill the prescribed capsules.

The steps used in calculating the proper capsule fill may be described as follows:

Step 1. Select an appropriate capsule size.
Step 2. Fill the capsule shell separately with each drug and diluent, and record the weights of each.
Step 3. Calculate the *diluent displacement weight* for each drug, as demonstrated in the following example problem.
Step 4. Calculate the amount of diluent required per capsule.
Step 5. Calculate the total quantities of each drug and the diluent needed to fill all of the capsules prescribed.

Note: Some pharmacists calculate for an extra capsule or two so as not to run short of fill due to any powder residue remaining in the mortar after the mixing process; this may not be done for "accountable" drugs, such as narcotics.

Table 17.1 ▼ **CAPSULE SIZES AND APPROXIMATE FILL CAPACITIES**

CAPSULE SIZE	APPROXIMATE VOLUME	APPROXIMATE POWDER WEIGHT
000	1.4 mL	430 mg–1.8 g
00	0.95 mL	390 mg–1.3 g
0	0.68 mL	325–900 mg
1	0.5 mL	227–650 mg
2	0.37 mL	200–520 mg
3	0.3 mL	120–390 mg
4	0.21 mL	100–260 mg
5	0.13 mL	65–130 mg

Example Calculation to Determine a Capsule Fill

Determine the total quantities of each drug and lactose required to fill the following prescription.

R̸   Drug A   20 mg
     Drug B   55 mg
     Lactose, q.s.
     M.ft. caps # 20

Step 1. For the purpose of this example, assume the pharmacist selected a size 1 capsule.
Step 2. The pharmacist filled a capsule individually with each ingredient, weighed them, and found:

     Capsule filled with drug A weighed   620 mg
     Capsule filled with drug B weighed   470 mg
     Capsule filled with lactose weighed   330 mg

Step 3. The *diluent displacement weights* for drugs A and B are calculated by ratio and proportion as follows:

For drug A:

$$\frac{620 \text{ mg (drug A in filled capsule)}}{330 \text{ mg (lactose in filled capsule)}} = \frac{20 \text{ mg (drug A per capsule)}}{x \text{ (lactose displacement)}}$$

x = 10.65 mg (diluent displacement by 20 mg of drug A)

For drug B:

$$\frac{470 \text{ mg}}{330 \text{ mg}} = \frac{55 \text{ mg}}{x}$$

x = 38.62 mg (diluent displacement by 55 mg of drug B)

Step 4. The diluent required per capsule:

330 mg − 49.27 mg (10.65 mg + 38.62 mg) = 280.73 mg lactose

Step 5. The total quantities of each drug and diluent needed to fill all the capsules prescribed:

Drug A = 20 mg × 20 (capsules) = 400 mg
Drug B = 55 mg × 20 (capsules) = 1100 mg
Lactose = 280.73 mg × 20 (capsules) = 5614.6 mg, *answers.*

Suppository Molding[7]

Pharmacists extemporaneously prepare suppositories by using a mold, such as that shown in Figure 17.3. The drug(s) prescribed and a suppository base are the components of any suppository.

As defined in Appendix B, *suppositories* are solid dosage forms intended for insertion into body orifices where they soften, melt, or dissolve, releasing their medications to the surrounding tissues. Any of a number of suppository bases can be used as vehicles for the medication; in extemporaneous compounding, cocoa butter (also termed theobroma oil) is commonly used. Cocoa butter is a solid at room temperature but melts at body temperatures.

▼ FIGURE 17.3 A partially opened 50-cell suppository mold. *(Courtesy of Chemical and Pharmaceutical Industry Co.)*

The calculations involved in preparing suppositories by molding are described by the following steps. Other methods are used and may be found in the cited reference.[8]

To calibrate the suppository mold:

Step 1. Fill all the cells of the suppository mold with melted base. After allowing time to cool and harden, extract the formed suppositories, weigh them, and determine the total and average suppository weights.

Step 2. Divide the total and average suppository weights by the density of the suppository base to determine the volume capacity of the suppository mold and the average volume of each cell.

To calculate and prepare medicated suppositories:

Step 1. Weigh the active ingredient for the preparation of a single suppository.

Step 2. Mix the single dose of active ingredient with a portion of melted base *insufficient* to fill one cell of the mold (based on information obtained by previously calibrating the mold).

Step 3. Pour the drug-base mixture into a cell, and add additional melted base to completely fill the cell.

Step 4. After the suppository cools and hardens, extract and weigh it.

Step 5. The weight of the base is determined by subtracting the amount of the drug from the weight of the molded suppository.

Step 6. The individual weights of the drug and base required to prepare the prescribed number of suppositories may then be determined by multiplying the amounts for a single suppository. The volume of base required may also be calculated, if desired, by the use of its known density.

Example Calculation to Prepare Suppositories by Molding

Calculate the quantities of drug A and cocoa butter needed to fill the following prescription.

R̸ Drug A   350 mg
 Cocoa Butter q.s.
 M. ft. rectal suppos. # 12

Step 1. 350 mg of drug A is weighed.

Step 2. Since a rectal suppository mold prepares suppositories weighing approximately 2 g, the amount of cocoa butter to use that would be *insufficient* to fill one cell may be estimated by:

2 g – 0.35 g (drug A) = 1.65 g (cocoa butter)

1.65 g ÷ 0.86 g/mL (density of cocoa butter) = 1.92 mL (approximate volume of melted cocoa butter, when added to drug A, to *completely* fill the cell)

By mixing the drug with 1 mL of melted cocoa butter, the pharmacist knows that this volume is *insufficient* to fill a cell.

Step 3. The mixture of 350 mg of drug A and 1 mL of melted cocoa butter is placed in a cell, and sufficient additional melted cocoa butter is used to completely fill the cell.

Step 4. The cooled and hardened suppository is extracted and is found to weigh 1.95 g.

Step 5. The weight of the cocoa butter in one suppository is calculated:

1.95 g – 0.35 g (drug A) = 1.6 g cocoa butter

Step 6. The total quantities of drug A and cocoa butter needed to fill the prescription are:

0.35 g × 12 (suppositories) = 4.2 g drug A

1.6 g × 12 (suppositories) = 19.2 g cocoa butter, *answers.*

Note: Some pharmacists calculate for an extra suppository or two so as not to run short of fill mixture. In filling the mold, each cell should be slightly overfilled to allow for contraction on cooling.

Compounding Specialized Formulas

Not all commercially available products are suitable for every patient. On occasion, a pharmacist must modify an existing product or prepare an original formulation to meet the requirements of a patient.

In their compounding practices, pharmacists may develop their own formulas, or they may refer to contemporary formulas developed and published by colleagues.[9] To facilitate the practice of compounding, some manufacturers make available resource materials, formulas, and a variety of compounding adjuncts, including ointment and suppository bases, oral suspending and syrup vehicles, rectal/vaginal vehicles, and other nonmedicated products to which medications may be added.[10]

The student should be aware that for each of the specialized formulas presented in this chapter, the reference given provides a step-by-step compounding process. Examples of methods of compounding are included with practice problems (59–63) at the end of this chapter for the purpose of demonstration.

Example Calculations of Specialized Formulas

Calculate the number of tablets containing the combination of spironolactone 25 mg and hydrochlorothiazide 25 mg that must be used to prepare the following formula using ORA-PLUS *as the oral suspending vehicle.*[11]

Spironolactone	*5 mg/mL*
Hydrochlorothiazide	*5 mg/mL*
ORA-PLUS ad	*120 mL*

Spironolactone/hydrochlorothiazide:

5 mg of each drug/mL × 120 mL = 600 mg of each drug

600 mg (of each drug) ÷ 25 mg (of each drug/tablet) = 24 tablets, *answer.*

Calculate the amount of FATTIBASE, a suppository base, required to prepare 200 suppositories from the following formula for one progesterone vaginal suppository.[12]

> Progesterone, micronized   25 mg
> Silica Gel, micronized   20 mg
> FATTIBASE ad   2 g

> 25 mg (progesterone) + 20 mg (silica gel) = 45 mg
> 2 g − 0.045 g = 1.955 g
> 1.955 g × 200 (suppositories) = 391 g FATTIBASE, *answer.*

CASE IN POINT 17.4[a] A pharmacist receives a telephone call from a pediatrician who has an 8.8-lb. 1-month-old patient with an acid reflux condition. The infant was started on ranitidine (ZANTAC) syrup, 15 mg/mL, at a dose of 10 mg/kg/day, and has shown improvement. However, because of the flavor (peppermint) and alcohol content (7.5%), the baby frequently rejects the medication.

The pharmacist suggests preparing a sugar-free and alcohol-free syrup/suspension with a fruity odor and taste. The physician agrees and prescribes ranitidine syrup/suspension, 60 mL, at a dose of 10 mg/kg/day, divided into two 0.5-mL doses.

The pharmacist uses finely crushed 75-mg ranitidine tablets as the source of the drug and ORA-SWEET SF as the vehicle.

How many 75-mg ranitidine tablets are required?

---
[a]Problem courtesy of Warren Beach, Department of Pharmaceutical and Biomedical Sciences, College of Pharmacy, The University of Georgia, Athens, GA.

PRACTICE PROBLEMS

Calculations for the Constitution of Dry Powders for Oral Administration

1. After constitution of a dry powder, each 5 mL of ampicillin for oral suspension contains 250 mg of ampicillin in package sizes to prepare 100 mL, 150 mL, or 200 mL of suspension. Which package size should be dispensed for a 20-kg child who is to take 50 mg/kg/day total, q.i.d. in equally divided and spaced doses for 10 days?

2. Manufacturer's directions call for the addition of 90 mL of water to constitute a 150-mL container of cefaclor to yield a strength of 250 mg of cefaclor per 5 mL. If 60 mL of water were mistakenly added in constituting the product, calculate the resultant milligrams of cefaclor per 5 mL.

3. The label on a bottle of dry powder mix for constitution states that when 128 mL of water are added, 150 mL of an oral suspension containing 250 mg of ampicillin in each 5 mL results.

   (a) How many milliliters of water should be added to the dry powder mix if a strength of 150 mg of ampicillin per 5 mL is desired?

   (b) If the dose of ampicillin is 5 mg/kg of body weight, how many milliliters of water should be added to the dry powder mix so that a child weighing 66 lb. would receive the proper dose in each 5 mL of the suspension?

4. Amoxicillin/clavulanate potassium (AUGMENTIN) powder for oral suspension is prepared prior to dispensing by adding 134 mL of purified water to the contents of the container to prepare 150 mL of suspension. If each teaspoonful of suspension contains 125 mg of amoxicillin and 31.25 mg of clavulanate potassium, how much of each of these agents is contained in the dry powder prior to reconstitution?

5. If, in the above problem, a pharmacist wished to use the dry product to prepare an oral suspension containing 200 mg of amoxicillin and 50 mg of clavulanate potassium/5 mL of suspension, how many milliliters of purified water should be used for reconstitution?

6. Clarithromycin for oral suspension is available in bottles containing dry granules intended for constitution with water to prepare a suspension. The package insert instructs a pharmacist to add 27 mL of water to prepare 50 mL of suspension for a clarithromycin concentration of 125 mg/5 mL. Calculate (a) the weight, in milligrams, of the dry clarithromycin in the product. If the pediatric dose is 7.5 mg/kg every 12 hours, calculate the dose, in milliliters, for (b) a child weighing 16.7 kg, and (c) another child weighing 55 lb.

Calculations Applied to Compounding for Parenteral Administration

7. A vial contains 5 g of a powdered drug for reconstitution prior to use in an infusion. The label states that when 9.6 mL of diluent are added, the solution which results contains a drug concentration of 500 mg/mL. A medication order calls for a drug concentration of 200 mg/mL. How many milliliters of diluent should be added to the vial?

8. A hospital pharmacist constitutes a vial containing 2 g of piperacillin sodium to 10 mL with sterile water for injection. This solution is then diluted by adding it to 100 mL of 5% dextrose injection for administration by infusion. What is the concentration, in milligrams per milliliter (mg/mL), of piperacillin sodium in the infusion solution?

9. A vial of cefazolin injection contains 1 g of drug. When 2.5 mL of diluent are added, 3 mL of injection are prepared. If 1.6 mL of the injection are diluted to 200 mL with sodium chloride injection, how many milliliters of the dilution should be administered daily to a child weighing 40 lb. if the daily dose is 25 mg/kg of body weight?

10.[7] Medication Order: Piperacillin, 1500 mg every 6 hours.
Product: 3-g vial, piperacillin.
Pharmacy operations: Reconstitute vial with 14 mL of sterile water for injection to prepare 15 mL of injection. Add portion required to 50 mL of sodium chloride injection.
Administer: 20-minute IV infusion.

(a) How many milliliters of solution from the reconstituted vial should be used?

(b) What should be the infusion rate in milliliters per hour?

(c) With a drop factor of 20 drops per milliliter, calculate the infusion rate in drops per minute.

11. A medication order calls for 400 mg of cefazolin sodium to be administered IM to a patient every 12 hours. Vials containing 500 mg, 1 g, and 10 g of cefazolin sodium are available. According to the manufacturer's directions, dilutions may be made as follows:

Vial Size	Solvent to Be Added	Final Volume
500 mg	2 mL	2.2 mL
1 g	2.5 mL	3 mL
10 g	45 mL	51 mL

Explain how the prescribed amount of cefazolin sodium could be obtained.

12. Using the vial sizes in Problem 11 as the source of cefazolin sodium, how many milliliters of the diluted 500-mg vial should be administered to a 40-lb. child who is to receive 8 mg of cefazolin sodium per kilogram of body weight?

13. Using cefazolin sodium injection in a concentration of 125 mg/mL, complete the following table representing a *Pediatric Dosage Guide:*

Weight		Dose (25 mg/kg/day divided into 3 doses)	
		approximate single	mL of dilution
lb.	kg	dose (mg/q8h)	(125 mg/mL) needed
10	4.5	37.5 or 38 mg	0.3 mL
20	_____	_____	_____
30	_____	_____	_____
40	_____	_____	_____
50	_____	_____	_____

14. A vial contains 1 g of ceftazidime. Express the concentrations of the drug, in milligrams per milliliter, following constitution with sterile water for injection to the following volumes: (a) 2.2 mL, (b) 4.5 mL, and (c) 10 mL.

15. Acetazolamide sodium is available in 500-mg vials to be constituted to 5 mL with sterile water for injection before use. The dose of the drug for children is 5 mg/kg of body weight. How many milliliters of the injection should be administered to a child weighing 25 lb.?

16. An intravenous infusion for a child weighing 60 lb. is to contain 20 mg of vancomycin hydrochloride per kilogram of body weight in 200 mL of sodium chloride injection. Using a 10-mL vial containing 500 mg of vancomycin hydrochloride (dry powder), explain how you would obtain the amount needed in preparing the infusion.

Calculations for the Use of Prefabricated Dosage Forms in Compounding

17. ℞ Potassium Perman-
        ganate Solution   500 mL
        1:10,000
        Sig. Use as directed.

Using tablets, each containing 0.3 g of potassium permanganate, explain how you would obtain the amount of potassium permanganate needed for the prescription.

18. ℞ Estropipate   0.0125% w/w
        Cream Base   ad 60 g
        Sig. Vaginal Cream.

How many 0.75-mg tablets of estropipate may be used to prepare the prescription?

19[a]. ℞ Testosterone   10 mg/0.25 mL
        Sucralose   0.15 g
        BHT   0.01 g
        Flavor   0.3 mL
        Almond oil, ad   30   mL

How many 30-mg tablets of testosterone are needed to fill the prescription?

20. ℞ Phenacaine Hydrochloride
        Solution 1%   7.5 mL
        Scopolamine Hydro-
          bromide Solution
          0.2%   7.5 mL
        Sig. For the eye.

How many tablets, each containing 600 μg of scopolamine hydrobromide, should be used in preparing the prescription?

21. ℞ Hexachlorophene
        Hydrocortisone aa   0.25%
        Coal Tar Solution   30 mL
        Hydrophilic Ointment
          ad   120 g
        Sig. Apply.

How many tablets, each containing 20 mg of hydrocortisone, should be used in preparing the prescription?

22. How many milliliters of an injection containing 40 mg of a drug per milliliter would provide the amount of the drug needed to prepare 120 mL of a 0.2% suspension?

23. ℞ Allopurinol   65 mg/5 mL
        Cologel   40 mL
        Syrup ad   150 mL
        M. ft. susp.
        Sig. As directed.

How many scored 100-mg allopurinol tablets may be used in preparing the prescription?

24. ℞ Enalapril   7.5 mg
        Lactose ad   200   mg
        DTD Caps # 40
        Sig. Take one capsule each
          morning.

How many 20-mg tablets of enalapril, each weighing 120 mg, and how many grams of lactose would be needed to prepare the prescription?

25. How many tablets for topical solution, each containing 300 mg of potassium permanganate, should be added to 1 gallon of purified water to provide a concentration of 0.012% w/v?

26. A prescription for 240 mL of a cough mixture calls for 2 mg of hydrocodone bitartrate per teaspoonful. How many tablets, each containing 5 mg of hydrocodone bitartrate, should be used in preparing the cough mixture?

27. ℞ Dantrolene Sodium   5 mg/mL
        Citric Acid   150 mg
        Purified Water   10 mL
        Syrup ad   125 mL
        M. ft. susp.
        Sig. As directed.

If the only source of dantrolene sodium is 100-mg capsules, each containing 200 mg of drug-diluent powder mix, (a) how many capsules must be opened, and (b) how many milligrams of the powder mix should be used in preparing the prescription?

28. ℞[13] Ketorolac Trome-
              thamine   7.5 mg/5 mL
           Suspension Vehicle
              ad   120 mL
           Sig. 1 tsp q6h

How many 10-mg ketorolac tromethamine (Toradol) tablets may be used to prepare this prescription?

---

[a]Problem courtesy of Deborah Elder, Department of Pharmaceutical and Biomedical Sciences, College of Pharmacy, The University of Georgia, Athens, GA.

29. How many DANTRIUM capsules, each containing 25 mg of dantrolene, are needed to prepare 100 mL of a pediatric suspension containing 5 mg of dantrolene per milliliter?

30. The following is a formula for a diazepam rectal gel.[14] How many 10-mL vials of VALIUM Injection containing 5 mg/mL of diazepam would be needed to compound the formula?

Diazepam	100 mg
Methylcellulose	
(1500 cps)	2.5 g
Methylparaben	100 mg
Glycerin	5 g
Purified Water ad	100 mL

31. How many tablets, each containing 25 mg of spironolactone, are needed to prepare 200 mL of a pediatric suspension to contain 5 mg of spironolactone per milliliter?

32. A physician prescribes 30 capsules, each containing 300 mg of ibuprofen, for a patient. The pharmacist has on hand 400-mg and 600-mg ibuprofen tablets. How many each of these tablets could be used to obtain the amount of ibuprofen needed in preparing the prescription?

33. ℞ Indomethacin Powder 1%
    Carbopol 941 Powder 2%
    Purified Water 10%
    Alcohol ad 90 mL
    Sig. Use as directed.

    How many 75-mg capsules of indomethacin should be used in preparing the prescription?

34. ℞ Minoxidil 0.3%
    Vehicle/N ad 50 mL
    Sig. Apply to affected areas of the scalp b.i.d.

    Tablets containing 2.5 mg and 10 mg of minoxidil are available. Explain how you would obtain the amount of minoxidil needed in preparing the prescription, using the available sources of the drug.

35. If a pharmacist used one 50-mg tablet of a drug to prepare 30 mL of an otic suspension in sweet oil, calculate the percentage strength of the preparation.

36. ℞ Aminophylline 500 mg
    Sodium Pentobarbital 75 mg
    Carbowax Base ad 2 g
    Ft. suppos. no. 12
    Sig. Insert one at night.

    How many capsules, each containing 100 mg of sodium pentobarbital, should be used to provide the sodium pentobarbital needed in preparing the prescription?

37. A starting pediatric dose of phenytoin sodium (DILANTIN Sodium) is 6 mg/kg/d, administered in three equally divided doses. Using tablets containing 50 mg of phenytoin sodium, a pharmacist prepared a suspension such that each 1 mL, delivered from a calibrated dropper, contained a single dose for a 44-lb. child. How many tablets should be used to prepare 30 mL of the suspension?

38. ℞ CARAFATE 400 mg/5 mL
    Cherry Syrup 40 mL
    Sorbitol Solution 40 mL
    Flavor q.s.
    Purified Water ad 125 mL
    Sig. 5 mL t.i.d.

    How many 1-g CARAFATE tablets should be used in preparing the prescription?

Calculations Used in Capsule Filling and Suppository Molding

39.[7] A pharmacist needs to prepare 50 capsules, each containing 4 mg of estriol and 1 mg of estradiol. A size 3 capsule is selected for use. Capsule shells are individually filled with each drug and lactose and the weights recorded as follows:

Estriol	250 mg
Estradiol	190 mg
Lactose	320 mg

(a) How many milligrams of each component will be needed to fill all the capsules?

(b) How many milligrams should the content of each capsule weigh?

40.[7] A pharmacist prepares six suppositories using a polyethylene glycol base, density 1.18 g/mL. The total weight of the suppositories is found to be 13.81 g. Calculate the volume of the mold per cell.

41.[7,15] ℞ Fluconazole   200 mg
        PEG base, q.s.
        M. ft. suppos # 20

(a) How many grams of fluconazole are needed?

(b) If a trial molded suppository weighs 2.4 g, how many grams of PEG base are needed to compound the prescription?

Calculations of Specialized Formulas

42. The following is a formula for an oral ulceration mouthwash.[16]

Hydrocortisone	55.2 mg
Lidocaine HCl	2.4 g
Erythromycin Stearate	1.5 g
Diphenhydramine HCl	150 mg
Nystatin	2,000,000 units
Xanthan Gum	240 mg
Stevia Powder Extract	280 mg
Sodium Saccharin	120 mg
Flavor	1 mL
Simple Syrup or Sorbitol Solution (70%) ad	120 mL

(a) Calculate the percentage strength of hydrocortisone in the formula.

(b) If nystatin is available as a powder containing 5225 units/mg, calculate the quantity required, in milligrams, to compound the formula.

(c) Calculate the concentration of erythromycin stearate, in mg/mL, in the formula.

43. Misoprostol and Lidocaine in Glycerin Mouth Paint[17]

Misoprostol 200-mcg tablets	12 tablets
Lidocaine HCl	1 g
Glycerin qs ad	100 mL

How many micrograms of misoprostol would be present in each milliliter of mouth paint?

44. Progesterone Liquid Fill Capsules.[18]

Progesterone, micronized	10 g
Sesame Oil qs ad	30 mL
To make 100 capsules	

How many (a) micrograms of progesterone and (b) microliters of the formula would be contained in each capsule?

45. Tri-Est Aqueous Injection[19]

Estriol	200	mg
Estrone	25	mg
Estradiol	25	mg
Polysorbate 80	0.2	mL
Benzyl Alcohol	1	mL
Sterile Water for Injection ad	100	mL

How many milliliters of the injection should be used to deliver 1.75 mg of total estrogens?

46. Intracavernosal Injection[20]

Prostaglandin E	5.9 μg/mL
Papaverine HCl	17.6 mg/mL
Phentolamine Mesylate	0.6 mg/mL
Sterile Water for Injection ad	1.5 mL

How many milligrams of each ingredient should be used in preparing 12 syringes, each containing 1.5 mL of injection?

47. Progesterone Nasal Spray[21]

Progesterone	20 mg
Dimethyl-β-cyclodextrin	62 mg
Purified Water ad	1 mL

How many milligrams each of progesterone and dimethyl-β-cyclodextrin would be delivered in each 0.05 mL spray of solution?

48. Triple Estrogen Slow-Release Capsules[22]

    For 100 capsules:

Estriol	200	mg
Estrone	25	mg
Estradiol	25	mg
Methocel E4M premium	10	g
Lactose	23.75 g	

    Calculate the weight, in milligrams, of the formula in each capsule.

49. Nail Fungus Solution[23]

NIZORAL, 200-mg tablets	10 tablets
Clotrimazole	900 mg
Ethyl Alcohol, 95%	5 mL
Polyethylene Glycol 300	67 mL
Dimethyl Sulfoxide	23 mL

    If the formula prepares 98 mL, what is the percent concentration of NIZORAL in the solution?

50.[a] ℞

Menthol	2	% w/w
Camphor	1	% w/w
Urea	10	% w/w
Potassium Sorbate	0.1%	w/w
Absorbent ointment base, ad	30	g

    If a 1% w/v potassium sorbate solution (sp. gr. 0.96) is used as the source of potassium sorbate, how many grams of the absorbent ointment base are required to fill the prescription?

51.[a] A pharmacist compounds 45 g of a transdermal gel to contain 50 mg/g of promethazine hydrochloride. The promethazine hydrochloride is dissolved in a sufficient quantity of 20% Pluronic F-127 in water, representing 80% w/w of the gel (aqueous phase), with the remainder being lecithin-isopropyl palmitate (oil phase). How many grams of each of the three ingredients are required?

52. Migraine Headache Suppositories[28]

Ergotamine Tartrate	2	mg
Caffeine	100	mg
Hyoscyamine Sulfate	0.25 mg	
Pentobarbital Sodium	60	mg
FATTIBASE ad	2	g

    The formula is for one suppository. If the specific gravity of FATTIBASE is 0.89, how many milliliters of the melted base (assuming no volume change due to heat) may be used to prepare 36 suppositories?

53. Veterinary Dexamethasone Ophthalmic Ointment[25]

Dexamethasone Sodium Phosphate	39.6 mg
Bacteriostatic Water for Injection	0.4 mL
Polysorbate 80	0.3 mL
Lacri-Lube qs	30 g

    Calculate the percentage strength of dexamethasone (base) in the formula if 1 mg of dexamethasone (base) is equivalent to 1.32 mg of dexamethasone sodium phosphate.

54. The following is a formula for a captopril oral liquid.[10]

    ℞
Captopril	100-mg tablet
ORA-SWEET ad	134 mL

    How many milliliters of the oral liquid would provide 0.75 mg of captopril?

55. The following is a formula for a rifampin oral liquid.[10]

    ℞
Rifampin	25 mg/mL
ORA-PLUS ad	120 mL

    How many 300-mg tablets of rifampin should be used?

---

[a] Problem courtesy of Deborah Elder, Department of Pharmaceutical and Biomedical Sciences, College of Pharmacy, The University of Georgia, Athens, GA.

56. The following is a formula for fluco-
    nazole topical cream.[10]

    ℞ Fluconazole   10   g
       Glycerin   18.75 g
       DERMABASE ad   100 g

    How many milliliters of glycerin
    should be used (sp. gr. 1.25)?

57. The following is a formula for a
    clotrimazole topical preparation.[10]

    ℞ Clotrimazole, powder   1%
       DERMABASE ad   30 g

    How many grams of DERMABASE
    are required?

58.[a] A pharmacist receives a prescription
    for 45 mL of a 50% castor oil emul-
    sion. A mixture of two emulsifying
    agents is used, 5.4 parts of Tween
    80 and 1 part of Span 20. If a total
    of 5% emulsifying agents is used in
    compounding the prescription, how
    many grams each of Tween 80 and
    Span 20 are used?

Miscellaneous Compounding Calculations with Methods of Preparation[b]

59.[26] Fluconazole 2% Topical
    Microemulsion

Fluconazole	2 g
Lauryl Alcohol	10 g
Labrasobalcohol (50%)	20 g
Purified Water qs, ad	100 mL

    Method of Preparation:

    1. *Calculate the required quantity of
       each ingredient for the total amount
       to be prepared.*
    2. *Weigh and/or measure each ingre-
       dient accurately.*
    3. *Mix the lauryl alcohol with the labra-
       sobalcohol mixture until uniform.*
    4. *Incorporate the fluconazole slowly
       and mix well.*
    5. *Incorporate sufficient purified water
       slowly and with continuous stirring
       to volume and mix well.*

Calculate:

(a) Lauryl alcohol has a specific gravity
    of 0.83. Calculate the milliliters of
    lauryl alcohol used in the formula.
(b) Lauryl alcohol dissolves about
    14.25 mg of fluconazole per mil-
    liliter. Calculate the fluconazole
    to lauryl alcohol ratio (mg/mL) in
    the formula.
(c) Based on (b), would fluconazole
    be in suspension or solution?

60.[27] Rufinamide 40-mg/mL Oral
    Suspension

Rufinamide	4 g
Ora-Plus	50 mL
Ora Sweet, ad	100 mL

    Method of Preparation:

    1. *Calculate the required quantity of
       each ingredient for the total amount
       to be prepared.*
    2. *Weigh and/or measure each ingre-
       dient accurately.*
    3. *Pulverize the required number of
       rufinamide tablets to a fine powder.*
    4. *Add about 25 mL of Ora-Plus
       (suspending agent) and mix to form
       a smooth paste.*
    5. *Add the remainder of the Ora-Plus
       and mix well.*
    6. *Add sufficient Ora-Sweet (flavoring
       vehicle) to final volume and mix well.*

Calculate:

(a) How many 200-mg rufinamide
    tablets would be required to
    compound the formula?
(b) If treatment with rufinamide is
    initiated for a 55-lb child at a
    daily dose of 10 mg/kg/day and
    increased by 10 mg/kg/day on
    the third day, how many millili-
    ters of the formula would remain
    after the first week of treatment if
    100 mL were dispensed?

---

[a]Problem courtesy of Deborah Elder, Department of Pharmaceutical and Biomedical Sciences, College of Pharmacy, The University of Georgia, Athens, GA.

[b]Formulas and methods of preparation reproduced with permission of Loyd V. Allen Jr, Editor- in-Chief, *International Journal of Pharmaceutical Compounding*. Edmond, OK.

61.[28] Topiramate 6-mL/mL Oral Suspension

Topiramate	600 mg
Ora-Plus	50 mL
Ora-Sweet, ad	100 mL

Method of Preparation:

1. *Calculate the required quantity of each ingredient for the total amount to be prepared.*
2. *Weigh and/or measure each ingredient accurately.*
3. *Obtain the topiramate as the 100-mg tablets and pulverize to a fine powder.*
4. *Incorporate the Ora-Plus (suspending agent) slowly and mix until uniform and smooth.*
5. *Incorporate sufficient Ora-Sweet (flavoring vehicle) slowly to volume and mix well.*

Calculate:

(a) Calculate the number of topiramate tablets needed to prepare the formula.
(b) For adult prophylaxis of migraine headache, the dose is gradually increased from 25 mg/day during week 1, to 25 mg twice a day during week 2, to 25 mg in the AM and 50 in the PM each day during the third week. How many milliliters of the formula would be required for the first 3 weeks of treatment?

62.[29] Acyclovir 200-mg/5-mL oral suspension (from the injection)

Acyclovir sodium	4 g
Ora-Plus	50 mL
Ora-Sweet, ad	100 mL

Method of Preparation:

1. *Calculate the required quantity of each ingredient for the total amount to be prepared.*
2. *Weigh and/or measure each ingredient accurately.*
3. *Reconstitute the acyclovir sodium vial with the smallest quantity of purified water required to allow withdrawal from the vial. Note: It does not have to all be in solution.*
4. *Place in a suitable calibrated container.*
5. *Add the Ora-Plus geometrically and mix well.*
6. *Add sufficient Ora-Sweet to volume and mix well.*

Calculate:

(a) Acyclovir sodium is available as a sterile lyophilized powder for reconstitution with sterile water for injection in vials containing 1000 mg of acyclovir. If a pharmacist used 6 mL of diluent to prepare 7 mL of injection from each vial required, how many milliliters of Ora-Sweet would be needed to compound the formula?
(b) If the dose prescribed for a 60-lb child for the treatment of chickenpox was 20 mg/kg per dose orally, four times daily for 5 days, what volume of formula would be needed?

63.[30] Dexpanthenol 5% Gel-Cream

Dexpanthenol	5 g
Mineral oil, light	10 mL
Polyethylene glycol 400	15 mL
Pluronic F-127	20 g
Purified water, ad	100 g

Method of Preparation:

1. *Calculate the required quantity of each ingredient for the total amount to be prepared.*
2. *Weigh and/or measure each ingredient accurately.*
3. *Dissolve the dexpanthenol and PEG 400 in about 50 mL of purified water.*
4. *Add the mineral oil and stir, heating to 60 to 70°C.*
5. *Incorporate the Pluronic F-127 slowly and stir until dissolved.*
6. *Cool to room temperature.*
7. *Add sufficient purified water to final weight and mix well.*

Calculate:

(a) If the mineral oil has a specific gravity of 0.82 and the polyethylene glycol has a specific gravity of 1.14, what would be the expected weight of the mixture in above-steps 3 and 4?

(b) How many milliliters of purified water are needed to compound the formula?

CALCQUIZ

17.A. Due to incompletely developed renal function in neonates and infants less than 3 months old, which affects the elimination of amoxicillin, the upper dose is considered 30 mg/kg/day, divided and administered every 12 hours. A pharmacist receives a medication order for a 12-week-old infant weighing 15 lb with a mild upper respiratory infection. A bottle of amoxicillin pediatric drops is prescribed. When this is reconstituted with the addition of 23 mL of water, a 30-mL suspension of amoxicillin, 50 mg/mL, is prepared. Calculate (a) the volume occupied by the dry amoxicillin content, (b) the daily dose of amoxicillin for the infant at 20 mg/kg/day in two divided doses, (c) the daily dose of suspension required, and (d) the single dose, in drops, using a calibrated dropper delivering 20 drops/mL.

17.B. A package contains 1250 mg of the antibiotic clarithromycin. When reconstituted with 27 mL of water, 50 mL of oral suspension may be prepared. The pediatric dose for a 20-lb child is determined to be 62.5 mg. How many milliliters of water should be used to reconstitute the antibiotic such that the dose may be administered by 5 mL of oral suspension?

17.C. A vial contains 1 g of capreomycin in a 10-mL vial for reconstitution prior to injection. According to the package insert, when 2.15 mL of diluent is added, 2.85 mL of injection is prepared and when 3.3 mL of diluent is added, 4 mL of injection is prepared. How many milliliters of diluent should be added to prepare an injection containing capreomycin, 300 mg/mL?

17.D. An injection of epoprostenol sodium (FLOLAN) is prepared by dissolving the contents of one 0.5 mg vial with 5 mL of the copackaged sterile diluent. Then, prior to intravenous infusion, 3 mL is withdrawn from the vial to prepare 100 mL of injection. Calculate (a) the concentration of epoprostenol sodium in ng/mL in the injection and (b) if the injection is to infused at a rate of 8 ng/kg/min, calculate the infusion delivery rate in mL/h for a patient weighing 176 lb.

17.E.[a] A compounding pharmacist receives a prescription for 14 medicated chewable gummy bears for a pediatric patient. Each gummy bear is to contain 10 mg of hydroxyzine. The pharmacist decides to use three 50-mg capsules of hydroxyzine as the drug source and determines their combined contents to weigh 625 mg. If each cell of the gummy bear mold holds a calibrated 1.56 g, and if the gummy gel base has the following general formula,[31] how much of each ingredient is required to fill the prescription?

Gelatin	43.4 g
Glycerin	155 mL (sp. gr. 1.25)
Purified water	21.6 mL

[a]Problem courtesy of Deborah Elder, Department of Pharmaceutical and Biomedical Sciences, College of Pharmacy, The University of Georgia, Athens, GA.

ANSWERS TO "CASE IN POINT" AND PRACTICE PROBLEMS

Case in Point 17.1

Calculate the amount of amoxicillin in container:

$$\frac{250 \text{ mg (amoxicillin)}}{5 \text{ mL}} = \frac{x \text{ mg (amoxicillin)}}{100 \text{ mL}}$$

x = 5000 mg amoxicillin in container

Calculate volume that can be prepared from 5000 mg at 200 mg/5 mL:

$$\frac{200 \text{ mg}}{5 \text{ mL}} = \frac{5000 \text{ mg}}{x \text{ ml}};$$

x = 125 mL of oral suspension can be prepared

Calculate volume of amoxicillin powder in container:

100 mL − 68 mL (water added by label instructions) = 32 mL (volume of powder)

Calculate water requirement for new concentration:

125 mL − 32 mL = 93 mL of water required, *answer.*

Proof: 5000 mg amoxicillin per 125 mL = 200 mg amoxicillin per 5 mL

Case in Point 17.2

(a) $750 \text{ mg} \times \dfrac{1 \text{ mL}}{500 \text{ mL}} = 1.5 \text{ mL}$ of reconstituted solution, *answer.*

(b) Infusion time: 30 minutes
Infusion volume: 101.5 mL
Infusion rate per hour:

$$60 \text{ min} \frac{101.5 \text{ mL}}{30 \text{ min}} = 203 \text{ mL, infusion}$$

rate per hour, *answer.*

(c) 101.5 mL (infusion volume)

$$\times \frac{10 \text{ drops}}{1 \text{ mL}} = 1015 \text{ drops}$$

$$\frac{1015 \text{ drops}}{30 \text{ min}} = 33.8 \text{ or } 34 \text{ drops per}$$

minute, *answer.*

Case in Point 17.3

(a) A 30-kg patient weighs 66 lb (30 kg × 2.2 lb/kg)

According to the guideline, a 66-lb patient should receive 50 mL of oral suspension.

According to the specification, the oral suspension should have a drug concentration of 15 mg/mL.

15 mg/mL × 50 mL (oral suspension) = 750 mg TAMIFLU needed.

750 mg/75 mg per capsule = 10 TAMIFLU capsules required, *answer.*

(b) 60 mg (dose)/15 mg per mL = 4 mL daily dose, *answer.*

Case in Point 17.4

Calculate milligrams of ranitidine required per 0.5-mL dose:

$$\frac{8.8 \text{ lb.}}{2.2 \text{ lb./kg}} = 4 \text{ kg (weight of child)}$$

4 kg × 10 mg/kg/day = 40 mg/day

40 mg ÷ 2 doses/day = 20 mg/dose; thus, 20 mg/0.5-mL dose

Calculate milligrams of ranitidine required in 60-mL prescription:

$$\frac{20 \text{ mg}}{0.5 \text{ mL}} = \frac{x \text{ mg}}{60 \text{ mL}};$$

x = 2400 mg ranitidine required

Calculate number of 75-mg ranitidine tablets needed to provide 2400 mg

2400 mg ÷ 75 mg/tablet = 32 tablets, *answer.*

Practice Problems

1. 200 mL
2. 312.5 mg cefaclor
3. (a) 228 mL water
   (b) 228 mL water
4. 3750 mg amoxicillin
   937.3 mg clavulanate potassium
5. 77.75 mL purified water

6. (a) 1.25 g clarithromycin
   (b) 5-mL dose
   (c) 7.5-mL dose

7. 24.6-mL diluent

8. 18.18 mg/mL piperacillin

9. 170.5 mL

10. (a) 7.5 mL
    (b) 172.5 mL/h
    (c) 57.5 or 58 drops/min

11. Dilute and use 1.767 mL of the 500-mg vial, or
    dilute and use 1.2 mL of the 1-g vial, or
    dilute and use 2.04 or 2 mL of the 10-g vial

12. 0.64 mL

13.
20	9.1 kg	75.8 mg	0.61 mL
30	13.6 kg	113.3 mg	0.91 mL
40	18.2 kg	151.7 mg	1.21 mL
50	22.7 kg	189.2 mg	1.51 mL

14. (a) 454.55 mg/mL
    (b) 222.22 mg/mL
    (c) 100   mg/mL

15. 0.57 mL acetazolamide sodium injection

16. 545 mg needed. Use 1 vial + 10 mL of sterile diluent to a second vial to make 10 mL, and use 0.9 mL of the dilution.

17. Dissolve 1 tablet in enough distilled water to make 60 mL, and take 10 mL of the dilution.

18. 10 tablets estropipate

19. 40 tablets testosterone

20. 25 tablets scopolamine hydrobromide

21. 15 tablets hydrocortisone

22. 6-mL injection

23. 19.5 tablets allopurinol

24. 15 tablets enalapril
    6.2 g lactose

25. 1.5 tablets potassium permanganate

26. 19.2 tablets hydrocodone bitartrate

27. (a) 7 capsules dantrolene sodium
    (b) 1250 mg powder

28. 18 tablets Toradol

29. 20 capsules DANTRIUM

30. 2 vials VALIUM Injection

31. 40 tablets spironolactone

32. 22.5 tablets (400 mg each) ibuprofen, or 15 tablets (600 mg each) ibuprofen

33. 12 capsules indomethacin

34. 60 tablets (2.5 mg each) minoxidil, or 15 tablets (10 mg each) minoxidil

35. 0.167%

36. 9 capsules sodium pentobarbital

37. 24 tablets phenytoin sodium

38. 10 tablets CARAFATE

39. (a) 200 mg estriol
       50 mg estradiol
       15,660 mg lactose
    (b) 318.2 mg

40. 1.95 mL

41. (a) 4 g fluconazole
    (b) 44 g PEG base

42. (a) 0.046% hydrocortisone
    (b) 382.78 mg nystatin
    (c) 12.5 mg/mL erythromycin stearate

43. 24 μg misoprostol

44. (a) 100,000 μg progesterone
    (b) 300 μL

45. 0.7 mL injection

46. 0.106 mg prostaglandin E
    316.8 mg papaverine HCl
    10.8 mg phentolamine mesylate

47. 1 mg progesterone
    3.1 mg dimethyl-β-cyclodextrin

48. 340 mg

49. 2.04% NIZORAL

50. 23.22 g absorbent ointment base

51. 2.25 g promethazine hydrochloride
    33.75 g Pluronic F-127 in water (20%)
    9 g lecithin-isopropyl palmitate

52. 74.34 mL FATTIBASE

53. 0.1% dexamethasone

54. 1 mL oral liquid

55. 10 tablets rifampin

56. 15 mL glycerin

57. 29.7 g DERMABASE

58. 1.89 or 1.9 g Tween 80
    0.35 g Span 20

59. (a) 12.05 mL lauryl alcohol
    (b) 165.9 mg/mL fluconazole/lauryl
        alcohol
    (c) suspension

60. (a) Twenty 200-mg rufinamide tablets
    (b) 25 mL

61. (a) Six 100-mg topiramate tablets
    (b) 175 mL

62. (a) 22 mL Ora-Sweet
    (b) 272.73 mL

63. (a) 30.3 g
    (b) 49.7 mL purified water

References

1. Pharmacy Compounding Accreditation Board. Available at: http://pcab.org. Accessed August 3, 2011.
2. International Academy of Compounding Pharmacists. Available at: http://www.iacprx.org. Accessed August 3, 2011.
3. United States Pharmacopeia 32—National Formulary 27, Rockville, MD: United States Pharmacopeial Convention, Inc. 2009.
4. Craig GP. *Clinical Calculations Made Easy.* Baltimore, MD: Lippincott Williams & Wilkins, 2001:196.
5. Allen LV Jr, Editor-in-Chief. Compounding with manufactured products. *International Journal of Pharmaceutical Compounding* 2010;14:448.
6. Directions for the emergency compounding of an oral suspension from TAMIFLU capsules. Available at: http://www.tamiflu.com/hcp/prescribing/hcp prescribe mix.jsp. Accessed August 5, 2011.
7. Prince SJ, Ansel HC, Prince SJ. *Pharmaceutical Calculations: The Pharmacist's Handbook.* Baltimore, MD: Lippincott Williams & Wilkins, 2004:96–105.
8. Allen LV Jr, Popovich NG, Ansel HC. *Pharmaceutical Dosage Forms and Drug Delivery Systems.* 9th Ed. Baltimore, MD: Lippincott Williams & Wilkins, 2010:320–322.
9. Allen LV Jr. *Allen's Compounded Formulations.* 2nd Ed. Washington, DC: American Pharmacist's Association, 2004.
10. Paddock Laboratories. Compounding. Available at: http://www.paddocklabs.com. Accessed August 8, 2011.
11. Anon. *International Journal of Pharmaceutical Compounding* 1997;1:183.
12. Anon. *International Journal of Pharmaceutical Compounding* 1998;2:65.
13. Prince SJ. Calculations. *International Journal of Pharmaceutical Compounding* 1998;2:164.
14. Allen LV Jr. Diazepam dosed as a rectal gel. *US Pharmacist* 2000;25:98.
15. Allen LV Jr. *The Art, Science, and Technology of Pharmaceutical Compounding.* Washington, DC: American Pharmacist's Association, 1997:140.
16. Allen LV Jr. Oral ulceration mouthwash. *International Journal of Pharmaceutical Compounding* 1999;3:10.
17. Ford PR. Misoprostol 0.0024% and lidocaine 1% in glycerin mouth paint. *International Journal of Pharmaceutical Compounding* 1999;3:48.
18. Allen LV Jr. Progesterone liquid fill capsules. *International Journal of Pharmaceutical Compounding* 1999;3:294.
19. Allen LV Jr. Tri-est 2.5 mg/mL aqueous injection. *International Journal of Pharmaceutical Compounding* 1999;3:304.
20. Preckshot J. Medication combinations for penile injections. *International Journal of Pharmaceutical Compounding* 1999;3:81.
21. Allen LV Jr. Progesterone nasal spray (2%). *International Journal of Pharmaceutical Compounding* 1998;2:56.
22. Allen JV Jr. triple estrogen 2.5 mg slow-release capsules. *International Journal of Pharmaceutical Compounding* 1998;2:56.
23. Nelson JL. Nail fungus solution. *International Journal of Pharmaceutical Compounding* 1998;2:277.

24. Allen LV Jr. Ergotamine tartrate, caffeine, hyoscyamine sulfate and pentobarbital sodium suppositories. *International Journal of Pharmaceutical Compounding* 1998;2:151.

25. Allen LV Jr. Veterinary dexamethasone ophthalmic ointment. *International Journal of Pharmaceutical Compounding* 1998;2:206.

26. Anon. Fluconazole 2% topical microemulsion. *International Journal of Pharmaceutical Compounding* 2009;13:555.

27. Anon. Rufinamide 40-mg/mL oral suspension. *International Journal of Pharmaceutical Compounding* 2010;14:426.

28. Anon. Topiramate 6-mg/mL oral suspension. *International Journal of Pharmaceutical Compounding* 2009;13:560.

29. Anon. Acyclovir 200 mg/5-mL oral suspension (from the injection). *International Journal of Pharmaceutical Compounding* 2010;14:151.

30. Anon. Dexpanthenol 5% gel-cream. *International Journal of Pharmaceutical Compounding* 2010;14:155.

31. Anon. Pediatric chewable gummy gel base. *International Journal of Pharmaceutical Compounding* 1997;1:106.

Selected Calculations Involving Veterinary Pharmaceuticals

18

Objectives

Upon successful completion of this chapter, the student will be able to:

• Calculate doses applicable to pharmaceuticals used in veterinary medicine.
• Calculate doses for cats and dogs based on weight conversion to body surface area.
• Apply relevant calculations to the compounding of veterinary pharmaceuticals.

Veterinary medicine, like human medicine, uses pharmaceuticals of various dosage forms and strengths in the diagnosis, prevention, treatment, and cure of disease and illness. Animals suffer from many of the same diseases and illnesses affecting humans, such as anemias, cardiovascular disease, infectious disease, and cancer.[1-2] Thus, many of the medications used in human medicine also apply in veterinary medicine. In addition, however, there are diseases that are specific to various animal species that require medications developed expressly for veterinary use.

Diseases that are unique to a specific species of animal require medications developed for that purpose. Veterinary drugs gain approval for specific uses in an intended animal species through the Center for Veterinary Medicine (CVM) of the Food and Drug Administration (FDA).[3-4] In addition to the use of veterinary drugs for FDA-approved uses, veterinarians also are permitted to prescribe both human- and animal-approved drugs for *extralabel* uses in animals—that is, for uses *not* specified in the approved labeling, so long as the drug is used within the context of a "veterinarian-client-patient relationship."[5-6] This permits greater flexibility for using a wide range of approved drugs in animal care.

The dosage forms used in veterinary medicine are like those used in human medicine—for example, tablets (as chewable tablets), capsules, oral liquids, injections, eye drops, and topical applications. However, specialized drug delivery devices commonly are used to administer the dosage forms. This includes esophageal syringes, drench guns, and oral tubes designed to deliver medication directly into an animal's stomach; pole-mounted syringes and projectile delivery systems, which allow injections to be administered from a safe distance; mastitis syringes, for inserting a drug formulation directly into the mammary gland; and others.[7]

The most obvious and striking difference between veterinary medicine and human medicine is the nature of the patient. Whereas humans *do* differ from one another in many respects, the differences are relatively minor compared with the wide-ranging differences among veterinary patients.

The various species of animals differ quite dramatically in size, structure, physical appearance, physiologic and biochemical characteristics, and in many other respects, including intelligence, temperament, and natural habitat.[8-10] There are at least 24,000 species of fish, 9,000 species of birds, 4,000 kinds of mammals, and 40,000 species of vertebrates.[10] Thus, the range of veterinary patient varies widely from birds, fish, and small domestic pets to various farm animals, the thoroughbred horse, and the exotic animal species of the jungle or zoological park.

Today's veterinarian specializes not only in small- and large-animal medicine, but also in various subspecialties, such as avian medicine, wildlife disease, *zoonoses* (animal diseases that can be transmitted to humans), and others. Community pharmacists, as well as those who practice in veterinary clinics and hospitals, fill the prescription orders of veterinarians.

Of special importance in animal medicine is the calculation of dosage based on an animal's weight, since this is such an important variable among animals. Consider this contrast: a pet cockatiel may weigh less than 100 grams, a kitten several pounds, a race horse 1,000 pounds, and an elephant 12,000 pounds or more. Even among pet dogs, the range is dramatic, from the small "toy" dogs—the Chihuahua that may weigh 2 pounds—to one of the heaviest dogs, the Saint Bernard that may weigh up to 180 pounds. In some instances, an animal's body surface area (BSA) is the factor used in determining drug dosage (Table 18.1). Species

Table 18.1 ▼ WEIGHT TO BODY SURFACE AREA CONVERSION FOR DOGS AND CATS

BODY SURFACE AREA (BSA) IN SQUARE METERS = K × (BODY WT IN GRAMS$^{2/3}$) × 10^{-4}
K = CONSTANT (10.1 FOR DOGS AND 10.0 FOR CATS)

DOGS				CATS	
BODY WT (kg)	BSA (m²)	BODY WT (kg)	BSA (m²)	BODY WT (kg)	BSA (m²)
0.5	0.06	26	0.88	0.5	0.06
1	0.10	27	0.90	1	0.10
2	0.15	28	0.92	1.5	0.12
3	0.20	29	0.94	2	0.15
4	0.25	30	0.96	2.5	0.17
5	0.29	31	0.99	3	0.20
6	0.33	32	1.01	3.5	0.22
7	0.36	33	1.03	4	0.24
8	0.40	34	1.05	4.5	0.26
9	0.43	35	1.07	5	0.28
10	0.46	36	1.09	5.5	0.29
11	0.49	37	1.11	6	0.31
12	0.52	38	1.13	6.5	0.33
13	0.55	39	1.15	7	0.34
14	0.58	40	1.17	7.5	0.36
15	0.60	41	1.19	8	0.38
16	0.63	42	1.21	8.5	0.39
17	0.66	43	1.23	9	0.41
18	0.69	44	1.25	9.5	0.42
19	0.71	45	1.26	10	0.44
20	0.74	46	1.28		
21	0.76	47	1.30		
22	0.78	48	1.32		
23	0.81	49	1.34		
24	0.83	50	1.36		
25	0.85				

Adapted, with permission, from Rosenthal RC. Chemotherapy. In: Ettinger SJ, Feldman EC, eds. *Textbook of Internal Medicine, Diseases of the Dog and Cat.* 4th Ed. Philadelphia: W.B. Saunders Company, 1995.

variation is another important consideration, as each species presents unique physiologic and pharmacokinetic characteristics. This includes *blood serum chemistry* values for animals that differ species to species.

Special Considerations in Compounding Veterinary Pharmaceuticals

Compounded prescriptions for veterinary use have the same benefits and restrictions as do counterpart compounded prescriptions for human use. The primary benefit is the ability of a pharmacist to compound a preparation that meets the specific requirements of the patient in terms of strength or dose and/or dosage form, when a similar commercially prepared product is unavailable. Specific guidance for compounding for animal patients may be found in the cited references.[6,11–14] In essence, the following apply:

* a valid veterinarian-client patient relationship must exist;
* failure to treat may result in adverse consequences to the animal;
* the compounded prescription must meet standards of safety, effectiveness, and stability;
* no FDA-approved human or animal drug in desired dosage form and/or strength is commercially available;
* the compounded dosage form must be prepared from an FDA-approved commercially available human or animal drug;
* the product must be compounded by a licensed pharmacist upon order from a licensed veterinarian or by a veterinarian within the scope of professional practice;
* the scale of the compounding must be commensurate with the need of the individual client-patient;
* compounded products intended for food animals must address special concerns of food safety including the avoidance of remaining tissue residues of drug; and
* all relevant federal and state laws relating to the compounding of drugs for use in animals must be followed including the regulations of the state Board of Pharmacy having jurisdiction.

The doses and treatments used in the "Practice Problems" that follow were derived from the referenced sources.[15,16] The problems may be solved using the calculation techniques described in previous chapters. It should be noted that the prescription abbreviation "sid," meaning "once a day," finds particular application in veterinary prescriptions.

CALCULATIONS CAPSULE

Veterinary Dosing

While most veterinary dosing parallels that for human dosing in the considerations of age, weight, pathological condition, concomitant therapy, and the diagnostic skill and experience of the prescriber, species variation is a special consideration in the treatment of animals. In addition, there is a unique equation for the determination of the body surface area (BSA) in dosage calculations for dogs and cats[15]:

$$BSA\ (m^2) = K \times (Body\ weight\ [grams])^{2/3} \times 10^{-4}$$

where K is the constant 10.1 for dogs and 10.0 for cats.

CASE IN POINT 18.1 A pharmacist received a prescription for the drug allopurinol for a pet parakeet in the treatment of gout. The veterinarian prescribed 0.5 mg to be administered by oral drops four times a day.

The pharmacist has 100-mg tablets and a dropper that has been calibrated to deliver 20 drops/mL. The pharmacist decides to crush a tablet, mix it with a sufficient quantity of water and make a suspension such that the pet's owner can conveniently administer the doses to the parakeet.

(a) How many milliliters of suspension should be prepared from the crushed 100-mg allopurinol tablet?

(b) How many drops should be administered to the parakeet per dose?

PRACTICE PROBLEMS

1. The drug pimobendan (VETMEDIN) is used in the treatment of CHF in dogs at a daily dose of 0.5 mg/kg. Scored, chewable tablets are commercially available containing 1.25 mg and 5 mg per tablet. Which of the following would best approximate the daily dose for a 16.5-lb. dog?

   (a) one-half 5-mg tablet
   (b) two 1.25-mg-tablets
   (c) two and a half 1.25-mg tablets
   (d) three 1.25-mg tablets

2. A 0.12% solution of chlorhexidine gluconate may be used as an oral cleansing solution to clean pets' teeth. Calculate the quantity of a 2% concentrate required to prepare a pint of the diluted solution.

3. Albuterol sulfate is administered orally to horses for bronchospasm at a dose of 8 mcg/kg. Calculate the number of milliliters of an 0.083% solution of albuterol sulfate to administer to a 900-lb. horse.

4.[a] A veterinarian writes a prescription for metronidazole, 20 mg/kg, for an 1100-lb. horse to be administered every 8 hours for 10 days. The pharmacist has 250-mg metronidazole tablets. How many tablets should be (a) administered per dose and (b) dispensed?

5. What fraction of a 50-mg aspirin suppository should be administered as an antipyretic to a 5.5-lb. cat if the veterinary dose is 10 mg/kg?

6. The dose of methotrexate sodium for neoplastic disease in cats is 2.5 mg/m² po twice weekly. If a 2-kg cat is determined to have a BSA of 0.15 m², calculate the single dose.

7. Phenylbutazone, an anti-inflammatory agent, may be administered to horses by intravenous injection at an average dose of 1.5 g/450 kg for 5 consecutive days. The usual injection contains phenylbutazone 200 mg/mL.

   How many milliliters of injection would be required in treating a 990-lb. horse?

8.[a] How many milliliters of a gentamicin injection, 100 mg/mL, should be administered to a 1250-lb. horse for a dose of 6.6 mg/kg?

9. The maximum dose of doxorubicin in canine chemotherapy is 200 mg/m². Using Table 18.1, calculate the maximum dose for a dog weighing 20 kg.

---

[a]Problem courtesy of H. Lindell, Veterinary Teaching Hospital Pharmacy, Athens, GA: University of Georgia.

10. Furosemide in the treatment of CHF in animals is used as a maintenance dose of 0.5 mg/kg sid. Calculate the dose for a 15-lb. dog.

11. Which strength tablets of enalapril maleate (ENACARD) would be most convenient to dispense in the treatment of an 11-lb. dog at a daily dose of 0.5 mg/kg?

    (a) 1-mg tablets
    (b) 2.5-mg tablets
    (c) 5-mg tablets
    (d) 10-mg tablets
    (e) 20-mg tablets

12. The dose of digoxin in dogs is 0.005 to 0.01 mg/kg po. Calculate the dosage range for a dog weighing 15 lb.

13. For large-breed dogs, the dose of digoxin is 0.22 mg/m². Using Table 18.1, calculate the dose for a dog weighing 22 kg.

14. A cockatiel may be given 6 mg of ketamine intramuscularly for anesthesia. Calculate the dose, on a mg/kg basis, for an 85-g cockatiel.

15. Some veterinarians treat seizures in dogs with potassium bromide, administering a loading dose of 90 mg/kg/day for 5 days concurrently with a maintenance dose of 30 mg/kg/day, the latter continued after the initial 5-day period. Calculate: (a) the daily dose (each day for days 1 to 5) for a 12-lb. dog; (b) the maintenance dose; (c), the quantity of potassium bromide needed to prepare one pint of a solution containing 250 mg of potassium bromide per milliliter; and (d), the number of milliliters of the solution needed to provide the maintenance dose.

16.[a] A veterinarian is treating a 66-lb. dog for ascarids with fenbendazole, 50 mg/kg/day orally for 3 days. How many milliliters of a 10% w/v suspension of fenbendazole should the pharmacist dispense?

17.[17] Cimetidine may be administered in the treatment of feline stomatitis at a dose of 5 to 10 mg/kg by mouth every 6 to 8 hours. Calculate (a) the dosage range for a cat weighing 9.4 lb and (b) the corresponding dosage range for an oral solution containing cimetidine, 300 mg/5 mL.

CALCQUIZ

18.A. Actinomycin is one of the chemotherapeutic agents used in veterinary medicine. The dose used is generally 0.7 to 1 mg/m² intravenously every 2 to 3 weeks. The drug is available as a lyophilized powder, 500 μg per vial, for reconstitution with sterile water for injection prior to use.

(a) Using the information in this chapter for conversion of weight to body surface area, and a 0.85 mg/m² dose of actinomycin, calculate the dose, in milligrams, for a 33-lb dog.
(b) If the drug in the vial results in a drug concentration of 0.5 mg/mL when reconstituted, calculate the volume of injection prepared.
(c) Calculate the dose of injection, in milliliters, applicable to the dog described in (a).

(continued)

---

[a]Problem courtesy of H. Lindell. Veterinary Teaching Hospital Pharmacy. Athens, GA: University of Georgia.

CALCQUIZ (continued)

18.B. Amlodipine besylate, an antihypertensive agent, has been administered orally to cats at a once daily dose of 0.625 mg by the formula[18]:

R: Amlodipine besylate   100 mg
      Fish Flavor, qs
      Cod liver oil, ad   100 mL

Calculate, the daily dose of amlodipine besylate for a 5.5-lb cat on the basis of:

(a) mg/kg
(b) mg/BSA in m^2, and
(c) milliliters of prescription.

18.C. A method of producing intravenous anesthesia in large animals utilizes an intravenous injection of diazepam (0.05 to 0.1 mg/kg) immediately prior to an intravenous infusion of the following[19]:

Ketamine   2.2   mg/kg
Xylazine   500   mg
Guaifenesin   5%
D5W, ad   1000 mL

The infusion is administered at a rate of 1 mL/kg/h.

For a horse weighing 980-lb, calculate:

(a) The dosage range for diazepam.
(b) The quantity of ketamine, in milligrams, to use in the infusion.
(c) The quantity of xylazine administered in mg/min.
(d) The quantity, in milliliters, of infusion remaining after 60 minutes.

18.D.[20] Captopril is used in dogs to treat hypertension and congestive heart failure at an initial dose of 1 mg/kg orally, three times daily. The pharmacist plans to prepare a 30-day supply of a suspension for a 12-lb dog such that a teaspoonful provides each dose. The source of captopril is 50-mg tablets.

(a) How many milligrams of captopril are required?
(b) How many milliliters of suspension are required?
(c) How many whole captopril tablets are required?
(d) If the required tablets are crushed and weigh a total of 1.2 g, what weight of the powder would be used in the suspension?

ANSWERS TO "CASE IN POINT" AND PRACTICE PROBLEMS

Case in Point 18.1

(a) For the pet owner's convenience, the pharmacist arbitrarily decided that the 0.5-mg dose of allopurinol should be contained in each drop of the suspension. Working backward in the calculation:

$$\frac{0.5 \text{ mg}}{1 \text{ drop}} = \frac{x \text{ mg}}{20 \text{ drops}} \quad x = 10 \text{ mg}$$

allopurinol (in 20 drops or 1 mL)

then, $\dfrac{10 \text{ mg}}{1 \text{ mL}} = \dfrac{100 \text{ mg (tablet)}}{x \text{ mL}}$

x = 10 mL suspension, *answer*.

(b) 1 drop/dose (predetermined), *answer*.

Practice Problems

1. (d) Three 1.25 mg tablets pimobendan
2. 28.4 mL chlorhexidine gluconate concentrate
3. 3.94 mL albuterol sulfate solution
4. (a) 40 metronidazole tablets
   (b) 1200 metronidazole tablets
5. ½ aspirin suppository
6. 0.375 mg methotrexate sodium
7. 37.5 mL phenylbutazone injection
8. 37.5 mL gentamicin injection
9. 148 mg doxorubicin
10. 3.4 mg furosemide
11. (b) 2.5 mg enalapril maleate tablets
12. 0.034 to 0.068 mg digoxin
13. 0.17 mg digoxin
14. 70.6 mg/kg ketamine
15. (a) 655 mg
    (b) 164 mg
    (c) 118.25 g potassium bromide
    (d) 0.66 mL
16. 45 mL fenbendazole
17. (a) 21.36 to 42.73 mg cimetidine
    (b) 0.36 to 0.71 mL

References

1. *The Merck Veterinary Manual*. 10th Ed. Whitehouse Station, NJ: Merck Sharpe & Dohme, 2010.
2. Plumb DC. *Plumb's Veterinary Drug Handbook*. 7th Ed. Hoboken, NJ: Wiley, 2011.
3. Code of Federal Regulations, Title 21, Part 514. *New Animal Drug Applications 2011*. Available at: http://www.accessdata.fda.gov/scripts/cdrh/cfdocs/cfcfr/CFRSearch.cfm?CFRPart=514. Accessed August 17, 2011.
4. Center for Veterinary Medicine, Food and Drug Administration. Available at: http://www.fda.gov/AboutFDA/CentersOffices/CVM/default.htm. Accessed August 17, 2011.
5. Extra-label drug use in animals. *Federal Register* 61:57731–57746. Accessed November 7, 1996.
6. Comyn G. Extra-label drug use in veterinary medicine. Available at: http://www.fda.gov/AnimalVeterinary/NewsEvents/FDAVeterinarianNewsletter/ucm100268.htm. Accessed August 17, 2011.
7. Animal drug delivery systems. *International Journal of Pharmaceutical Compounding* 1997;1:229. Adapted from: Blodinger J. *Formulation of Veterinary Dosage Forms*. New York: Marcel Dekker, 1983.
8. Jordan DG. Compounding for animals—a bird's eye view. *International Journal of Pharmaceutical Compounding* 1997;1:222–227.
9. Compounding for veterinary patients: pharmaceutical, biopharmaceutical, and physiologic considerations. *International Journal of Pharmaceutical Compounding* 1997;1:233–234.
10. *Concise Encyclopedia*. Buckinghamshire, GB: DK Publishing, 1999.
11. Lust E. Compounding for animal patients: contemporary issues. *Journal of the American Pharmacists Association* 2004;44:375–386.
12. *Pharmacy Today* June 2004:43.
13. Animal medicinal drug use clarification act of 1994 (AMDUCA). Available at: http://www.fda.gov/cvm/amducatoc.htm. Accessed January 4, 2008.
14. http://www.avma.org/issues/drugs/compounding/veterinary_compounding.asp. Accessed January 4, 2008.

15. Rosenthal RC. Chemotherapy. In: Ettinger SJ, Feldman EC, eds. *Textbook of Internal Medicine, Diseases of the Dog and Cat*. 4th Ed. Philadelphia, PA: W.B. Saunders, 1995.

16. Crabbe B. *The Comprehensive Guide to Equine Veterinary Medicine*. New York: Sterling Publishing Company, 2007.

17. Stockton SJ. *International Journal of Pharmaceutical Compounding* 2010;14:419.

18. Anon. *International Journal of Pharmaceutical Compounding* 2009;13:429.

19. Davidson G. Equine anesthesia: TRIPLE DRIP. *International Journal of Pharmaceutical Compounding* 2008;5:402.

20. Prince SJ. *International Journal of Pharmaceutical Compounding* 1999;3:234.

Selected Calculations Associated with Plant Extractives 19

Objectives

Upon successful completion of this chapter, the student will be able to:

- Perform calculations demonstrating the difference in drug content between *extracts, fluidextracts, and tinctures* of a medicinal plant.
- Perform calculations related to the concentration and dose of extracted botanicals.
- Perform calculations related to the concentration and dose of botanic dietary supplements.

Currently, the consuming public has renewed interest in the use of botanicals and dietary supplements. These products are widely available to consumers, and a variety of governmental agencies are trying to ensure their safety by setting appropriate quality standards.[1] The *United States Pharmacopeia—National Formulary* (USP/NF) includes official monographs, general tests, assays, and standards for a number of botanicals and dietary supplements.[2] Included among the official monographs for botanicals are those for echinacea, feverfew, garlic, ginkgo, ginseng, goldenseal, hawthorn, Saint John's wort, saw palmetto, and valerian. Dosage forms may be prepared from the dried and pulverized plant parts (e.g., leaves) containing the desired components.

Other pharmaceutical preparations are made by the process of *extraction*—that is, by removing desired constituents from plant materials through the use of select solvents. The plant materials (termed *crude drugs*) include seeds, leaves, bark, or other plant parts that contain known or suspected *active therapeutic ingredients* (ATIs) or *active ingredients* (AIs), including alkaloids, glycosides, or other pharmacologically active complex organic molecules.

Two major processes are used for the extraction of active constituents from plant materials, namely *maceration* and *percolation*.

The term *maceration* comes from the Latin *macerare*, meaning "to soak." By this process, comminuted crude drug is placed in a suitable vessel and allowed to soak in a solvent or mixture of solvents (termed the *menstruum*) for a sufficient period to soften the botanic material and effect the extraction of the soluble constituents. The menstruum selected is based on the solubility characteristics of the desired constituents. Hydroalcoholic mixtures commonly are employed. The dissolved constituents are separated from the exhausted crude drug by straining or filtration.

The term *percolation* is derived from the Latin *per*, meaning "through," and *colare*, meaning "to strain." By this process, comminuted crude drug is extracted of its soluble constituents by the slow passage of a menstruum through a column of the botanic material. The crude drug is carefully packed in an extraction apparatus (termed a *percolator*) and allowed to macerate for a prescribed period of time prior to percolation. Percolators are of various sizes and construction. Small-glass percolators, cone- or cylindrical-shaped, several inches in diameter, and about 12 inches in height, are available for laboratory use. In contrast, large stainless-steel percolators for industrial use may be six to eight feet in diameter and 12 to 18 feet in height. An orifice at the bottom of a percolator permits the convenient removal of the extractive (termed the **percolate**).

The primary dosage forms of plant extractives are extracts, fluidextracts, and tinctures. Frequently, however, the active therapeutic ingredient(s) are separated and used as single therapeutic agents in various dosage forms (e.g., tablets, capsules, elixirs, syrups). In some instances, synthetic replicas of the ATIs, or chemical congeners of them, are prepared and used in pharmaceutical products rather than the naturally occurring therapeutic agents.

Extracts, Fluidextracts, and Tinctures

Extracts are concentrated preparations of vegetable (or animal) drugs. Most extracts are prepared by percolation followed by the evaporation of all or nearly all the menstruum, yielding a powdered or ointment-like product of extracted drug in concentrated form. On a weight-for-weight basis, extracts commonly are two to six times as potent as the crude drug. In other words, 1 gram of extract may be equivalent in active constituents to 2 to 6 grams of the crude drug. Thus, an extract may be described as a "2 ×" (or other multiple) or as a "200%" (or other %) extract. Among the extracts in the USP/NF are: *Belladonna Extract, Cascara Sagrada Extract, Powdered Echinacea pallida Extract, Powdered Ginkgo Extract,* and *Powdered Asian Ginseng Extract.*[3]

Fluidextracts are liquid extractives of plant materials adjusted for drug content so that each milliliter of fluidextract is equivalent in constituents to 1 gram of the crude drug that it represents. Among the fluidextracts in the USP/NF are: *Cascara Sagrada Fluidextract, Garlic Fluidextract, Licorice Fluidextract,* and *Senna Fluidextract.*[3]

Tinctures are alcoholic or hydroalcoholic solutions prepared from plant materials. (Tinctures also may be prepared from chemical substances [e.g., iodine tincture].) Among the botanical tinctures in the USP/NF are: *Belladonna Tincture, Compound Cardamom Tincture, Opium Tincture, Sweet Orange Peel Tincture,* and *Tolu Balsam Tincture.*[3] Although there is no set strength for tinctures, those prepared from plant materials traditionally have used the following quantities of crude drug in the preparation of each 100 mL of tincture:

Potent drug (e.g., belladonna leaf)	10 g crude drug
Nonpotent drug (e.g., tolu balsam)	20 g crude drug
Fruit/Flavor (e.g., sweet orange peel)	50 g crude drug

The relative strengths of extracts, fluidextracts, and tinctures are depicted in Figure 19.1, which shows an example of the quantity of each that may be prepared from a quantity of crude drug. In terms of equivalency:

1 g =	1 mL =	0.25 g =	10 mL
crude drug	fluidextract	"400%" extract	"potent" tincture

Examples of calculations pertaining to plant extractives are as follows.

Example Calculations of Extracted Botanicals

If 1 mg of active ingredient (AI) is present in each gram of a crude drug, determine the concentration, in mg/g or mg/mL, of AI in the corresponding (a) fluidextract, (b) "400%" extract, and (c) potent tincture.

1000 mL Tincture   100 mL Fluidextract   25 g Extract

▼ FIGURE 19.1 Depiction of the relative concentrations of a potent tincture, a fluidextract, and an extract using as the example a "10%" tincture and a "400%" extract (see text for further explanation).

(a) Since, by definition, 1 mL of fluidextract is equivalent in active ingredient to 1 g of crude drug, 1 mg of active ingredient would be present in 1 mL of fluidextract.

$$1 \text{ mg AI/mL, } answer.$$

(b) A "400%" extract represents, in each gram, 4 g of crude drug. Thus:

$$\frac{1 \text{ g crude drug}}{4 \text{ g crude drug}} = \frac{1 \text{ mg AI}}{\text{x mg AI}}; \text{x} = 4 \text{ mg AI/g crude drug, } answer.$$

(c) Since a "potent tincture" represents in each 100 mL, the AI from 10 g of crude drug, 0.1 g of crude drug would be needed to prepare 1 mL of tincture. Thus:

$$\frac{1 \text{ g crude drug}}{0.1 \text{ g crude drug}} = \frac{1 \text{ mg AI}}{\text{x mg AI}}; \text{x} = 0.1 \text{ mg AI/mL tincture, } answer.$$

If the dose of belladonna tincture is 0.6 mL, determine the equivalent corresponding dose of (a) belladonna leaf, (b) belladonna fluidextract, and (c) an extract (200%) of belladonna.

(a) Since a potent tincture contains in each 100 mL, the AI from 10 g of crude drug is:

$$\frac{100 \text{ mL tr.}}{0.6 \text{ mL tr.}} = \frac{10 \text{ g crude drug}}{\text{x g crude drug}}; \text{x} = 0.06 \text{ g, } answer.$$

(b) Since 1 mL of fluidextract contains the AI from 1 g of crude drug:

$$\frac{1 \text{ g crude drug}}{0.06 \text{ g crude drug}} = \frac{1 \text{ mL fluidextract}}{\text{x mL fluidextract}}; \text{x} = 0.06 \text{ mL fluidextract, } answer.$$

Or, since a fluidextract is 10 times as concentrated as a potent tincture, its dose would be ¹⁄₁₀ that of a corresponding tincture:

$$\text{¹⁄₁₀ of } 0.6 \text{ mL} = 0.06 \text{ mL, } answer.$$

(c) Since a "400%" extract has four times the AI content as the crude drug, and since the dose of the crude drug as calculated above is 0.06 g, the dose of the extract would be ¼ of that dose:

$$0.06 \text{ g} \times ¼ = 0.015 \text{ g or } 15 \text{ mg, } \textit{answer.}$$

CASE IN POINT 19.1 An industrial pharmacist is charged with preparing a "400%" extract of cascara sagrada from 100 kg of crude drug.

(a) How many kilograms of the extract would be expected to be prepared?
(b) If the crude drug is assayed to contain 11% hydroxyanthracenes, what would be the expected percentage strength of the resultant extract?

Botanic Dietary Supplements

The official monographs (USP/NF) for botanic dietary supplements include quality standards for the content of their active constituents including, for example[2]:

Asian ginseng	NLT 0.2% ginsenoside Rg_1
	NLT 0.1% ginsenoside Rb_1
American ginseng	NLT 4% ginsenosides
Black cohosh	NLT 0.4% triterpene glycosides
Echinacea pallida	NLT 0.5% phenols (caftaric acid, chicoric acid, chlorogenic acid, and echinacoside)
Eleuthero	NLT 0.8% eleutheroside and eleutheroside E
Ginkgo	NLT 0.1% terpene lactones
Garlic	NLT 0.5% alliin
Goldenseal	NLT 2% hydrastine
	NLT 2.5% berberine
Red clover	NLT 0.5% isoflavones
Saint John's wort	NLT 0.3% hypericin extract
Valerian	NLT 0.8% valeric acid

The following are examples of calculations applicable to botanic dietary supplements.

Example Calculations of Botanic Supplements

A batch of garlic is determined to contain 10 mg of allicin in a 4-g sample. How many micrograms of allicin would be present in a 500-mg dose of garlic from this batch?

$$10 \text{ mg} = 10,000 \text{ } \mu g$$
$$500 \text{ mg} = 0.5 \text{ g}$$

$$\frac{4 \text{ g}}{0.5 \text{ g}} = \frac{10,000 \text{ } \mu g}{x \text{ } \mu g}; \quad x = 1250 \text{ } \mu g, \textit{ answer.}$$

The herb feverfew, when standardized as a powdered leaf, contains 0.2 percent of the agent parthenolide. How many milligrams of parthenolide would be present in a capsule containing 125 mg of powdered feverfew?

$$125 \text{ mg} \times 0.2\% = 0.25 \text{ mg, } \textit{answer.}$$

PRACTICE PROBLEMS

1. How many milliliters of a fluidextract would be equivalent in active ingredient to the following?

    (a) 10 g of crude drug
    (b) 10 mL of a "potent" tincture
    (c) 10 g of a "300%" extract

2. How many milliliters of a "potent" tincture may be prepared from the following?

    (a) 10 mL of a fluidextract
    (b) 10 g of a "400%" extract
    (c) 10 g of a "2X" extract

3. Cascara sagrada (bark) USP contains 7% of hydroxyanthracene derivatives, whereas the cascara sagrada extract USP contains 11 grams of hydroxyanthracene derivatives in each 100 g. Calculate the "%" of the extract relative to the crude drug (e.g., "250%").

4. How many milliliters of a cascara sagrada fluidextract can be prepared from a pound of cascara sagrada bark?

5. Powdered opium USP contains 10.25% of anhydrous morphine. How many grams of powdered opium should be used to prepare 100 mL of opium tincture USP, which contains 10 mg/mL of anhydrous morphine?

6. If senna leaves contain 25 mg of sennosides per gram of leaves, how many milligrams of sennosides would be contained in a formula for 1000 mL of a senna syrup that contains 250 mL of senna fluidextract?

7. SENOKOT syrup, a laxative, contains 1.7 mg standardized sennosides per milliliter. The maximum adult dose is 15 mL twice daily. How many milligrams of sennosides would a patient receive by taking the maximum dose?

8. If ginkgo biloba contains 24% of ginkgo heterosides, and if 120 mg are taken daily in three divided doses, how many milligrams of the ginkgo heterosides are contained in each of the divided doses?

9. If milk thistle is standardized to contain 70% of silymarin, how many milligrams of this substance are contained in a 200-mg dose of milk thistle?

10. If Saint John's wort is standardized to contain 0.3% of hypericin extract, how many milligrams of the extract would be taken daily when Saint John's wort is administered as a 300-mg capsule taken three times a day?

11. The herb valerian is administered as an extract containing 0.8% valeric acid. How many milligrams of valeric acid would be contained in each 300-mg dose of valerian extract?

CALCQUIZ

19.A.[4] Belladonna and opium rectal suppositories each weigh 2 g and contain 16.2 mg of powdered belladonna extract and 30 mg of powdered opium.

   (a) If powdered belladonna extract contains, in each 100 g, between 1.15 and 1.35 g of the alkaloids of belladonna leaf, calculate the range of alkaloids in each suppository.
   (b) Calculate the average percent concentration of belladonna alkaloids in the suppositories.
   (c) If the powdered opium used in preparing the suppositories contained 10.25% w/w of anhydrous morphine, calculate the percent strength of anhydrous morphine in the suppositories.

ANSWERS TO "CASE IN POINT" AND PRACTICE PROBLEMS

Case in Point 19.1

By definition, a 400% extract represents four times the potency of the corresponding crude drug. Thus:

(a) 100 kg ÷ 4 = 25 kg extract, *and*

(b) 11% × 4 = 44% hydroxyanthracenes, *answers*.

Practice Problems

1. (a) 10 mL
   (b) 1 mL
   (c) 30 mL

2. (a) 100 mL
   (b) 400 mL
   (c) 200 mL

3. "157%" extract

4. 454 mL cascara sagrada fluidextract

5. 9.76 g powdered opium

6. 6250 mg sennosides

7. 51 mg sennosides

8. 9.6 mg ginkgo heterosides

9. 140 mg silymarin

10. 2.7 mg hypericin

11. 2.4 mg valeric acid

· ·

References

1. Grauds C. Dietary supplements: new rules ensure quality. *Pharmacy Today* 2007;13:25.
2. *United States Pharmacopeia 32-National Formulary* 27. Rockville, MD: United States Pharmacopeial Convention, 2009;1:961–1136.
3. *United States Pharmacopeia 32-National Formulary* 27. Rockville, MD: United States Pharmacopeial Convention, 2009:1–3.
4. Stockton SJ. Calculations. *International Journal of Pharmaceutical Compounding* 2010;14:230.

Calculation of Active Drug Moiety 20

Objectives

Upon successful completion of this chapter, the student will be able to:

- Calculate the percentage composition of a chemical compound.
- Calculate the active drug moiety portion of a chemical compound.
- Perform calculations using active drug moiety in compounding procedures.

A pharmacist must be able to calculate the pharmacologically active drug (chemical) moiety when present in salt, ester, hydrated, or complex chemical form. Such calculations are essential when quantitatively comparing products of the same drug moiety but differing in chemical form. The calculations are applied in compounding procedures in which a different form of a drug is used to satisfy formulation requirements while the quantity of the pharmacologically active drug moiety is maintained at the desired therapeutic dose or concentration.

Atomic and Molecular Weights

A Table of Atomic Weights is included at the back of this book for reference.

Example Calculations of Atomic and Molecular Weights

Calculate the percentage composition of anhydrous dextrose, $C_6H_{12}O_6$.

$$
\begin{array}{ccccc}
C_6 & & H_{12} & & O_6 \\
(6 \times 12.01) & + & (12 \times 1.008) & + & (6 \times 16.00) & = \\
72.06 & + & 12.096 & + & 96.00 & = 180.16
\end{array}
$$

$$\frac{180.16}{72.06} = \frac{100\,(\%)}{x\,(\%)}$$

$$x = 40.00\% \text{ of carbon, } and$$

$$\frac{180.16}{12.096} = \frac{100\,(\%)}{y\,(\%)}$$

$$y = 6.71\% \text{ of hydrogen, } and$$

$$\frac{180.16}{96.00} = \frac{100\,(\%)}{z\,(\%)}$$

$$z = 53.29\% \text{ of oxygen, } answers.$$

Check: $40.00\% + 6.71\% + 53.29\% = 100\%$

Calculate the percentage of lithium (Li) in lithium carbonate, Li_2CO_3.

Molecular weight of lithium carbonate = 74
Atomic weight of lithium = 7

$$\frac{74}{2 \times 7} = \frac{100\ (\%)}{x\ (\%)}$$

$$x = 18.9\%,\ \textit{answer}.$$

A ferrous sulfate elixir contains 220 mg of ferrous sulfate ($FeSO_4 \cdot 7H_2O$) per teaspoonful dose. How many milligrams of elemental iron are represented in the dose?

Molecular weight of $FeSO_4 \cdot 7H_2O$ = 278
Atomic weight of Fe = 56

$$\frac{278}{56} = \frac{220\ (\text{mg})}{x\ (\text{mg})}$$

$$x = 44.3\ \text{or}\ 44\ \text{mg},\ \textit{answer}.$$

How many milligrams of sodium fluoride will provide 500 μg of fluoride ion?

$$\begin{array}{cc} \text{Na} & \text{F} \\ 23\ + & 19 = 42 \end{array}$$

$$\frac{19}{42} = \frac{500\ (\mu g)}{x\ (\mu g)}$$

$$x = 1105\ \mu g\ \text{or}\ 1.1\ \text{mg},\ \textit{answer}.$$

Chemically Equivalent Quantities

Example Calculations of Chemically Equivalent Quantities

The formula for magnesium citrate oral solution calls for 27.4 g of anhydrous citric acid ($C_6H_8O_7$) in 350 mL of the product. How many grams of citric acid monohydrate ($C_6H_8O_7 \cdot H_2O$) may be used in place of the anhydrous salt?

$$\text{Molecular weights}:$$
$$C_6H_8O_7 \cdot H_2O = 210 \qquad C_6H_8O_7 = 192$$

$$\frac{192}{210} = \frac{27.4\ (\text{g})}{x\ (\text{g})}$$

$$x = 29.97\ \text{or}\ 30\ \text{g},\ \textit{answer}.$$

Active Drug Moiety Equivalence

In pharmacotherapeutics, it is the pharmacologically active moiety of a drug compound that is responsible for the therapeutic response. To accommodate such diverse factors as drug solubility, drug absorption, and formulation/dosage form considerations, an active drug moiety may be developed into a salt, ester, or other complex chemical form.

Table 20.1 ▼ **EXAMPLES OF ACTIVE DRUG MOIETY PORTION OF SOME DRUG COMPOUNDS**

| | | MOLECULAR WEIGHT | |
| | | COMPOUND | ACTIVE DRUG MOIETY (FREE BASE) |
DRUG	EMPIRICAL FORMULA		
Cinacalcet HCl (SENSIPAR)	$C_{22}H_{22}F_3N \cdot HCl$	393.90	357.40
Escitalopram oxalate (LEXAPRO)	$C_{20}H_{21}FN_2O \cdot C_aH_2O_4$	414.40	336.38
Fluoxetine HCl (PROZAC)	$C_{17}H_{18}F_3NO \cdot HCl$	345.79	309.29
Metaproterenol sulfate (ALUPENT)	$(C_{11}H_{17}NO_3)_2 \cdot H_2SO_4$	520.59	211.26
Nelfinavir mesylate (VIRACEPT)	$C_{32}H_{45}N_3O_4S \cdot CH_4O_3S$	663.90	567.79
Rosiglitazone maleate (AVANDIA)	$C_{18}H_{19}N_3O_3S \cdot C_4H_4O_4$	473.52	357.44
Sumatriptan succinate (IMITREX)	$C_{14}H_{21}N_3O_2S \cdot C_4H_6O_4$	413.50	295.40

Prefabricated dosage forms that contain such chemical forms of a therapeutic entity frequently are labeled to indicate the product's drug composition, as for example, "each mL contains 1 mg of albuterol sulfate equivalent to 0.83 mg of albuterol."

In contemporary practice, the pharmacist may need to calculate the active drug moiety in a given preparation and/or compare the content between products.

Calculations of Active Drug Moiety in Compounding Procedures

The USP provides the following formula to calculate the theoretical weight of an ingredient in a compounded preparation[1]:

$$W = ab/de$$

Where:

W = *amount of substance to be weighed*
 a = *prescribed or calculated weight of active moiety*
 b = *chemical or formula weight of the ingredient (a) including any water of hydration*
 d = *decimal fraction of dry weight (from known moisture content)*
 e = *formula weight of active drug moiety*

Example Calculations of Active Drug Moiety Equivalence

What is the percentage strength of methadone (m.w. 313) in a solution containing 10 mg of methadone hydrochloride (m.w. 349) in each milliliter?

$$\frac{10 \text{ mg methadone HCl} \times 313 \text{ g/mole}}{349 \text{ g/mole}} = 8.97 \text{ mg, methadone equivalent;}$$

and, since 8.97 mg ≅ 0.009 g;

$$\frac{1 \text{ mL}}{100 \text{ mL}} = \frac{0.009 \text{ g}}{x \text{ g}}; \ x = 0.9 \text{ g/100 mL} = 0.9\%, \ answer.$$

How many milligrams of aminophylline (theophylline ethylenediamine) USP should be weighed to obtain 250 mg of anhydrous theophylline? The molecular weight of aminophylline dihydrate is

CALCULATIONS CAPSULE

Active Drug Moiety

To calculate the portion of a drug compound that is the active drug moiety, the following equation may be used:

$$\frac{Drug\ moiety\ (g/mole)}{Drug\ compound\ (g/mole)} = Drug\ moiety\ (fraction)$$

456, and the container indicates the presence of 0.4% w/w adsorbed moisture. The molecular weight of theophylline is 180, with 2 molecules present in aminophylline. By applying the above formula:

$$W = \frac{250\ mg \times 456\ g/mole}{0.994 \times 360\ g/mole} = 318.578\ or\ 319\ mg,\ answer.$$

If a prescription calls for the preparation of 30 mL of a 1% solution of lidocaine (m.w. 234), but for the purposes of solubility the pharmacist used lidocaine hydrochloride (m.w. 288), how many milligrams of the latter should be used?

$$30\ mL \times 1\%\ w/v = 0.3\ g\ or\ 300\ mg\ (lidocaine\ required)$$

$$W = \frac{300\ mg \times 288\ g/mole}{1 \times 234\ g/mole} = 369\ mg,\ answer.$$

CASE IN POINT 20.1[a] A pediatrician wishes to prescribe the drug metronidazole (m.w. 171) for a pediatric patient in the oral treatment of amebiasis. The patient is unable to swallow solid dosage forms, and an oral suspension of the drug would be extremely bitter. An alternative would be for the pharmacist to compound an oral suspension using metronidazole benzoate (m.w. 275), which has a low water solubility and thus little taste.

If the pediatric dosage range of metronidazole in the treatment of amebiasis is 35 to 50 mg/kg/day, calculate the dosage range of metronidazole benzoate.

[a]Problem courtesy of Warren Beach, Pharmaceutical and Biomedical Sciences, College of Pharmacy, University of Georgia, Athens, GA.

PRACTICE PROBLEMS

1. What is the percentage composition of dibasic sodium phosphate USP, $Na_2H\ PO_4 \cdot 7H_2O$?

2. Calculate the percentage of water in dextrose, $C_6H_{12}O_6 \cdot H_2O$.

3. What is the percentage of calcium in calcium gluconate, $C_{12}H_{22}CaO_{14}$?

4. A commercially available tablet contains 0.2 g of $FeSO_4 \cdot 2H_2O$. How many milligrams of elemental iron are represented in a daily dose of three tablets?

5. A certain solution contains 110 mg of sodium fluoride, NaF, in each 1000 mL. How many milligrams of fluoride ion are represented in each 2 mL of the solution?

6. How many grams of epinephrine bitartrate (m.w. 333) should be used in preparing 500 mL of an ophthalmic

solution containing the equivalent of 2% of epinephrine (m.w. 183)?

7. From the molecular weight (385.8) of ciprofloxacin hydrochloride, $C_{17}H_{18}FN_3$ $O_3 \cdot HCl \cdot H_2O$, calculate the molecular weight of ciprofloxacin base.

8. If 600 mg of glucosamine hydrochloride is equivalent to 500 mg of glucosamine (m.w. 179.2), calculate the molecular weight of glucosamine hydrochloride.

9. How many milligrams of betamethasone dipropionate (m.w. 504) should be used to prepare a 50-g tube of ointment labeled to contain the equivalent of 0.5 mg of betamethasone (m.w. 392) base per gram?

10. Sertraline Hydrochloride Capsules[2]:

    ℞: Sertraline Hydrochloride
       (ZOLOFT tablets,
       100 mg)   3 tablets
       Silica Gel   6 g
       Calcium Citrate   4 g
       M.ft. caps no. 40
       Sig. Use as directed.

    Calculate the grams of calcium in the formula derived from calcium citrate, $C_{10}H_{10}Ca_3O_{14} \cdot 4H_2O$ (m.w. 570.5).

11. Fentanyl Inhalation[3]:

    ℞: Fentanyl Citrate   4.71 mg
       Sterile Sodium Chloride
          Inhalation ad   60 mL
       Sig. Use as directed.

    Fentanyl citrate has a molecular weight of 528. Calculate the milligrams of the active drug moiety, fentanyl (m.w. 336), in the prescription.

12. A pediatric suspension of erythromycin ethylsuccinate (m.w. 862) contains the equivalent of 200 mg of erythromycin (m.w. 734) per 5-mL dose. Calculate the milligrams of erythromycin ethylsuccinate contained in 100 mL of the suspension.

13. A sterile ophthalmic suspension of BETOPTIC S contains 0.25% of betaxolol base (m.w. 307), present as the hydrochloride salt (m.w. 344). Calculate the percentage of betaxolol hydrochloride in the suspension.

14. If the molecular weight of the HIV protease inhibitor nelfinavir is 568 and that of nelfinavir mesylate is 664, calculate the milligrams of the latter in each tablet labeled to contain the equivalent of 250 mg of nelfinavir.

15. An ophthalmic solution is labeled to contain the equivalent of 0.3% of ciprofloxacin base (m.w. 332). How many milligrams of ciprofloxacin hydrochloride (m.w. 386) may be used to prepare each 5 mL of the solution?

16. The molecular weight of albuterol sulfate is 576, and the empirical formula is $(C_{13}H_{21}NO_3)_2 \cdot H_2SO_4$. If each actuation of an inhalation aerosol delivers 108 μg of albuterol sulfate, calculate the quantity of albuterol base delivered.

17. An injection contains 20 mg/mL of dolasetron mesylate monohydrate in 0.625-mL vials. The molecular weight of the drug is 438.5. Approximately 74% of dolasetron mesylate monohydrate is dolasetron base. Calculate the quantity of dolasetron base administered by 0.6 mL of injection.

CALCQUIZ

20.A. DIPROLENE ointment has a potency expressed as the equivalent of "0.05% beta-methasone." Betamethasone dipropionate is actually used in the formulation. The molecular weight of betamethasone is 392.4 and that of betamethasone dipropionate is 504.6.

   (a) Calculate the percent strength of betamethasone dipropionate in the ointment.
   (b) Calculate the quantity of betamethasone dipropionate, in mg/g, in a 15-g tube of the ointment.
   (c) If a pharmacist received an order to prepare an ointment containing 0.02% betamethasone, how many grams of ointment base would need to be mixed with a 15-g tube of DIPROLENE ointment?
   (d) If the manufacturer decided to prepare ointments containing 0.075% betamethasone, how many *additional* milligrams of betamethasone dipropionate would be needed in each 15-g tube of DIPROLENE ointment?

20.B. AVELOX IV contains in each 250-mL bag, moxifloxacin hydrochloride (equivalent to 400 mg of moxifloxacin) and 0.8% sodium chloride. The molecular weight of moxifloxacin hydrochloride is 437.9.

   (a) Calculate the quantity, in mg/mL, of moxifloxacin hydrochloride in the injection.
   (b) Calculate the milligrams and mEq of sodium in the IV solution.

ANSWERS TO "CASE IN POINT" AND PRACTICE PROBLEMS

Case in Point 20.1

$$\frac{171 \text{ (m.w.)}}{275 \text{ (m.w.)}} = \frac{35 \text{ mg/kg/day}}{x};$$

$x = 56.29$ mg/kg/day, *and*

$$\frac{171 \text{ (m.w.)}}{275 \text{ (m.w.)}} = \frac{50 \text{ mg/kg/day}}{x};$$

$x = 80.41$ mg/kg/day, *answers.*

Practice Problems

1. Na: 17.16%
   H: 5.60%
   P: 11.57%
   0: 65.67%
2. 9.1% water
3. 9.3% calcium

4. 178.5 or 179 mg elemental iron
5. 0.1 mg fluoride ion
6. 18.2 g epinephrine bitartrate
7. 331.3
8. 215
9. 32.1 mg betamethasone dipropionate
10. 0.842 g calcium
11. 2.99 or 3 mg fentanyl
12. 4697.5 or 4698 mg erythromycin ethylsuccinate
13. 0.28% betaxolol hydrochloride
14. 292.3 mg nelfinavir mesylate
15. 17.4 mg ciprofloxacin hydrochloride
16. 89.6 μg albuterol base
17. 8.88 mg dolasetron base

References

1. *United States Pharmacopeia 32—National Formulary 27.* Rockville, MD: United States Pharmacopeial Convention, 2008;1:676.
2. Allen LV Jr. Sertraline 7.5 mg capsules. *International Journal of Pharmaceutical Compounding* 1998;2:443.
3. Allen LV Jr. Fentanyl 300-mcg/6-mL inhalation. *International Journal of Pharmaceutical Compounding* 1998;2:153.

Selected Calculations Involving Radiopharmaceuticals 21

Objectives

Upon successful completion of this chapter, the student will be able to:

- Convert units of radioactivity within and between the *curie-* and *becquerel-*systems.
- Calculate radioactive decay and half-life.
- Perform dose and activity calculations of radiopharmaceuticals.

Radioisotopes

The atoms of a given element are not necessarily alike. In fact, certain elements actually consist of several components, called *isotopes*, that are chemically identical but physically may differ slightly in mass. Isotopes, then, may be defined as atoms that have the same nuclear charge, and hence the same atomic number, but different masses. The mass number physically characterizes a particular isotope.

Isotopes can be classified as stable and unstable. Stable isotopes never change unless affected by some outside force; unstable isotopes are distinguishable by radioactive transformations and hence are said to be radioactive. The radioactive isotopes of the elements are called *radioisotopes* or *radionuclides*. They can be divided into two types: naturally occurring and artificially produced radionuclides.

The branch of medicine that utilizes radioisotopes and radiation in the diagnosis and treatment of disease is *nuclear medicine*. Pharmacists who prepare radioactive pharmaceuticals or *radiopharmaceuticals* for use in patient care, practice *nuclear pharmacy* and are referred to as *nuclear pharmacists*.

The medical uses of nuclear materials may be described as

(a) *diagnostic*, as in body imaging and organ and tissue uptake of radiolabeled drugs to determine metabolic or other physiologic parameters;
(b) *therapeutic*, in the delivery of palliative or therapeutic doses of radiation to specific tissues or body areas, as in the treatment of cancer;
(c) *clinical research*, as in the study of a subject's response to a new radioactive drug or device; and
(d) *in vitro diagnostic testing* kits.

The United States Pharmacopeia/National Formulary devotes a chapter to the compounding of radiopharmaceuticals for positron emission tomography (PET).[1] Radiopharmaceuticals administered for PET procedures typically incorporate radionuclides, which have very short half-lives, as technetium-99m, gallium-67, and thallium-201. The radioisotope used in about 80 percent of nuclear diagnostic procedures is Tc-99m (the *m* standing for metastable).[2] It has a half-life of about 6 hours.

A list of some radiopharmaceuticals official in the USP/NF is presented in Table 21.1.

Table 21.1 ▼ EXAMPLES OF SOME RADIOPHARMACEUTICALS OFFICIAL IN THE USP/NF[a]

Chromic Phosphate P 32 Suspension
Chromium Cr 51 Edetate Injection
Cyanocobalamin Co 57 Capsules
Fludeoxyglucose F 18 Injection
Flumazenil C 11 Injection
Fluorodopa F 18 Injection
Indium In 111 Pentetate Injection
Iobenguane I 123 Injection
Iodinated I 131 Albumin Injection
Iodohippurate Sodium I 131 Injection
Methionine C 11 Injection
Rose Bengal Sodium I 131 Injection
Rubidium Chloride Rb 82 Injection
Sodium Acetate C 11 Injection
Sodium Chromate Cr 51 Injection
Sodium Fluoride F 18 Injection
Sodium Iodide I 123 Solution
Technetium Tc 99m Albumin Injection
Technetium Tc 99m Etidronate Injection
Technetium Tc 99m Gluceptate Injection
Technetium Tc 99m Mebrofenin Injection
Technetium Tc 99m Pentetate Injection
Technetium Tc 99m Pyrophosphate Injection
Technetium Tc 99m Sulfur Colloid Injection
Thallous Chloride TI 201 Injection
Xenon Xe 133 Injection

[a]*United States Pharmacopeia 32—National Formulary 27*. Rockville, MD: United States Pharmacopeial Convention, 2009.

Radioactivity

The breakdown of an unstable isotope is characterized by radioactivity. In the process of radioactivity, an unstable isotope undergoes changes until a stable state is reached, and in the transformation, it emits energy in the form of radiation. This radiation may consist of *alpha particles*, *beta particles*, and *gamma rays*. The stable state is reached as a result of *radioactive decay*, which is characteristic of all types of radioactivity. Individual radioisotopes differ in the rate of radioactive decay, but in each case, a definite time is required for half the original atoms to decay. This time is called the *half-life* of the radioisotope. Each radioisotope, then, has a distinct half-life.

▼ FIGURE 21.1 Illustration of the decay rate/half-life of radioisotopes. *(From U.S. Department of Health and Human Services: Radiation Event Medical Management. Available at: http://remm.nlm.gov/halflife.htm. Accessed August 20, 2011.)*

An illustration of the decay rate/half-life of radioisotopes is shown in Figure 21.1 and a list of the half-lives of some commonly used radioisotopes is presented in Table 21.2.

The rate of decay is always a constant fraction of the total number of undecomposed atoms present. Mathematically, the rate of disintegration may be expressed as follows:

$$-\frac{dN}{dt} - \lambda N \qquad \text{(Equation 1)}$$

in which N is the number of undecomposed atoms at time t, and λ is the decay constant or the fraction disintegrating per unit of time.

The constant may be expressed in any unit of time, such as reciprocal seconds, minutes, or hours, among others. The numeric value of the decay constant will be 24 times as great when expressed in days, for example, as when expressed in hours. This equation may be integrated to give the expression of the *exponential decay law*, which may be written,

$$N = N_o e^{-\lambda t} \qquad \text{(Equation 2)}$$

in which N is the number of atoms remaining at elapsed time t, N_0 is the number of atoms originally present (when t = 0), λ is the decay constant for the unit of time in terms of which the interval t is expressed, and e is the base of the natural logarithm 2.71828.

Because the rate of decay can also be characterized by the half-life ($T_{1/2}$), the value of N in equation 2 at the end of a half period is $\frac{1}{2}N_0$. The equation then becomes,

$$\tfrac{1}{2}N_o = N_o{}^{-\lambda T_{1/2}} \qquad \text{(Equation 3)}$$

Table 21.2 ▼ HALF-LIVES OF SOME
RADIOISOTOPES

RADIOISOTOPE	HALF-LIFE
^{198}Au	2.70 days
^{14}C	5,700 years
^{45}Ca	180 days
^{57}Co	270 days
^{60}Co	5.27 years
^{51}Cr	27.8 days
^{59}Fe	45.1 days
^{67}Ga	78.3 hours
^{203}Hg	46.6 days
^{123}I	13.2 hours
^{125}I	60 days
^{131}I	8.08 days
^{111}In	2.83 days
^{42}K	12.4 hours
^{81m}Kr	13.1 seconds
^{99}Mo	2.6 years
^{22}Na	2.6 years
^{24}Na	15.0 hours
^{32}P	14.3 days
^{35}S	87.2 days
^{75}Se	120 days
^{85}Sr	64 days
^{99m}Tc	6.03 hours
^{201}Tl	73.1 hours
^{133}Xe	5.24 days
^{169}Yb	32.0 days

Solving equation 3 by natural logarithms results in the following expression:

$$\ln \tfrac{1}{2} = -\lambda T_{1/2}$$

$$\text{or} \quad \lambda T_{1/2} = \ln 2$$

$$\text{then} \quad \lambda T_{1/2} = 2.303 \log 2$$

$$\text{and} \quad T_{1/2} = \frac{0.693}{\lambda} \qquad \text{(Equation 4)}$$

The half-life ($T_{1/2}$) is thus related to the disintegration constant λ by equation 4. Hence, if one value is known, the other can be readily calculated. The term "disintegration" is widely used; however, the alternative term "transformation" is used in some literature references.

Units of Radioactivity

The quantity of activity of a radioisotope is expressed in absolute units (total number of atoms disintegrating per unit time). The basic unit is the *curie* (Ci), which is defined as that

Table 21.3 ▼ **CONVERSION EQUIVALENTS**[a]

NUMBER OF ATOMS TRANSFORMING PER SECOND	SI UNIT: BECQUEREL (Bq)	HISTORICAL UNIT: CURIE (Ci)
1	1 Bq	27 picocurie (pCi)
1000	1 kilobecquerel (kBq)	27 nanocurie (nCi)
1×10^6	1 megabecquerel (MBq)	27 microcurie (μCi)
1×10^9	1 gigabecquerel (GBq)	27 millicurie (mCi)
37	37 Bq	1 (nCi)
37,000	37 kBq	1 (μCi)
3.7×10^7	37 MBq	1 (mCi)
3.7×10^{10}	37 GBq	1 Ci

[a]Source: World Health Organization, Radiopharmaceuticals. Document QAS/08.262/FINAL, adopted at the Forty-third WHO Expert Committee on Specifications for Pharmaceutical Preparations in October 2008 for addition to the 4th edition of *The International Pharmacopoeia*. Available at: http://www.who.int/medicines/publications/pharmacopoeia/Radgenmono.pdf. Accessed August 20, 2011.

quantity of a radioisotope in which 3.7×10^{10} (37 billion) atoms disintegrate per second. The *millicurie* (mCi) is one thousandth of a curie, and the *microcurie* (μCi) is one millionth of a curie. The *nanocurie* (nCi), also known as the *millimicrocurie*, is one billionth of a curie (10^{-9} Ci).

The International System (SI; see Chapter 2) unit for radioactivity is the *becquerel* (Bq), which is defined as 1 disintegration per second. Because the becquerel is so small, it is more convenient to use multiples of the unit, such as the *kilobecquerel* (kBq), which is equal to 10^3 disintegrations per second; the *megabecquerel* (MBq), which is equal to 10^6 disintegrations per second; and the *gigabecquerel* (GBq), which is equal to 10^9 disintegrations per second.

The *United States Pharmacopeia* has adopted the becquerel to eventually replace the long-familiar curie as a matter of international agreement. For the present, both units are used to label radioactivity, and the doses of many radiopharmaceuticals are expressed in megabecquerels as well as in millicuries and/or microcuries.

Table 21.3 provides equivalents for conversion from the curie (and its subunits) to the becquerel (and its multiples), and vice versa.

Example Calculations of Radioactivity Unit Conversion

A thallous chloride Tl 201 injection has a labeled activity of 550 microcuries (μCi). Express this activity in terms of megabecquerels.

$$550\ \mu Ci = 0.55\ mCi$$
$$1 mCi = 37\ MBq$$
$$\frac{1\ (mCi)}{0.55\ (mCi)} = \frac{37\ (MBq)}{x\ (MBq)}$$
$$x = 20.35\ MBq,\ answer.$$

Sodium chromate Cr 51 injection is administered in a dose of 3.7 MBq for the determination of blood volume. Express this dose in terms of microcuries.

$$1 \text{ MBq} = 0.027 \text{ mCi}$$

$$\frac{1 \text{ (MBq)}}{3.7 \text{ (MBq)}} = \frac{0.027 \text{ (mCi)}}{x \text{ (mCi)}}$$

$$x = 0.1 \text{ mCi}$$

$$= 100 \text{ } \mu Ci, \text{ } answer.$$

Example Calculations of Half-Life and Disintegration Constant

The disintegration constant of a radioisotope is 0.02496 day⁻¹. Calculate the half-life of the radioisotope.

$$T_{1/2} = \frac{0.693}{\lambda}$$

$$\text{Substituting, } T_{1/2} = \frac{0.693}{0.02496 \text{ day}^{-1}}$$

$$T_{1/2} = 27.76 \text{ or } 27.8 \text{ days, } answer.$$

The half-life of ^{198}Au is 2.70 days. Calculate its disintegration constant.

$$T_{1/2} = \frac{0.693}{\lambda}$$

$$\text{Substituting, } 2.70 \text{ days} = \frac{0.693}{\lambda}$$

$$\lambda = \frac{0.693}{2.70 \text{ days}} = 0.2567 \text{ day}^{-1}, \text{ } answer.$$

The original quantity of a radioisotope is given as 500 μCi (18.5 MBq)/mL. If the quantity remaining after 16 days is 125 μCi (4.625 MBq)/mL, calculate (a) the disintegration constant and (b) the half-life of the radioisotope.

(a) Equation 2, written in logarithmic form, becomes

$$\ln \frac{N}{N_o} = -\lambda t$$

or

$$\lambda = \frac{2.303}{t} \log \frac{N_0}{N}$$

Substituting:

$$\lambda = \frac{2.303}{16} \log \frac{500}{125} \text{ or, } \frac{2.303}{16} \log \frac{18.5 \text{ (MBq)}}{4.625 \text{ (MBq)}}$$

$$\lambda = \frac{2.303}{16} (0.6021)$$

$$\lambda = 0.08666 \text{ day}^{-1}, \text{ } answer.$$

(b) Equation 4 may now be used to calculate the half-life.

$$T_{1/2} = \frac{0.693}{\lambda}$$

Substituting, $T_{1/2} = \dfrac{0.693}{0.08666 \, \text{day}^{-1}} = 8.0 \, \text{days,}$ *answer.*

Pharmacists may find it useful to corroborate their complex calculations by referring to one of many Web sites that offer radioactive decay calculators, such as the one referenced.[3]

CALCULATIONS CAPSULE

Half-Life

The half-life equation is:

$$T_{1/2} = \frac{0.693}{\lambda}$$

λ = Half-life coefficient or disintegration constant

Example Calculations of Remaining Activity Over Time

A sample of ^{131}I has an initial activity of 30 μCi (1.11 MBq). Its half-life is 8.08 days. Calculate its activity, in microcuries (megabecquerels), at the end of exactly 20 days.

By substituting $\lambda = \dfrac{0.693}{T_{1/2}}$ and $e^{-0.693} = \frac{1}{2}$

In Equation 2, the activity of a radioactive sample decreases with time according to the following expression:

$$N = N_0 \left(2^{-t/T_{1/2}} \right) = N_0 \left(\frac{1}{2^{t/T_{1/2}}} \right)$$

Since $t/T \frac{1}{2} = \dfrac{20}{8.08} = 2.475$

then $N = 30 \left(\dfrac{1}{2^{2.475}} \right)$

Solving by logarithms, $\log N = \log 30 - \log 2 \, (2.475)$
$$= 1.4771 - 0.7450$$
$$\log N = 0.7321$$
$$N = 5.39 \text{ or } 5.4 \text{ μCi, } answer.$$

Or, using megabecquerel units:

$$N = 1.11 \left(\frac{1}{2^{2.475}} \right)$$

Solving by logarithms, log N = log 1.11 − log 2 (2.475)

$$= 0.0453 - 0.7450$$

$$\log N = -0.6997$$

$$N = 0.1997 \text{ or } 0.2 \text{ MBq, } answer.$$

A vial of sodium phosphate P 32 solution has a labeled activity of 500 µCi (18.5 MBq)/mL. How many milliliters of this solution should be administered exactly 10 days after the original assay to provide an activity of 250 Ci (9.25 MBq)? The half-life of ^{32}P is 14.3 days.

The activity exactly 10 days after the original assay is given by

$$N = N_0 \left(\frac{1}{2^{t/T_{1/2}}} \right)$$

Since $t/T_{1/2} = \dfrac{10}{14.3} = 0.6993$

then $N = 500 \left(\dfrac{1}{2^{0.6993}} \right)$

$$\log N = \log 500 - \log 2 \,(0.6993)$$

$$= 2.6990 - 0.2105$$

$$\log N = 2.4885$$

$$N = 308 \ \mu Ci/mL, \text{ activity after radioactive decay}$$

$$\frac{308 \ (\mu Ci)}{250 \ (\mu Ci)} = \frac{1 \ (mL)}{x \ (mL)}$$

$$x = 0.81 \text{ mL, } answer.$$

Or, using megabecquerel units:

$$N = 18.5 \left(\frac{1}{2^{0.6993}} \right)$$

$$\log N = \log 18.5 - \log 2 \,(0.6993)$$

$$= 1.2672 - 0.2105$$

$$\log N = 1.0567$$

$$= 11.39 \text{ MBq/mL, activity after radioactive decay}$$

$$\frac{11.39 \ (MBq)}{9.25 \ (MBq)} = \frac{1 \ (mL)}{x \ (mL)}$$

$$x = 0.81 \text{ mL, } answer.$$

CASE IN POINT 21.1[a] The Nuclear Pharmacy receives an order for a 25-mCi technetium Tc 99m MDP (bone scan dose) to be administered at 10:00 AM (1000 hours). The pharmacist has prepared an MDP bone kit with the concentration of 50 mCi/mL at 0600. What volume of the kit should be dispensed to provide the dose as ordered? The half-life of technetium Tc 99m is 6.03 hours.

[a]Problem courtesy of Kenneth M. Duke, Clinical and Administrative Pharmacy, College of Pharmacy, University of Georgia, Athens, GA.

PRACTICE PROBLEMS

1. Cyanocobalamin Co 57 capsules are administered in doses of 0.5 to 1.0 μCi in a test for pernicious anemia. Express this dosage range in terms of becquerel units.

2. If 1 mCi of radioactivity is equivalent to 37 MBq in activity, how many becquerels of radioactivity would be the equivalent of 1 Ci?

3. A gallium citrate Ga 67 injection has a labeled activity of 366 MBq. Express this activity in terms of millicuries.

4. If 1.85 MBq of radioactivity is equivalent to 50 μCi, how many millicuries would be represented in 7.4 MBq?

5. If 50 μCi of radioactivity is equivalent to 1.85 MBq of activity, how many megabecquerels of radioactivity would be the equivalent of 10 mCi?

6. Express an administered dose of 5 mCi sodium phosphate P 32 solution in terms of megabecquerels.

7. Calculate the half-life of a radioisotope that has a disintegration constant of 0.00456 day^{-1}.

8. Calculate the half-life of ^{203}Hg, which has a disintegration constant of 0.0149 day^{-1}.

9. Calculate the disintegration constant of ^{64}Cu, which has a half-life of 12.8 hours.

10. Calculate the disintegration constant of ^{35}S, which has a half-life of 87.2 days.

11. The original quantity of a radioisotope is given as 100 mCi (3700 MBq). If the quantity remaining after 6 days is 75 mCi (2775 MBq), calculate the disintegration constant and the half-life of the radioisotope.

12. A series of measurements on a sample of a radioisotope gave the following data:

Days	Counts per Minute
0	5600
4	2000

Calculate the disintegration constant and the half-life of the radioisotope.

13. The original activity of a radioisotope is given as 10 mCi (370 MBq) per 10 mL. If the quantity remaining after exactly 15 days is 850 μCi (31.45 MBq)/mL, calculate the disintegration constant and the half-life of the radioisotope.

14. If the half-life of a radioisotope is 12 hours, what will be the activity after 4 days of a sample that has an original activity of 1 Ci (37,000 MBq)? Express the activity in terms of microcuries (megabecquerels).

15. Sodium iodide I 131 capsules have a labeled potency of 100 μCi (3.7 MBq). What will be their activity exactly 3 days after the stated assay date? The half-life of ^{131}I is 8.08 days.

16. A sodium chromate Cr 51 injection has a labeled activity of 50 mCi (1850 MBq) at 5:00 PM on April 19. Calculate its activity at 5:00 PM on May 1. The half-life of ^{51}Cr is 27.8 days.

17. Iodinated I 125 albumin injection contains 0.5 mCi (18.5 MBq) of radioactivity per milliliter. How many milliliters of the solution should be administered exactly 30 days after the original assay to provide an activity of 60 μCi (2.22 MBq)? The half-life of ^{125}I is 60 days.

18. An ytterbium Yb 169 pentetate injection has a labeled radioactivity of 5 mCi (185 MBq)/mL. How many milliliters of the injection should be administered 10 days after the

original assay to provide an activity of 100 μCi (3.7 MBq)/kg of body weight for a person weighing 110 lb? The half-life of ^{169}Yb is 32.0 days.

19. A sodium pertechnetate Tc 99m injection has a labeled activity of 15 mCi (555 MBq)/mL. If the injection is administered 10 hours after the time of calibration, (a) what will be its activity, and (b) how many milliliters

of the injection will be required to provide a dose of 15 mCi (555 MBq)? The half-life of ^{99m}Tc is 6.0 hours.

20. A sodium phosphate P 32 solution contains 1 mCi (37 MBq)/mL at the time of calibration. How many milliliters of the solution will provide an activity of 500 μCi (18.5 MBq) 1 week after the original assay? The half-life of ^{32}P is 14.3 days.

CALCQUIZ

21.A.[a] An iodine I 131 capsule has been ordered for administration on Tuesday, November 11, at 12 noon. The requested dose is 25 mCi. If the patient is unable to make the appointment on November 11, what dose remains for a 12 noon appointment on Thursday, November 13? The half-life of iodine I 131 is 8 days.

21.B.[a] An order is received for a 100-mCi vial of technetium Tc 99m pertechnetate calibrated for 8:00 AM (0800 hours) to be used as a linearity source for dose calibrator testing at one of the nuclear medicine accounts. The pharmacy must prepare the dose for delivery at 0500. What activity should be dispensed at 0500 to deliver the desired activity? The half-life of technetium Tc 99m pertechnetate is 6.02 hours.

21.C.[4] A pharmacist receives an order for an 8-μCi dose of ^{99m}Tc-mertiatide for a study to be performed at 10:30 AM. At 6:00 AM, the morning of the study, the pharmacist prepares the dose. The standard decay equation yields a fraction of 0.596 of the initial activity remaining after 4.5 hours. How many μCi are needed at 6:00 AM to obtain the correct dose at 10:30 AM?

[a]Problem courtesy of Kenneth M. Duke, Clinical and Administrative Pharmacy, College of Pharmacy, University of Georgia, Athens, GA.

ANSWERS TO "CASE IN POINT" AND PRACTICE PROBLEMS

Case in Point 21.1

Solving first for the half-life coefficient, lambda (λ), for Tc 99m:

$\lambda = 0.693/T_{1/2}$
$\lambda = 0.693/6$ (hours)
$\lambda = 0.1155$ hours^{-1}

Since the stock solution was compounded to contain 50 mCi/mL at 0600, we can decay this concentration to the 1000 dosage time and solve as a proportion problem.

Using the decay formula: $A = A_0 e^{-\lambda t}$

A = Final activity
A_0 = Initial activity
t = Decay time
$A = 50\ e^{-(0.1155)4}$
$A = 50\ (0.63)$
$A = 31.5$ mCi/mL

Required dose = 25 mCi

Volume to dispense = 25mCi/31.5 mCi/mL
= 0.79 mL, *answer*.

Practice Problems

1. 18,500 to 37,000 Bq
2. 3.7×10^{10} Bq
3. 9.9 mCi
4. 0.2 mCi
5. 370 MBq
6. 185 MBq
7. 152 days
8. 46.5 days
9. 0.0541 hour^{-1}
10. 0.00795 hour^{-1}
11. $\lambda = 0.04794$ day^{-1}
    $T_{1/2} = 14.5$ days
12. $\lambda = 0.2574$ day^{-1}
    $T_{1/2} = 2.7$ days
13. $\lambda = 0.01084$ day^{-1}
    $T_{1/2} = 64$ days
14. 3907 µCi (144.5 MBq)
15. 77.3 µCi (2.86 MBq)
16. 37.1 mCi (1372.7 MBq)
17. 0.17 mL
18. 1.24 mL
19. (a) 4.7 mCi (174.8 MBq)
    (b) 3.2 mL
20. 0.7 mL

References

1. *United States Pharmacopeia 32—National Formulary 27*. Rockville, MD: United States Pharmacopeial Convention, 2009;365–369.
2. The regulation and use of radioisotopes in today's world. U.S. Nuclear Regulatory Commission. Available at: http://www.nrc.gov/reading-rm/doc-collections/nuregs/brochures/br0217/. Accessed August 20, 2011.
3. Radioactive Decay Calculator. University of Washington, Environmental Health & Safety. Available at: http://www.ehs.washington.edu/rso/calculator/activity_calc.shtm. Accessed August 22, 2011.
4. Basmadjian N. Prescription preparation in nuclear pharmacy: three case studies. *International Journal of Pharmaceutical Compounding* 1998;2:429–431.

Selected Bioavailability and Pharmacokinetic Calculations

Objectives

Upon successful completion of this chapter, the student will be able to:

- Perform basic calculations of bioavailability and bioequivalence.
- Perform basic calculations of elimination half-life and volume of distribution.

The availability to the biologic system of a drug substance formulated into a pharmaceutical product is integral to the goals of dosage form design and paramount to the effectiveness of the medication.

Before a drug substance can be absorbed by the biologic system, it must be released from its dosage form (e.g., tablet) or drug delivery system (e.g., transdermal patch) and dissolved in the physiologic fluids. Several factors play a role in a drug's biologic availability, including the physical and chemical characteristics of the drug itself, such as its particle size and solubility, and the features of the dosage form or delivery system, such as the nature of the formulative ingredients and the method of manufacture. The area of study that deals with the properties of drug substances and dosage forms that influence the release of the drug for biologic activity is termed *biopharmaceutics*. The term *bioavailability* refers to the *relative amount* of drug from an administered dosage form that enters the systemic circulation.

Pharmacokinetics is the study and characterization of the time course of the absorption, distribution, metabolism, and elimination (ADME) of drugs. *Drug absorption* is the process of uptake of the compound from the site of administration into the systemic circulation. *Drug distribution* refers to the transfer of the drug from the blood to extravascular fluids and tissues. *Drug metabolism* is the enzymatic or biochemical transformation of the drug substance to (usually less toxic) metabolic products, which may be eliminated more readily from the body. *Drug elimination* is the removal of the drug substance or its metabolites from the body, such as through the kidney (urine), intestines (feces), skin (sweat), saliva, and/or milk.

The relationship among the processes of absorption, distribution, metabolism, and elimination influences the therapeutic and toxicologic effects of drugs. The application of pharmacokinetic principles in the treatment of individual patients in optimizing drug therapy is referred to as *clinical pharmacokinetics*.

Drug Availability from Dosage Forms and Delivery Systems

The availability of a drug from a dosage form or delivery system is determined by measuring its dissolution characteristics *in vitro* (outside the biologic system) and/or its absorption patterns *in vivo* (within the biologic system). Generally, data are collected that provide information on both *rate* and *extent* of drug dissolution and/or absorption. The data collected may be plotted on graph paper to depict concentration versus time curves for the drug's dissolution and/or absorption.

Plotting and Interpreting Drug Dissolution Data

Drug dissolution data are obtained in vitro for tablets or capsules using the USP Dissolution Test, which defines the apparatus and methods to be used.[1] The data obtained may be presented in tabular form and depicted graphically, as in the following example.

The following dissolution data were obtained from a 250-mg capsule of ampicillin. Plot the data on graph paper and determine the approximate percentage of ampicillin dissolved following 15, 30, and 45 minutes of the study.

Period (minutes)	Ampicillin Dissolved (mg)
5	12
10	30
20	75
40	120
60	150

Plotting the data:

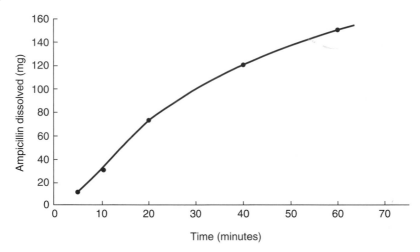

Determining the intercepts at 15, 30, and 45 minutes:

At 15 minutes, approximately 50 mg or 20% of the ampicillin,
At 30 minutes, approximately 100 mg or 40% of the ampicillin,
At 45 minutes, approximately 125 mg or 50% of the ampicillin, *answers.*

Example Calculations of Bioavailability and Bioequivalence

Amount of Drug Bioavailable from a Dosage Form

If drug dissolution or drug absorption studies demonstrate consistently that only a portion of a drug substance in a dosage form is "available" for biologic absorption, the drug's bioavailability factor (F), which represents the decimal percentage of a drug substance available, may be used to calculate bioavailability. The value of F may be zero, indicating no absorption, to a maximum of a value of 1, indicating complete absorption.

If the bioavailability factor (F) for a drug substance in a dosage form is 0.60, how many milligrams of drug would be available for absorption from a 100-mg tablet of the drug?

The bioavailability factor (F) indicates that only 60% of the drug present in the dosage form is available for absorption. Thus:

$$100 \text{ mg} \times 0.60 = 60 \text{ mg}, \textit{answer.}$$

The administration of medication with food can affect bioavailability.

The oral bioavailability of 10-mg alendronate tablets is stated as 0.59%. Concomitant administration with coffee or orange juice reduces the bioavailability by approximately 60%. Calculate the quantity of alendronate bioavailable, in milligrams, following a 10-mg dose swallowed with orange juice.

$$10 \text{ mg} \times 0.59\% = 0.059 \text{ mg}$$
$$0.059 \text{ mg} \times 40\% = 0.0236 \text{ mg}, \textit{answer.}$$

"Bioequivalent" Amounts of "Bioinequivalent" Dosage Forms

The bioavailability of a given drug substance may vary when in different dosage forms or in the same dosage form but from a different manufacturer. Thus, it may be desired to calculate the equivalent doses for two *bioinequivalent* products.

If the bioavailability (F) of digoxin in a 0.25-mg tablet is 0.60 compared to the bioavailability (F) of 0.75 in a digoxin elixir (0.05 mg/mL), calculate the dose of the elixir equivalent to the tablet.

First, calculate the amount of "bioavailable" digoxin in the tablet:

$$0.25 \text{ mg} \times 0.60 = 0.15 \text{ mg}, \text{ bioavailable amount of digoxin in the tablet}$$

Next, calculate the amount of "bioavailable" digoxin per milliliter of the elixir:

$$0.05 \text{ mg} \times 0.75 = 0.0375 \text{ mg}, \text{ bioavailable amount of digoxin per milliliter of the elixir}$$

Finally, determine the quantity of elixir that will provide 0.15 mg of "bioavailable" digoxin: By proportion:

$$\frac{0.0375 \text{ (mg)}}{0.15 \text{ (mg)}} = \frac{1 \text{ (mL)}}{x \text{ (mL)}}$$
$$x = 4 \text{ mL}, \textit{answer.}$$

A newly admitted hospital patient has been taking a brand of digoxin tablets, 250 μg, that are 60% bioavailable. The hospitalist wishes to administer a comparable IV dose using an injection containing digoxin, 0.5 mg/2 mL. What is the comparable dose?

$$250 \text{ μg} \times 60\% = 150 \text{ μg (effective or absorbed dose)}$$
$$\text{Injection} = 0.5 \text{ mg/2 mL} = 500 \text{ μg/2 mL}$$
$$150 \text{ μg} \times \frac{2 \text{ mL}}{500 \text{ μg}} = 0.6 \text{ mL digoxin injection, } \textit{answer.}$$

Plotting and Interpreting a Blood-Drug–Concentration-Time Curve

Following the administration of a medication, if blood samples are drawn from the patient at specific time intervals and analyzed for drug content, the resulting data may be plotted on ordinary graph paper to prepare a blood-drug–concentration-time curve. The vertical axis of this type of plot characteristically presents the concentration of drug present in the blood (or serum or plasma) and the horizontal axis presents the times the samples were obtained after administration of the drug. When the drug is first administered (time zero), the blood concentration of the drug should also be zero. As an orally administered drug passes into the stomach and/or intestine, it is released from the dosage form, fully or partially dissolves, and is absorbed. As the sampling and analysis continue, the blood samples reveal increasing concentrations of drug, until the maximum (peak) concentration (C_{max}) is reached. Then the blood level of the drug decreases progressively and, if no additional dose is given, eventually falls back to zero.

For conventional dosage forms, such as tablets and capsules, the C_{max} will usually occur at only a single time point, referred to as T_{max}. The amount of drug is usually expressed in terms of its concentration in relation to a specific volume of blood, serum, or plasma. For example, the concentration may be expressed as g/100 mL, μg/mL, mg/dL, or mg% (mg/100 mL). The quantity of a dose administered and its bioavailability, dissolution, and absorption characteristics influence the blood level concentration for a drug substance. The rate or speed of drug absorption determines the T_{max}, the time of greatest blood drug concentration after administration; the faster the rate of absorption, the sooner the T_{max}.

In a blood-drug–concentration-time curve, the area under the curve (AUC) is considered representative of the *total* amount of drug absorbed into systemic circulation. The area under the curve may be measured mathematically, using a technique known as the trapezoidal rule. The procedure may be found in other textbooks, references, and at various Web sites.

From the following data, plot a serum concentration-time curve and determine (a) the peak height concentration (C_{max}) and (b) the time of the peak height concentration (T_{max}).

Time Period (hours)	Serum Drug Concentration (mg/mL)
0.5	1.0
1.0	2.0
2.0	4.0
3.0	3.8
4.0	2.9
6.0	1.9
8.0	1.0
10.0	0.3
12.0	0.2

Plotting the data and interpretation of the curve:

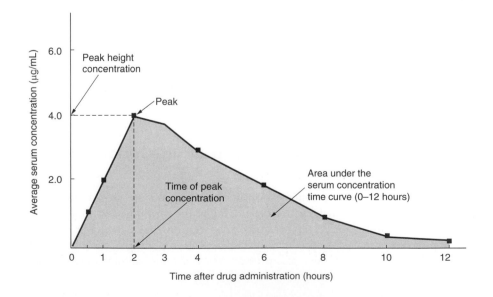

Determining the intercept for C_{max} and T_{max}:

$$C_{max} = 4.0 \ \mu g/mL$$
$$T_{max} = 2 \text{ hours, } answers.$$

Calculation of the bioavailability (F) of a drug may be determined by comparison of the AUC data for the particular dosage form against the intravenous form[3]:

$$F = \frac{AUC_{dosage \ form}}{AUC_{intravenous}}$$

It is recalled that the value *F* is the fraction of an administered dose that enters the systemic circulation. The intravenous route is the reference standard for comparison since the quantity of drug administered intravenously is considered to enter completely into the systemic circulation.[2]

If the AUC for an oral dose of a drug administered by tablet is 4.5 μg/mL and the intravenous dose is 11.2 μg/mL, calculate the bioavailability of the oral dose of the drug.[3]

$$F = \frac{AUC_{oral \ tablet}}{AUC_{IV}}$$

$$F = \frac{4.5 \ \mu g/mL}{11.2 \ \mu g/mL} = 0.4 \text{ or } 40\%, \ answer.$$

CASE IN POINT 22.1[3] A hospitalized patient has been receiving ranitidine (ZANTAC) 50 mg by intravenous injection every 8 hours. After discharge, the patient's physician wishes to continue treatment with a bioequivalent dose of the oral liquid form of ranitidine. From the literature, the community pharmacist determines that the oral liquid is 50% bioavailable. The product is available in a concentration of 75 mg/5 mL, to be taken twice a day. How many milliliters of the oral liquid should be indicated per dose on the prescription label?

INTRODUCTORY CONCEPTS AND CALCULATIONS INVOLVED IN PHARMACOKINETICS

As defined previously, pharmacokinetics is the study and characterization of the time course of absorption, distribution, metabolism, and elimination of drugs. Many of the calculations involved in pharmacokinetics are complex and the subject of advanced textbooks devoted to this important field. The intention in the following discussion is to define and describe some of the more introductory concepts and calculations.

Example Calculations of Selected Pharmacokinetic Parameters

Plasma Concentration of Unbound Versus Bound Drugs

Once absorbed into the circulation, a portion of the total drug plasma concentration (C_T) is bound to plasma proteins (usually albumin), and a portion remains unbound, or free. It is the unbound drug (C_U) that is available for further transport to its site of action in the body. The fraction of unbound drug compared with bound drug (C_B) is primarily a function of the affinity of the drug molecules for binding to the plasma proteins and the concentration of the latter (some patients may have a reduced or elevated serum albumin concentration). Some drug molecules may be more than 90% bound to plasma proteins, whereas others may be bound only slightly. Any change in the degree of binding of a given drug substance can alter its distribution and elimination and thus its clinical effects.

The fraction of unbound drug in the plasma compared with the total plasma drug concentration, bound and unbound, is termed *alpha* (or α).

Thus,

$$\alpha = \frac{C_U}{C_U + C_B} = \frac{C_U}{C_T}$$

If one knows the value of α for a drug and the total plasma concentration (C_T), the concentration of free drug in the plasma may be determined by a rearranged equation:

$$C_U = \alpha \times (C_T)$$

If the alpha (α) value for the drug digoxin is 0.70, what would be the concentration of free drug in the plasma if the total plasma concentration of the drug were determined to be 0.7 ng/mL?

$$C_U = (0.70) \times (0.7 \text{ ng/mL})$$
$$= 0.49 \text{ ng/mL, } answer.$$

Apparent Volume of Distribution of a Drug Substance

The apparent volume of distribution for a drug is not a "real" volume but rather a hypothetical volume of body fluid that would be required to dissolve the total amount of drug at the same concentration as that found in the blood. The volume of distribution is an indicator of the extent of a drug's distribution throughout the body fluids and tissues. The information is useful in understanding how the body processes and distributes a given drug substance. After a dose of a drug is administered intravenously, a change in the concentration of the drug in the blood means a corresponding change in the drug's concentration in another body fluid or tissue. This sequence allows an understanding of the pattern of the drug's distribution.

It may be useful in understanding the concept of volume of distribution to imagine a 100-mg amount of a drug substance dissolved in an undetermined volume of water. If the analysis of a sample of the resultant solution revealed a drug concentration of 20 mg per liter, it can be seen that the total volume of water in which the drug was dissolved equaled 5 liters; that is:

$$\frac{20 \text{ (mg)}}{100 \text{ (mg)}} = \frac{1 \text{ (liter)}}{x \text{ (liters)}}$$
$$x = 5 \text{ liters}$$

Different drugs administered in the same amount will show different volumes of distribution because of different distribution characteristics. For example, drugs that remain in the blood after intravenous administration because of drug binding to plasma proteins or to blood cells show high blood concentrations and low volumes of distribution. Conversely, drugs that exit the circulation rapidly and diffuse into other body fluids and tissues show low blood concentrations and high volumes of distribution.

If the volume of distribution in an adult is 5 liters, the drug is considered confined to the circulatory system, as it would be immediately after a rapid intravenous injection (IV bolus). If the volume of distribution is between 10 and 20 liters, or between 15% and 27% of the body weight, it is assumed that the drug has been distributed into the extracellular fluids; if it is between 25 and 30 liters, or between 35% and 42% of body weight, it is assumed that the drug has been distributed into the intracellular fluid; if it is about 40 liters, or 60% of the body weight, the assumption is that the drug has been distributed in the whole body fluid.[4] If the apparent volume of distribution actually exceeds the body weight, it is assumed that the drug is being stored in body fat, bound to body tissues, or is distributed in peripheral compartments.

The equation for determining the volume of distribution (Vd) is:

$$Vd = \frac{D}{C_P}$$

in which D is the total amount of drug in the body, and C_p is the drug's plasma concentration. The apparent volume of distribution may be expressed as a simple volume or as a percentage of body weight.

A patient received a single intravenous dose of 300 mg of a drug substance that produced an immediate blood concentration of 8.2 μg of drug per milliliter. Calculate the apparent volume of distribution.

$$Vd = \frac{D}{C_P}$$
$$= \frac{300 \text{ mg}}{8.2 \text{ } \mu g/mL} = \frac{300 \text{ mg}}{8.2 \text{ mg/L}}$$
$$= 36.6 \text{ L, } answer.$$

Calculate the volume of distribution for the drug levofloxacin (LEVAQUIN) which, following an oral dose of 500 mg, resulted in a peak plasma concentration of 5.7 μg/mL in 90 minutes.

$$V_d = \frac{D}{C_P}$$

$$= \frac{500 \text{ mg}}{5.7 \text{ } \mu cg/mL} = \frac{500 \text{ mg}}{5.7 \text{ mg/L}}$$
$$= 87.7 \text{ L, } answer.$$

Total Amount of Drug Given Volume of Distribution and Plasma Concentration

Calculating the total amount of drug in a body, given the volume of distribution and the plasma drug concentration, involves the following.

Four hours following the intravenous administration of a drug, a patient weighing 70 kg was found to have a drug blood level concentration of 10 μg/mL. Assuming the apparent volume of distribution is 10% of body weight, calculate the total amount of drug present in body fluids 4 hours after the drug was administered.

$$Vd = \frac{D}{C_P} \qquad D = (Vd) \times (C_P)$$
$$Vd = 10\% \text{ of } 70 \text{ kg} = 7 \text{ kg} = 7 \text{ L}$$

$$C_P = 10 \ \mu g/mL = 10 \ mg/L$$
$$7 \ L = \frac{D}{10 \ mg/L}$$
$$D = (7 \ L) \times (10 \ mg/L)$$
$$= 70 \ mg, \textit{answer.}$$

Elimination Half-Life and Elimination Rate Constant

The elimination phase of a drug from the body is reflected by a decline in the drug's plasma concentration. The ***elimination half-life*** ($t\frac{1}{2}$) is the time it takes for the plasma drug concentration (as well as the amount of drug in the body) to fall by one half. For example, if it takes 3 hours for the plasma concentration of a drug to fall from 6 to 3 mg/L, its half-life would be 3 hours. It would take the same period of time (3 hours) for the concentration to fall from 3 to 1.5 mg/L, or from 1.5 to 0.75 mg/L. Many drug substances follow first-order kinetics in their elimination from the body, meaning that the rate of drug elimination per unit of time is proportional to the amount present at that time. As demonstrated previously, the elimination half-life is independent of the amount of drug in the body, and the amount of drug eliminated is less in each succeeding half-life. After five elimination half-lives, it may be expected that virtually all of a drug (97%) originally present will have been eliminated. The student might wish to examine this point, starting with a 100-mg dose of a drug (after first half-life, 50 mg, etc.).

Blood level data from a drug may be plotted against time on regular graph paper to obtain an exponential curve, or it may be plotted on semilogarithmic graph paper to obtain a straight line. From the latter, the elimination half-life may be determined, as shown in the example that follows in this section.

The elimination rate constant (K_{el}) characterizes the elimination process and may simply be regarded as the *fractional rate of drug removal per unit time, expressed as a decimal fraction* (e.g., 0.01 min^{-1}, meaning 1% per minute). The elimination rate constant for a first-order process may be calculated using the equation:

$$K_{el} = \frac{0.693}{t_{1/2}}$$

The derivation of this equation is described for the exponential decay of radioisotopes (see Chapter 21).

A patient received 12 mg of a drug intravenously and blood samples were drawn and analyzed at specific time intervals, resulting in the following data. Plot the data on semilogarithmic graph paper and determine the elimination half-life of the drug.

Plasma Drug Level Concentration ($\mu g/100 \ mL$)	Time (hours)
26.5	1
17.5	2
11.5	3
7.6	4
5.0	5
3.3	6

Plotting the data:

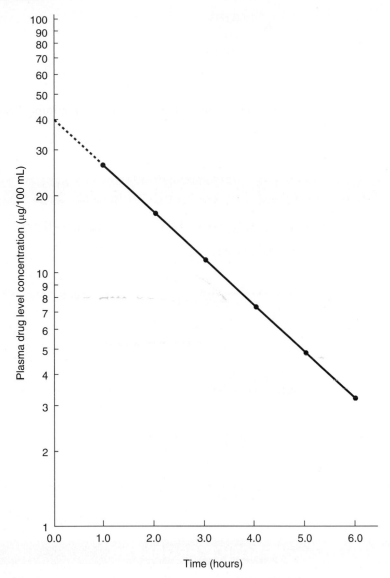

Time (hours)

From the plotted data, the straight line may by extrapolated to time zero to determine the initial plasma drug concentration, which is found to be 40 µg/100 mL. The time it takes to reduce that level to one-half, or 20 µg/100 mL, is the elimination half-life. The 20 µg/100 mL concentration intersects the straight line at 1.7 hours.

Therefore, the elimination half-life is 1.7 hours, *answer*.

Note: The same answer may be obtained by selecting any plasma drug concentration (for example, 10 µg/100 mL), determining the time of that plasma level from the intercept, repeating the process for one-half of that drug level (5 µg/100 mL), and determining the elapsed time by subtraction to obtain the elimination half-life.

Calculate the elimination rate constant for a drug that has an elimination half-life of 50 minutes.

$$K_{el} = \frac{0.693}{t_{1/2}}$$

$$= \frac{0.693}{50 \text{ min}}$$

$$= 0.0139 \text{ min}^{-1}, \text{ } answer.$$

Additional related calculations, such as drug dosage based on creatinine clearance, may be found in Chapter 10.

CALCULATIONS CAPSULE

Selected Bioavailability and Pharmacokinetics

Bioavailability factor (F) for a dosage form:

$$F = \frac{AUC_{dosage \text{ } form}}{AUC_{intravenous}}$$

Volume of distribution (Vd):

$$Vd = \frac{D}{C_P}$$

D = total administered (IV) amount of drug
C_P = blood/plasma concentration of drug

Elimination rate constant (K_{el}):

$$K_{el} = \frac{0.693}{t_{1/2}}$$

PRACTICE PROBLEMS

Calculations of Bioavailability and Bioequivalence

1. If the bioavailability factor (F) for a 100-mg tablet of a drug is 0.70 compared with the bioavailability factor of 1.0 for an injection of the same drug, how many milliliters of the injection containing 40 mg/mL would be considered bioequivalent to the tablet?

2. If 5 mL of an elixir containing 2 mg mL of a drug is bioequivalent to a 15-mg tablet having a bioavailability factor of 0.60, what is the bioavailability factor (F) of the elixir?

3. If 500 mg of a drug are administered orally and 300 mg are absorbed into the circulation, calculate the bioavailability factor (F).

4.[3] A drug is 40% bioavailable by the oral route and 58% bioavailable by the transdermal route. If a patient is taking a 2.5-mg oral dose twice a day and is switched to the counterpart 2% ointment, how many grams of the

PRACTICE PROBLEMS

ointment should be administered to provide the equivalent dose of the drug?

5.[3] A drug used to treat asthma is 55% bioavailable as 5-mg tablets. If a patient is switched to the inhalant form of the drug, which is 87% bioavailable, how many metered 500-µg sprays should the patient administer every 12 hours to receive an equivalent drug dose?

Calculations of Bound Drug, Elimination Half-Life, and Volume of Distribution

6.[3] If a 6-mg dose of a drug is administered intravenously and produces a blood concentration of 0.4 µg mL, calculate its apparent volume of distribution.

7. If at equilibrium, two thirds of the amount of a drug substance in the blood is bound to protein, what would be the alpha (α) value of the drug?

8. The alpha (α) value for a drug in the blood is 0.90, equating to 0.55 ng/mL. What is the concentration of total drug in the blood?

9. A patient received an intravenous dose of 10 mg of a drug. A blood sample was drawn, and it contained 40 µg/100 mL. Calculate the apparent volume of distribution for the drug.

10. The volume of distribution for a drug was found to be 10 liters with a blood level concentration of 2 µg/mL. Calculate the total amount of drug present in the patient.

11. Calculate the elimination rate constant for a drug having an elimination half-life of 1.7 hours.

12. Plot the following data on semilogarithmic graph paper and determine (a) the elimination half-life of the drug and (b) the elimination rate constant.

Plasma Drug Concentration (µg/100 mL)	Time (hours)
8.5	0.5
6.8	1.0
5.4	1.5
4.0	2.0
3.2	2.5
2.5	3.0

13. What percentage of an originally administered intravenous dose of a drug remains in the body following three half-lives?

14. If the half-life of a drug is 4 hours, approximately what percentage of the drug administered would remain in the body 15 hours after administration?

15. If 100 mg of a drug are administered intravenously, and the resultant drug plasma concentration is determined to be 2.5 µg/mL, calculate the apparent volume of distribution.

16. If a dose of 1 g of a drug is administered intravenously to a patient and the drug plasma concentration is determined to be 65 µg/mL, calculate the apparent volume of distribution.

17. The volume of distribution for chlordiazepoxide has been determined to be 34 liters. Calculate the expected drug plasma concentration of the drug, in micrograms per deciliter, immediately after an intravenous dose of 5 mg.

18. In normal subjects, blood makes up about 7% of the body weight.

    (a) Calculate the approximate blood volume, in liters, for a man weighing 70 kg.

    (b) If the drug ZANTAC reached peak blood levels of about 500 ng/mL 2 to 3 hours after an oral dose, calculate the total amount of the drug, in milligrams, in the blood of the patient described in (a) when peak blood levels are achieved.

CALCQUIZ

22.A. A package insert for cefdinir capsules and oral suspension states that following oral administration, the bioavailability of cefdinir suspension is 120% relative to the capsules. The bioavailability of cefdinir capsules is stated as 21% following the administration of a 300-mg capsule dose and 16% following the administration of a 600-mg capsule dose. Calculate the bioavailable quantity of cefdinir, in milligrams, following the administration of a dose of the oral suspension containing 300 mg of cefdinir.

22.B.[a] The drug aminophylline is 80% theophylline. A patient to be discharged from the hospital has been receiving aminophylline 40 mg/h by IV infusion. Upon discharge, the physician orders oral theophylline tablets. The pharmacist recognizes that the prescribed tablets have 85% bioavailability. What oral daily dose, in milligrams of theophylline, should the patient receive by tablets?

22.C. Following the subcutaneous injection of 100 μg of the drug octreotide acetate, a peak plasma concentration of 5.2 ng/mL is reached in 24 minutes. Calculate the apparent volume of distribution. If the drug's half-life is stated in the literature as 1.8 hours, calculate the elimination rate constant.

[a]Problem courtesy of Flynn Warren, Bishop, GA.

ANSWERS TO "CASE IN POINT" AND PRACTICE PROBLEMS

Case in Point 22.1

IV daily dose

$$= \frac{50 \text{ mg}}{1 \text{ dose}} \times \frac{3 \text{ doses}}{1 \text{ day}} = 150 \text{ mg/day}$$

F for the IV route = 1 or 100%

$100\% \times 150 \text{ mg/day} = 50\% \times \text{Dose}_{oral}$

$\text{Dose}_{oral} = 300 \text{ mg/day}$

$$\frac{300 \text{ mg}}{1 \text{ day}} \times \frac{1 \text{ day}}{2 \text{ doses}} = 150 \text{ mg/dose}$$

$$\frac{150 \text{ mg}}{1 \text{ dose}} \times \frac{5 \text{ mL}}{75 \text{ mg}} = 10 \text{ mL/dose}, \text{ } answer.$$

Practice Problems

1. 1.75 mL injection
2. 0.9
3. 0.6
4. 0.17 g ointment
5. 3.16 or 3 sprays
6. 15 L
7. 0.33
8. 0.61 mg/mL
9. 25 L
10. 20 mg
11. 0.408 hr^{-1}
12. graph
13. 12.5%
14. 7.43%
15. 40 L
16. 15.4 L
17. 14.7 μg/dL chlordiazepoxide
18. (a) 4.9 L
    (b) 2.45 mg ZANTAC

. . . .

References

1. *United States Pharmacopeia 32—National Formulary 27*. Rockville, MD: United States Pharmacopeial Convention, 2009;1:263–270.
2. Chereson R. Bioavailability, bioequivalence, and drug selection. Available at: http://www.pharmacyonline. creighton.edu/pha443/pdf/pkin08.pdf. Accessed September 25, 2008.
3. Prince SJ. In: Ansel HC, Prince SJ. *Pharmaceutical Calculations: The Pharmacist's Handbook*. Baltimore: Lippincott Williams & Wilkins, 2004:150–164.
4. Ritschel WA. *Handbook of Basic Pharmacokinetics*. 2nd ed. Hamilton, IL: Drug Intelligence Publications, 1982:219.

Objectives

Upon successful completion of this chapter, the student will be able to:

- Differentiate between the pharmacoeconomic methods: *cost-benefit analysis*, *cost-effectiveness analysis*, and *cost-minimization analysis* and perform example calculations of each.
- Perform cost-differential calculations between branded drug products and generic equivalents.
- Perform cost-differential calculations between dosage forms and routes of administration.
- Perform cost-differential calculations based on dosing regimens.
- Perform cost-differential calculations based on alternative treatment plans.
- Perform cost-differential calculations based on patient conversions.

In the broad context, the term ***pharmacoeconomics*** refers to all aspects of costs and therapeutic outcomes associated with the use of pharmaceuticals in health care. It encompasses many considerations including drug acquisition costs, cost/benefit relationships of drug therapy decisions, nondrug treatment alternatives, and health outcomes; factors associated with drug product selection and drug formulary decisions; cost/benefit of pharmacist-provided medication therapy management (MTM) services; the impact of proper drug utilization on incidence of hospitalization and length of stay; economic and health consequences of patient noncompliance, drug misuse, and adverse drug reactions; and the demographics of medication use by patients of various age groups, gender, and socioeconomic status, among other factors.

Pharmacoeconomics is the subject of much current research, with a broad array of information available in the primary literature and through various references and textbooks dedicated to the topic. The scope of this chapter necessarily is limited to the presentation of some introductory calculations. Calculations pertaining to drug acquisition costs, mark-up, selling price, discounts, and methods of prescription pricing may be found in earlier editions of this textbook.

Pharmacoeconomic Methods of Analysis

There are a number of established methods of pharmacoeconomic analysis, including *cost-benefit analysis (CBA)*, *cost-effectiveness analysis (CEA)*, and *cost-minimization analysis (CMA)*.[1-3]

Example Calculations for Pharmacoeconomic Methods of Analysis

Cost-Benefit Analysis (CBA)

Cost-benefit analysis involves identifying and measuring all the costs of providing a program or treatment and comparing those costs with the benefits that result. The analysis is expressed through a *benefit-to-cost ratio, that is:*

$$\text{Benefit-to-cost ratio} = \frac{\text{Benefits (\$)}}{\text{Costs (\$)}}$$

Obviously, if the data inserted in the ratio yield a number greater than 1, the benefits exceed the costs, and the program or treatment is considered beneficial.

Determine the benefit-to-cost ratio for a program in which the cost of pharmacist intervention was determined to be $12,000 and the benefits accrued to be $26,000.

$$\text{Benefit-to-cost ratio} = \frac{\$26,000}{\$12,000} = 2.167 \text{ or } 2.2, \textit{ answer.}$$

Cost-Effectiveness Analysis (CEA)

Cost-effectiveness analysis may be used to compare treatment alternatives with cost measured in dollars and treatment outcomes expressed in terms of the therapeutic objective (as the lowering of blood cholesterol). The results are expressed through a *cost-to-effectiveness (C/E) ratio*, that is:

$$\text{Cost-to-effectiveness ratio} = \frac{\text{Costs (\$)}}{\text{Therapeutic effect (in measurable units)}}$$

Determine the cost-effectiveness ratios for two 12-month treatments for the lowering of systolic blood pressure. Treatment A cost $1200 and lowered systolic blood pressure by an average of 5 mm of mercury. Treatment B cost $800 and lowered systolic blood pressure by an average of 8 mm of mercury.

$$\text{Treatment A} : \text{C/E ratio} = \frac{\$1200}{5 \text{ mm Hg}} = 240 \, (\$/\text{mm Hg}), \textit{ and}$$

$$\text{Treatment B} : \text{C/E ratio} = \frac{\$800}{8 \text{ mm Hg}} = 100 \, (\$/\text{mm Hg}), \textit{ answers.}$$

Cost-Minimization Analysis (CMA)

Cost-minimization analysis involves the comparison of two or more treatment alternatives, the outcomes of which are assumed or determined to be equivalent. The cost of each treatment alternative is expressed in dollars, and the costs are compared.

If cost minimization analyses demonstrate that two alternative treatments cost $1120 (treatment A) and $1450 (treatment B), respectively, calculate the cost benefit of treatment A compared with treatment B.

$$\$1450 - \$1120 = \$330, \textit{ answer.}$$

Cost Considerations of Drug and Drug Product Selection

Drug therapy and other means of treatment (e.g., surgery) are intended to serve the health care interests of the patient while being cost effective. In prescribing drug therapy, clinical as well as economic factors are important considerations in the selection of the drug substance and drug product. For example, if an expensive drug reduces morbidity and hospitalization time, it is considered both therapeutically advantageous and cost effective. If, however, a less expensive drug would provide therapeutic benefit comparable to the more expensive drug, the less costly drug is likely to be selected for use. Interventions by pharmacists in pharmaceutical care decisions have been shown to be cost effective and can enhance therapeutic outcomes.

In general, new drug entities and/or novel dosage forms that are protected by patents and are available from only a single source are more expensive than older, off-patent drugs available from multiple manufacturers or distributors. *Multisource pharmaceuticals* generally are lower priced because, unlike the innovator product, they do not bear the original research costs incurred in developing and bringing the new drug to market. Multisource pharmaceuticals generally are available to the pharmacist both as brand name and generic products and at a range of prices. For economic reasons, the prescribing physician, patient, health care institution, state or federally sponsored program, or other third-party payer may request or reimburse only for the dispensing of a generic product, when available. Whereas the term *generic equivalent* is used to describe FDA-approved subsequent versions of innovator small-molecule drugs, the term *biosimilars* is used for approved subsequent versions of innovator biopharmaceutical products.

It is common practice for drug use decision makers, such as drug formulary committees at hospitals, to establish a list of drugs approved for use and funding that balances therapeutic outcome and cost containment goals. Drug and drug product selection choices may be presented to prescribers on the basis of cost per day or cost per course of treatment.

Programs that are directed toward changing a patient's current drug, drug product, or route of drug administration often are referred to as ***conversion programs***.

Example Calculations Based on Drug or Drug Product Selection

Cost Differential Between Therapeutic Agents

Often there is a substantial cost differential between therapeutic agents within a therapeutic category. The cost differential may be based on the newness, innovation, patent status, and/or the cost of development or production of some members of the therapeutic class compared with others. In general, newer agents introduced into the marketplace are more expensive than older counterpart drugs. *Therapeutic interchange* programs, which allow for the substitution of one drug for another while maintaining comparable therapeutic benefit, can result in cost savings.

Calculate the cost differential between the thrombolytic agents streptokinase (250,000 IU; $96.41) and the biotechnology derived drug alteplase (50 mg; $1,100) if the total amount proposed to be administered to a patient is either 1,500,000 IU of streptokinase or 90 mg of alteplase.

$$\text{Cost of streptokinase}: \quad \frac{250{,}000\,\text{IU}}{1{,}500{,}000\,\text{IU}} = \frac{\$96.41}{x}; \quad x = \$578.46,\ and$$

$$\text{Cost of alteplase}: \quad \frac{50\,\text{mg}}{90\,\text{mg}} = \frac{\$1100}{x}; \quad x = \$1980,\ and$$

$$\text{Cost differential}: \quad \$1980 - \$578.46 = \$1401.54,\ answer.$$

Cost Differential Between Branded Drug Products and Generic Equivalents

Drugs introduced to the marketplace as innovator, patented, and brand-name products often remain higher in price than generic equivalents, even after their patent protections expire. *Drug product selection* decisions may be made on this cost basis by health care providers, consumers, and insurance or health benefits managers.

The generic equivalent of a drug costs $12.40/100 tablets, whereas the innovator product costs $46.20/100 tablets. Calculate the drug cost differential for a 30-day supply if two tablets are taken daily.

Tablets required: 2 tablets (daily) × 30 (days) = 60 tablets

Cost of generic drug : $\dfrac{100\,\text{tablets}}{60\,\text{tablets}} = \dfrac{\$12.40}{x}$; x = $7.44, *and*

Cost of innovator drug : $\dfrac{100\,\text{tablets}}{60\,\text{tablets}} = \dfrac{\$46.20}{x}$; x = $27.72, *and*

Cost differential: $27.72 − $7.44 = $20.28, *answer*.

Cost Differential Between Dosage Forms and Routes of Administration

There is often a cost differential between dosage forms of the same therapeutic agent due to the costs of development or production. For instance, tablets are generally less expensive to develop and manufacture than are liquid forms, with injectable products and transdermal patches being among the most expensive. For patients receiving intravenous therapy, the associated costs are expanded greatly by the additional personnel and adjunctive materials and equipment needed to administer the medication. Many hospital cost containment programs encourage the conversion from parenteral medications to oral therapy as soon as feasible without compromising the desired therapeutic outcomes.

Verapamil 80-mg tablets are taken three times a day and cost $7.52/100 tablets. Extended-release capsules containing 240 mg of verapamil are taken once daily and cost $15.52/100 capsules. Calculate the treatment cost differential over a 30-day period.

80-mg tablets: $7.52 ÷ 100 (tablets) = $0.0752 (per tablet)
3 tablets (per day) × 30 (days) = 90 tablets
$0.0752 × 90 (tablets) = $6.768 or $6.77, *and*

240-mg capsules: $15.52 ÷ 100 (capsules) = $0.1552 (per capsule)
1 capsule (per day) × 30 (days) = 30 capsules
$0.01552 × 30 (capsules) = $4.656 or $4.66, *and*

Cost differential: $6.77 − $4.66 = $2.11, *answer*.

A hospitalized patient was switched from intravenous ciprofloxacin (400 mg q12h) to oral ciprofloxacin (500 mg q12h). Calculate the daily drug cost savings if the intravenous product cost is $12.00 per 200 mg and the oral product cost is $2.95 per 250-mg capsule.

Intravenous ciprofloxacin: 400 mg × 2 (times per day) = 800 mg
800 mg × $12.00/200 mg = $48.00, *and*

Oral ciprofloxacin: 500 mg × 2 (times per day) = 1000 mg
1000 mg × $2.95/250 mg = $11.80, *and*

Cost differential: $48.00 − $11.80 = $36.20, *answer*.

Cost Differential of Dosing Regimens

A dosing regimen for a specific drug may be changed to be more cost effective without affecting the desired therapeutic outcome.

A dosage interval adjustment was made in the intravenous administration of the drug ranitidine in a group of 23 hospitalized patients such that the number of doses per patient per treatment day was reduced from an average of 2.33 to 1.51 without sacrificing therapeutic outcomes. If the cost of each dose of ranitidine was $4.02, calculate the daily cost savings to the hospital.

Reduction in doses per patient per day:	2.33–1.51 = 0.82 doses
Reduction in doses in patient group:	0.82 dose × 23 (patients) = 18.86 doses
Cost savings:	$4.02 × 18.86 (doses) = $75.8172 or $75.82, *answer.*

Cost Differential of Drug Product Modification

One example of drug product modification for the purpose of economic advantage is the practice of tablet splitting in which tablets are prescribed and dispensed at twice the strength but in half the quantity.

A physician prescribed fifteen 80-mg tablets of simvastatin tablets and instructed the patient to split the tablets in half for a 30-day supply at a 40-mg daily dose. One hundred 80-mg tablets cost $12.50 and an equal number of 40-mg tablets cost $10.50. Calculate the patient's savings on a month's supply.

80-mg tablets: 15 tablets × $12.50/100 tablets = $1.88
40-mg tablets: 30 tablets × $10.50/100 tablets = $3.15
$3.15 – $1.88 = $1.27 savings, *answer.*

Cost Differential of Alternative Treatment Plans

Preventive medicine, drug therapy, surgery, radiation, and many other choices may be valid alternatives in maintaining health or in treating illness.

If the daily treatment of an ulcer patient with cimetidine prevents readmission to a hospital, calculate the potential savings over reoccurrence of hospitalization if the daily drug costs are $1.38 and the prior 5-day hospital bill was $4056.

Drug cost:	$1.38 × 5 (days) = $6.90
Potential savings:	$4056 – $6.90 = $4049.10, *answer.*

CASE IN POINT 23.1: A hospital's Pharmacy and Therapeutics Committee is determining the most economical of three drugs considered to be therapeutically equivalent. The least expensive drug, per patient treatment day, is to be added to the hospital's drug formulary.

Drug A: 0.5 g/mL, 5-mL vial; dose, 1 mL q6h; cost, $16.50/vial
Drug B: 1 g/mL, 10-mL vial; dose, 0.75 mL q8h; cost, $57.42/vial
Drug C: 1.5 g/mL, 1-mL ampul; dose, 1 mL q12h; cost, $15.94/ampul

Which drug is most economical, per patient treatment day, not taking into consideration any material or personnel costs?

Cost Differential in Delivering Medication Therapy Management Services

Medication therapy management (MTM) services involve pharmacist interventions and counseling services, which promotes and provides the safe and effective use of medications to achieve the targeted outcomes from medication therapy. The costs associated with such services include direct costs (e.g., pharmacist's salary) and indirect costs (e.g., all pharmacy operations overhead).[5] Costs include personnel expenses (salary, benefits, etc.) of the clerk who greets the patient, the pharmacy technician or pharmacy student who enters input into the patient's medication record, and the pharmacist who interprets the medication record, consults with the patient, and together with the patient formulates a plan to achieve the therapeutic outcomes.[5] One calculation of the many involved in providing MTM services involves personnel costs.

By one estimate, personnel expenses in the provision of a single MTM service includes the time and costs as follows: pharmacy clerk, 5 minutes @ $8.00/h; pharmacy technician 10 minutes @ $13.50/h; and pharmacist, 15 minutes @ $65/h. Calculate the personnel cost in delivering a single MTM service.[5]

Pharmacy clerk: 5 min × $8.00/60 min = $0.67
Pharmacy technician: 10 min × $13.50/60 min = $2.25
Pharmacist: 15 min × $65.00/60 min = $16.25
Total: $0.67 + $2.25 + $16.25 = $19.17, *answer.*

PRACTICE PROBLEMS

Pharmacoeconomic Methods of Analysis Calculations

1. Using the ratio for cost-benefit analysis, determine the numerical result of a program in which pharmacist intervention costing $8875 resulted in benefits valued at $14,200.

2. Using the ratio for cost-effectiveness analysis, determine the numerical difference between two drug therapies for total serum cholesterol reduction in which treatment A, costing $55, lowered total cholesterol by 5 dg/100 mL of serum, and treatment B, costing $98, lowered total cholesterol by 7 dg/100 mL of serum.

Drug and Drug Product Selection and Utilization Calculations

3. An antianginal drug is available in a three-times-a-day tablet at $42.50/100 tablets, in a twice-a-day tablet at $64.00/100 tablets, and in a once-a-day tablet at $80.20/100 tablets. Which form would be most economical to a compliant patient and at what cost?

4. A physician inquires of a pharmacist regarding the most economical of the following antihypertensive therapies: drug A, 30-mg tablets taken q.i.d. costing $0.33/tablet; drug B, 10-mg tablets taken t.i.d. costing $0.20/tablet; or drug C, 2.5-mg tablets taken b.i.d, costing $0.38/tablet. Indicate the most economical drug and the drug cost for a 30-day supply.

5. A physician offers a patient the option of prescribing 30 scored ZOLOFT 100-mg tablets (for the patient to break in half with a dose of one-half tablet) or 60 tablets containing

50 mg of the drug. Calculate the cost differential and indicate the most economical option for the patient if the 100-mg tablets cost $126.78 per 100 tablets and the 50-mg tablets cost $115.00 per 100 tablets.

6. Calculate the daily drug cost differential between a dose of a drug administered q8h and costing $6.25/dose and a counterpart drug administered once daily and costing $26.50/dose.

7. If 100 tablets of an innovator drug cost $114.50 and 60 tablets of a generic equivalent cost $27.75, calculate the cost differential for a 30-day supply.

8. A pharmacist can purchase 5-mg tablets of a drug at (a) $16.21 for a bottle of 100 tablets, (b) $73.41 for a bottle of 500 tablets, or (c) $124.25 for a bottle of 1000 tablets. Calculate the drug costs for each of the package sizes to fill a prescription for 60 tablets.

9. A hospital pharmacy recommended parenteral cefazolin (dose: 0.5 g q8h; cost: $1.80/g) over parenteral cefoxitin (dose: 1 g q6h; cost: $6.48/g) to balance therapeutic outcomes with cost containment. Calculate the difference in drug cost between these two treatments per patient day.

10. An anti-AIDS compound is commonly taken at an adult daily dose of 600 mg, in two or more divided doses. If 300-mg tablets cost $265 per 60, calculate the drug cost per year.

11. The drug hydralazine may be administered intravenously when needed to control hypertension at 20-mg doses in D5W every 12 hours for 48 hours, after which the patient is converted to oral dosage, 10-mg tablets four times per day for 2 days, then 25-mg tablets four times per day for the next 5 days. If the 20-mg IV ampul costs $6.00; 10-mg tablets, $18.00/100 tablets; 25-mg tablets, $26.00/100 tablets; and D5W, $10.00 per bottle, calculate the *average daily* costs of intravenous and oral therapy.

12. A physician has a choice of prescribing the following ACE inhibitor drugs to treat hypertension, with the pharmacist's cost of each, per 100 tablets, given in parentheses: drug A, 10 mg ($63.00); drug B, 25 mg ($59.00); drug C, 5 mg ($84.00); and drug D, 10 mg ($70.00). Each drug is once-a-day dosing except for drug B tablets, which are taken twice a day. Calculate the 30-day medication cost for each drug.

13. The cost to a hospital of a drug is $16.97 per 10-mg vial. If the drug is administered by intermittent injection at 0.15 mg/kg/hr for 24 hours, calculate the daily cost of the drug used for a 70-kg patient.

14. If the drug in the preceding problem may be administered to the same patient by continuous infusion (rather than by intermittent injection) with a 0.1 mg/kg loading dose and subsequent doses of 0.05 mg/kg for the next 23 hours, calculate the daily cost of the drug by this route of administration.

15. The intravenous dosing schedules and costs of the following cephalosporin antimicrobial agents are: cefazolin, 1 g every 8 hours ($3.00); cefoxitin, 1 g every 6 hours ($6.24); and Cefotan, 1 g every 24 hours ($31.39). Calculate the daily cost of each drug.

CALCQUIZ

23.A.[a] Colchicine and nonsteroidal anti-inflammatory drugs (NSAIDs) are included among the treatments of gout. Treatment with colchicine results in fewer adverse effects than does treatment with NSAIDs. The average monthly drug-only cost of colchicine may run 10 times the approximate $30 per month cost for NSAIDs. On the other hand, for the 1.8% to 1.9% of gout patients receiving NSAIDs who require hospitalization due to a serious adverse event, the cost of hospitalization at $____ per day for an average of 5 days is a serious factor to consider in drug selection.

Student research: obtain, and utilize in the calculations, information on the average daily hospitalization cost in the local community, region, or nation.

Calculate: the comparative monthly treatment costs for two hypothetical 100-patient treatment groups, one (NSAID) with average incidence of adverse effects, and the other group taking colchicine.

23.B.[b] Utilizing relevant information in this chapter, calculate the estimated average monthly cost of providing MTM services in a pharmacy which provides 120 individual occasions of MTM services per month utilizing:

    4 minutes of clerk-time/each MTM service
    5 minutes of pharmacy-student time/each MTM service
    13 minutes of pharmacist-time/each MTM service and
    $16.35/each MTM service for associated costs (materials, overhead, etc.)

23.C. A pharmacist-member of a hospital formulary committee compared the cost of 10 days of IV therapy with moxifloxacin hydrochloride (400 mg/250 mL IV once daily) against 4 days of IV therapy (400 mg/250 mL IV once daily) followed by 6 days of oral moxifloxacin hydrochloride therapy (400 mg tablets PO once daily).

Student research: obtain information on the usual pharmacy acquisition costs of the medications-dosage forms in the problem.

Calculate: the difference in the cost of 10 days of medication for the two treatments.

---

[a]Problem derived from data from Wertheimer et al.[4]
[b]Problem derived from data from Kupp.[5]

ANSWERS TO "CASE IN POINT" AND PRACTICE PROBLEMS

Case in Point 23.1

Drug A dose, in mL/day:
1 mL/dose × 4 doses/day = 4 mL/day

Cost/day:

$$\frac{5 \text{ mL}}{\$16.50} = \frac{4 \text{ mL}}{x} \quad x = \$13.20/\text{day}$$

Drug B dose, in mL/day:
0.75 mL/dose × 3 doses/day = 2.25 mL/day

Cost/day:

$$\frac{10 \text{ mL}}{\$57.42} = \frac{2.25}{x} \quad x = \$12.92/\text{day}$$

Drug C dose, in mL/day:
1 mL/dose × 2 doses/day = 2 mL/day

Cost/day:

$$\frac{1 \text{ mL}}{\$15.94} = \frac{2 \text{ mL}}{x} \quad x = \$31.84/\text{day}$$

Therefore, drug B is the least expensive per day, *answer*.

Practice Problems

1. 1.6
2. $3/dg
3. once-a-day tablet, $0.80/day
4. drug B, $18.00
5. $30.97, 100-mg tablets
6. $7.75
7. $20.47
8. (a) $9.73
   (b) $8.81
   (c) $7.46
9. $23.22
10. $3224.17
11. IV therapy, $32.00 per day, average oral therapy, $0.74 per day, average
12. drug A, $18.90
    drug B, $35.40
    drug C, $25.20
    drug D, $21.00
13. $427.64
14. $148.49
15. cefazolin, $9.00
    cefoxitin, $24.96
    cefotan, $31.39

References

1. Sanchez LA. Pharmacoeconomic principles and methods: an introduction for hospital pharmacists. *Hospital Pharmacy* 1994;29:774–779.
2. Gurnee MC, Sylvestri MF, Ortmeier BG. Understanding the basic principles of pharmacoeconomics. *Managed Care Pharmacy Practice* 1995;2:34–42.
3. Draugalis JR, Bootman JL, Larson LN, et al. Pharmacoeconomics. *Current Concepts* 1989;1–32.
4. Wertheimer AI, Davis MW, Lauterio TJ. A new perspective of the pharmacoeconomics of colchicine. *Current Medical Research and Opinion* 2011;27:931–937.
5. Rupp MT. Analyzing the costs to deliver medication therapy management services. *Pharmacy Today* 2011;17:56–64.

Appendices

Common Systems of Measurement and Intersystem Conversion

The International System of Units (SI) is the *official* system for weights and measures in the *United States Pharmacopeia—National Formulary*. However, other so-called *common systems of measurement* are encountered in pharmacy and must be recognized and understood. The **apothecaries' system of measurement** is the traditional system of pharmacy, and although it is now largely of historic significance, components of this system are occasionally found on prescriptions. The **avoirdupois system** is the common system of commerce, employed along with the SI in the United States. It is through this system that items are purchased and sold by the ounce and pound. This appendix defines these common systems, expresses their quantitative relationship to one another and to the SI, and provides the means for intersystem conversion. Conversion of temperature between the Fahrenheit and Celsius (or centigrade) scales, and alcohol conversion of proof strength are also included in this appendix.

Apothecaries' Fluid Measure

60 minims (♏) = 1 fluidrachm or fluidram (f℥ or ℥)[a]
8 fluidrachms (480 minims) = 1 fluidounce (f℥ or ℥)[a]
16 fluidounces = 1 pint (pt)
2 pints (32 fluidounces) = 1 quart (qt)
4 quarts (8 pints) = 1 gallon (gal)

This table may also be written:

gal	qt	pt	f℥	f℥	♏
1	4	8	128	1024	61440
	1	2	32	256	15360
		1	16	128	7680
			1	8	480
				1	60

Apothecaries' Measure of Weight

20 grains (gr) = 1 scruple (Ɵ)
3 scruples (60 grains) = 1 drachm or dram (ʒ)
8 drachms (480 grains) = 1 ounce (℥)
12 ounces (5760 grains) = 1 pound (℔)

This table may also be written:

℔	℥	ʒ	Ɵ	gr
1	12	96	288	5760
	1	8	24	480
		1	3	60
			1	20

---

[a] When it is clear that a liquid is to be measured, the *f* may be omitted in this symbol.

A typical set of Apothecaries' Weights consists of the following units:

ʒii   ʒi   ʒss   Ʒii   Ʒi   ƷSS   Ɵii   Ɵi   Ɵss

5-grain, 4-grain, 3-grain, 2-grain, 1-grain, ½-grain

Avoirdupois Measure of Weight

437½ or 437.5 grain (gr) = 1 ounce (oz.)
16 ounces (7000 grains) = 1 pound (lb.)

This table may also be written:

lb.	*oz.*	*gr*
1	16	7000
	1	437.5

Fundamental Operations and Calculations

The *grain* has a value common to the apothecaries' and avoirdupois systems of measuring weight.

Bulk or stock packages of powdered drugs and chemicals (and occasionally some liquids when they are sold by weight) are customarily provided to the pharmacist in avoirdupois units of weight by manufacturers and wholesalers. The pharmacist likewise sells bulk packages of nonprescription drug and chemical items by the avoirdupois system.

In contrast with the invariable use of *simple* quantities in the metric system, measurements in the common systems are recorded whenever possible in *compound quantities*, i.e., quantities expressed in two or more denominations. So, 20 fʒ; may be used during the process of calculating, but as a final result, it should be recorded as 1 pt 4 fʒ.

In days gone by, when prescriptions were written in the apothecaries' system, the following format was used, with Roman numerals placed after the abbreviations or symbols for the denominations.

℞	Codeine Sulfate	gr iv
	Ammonium Chloride	ʒ iss
	Cherry Syrup ad	fʒ iv
	Sig. ʒi as directed.	

Example Calculations in the Apothecaries' system

Usually, before a compound quantity can be used in a calculation, it must be expressed in terms of a single denomination. To do so, each denomination in the compound quantity must be reduced to the required denomination and the results added.

Reduce ʒss ʒii Ɵi to grains.

$$\begin{aligned}
\text{ʒss} &= \tfrac{1}{2} \times 480 \text{ gr} = 240 \text{ gr} \\
\text{ʒii} &= 2 \times 60 \ \text{ gr} = 120 \text{ gr} \\
\text{Ɵi} &= 1 \times 20 \ \text{ gr} = \underline{\ 20 \text{ gr}} \\
& \qquad\qquad\qquad\quad 380 \text{ gr, } answer.
\end{aligned}$$

Reduce fʒiv fʒiiss to fluidrachms.

$$\begin{aligned}
\text{fʒiv} &= 4 \times 8 \text{ fʒ} = 32 \quad \text{fʒ} \\
\text{fʒiiss} &= \underline{\ 2\tfrac{1}{2} \text{ fʒ}} \\
& \qquad\qquad\quad 34\tfrac{1}{2} \text{ fʒ, } answer.
\end{aligned}$$

Addition or Subtraction

To add or subtract quantities in the common systems, reduce to a common denomination, add or subtract, and reduce the result (unless it is to be used in further calculations) to a compound quantity.

A formula contains Əii of ingredient A, ʒi of ingredient B, ʒiv of ingredient C, and gr viiss of ingredient D. Calculate the total weight of the ingredients.

$$
\begin{aligned}
\text{Əii} &= 2 \times 20 \text{ gr} = 40 \quad \text{gr} \\
\text{ʒi} &= 1 \times 60 \text{ gr} = 60 \quad \text{gr} \\
\text{ʒiv} &= 4 \times 60 \text{ gr} = 240 \quad \text{gr} \\
\text{gr viiss} &= \underline{7\tfrac{1}{2} \text{ gr}} \\
& 347\tfrac{1}{2} \text{ gr} = 5 \ \text{ʒ} \ 2 \ \text{Ə} \ 7\tfrac{1}{2} \text{ gr, } \textit{answer.}
\end{aligned}
$$

A pharmacist had 1 gallon of alcohol. At different times, he dispensed f ʒiv, 2 pt, f ℥viii, and fʒiv. What volume of alcohol was left?

$$
\begin{aligned}
\text{fʒiv} & = 4 \quad \text{fʒ} \\
2 \text{ pt} &= 2 \times 16 \text{ fʒ} = 32 \quad \text{fʒ} \\
\text{f℥viii} & = 8 \quad \text{fʒ} \\
\text{fʒiv} & = \underline{\tfrac{1}{2} \quad \text{fʒ}} \\
& \phantom{= 2 \times 16 \text{ fʒ}} 44\tfrac{1}{2} \text{ fʒ, } \textit{total dispensed.} \\[4pt]
1 \text{ gal} &= 128 \quad \text{fʒ} \\
& \underline{- 44\tfrac{1}{2} \text{ fʒ}} \\
& 83\tfrac{1}{2} \text{ fʒ} = 5 \text{ pt } 3 \text{ fʒ } 4 \text{ fʒ, } \textit{answer.}
\end{aligned}
$$

Multiplication and Division

A *simple* quantity may be multiplied or divided by any *pure* number.

A prescription for 24 capsules calls for gr ¼ of ingredient A, Əss of ingredient B, and gr v of ingredient C in each powder. How much of each ingredient should be used in compounding the prescription?

$$
\begin{aligned}
24 \times \text{gr } \tfrac{1}{4} &= 6 \text{ gr of ingredient A,} \\
24 \times \tfrac{1}{2} \text{ Ə} &= 12 \text{ Ə, or } 4 \text{ ʒ of ingredient B,} \\
24 \times \text{gr v} &= 120 \text{ gr, or } 2 \text{ ʒ of ingredient C, } \textit{answers.}
\end{aligned}
$$

How many 15-minim doses can be obtained from a mixture containing f℥iii of one ingredient and fʒii of another?

$$
\begin{aligned}
\text{f℥iii} &= 3 \times 480 \text{ ♏} = 1440 \text{ ♏} \\
\text{fʒii} &= 2 \times 60 \text{ ♏} = \underline{120 \text{ ♏}} \\
& \phantom{= 2 \times 60 } 1560 \text{ ♏, } \textit{total.} \\
{}^{1560}/_{15} \text{ doses} &= 104 \text{ doses, } \textit{answer.}
\end{aligned}
$$

Relationship Between Avoirdupois and Apothecaries' Weights

As noted previously, the *grain* is the same in both the avoirdupois and apothecaries' systems of weight, but other denominations with the same names (the *ounce* and the *pound*) are not equal.

To convert from either system to the other, first reduce the given quantity to grains in the one system, and then reduce to any desired denomination in the other system.

The custom of buying chemicals by avoirdupois weight and compounding prescriptions by apothecaries' weight leads to problems, many of which can be most conveniently solved by proportion.

Example Calculations Involving the Avoirdupois System

Convert ℥ii ʒii to avoirdupois weight.

$$℥ii = 2 \times 480 \text{ gr} = 960 \text{ gr}$$
$$ʒii = 2 \times 60 \text{ gr} = \underline{120 \text{ gr}}$$
$$\text{Total:} \qquad\qquad 1080 \text{ gr}$$

$$1 \text{ oz} = 437.5 \text{ gr}$$
$$\frac{1080}{437.5} \text{ oz} = 2 \text{ oz, } 205 \text{ gr, } answer.$$

How many grains of a chemical are left in a 1-oz (avoir). bottle after ʒvii are dispensed from it?

$$1 \text{ oz} = 1 \times 437.5 \text{ gr} = 437.5 \text{ gr}$$
$$ʒvii = 7 \times 60 \text{ gr} \qquad = \underline{420.0 \text{ gr}}$$
$$\text{Difference:} \qquad\qquad 17.5 \text{ gr, } answer.$$

If a drug costs $8.75 per oz (avoir.), what is the cost of 2 ʒ?

$$1 \text{ oz} = 437.5 \text{ gr, and } 2 ʒ = 120 \text{ gr}$$
$$\frac{437.5 \text{ (gr)}}{120 \text{ (gr)}} = \frac{8.75 \text{ (\$)}}{x \text{ (\$)}}$$
$$x = \$2.40, \quad answer.$$

Intersystem Conversion

In pharmacy and medicine, the SI currently predominates in use over the common systems. Most prescriptions and medication orders are written in the SI, and labeling on prefabricated pharmaceutical products has drug strengths and dosages described in SI units. Manufacturing formulas are similarly expressed almost exclusively in SI units, replacing use of the common systems of measurement.

On occasion, however, it may be necessary to translate a weight or measurement from units of one system to units of another system. This translation is called *conversion*. The translation of a denomination of one system to that of another system requires a *conversion factor* or *conversion equivalent*.

Table A.1 presents both practical and precise conversion equivalents. In most pharmacy practice applications, the practical equivalents may be used. The precise equivalents show their derivation. *The practical equivalents should be memorized.*

Note that such equivalents may be used in two ways. For example, to convert a number of fluidounces to milliliters, *multiply* by 29.57; to convert a number of milliliters to fluidounces, *divide* by 29.57.

Some individuals prefer to set up a ratio of a known equivalent and solve conversion problems by proportion. For example, in determining the number of milliliters in 8 fluidounces,

Table A.1 ▼ PRACTICAL AND PRECISE CONVERSION EQUIVALENTS

UNIT	PRACTICAL PHARMACY EQUIVALENT	PRECISE EQUIVALENT[a]	
Conversion Equivalents of Length			
1 m	39.37 in	39.37008	in
1 in	2.54 cm (exact)		
Conversion Equivalents of Volume			
1 mL	16.23 ♏	16.23073	♏
1 ♏	0.06 mL	0.06161152	mL
1 fʒ	3.69 mL	3.696691	mL
1 f℥	29.57 mL	29.57353	mL
1 pt	473　mL	473.1765	mL
1 gal. (U.S)[b]	3785　mL	3785.412	mL
Conversion Equivalents of Weight			
1 g	15.432 gr	15.43236	gr
1 kg	2.20　lb (avoir.)	2.204623	lb (avoir).
1 gr	0.065 g (65 mg)	0.06479891	g
1 oz. (avoir.)	28.35　g	28.349523125	g
1 ℥	31.1　g	31.1034768	g
1 lb (avoir.)	454　g	453.59237	g
1 lb (apoth.)	373　g	373.2417216	g
Other Useful Equivalents			
1 oz. (avoir)	437.5 gr (exact)		
1 ℥	480 gr (exact)		
1 gal. (U.S.)	128 fʒ (exact)		

[a]Precise equivalents from the National Institute of Standards and Technology. Available at: http://ts.nist.gov/WeightsAndMeasures/Publications/appxc.cfm#1. Accessed March 15, 2011.
[b]The U.S. gallon is specified because the British imperial gallon and other counterpart measures differ substantially, as follows: British imperial gallon, 4545 mL; pint, 568.25 mL; fʒ, 28.412 mL; f℥, 3.55 mL; and ♏, 0.059 mL. Note, however, that the SI is used in both the *United States Pharmacopeia* and *British Pharmacopeia*.

an equivalent relating *milliliters to fluidounces is selected* (1 f℥ = 29.57 mL) and the problem is solved by proportion as follows:

$$\frac{1 \text{ (f℥)}}{8 \text{ (f℥)}} = \frac{29.57 \text{ (mL)}}{x \text{ (mL)}}$$

$$x = 236.56 \text{ mL, } answer.$$

In using the ratio and proportion method, the equivalent that contains both the units named in the problem is the best one to use. Sometimes, more than one equivalent may be appropriate. For instance, in converting grams to grains, or vice versa, the gram-to-grain relationship is found in the following basic equivalents, 1 g = 15.432 gr and 1 gr = 0.065 g, as well as in *derived equivalents*, such as 31.1 g = 480 gr and 28.35 g = 437.5 gr. It is best to use the basic equivalents when converting from one system to another and to select the equivalent that provides the answer most readily.

In response to the question, *must we round off results so as to contain no more significant figures than are contained in the conversion factor?*, the answer is *yes*. If we desire greater accuracy, we should use a more accurate conversion factor. But to the question, *If a formula includes the one-figure quantity 5 g, and we convert it to grains, must we round off the result to one significant figure?*, the answer is decidedly *no*. We should interpret the quantity given in a formula as expressing the precision we are expected to achieve in compounding—usually not less than three-figure accuracy. Hence, 5 g in a formula or prescription should be interpreted as meaning *5.00 g* or greater precision.

For prescriptions and all other problems stated in the apothecaries' or avoirdupois systems of measurement, it is recommended that all such quantities be converted to equivalent metric quantities before solving in the usual manner described in this text.

Conversion of Linear Quantities

Example Calculations of Linear Conversion

The fiber length of a sample of purified cotton is 6.35 mm. Express the length in inches.

$$6.35 \text{ mm} = 0.635 \text{ cm}$$
$$1 \text{ in} = 2.54 \text{ cm}$$

Solving by proportion:

$$\frac{1 \text{ (in)}}{x \text{ (in)}} = \frac{2.54 \text{ (cm)}}{0.635 \text{ (cm)}}$$
$$x = 0.250 \text{ in, or } \tfrac{1}{4} \text{ in, } answer.$$

Or, solving by dimensional analysis:

$$6.35 \text{ mm} \times \frac{1 \text{ cm}}{10 \text{ mm}} \times \frac{1 \text{ in}}{2.54 \text{ cm}} = 0.250 \text{ in, } answer.$$

A medicinal plaster measures 4½ in. by 6½ in. What are its dimensions in centimeters?

Assuming three-figure precision in the measurement,

$$4\tfrac{1}{2} \text{ or } 4.50 \times 2.54 \text{ cm} = 11.4 \text{ cm wide,}$$
$$6\tfrac{1}{2} \text{ or } 6.50 \times 2.54 \text{ cm} = 16.5 \text{ cm long, } answers.$$

Rulers are often calibrated in dual scale.

Conversion of Liquid Quantities

Example Calculations of Fluid Volume Conversions

Convert 2.5 L to fluidounces.

$$2.5 \text{ L} = 2500 \text{ mL}$$

Solving by proportion:

$$\frac{1 \text{ (f℥)}}{x \text{ (f℥)}} = \frac{29.57 \text{ (mL)}}{2500 \text{ (mL)}}$$
$$x = 84.5 \text{ f℥, } answer.$$

Or, solving by dimensional analysis:

$$2.5 \, L \times \frac{1000 \, mL}{1 \, L} \times \frac{1 \, f\zeta}{29.57 \, mL} = 84.5 \, f\zeta, \, answer.$$

Convert 2½ pt. to milliliters.

$$2\frac{1}{2} \, pt. = 2\frac{1}{2} \times 16 \, f\zeta = 40 \, f\zeta$$
$$40 \times 29.57 \, mL = 1182.8 \, or \, 1180 \, mL, \, answer.$$

Or, solving by dimensional analysis:

$$2\frac{1}{2} \, pt. \times \frac{16 f\zeta}{1 \, pt} \times \frac{29.57 \, mL}{1 \, f\zeta} = 1182.8 \, or \, 1180 \, mL, \, answer.$$

Conversion of Weights

Example Calculations of Weight Conversion

Convert 12.5 g to grains.

$$12.5 \times 15.432 \, gr = 192.9 \, or \, 193 \, gr, \, answer.$$

Alternate solution (about 0.5% less accurate):

$$\frac{12.5}{0.065} \, gr = 192.3 \, or \, 192 \, gr, \, answer.$$

Convert 5 mg to grains.

Solving by proportion:

$$\frac{1 \, (gr)}{x \, (gr)} = \frac{65 \, (mg)}{5 \, (mg)}$$
$$x = \frac{5}{65} \, gr = \frac{1}{13} \, gr, \, answer.$$

Convert 15 kg to avoirdupois pounds.

Solving by proportion:

$$\frac{1 \, (kg)}{15 \, (kg)} = \frac{2.2 \, (lb.)}{x \, (lb.)}$$
$$x = 33.0 \, lb., \, answer.$$

Convert 6.2 gr to milligrams.

$$6.2 \times 65 \, mg = 403 \, or \, 400 \, mg, \, answer.$$

Or, solving by dimensional analysis:

$$6.2 \, gr \times \frac{1 \, g}{15.432 \, gr} \times \frac{1000 \, mg}{1 \, g} = 401.8 \, or \, 400 \, mg, \, answer.$$

Convert 176 avoirdupois pounds to kilograms.

$$\frac{176}{2.2} \, kg = 80.0 \, kg, \, answer.$$

"Consumer Approximate" Measures

A pharmacy consumer may ask for a quantity of a product that differs from the system of measurement on the desired product's label. It is a simple matter to find a "consumer approximate" equivalent. For example, a requested "pint" of a mouthwash may be satisfied by a product labeled "500 mL." Similarly, a request for "an ounce" of a product would be satisfied with a 30-g size package if a solid or a 30-mL size package if a liquid. *"Consumer approximate" measures may not substitute for actual equivalent measures used in pharmaceutical calculations.*

Conversion of Temperatures

In 1709, the German scientist Gabriel Fahrenheit discovered that according to the scale he had marked on a thermometer, ice melted at 32° and water boiled at 212°, a difference of 180 degrees. In 1742, Anders Celsius, a Swedish astronomer, suggested the convenience of a thermometer with a scale having a difference of 100° between two fixed points, with 0° for the freezing point and 100° for the boiling point of water. Thus, the *Fahrenheit* and the *Celsius*, or *centigrade*, thermometers were established.

Because 100 degrees centigrade (°C) measures the same difference in temperature that is measured by 180 degrees Fahrenheit (°F), each degree centigrade is the equivalent of 1.8 or 9/5 the size of each degree Fahrenheit.

There are a number of different arithmetic methods for the conversion of temperatures from the centigrade scale to the Fahrenheit scale and vice versa, as described in an earlier edition of this text. One of these methods, as used in the *United States Pharmacopeia* (USP), is described by the following equations. It should be noted that temperatures in the USP are expressed in degrees centigrade.[1]

$$°F = \frac{9}{5}°C + 32, \text{ and}$$

$$°C = \frac{5}{9} \times (°F - 32)$$

Example Calculations of Temperature Conversions

Convert 26°C to corresponding degrees Fahrenheit.

$$°F = \frac{9}{5}(26°C) + 32 = 78.8°F, \text{ } answer.$$

Convert 98.6°F to corresponding degrees centigrade.

$$°C = \frac{5}{9} \times (98.6°F - 32) = 37°C, \text{ } answer.$$

Clinical Aspects of Thermometry

The instrument used to measure body temperature is termed a *clinical* or *fever thermometer*. Traditional clinical thermometers include (1) the *oral thermometer*, slender in the design of stem and bulb reservoir; (2) the *rectal thermometer*, having a blunt, pear-shaped, thick-bulb reservoir for both safety and to ensure retention in the rectum; and (3) a *universal or security thermometer*, which is stubby in design, for both oral or rectal use. In addition, *oral electronic digital fever thermometers* and *infrared emission detection (IRED) ear thermometers* are widely used. The oral electronic digital fever thermometer works by the absorption of heat from the point of body contact. Heat causes the expansion and rise of mercury in the thermometer and the response of the thermocouple. The infrared emission detection (IRED) ear thermometer measures heat radiated from the tympanic membrane without actually touching the membrane.

A recent innovation is a thermometry system of *single-use disposable* clinical thermometers that reduce the risk of passing harmful micro-organisms between patients.[2] These disposable thermometers are commercially available in both nonsterile and sterile units. The thermometers use a dot sensor matrix consisting of temperature-sensitive indicating dots. Each dot changes color at a specific temperature relative to the melting point of the specific chemical mixture in the dot. Each dot changes color at a temperature of 0.2°F or 0.1°C higher than the preceding dot. Body temperature is read from a numerical temperature scale. Clinically accurate oral body temperatures are obtained in 60 seconds and axillary temperatures in 3 minutes.

Specialized thermometers include *basal thermometers* and *low-reading thermometers*. The *basal temperature* is the body's normal resting temperature, generally taken immediately on awakening in the morning. In women, body temperature normally rises slightly because of hormonal changes associated with ovulation. Basal thermometers, calibrated in tenths of a degree, are designed to measure these slight changes in temperature. When charted over the course of a month, these changes are useful in assessing optimal times for conception. Other specialty thermometers include *neonatal digital thermometers, veterinary digital thermometers*, and *rapid response digital thermometers*, which reveal temperature readings in as little as 15 seconds.

Low-reading thermometers are required in diagnosing hypothermia. The standard clinical thermometer reads from 34.4°C (94°F) to 42.2°C (108°F), which is not fully satisfactory for measuring hypothermia, which may involve body temperatures of 35°C (95°F) or lower. A low-reading thermometer registers temperatures between 28.9°C (84°F) and 42.2°C (108°F). Examples of various thermometers are shown in Figure A.1.

In the past, the *normal* body temperature for healthy adults was accepted to be 37°C (98.6°F) based on studies performed over a century ago. The use of advanced electronic digital thermometers, however, has shown that normal adult temperature may vary widely between individuals (from 96.3°F to 99.9°F in one study).[3] Lowest body temperatures generally occur in the early morning and peak high temperatures in the late afternoon, with an average diurnal variation of approximately 0.9°F.

Pharmaceutical Aspects of Temperature

Temperature control is an important consideration in the manufacture, shipping, and storage of pharmaceutical products. Excessive temperature can result in chemical or physical instability of a therapeutic agent or its dosage form. For this reason, the labeling of pharmaceutical products contains information on the appropriate temperature range under which the product should be maintained. The *United States Pharmacopeia* provides the following definitions for the storage of pharmaceuticals.[1]

Freezer – between −25°C and − 10°C (− 13°F and 14°F)
Cold – not exceeding 8°C (46°F)
Refrigerator – between 2°C and 8°C (36°F and 46°F)
Cool – between 8°C and 15°C (46°F and 59°F)
Warm – between 30°C and 40°C (86°F and 104°F)
Excessive Heat – above 40°C (104°F)
Controlled Room Temperature – between 20°C and 25°C (68°F and 77°F)

▼ FIGURE A.1 Examples of various clinical thermometers. From top to bottom: oral fever thermometer; rectal thermometer; basal thermometer; oral digital fever thermometer. *(Courtesy of Becton Dickinson and Company.)*

Alcohol Proof Strength Conversions

Alcohol is commonly employed in the small- and large-scale manufacturing of pharmaceuticals. There are special terms associated with alcohol that require understanding for correct interpretation and conversion.

Proof spirit is an aqueous solution containing 50% v/v of *absolute alcohol* (100% v/v ethyl alcohol). Alcohols of other percentage strengths are said to be *above proof* or *below proof*, depending on whether they contain more or less than 50% v/v of absolute alcohol.

Proof strength is twice the percentage strength of alcohol and thus 50% v/v alcohol is 100 proof. In reverse then, alcohol that is 90 proof is equivalent to 45% v/v alcohol.

Alcohol for manufacturing use may be purchased by the *proof gallon*. A proof gallon is a gallon by measure of proof spirit; that is, a gallon of 100 proof or 50% v/v absolute alcohol.

Example Calculations Involving Proof Strength and Proof Gallons

To calculate the number of proof gallons contained in a given quantity of alcohol of specified strength, observe the following. Because a proof gallon has a percentage strength of 50% (v/v), the equivalent number of proof gallons may be calculated by the formula:

$$\text{Proof gallons} = \frac{\text{gallons} \times \text{Percentage strength of solution}}{50 \ (\%)}$$

Because proof strength is twice percentage strength, the formula may be revised as follows:

$$\text{Proof gallons} = \frac{\text{gallons} \times \text{Proof strength of solution}}{100 \ (\text{proof})}$$

How many proof gallons are contained in 5 gallons of 75% v/v alcohol?

First method:
1 proof gallon = 1 gallon of 50% v/v strength

$$\frac{5 \ (\text{gallons}) \times 75 \ (\%)}{50 \ (\%)} = 7.5 \ \text{proof gallons, } answer.$$

Second method:
75% v/v = 150 proof

$$\frac{5\ (\text{gallons}) \times 150\ (\text{proof})}{100\ (\text{proof})} = 7.5 \text{ proof gallons, } answer.$$

To calculate the number of gallons of alcohol of specified strength equivalent to a given number of proof gallons, observe the following.

$$\text{gallons} = \frac{\text{Proof gallons} \times 50\ (\%)}{\text{Percentage strength of solution}}$$

or,

$$\text{gallons} = \frac{\text{Proof gallons} \times 100\ (\text{proof})}{\text{Proof strength of solution}}$$

How many gallons of 20% v/v alcohol would be the equivalent of 20 proof gallons?

First method:
1 proof gallon = 1 wine gallon of 50% v/v strength

$$\frac{20\ (\text{proof gallons}) \times 50\ (\%)}{20\ (\%)} = 50 \text{ gallons, } answer.$$

Second method:
20% v/v = 40 proof

$$\frac{20\ (\text{proof gallons}) \times 100\ (\text{proof})}{40\ (\text{proof})} = 50 \text{ gallons, } answer.$$

To calculate the tax on a given quantity of alcohol of a specified strength, observe the following.

If the tax on alcohol is quoted at $13.50 per proof gallon, how much tax would be collected on 10 gallons of alcohol marked 190 proof?

$$\frac{10\ (\text{gallons}) \times 190\ (\text{proof})}{100\ (\text{proof})} = 19 \text{ proof gallons}$$
$$\$13.50 \times 19\ (\text{proof gallons}) = \$256.50, \ answer.$$

Note: when specific equations, as those described above, are difficult to recall, it is always an option to perform calculations in a stepwise and logical fashion. Although a greater number of steps may be required, the outcome is worth the time.

For example, in the previously-stated problem, *"How many proof gallons are contained in 5 gallons of 75% v/v alcohol?"* If one worked logically on the basis of the amount of absolute alcohol in 5 gallons of 75% v/v alcohol, the answer to the problem may be deduced as follows:

5 gallons × 75% v/v = 3.75 gallons of absolute alcohol (100% v/v)

then, it follows that:

3.75 gallons of absolute alcohol × 2 = 7.5 proof gallons, *answer.*

The student may wish to work the same problem in terms of milliliters (3785 mL/gallon) to arrive at the same answer.

PRACTICE PROBLEMS

Calculations of the Avoirdupois and Apothecaries' Systems

1. Reduce each of the following quantities to grains:
   (a) ℈ii ℈is.
   (b) ℥ii ℥iss.
   (c) ℥i ℥ss ℈i.
   (d) ℥i ℈i gr x.

2. Reduce 1 pint, f℥ii to fluidrachms.

3. According to product literature, each DONNATAL EXTENTAB tablet contains:

Phenobarbital, USP	3/4 gr
Hyoscyamine sulfate, USP	0.3111 mg
Atropine sulfate, USP	0.0582 mg
Scopolamine hydrobromide, USP	0.0195 mg

   Convert the quantity of phenobarbital to milligrams and the quantity of hyoscyamine sulfate to grains, expressed as a common fraction.

4. How many f℥ii-bottles of cough syrup can be obtained from 5 gallons of the cough syrup?

5. Low-dose aspirin tablets contain 1¼ grains of aspirin in each tablet. How many tablets can be prepared from 1 avoirdupois pound of aspirin?

6. How many $\frac{1}{400}$-gr tablets of nitroglycerin can a manufacturer prepare from a quantity of a trituration of nitroglycerin that contains ⅛ oz of the drug?

Intersystem Conversion Calculations

7. A brand of nitroglycerin transdermal patch measures 2.5 inches in diameter. Express this dimension in centimeters.

8. Urethral suppositories are traditionally prepared to the following lengths: 50 mm for females and 125 mm for males. Convert these dimensions to inches.

9. A pharmacist received a prescription calling for 30 capsules, each to contain $\frac{1}{200}$ gr of nitroglycerin. How many 0.4-mg nitroglycerin tablets would supply the amount required?

10. If a physician prescribed 4 grams of aspirin to be taken by a patient daily, about how many 5-grain tablets should the patient take each day?

11. ℞ Codeine Sulfate   30 mg
       Acetaminophen   325 mg
       M. ft. cap. D.T.D. no. 24
       Sig. One capsule t.i.d. for pain.

    How many grains each of codeine sulfate and acetaminophen would be contained in the prescription?

12. If a child accidentally swallowed 2 fluidounces of FEOSOL Elixir, containing 2/3 gr of ferrous sulfate per 5 mL, how many milligrams of ferrous sulfate did the child ingest?

13. Sustained-release tablets of nitroglycerin contain the following amounts of drug: 1/25 gr, 1/10 gr, and 1/50 gr. Express these quantities as milligrams.

14. The usual dose of colchicine for an acute gout attack is 1/120 gr every hour for 8 doses. How many milligrams of colchicine are represented in the usual dose?

15. If f℥i of a cough syrup contains 10 gr of sodium citrate, how many milligrams are contained in 5 mL?

16. A formula for a cough syrup contains ⅛ gr of codeine phosphate per teaspoonful (5 mL). How many grams of codeine phosphate should be used in preparing 1 pint of the cough syrup?

Temperature Conversions

17. Convert the following from centigrade to Fahrenheit:
    (a) 10°C
    (b) −30°C
    (c) 4°C
    (d) −173°C

18. Convert the following from Fahrenheit to centigrade:
    (a) 77°F
    (b) 240°F
    (c) 98.9°F
    (d) 227.1°F

19. A patient's rectal temperature reading is frequently 1°F higher than the oral temperature reading. Express this difference in degrees centigrade.

20. A woman charting her basal temperature finds that her body temperature on day 14 is 97.7°F and on day 18 is 98.6°F. Express this temperature range and the difference in degrees centigrade.

Proof Strength Conversions

21. If the tax on alcohol is $13.50 per proof gallon, how much tax must be paid on 5 gallons of alcohol, USP, which contains 94.9% v/v of pure alcohol?

22. On the first of the month, a hospital pharmacist had on hand a drum containing 54 gallons of 95% alcohol. During the month, the following amounts were used:
    • 10 gallons in the manufacture of bathing lotion
    • 20 gallons in the manufacture of medicated alcohol
    • 5 gallons in the manufacture of soap solution

    How many proof gallons of alcohol were on hand at the end of the month?

ANSWERS TO PRACTICE PROBLEMS

1. (a) 150 gr
   (b) 1050 gr
   (c) 530 gr
   (d) 90 gr

2. 144 f℥

3. 48.75 mg phenobarbital and ≈ 1/209 gr hyoscyamine sulfate

4. 320 tablets

5. 5600 tablets

6. 21,875 tablets

7. 6.35 cm

8. 1.97 in., 4.92 in.

9. 24.4 or 25 tablets

10. 12 tablets

11. 11 7/100 or 11.08 gr of codeine sulfate 120 gr of acetaminophen

12. 512.55 mg

13. 2.6 mg (1/25 gr)
    6.5 mg (1/10 gr)
    1.3 mg (1/50 gr)

14. 0.54 mg

15. 109.9 mg

16. 0.769 g

17. (a) 50°F
    (b) −22°F
    (c) 39.2°F
    (d) −279.4°F

18. (a) 25°C
    (b) 115.6°C
    (c) 37.2°C
    (d) 108.4°C

19. 0.56°C

20. 36.5° to 37°C
    0.5°C

21. $128.12

22. 361.1 proof gallons

References

1. United States Pharmacopeia 31st Rev. National Formulary 26. Rockville, MD: United States Pharmacopeial Convention, 2008;1:8, 905–906.
2. Tempa-Dot Thermometers. Available at: http://www.3m.com/product/information/Tempa-Dot-Thermometer.html. Accessed March 24, 2011.
3. Mackowiak PA, Wasserman SS, Levine MM. A critical appraisal of 98.6°F, the upper limit of the normal body temperature and other legacies of Carl Reinhold Wunderlich. *Journal of American Medical Association* 1992;268:1578.

Glossary of Pharmaceutical Dosage Forms and Drug Delivery Systems[a]

Aerosols. Pharmaceutical aerosols are products packaged under pressure that contain therapeutically active ingredients that are released as a fine mist, spray, or foam on actuation of the valve assembly. Some aerosol emissions are intended to be inhaled deep into the lungs (*inhalation aerosol*), whereas others are intended for topical application to the skin or to mucous membranes. Aerosols with metered valve assemblies permit a specific quantity of emission for dosage regulation.

Aromatic Waters. Aromatic waters are clear, saturated solutions of volatile oils or other aromatic substances in water. They are used orally, topically, or pharmaceutically for the characteristics of the aromatic material they contain.

Boluses. Boluses are large elongated tablets intended for administration to animals.

Capsules. Capsules are solid dosage forms in which one or more medicinal and/or inert substances are enclosed within small shells of gelatin. Capsule shells are produced in varying sizes, shapes, color, and hardness. *Hard-shell* capsules, which have two telescoping parts, are used in the manufacture of most commercial capsule products and in the extemporaneous filling of prescriptions. They are filled with powder mixtures or granules.

Soft-shell gelatin capsules, sometimes called *softgels*, are formed, filled, and sealed in a continuous process by specialized large-scale equipment. They may be filled with powders, semisolids, or liquids.

Capsules contain a specific quantity of fill, with the capsule size selected to accommodate that quantity. In addition to their medication content, capsules usually contain inert substances, such as fillers. When swallowed, the gelatin capsule shell is dissolved by gastrointestinal fluids, releasing the contents.

Delayed-release capsules are prepared in such a manner as to resist the release of the contents until the capsules have passed through the stomach and into the intestines.

Extended-release capsules are prepared in such a manner as to release the medication from the capsules over an extended period following ingestion.

Creams. Creams are semisolid preparations containing one or more drug substances dissolved or dispersed in a suitable base. Many creams are either oil-in-water emulsions or aqueous microcrystalline dispersions in a water-washable base. Compared to ointments, creams are easier to spread and remove. Creams are used for administering drugs to the skin and, to a lesser extent, to mucous membranes.

Drug Delivery Systems. Drug delivery systems are physical carriers used to deliver medications to site-specific areas. They include transdermal, ocular, and intrauterine systems.

Transdermal drug delivery systems support the passage of drug substances from the surface of the skin, through its various layers, and into the systemic circulation. These systems are sophisticated skin patches containing a drug formulation within a reservoir for the controlled delivery of drug.

Ocular drug delivery systems consist of drug-impregnated membranes that, when placed in the lower conjunctival sac, release medication at a constant rate over an extended period.

Intrauterine drug delivery systems consist of a drug-containing intrauterine device that releases medication over an extended period after insertion into the uterus.

Elixirs. Elixirs are sweetened, flavored, hydroalcoholic solutions intended for oral administration. They may be medicated or nonmedicated. Compared to syrups, elixirs are usually less sweet and less

---

[a]*Some portions of this Glossary have been abstracted from USP34-NF29, <1151>. Copyright 2010 The United States Pharmacopeial Convention. Permission Granted.*

viscous because they contain a lesser amount of sugar. Because of their hydroalcoholic character, elixirs are better able than are syrups to maintain both water-soluble and alcohol-soluble components in solution.

Emulsions. An emulsion is a type of system in which one liquid is dispersed throughout another liquid in the form of fine droplets. The two liquids, generally an oil and water, are immiscible and constitute two phases that would separate into layers without the presence of a third agent, an *emulsifier* or *emulsifying agent.* The latter facilitates the emulsification process and provides physical stability to the system.

If oil is the internal phase, then the emulsion is termed an oil-in-water, or o/w, emulsion. If water is the internal phase, then the emulsion is termed a water-in-oil, or w/o, emulsion. The type of emulsion produced is largely determined by the emulsifying agent, with hydrophilic agents generally producing oil-in-water emulsions and lipophilic agents generally producing water-in-oil emulsions. Emulsifying agents may have both hydrophilic and lipophilic characteristics, hence the term hydrophilic-lipophilic balance (HLB).

Depending on their formulation, emulsions may be administered orally, topically, or by intravenous injection.

Extracts. Extracts are concentrated preparations of vegetable or animal drugs prepared by extracting the constituents from the natural source and drying the extractive to the desired pilular or powdered form.

Fluidextracts. Fluidextracts are liquid extractives of vegetable drugs generally prepared such that 1 mL represents the active constituents from 1 g of the vegetable drug.

Gels. Gels are semisolid systems consisting of either suspensions of small inorganic particles or large organic molecules interpenetrated by a liquid.

Implants or Pellets. Implants or pellets are small, sterile, solid dosage forms containing a concentrated drug for subcutaneous implantation in the body where they continuously release their medication over prolonged periods.

Inhalations. Inhalations are finely powdered drug substances, solutions, or suspensions of drug substances administered by the nasal or oral respiratory route for local or systemic effects. Special devices are used to facilitate their administration. *Metered-dose inhalers (MDIs)* are propellant-driven drug suspensions or solutions in liquefied gas propellant, intended to deliver metered doses of drug to the respiratory tract. MDIs are packaged to contain multiple doses (often several hundred) with each valve actuation delivering controlled volumes ranging from 25 to 100 μL.

Injections. Injections are sterile preparations intended for parenteral administration by needle or pressure syringe. Drugs may be injected into most any vessel or tissue of the body, but the most common routes are intravenous (IV), intramuscular (IM), and subcutaneous (SC). Injections may be solutions or suspensions of a drug substance in an aqueous or nonaqueous vehicle. They may be small-volume injections, packaged in ampuls for single-dose administration, or vials for multiple-dose injections. Large-volume parenterals, containing 100 mL to 1 liter of fluid, are intended for the slow intravenous administration (or infusion) of medications and/or nutrients in the institutional or home care setting.

Irrigations. Irrigations are sterile solutions intended to bathe or flush open wounds or body cavities. They are not intended for injection.

Liniments. Liniments are alcoholic or oleaginous solutions, suspensions, or emulsions of medicinal agents intended for external application to the skin, generally by rubbing. Liniments have application both in human and veterinary medicine.

Lotions. Lotions are liquid preparations intended for external application to the skin. They are generally suspensions or emulsions of dispersed solid or liquid materials in an aqueous vehicle. Their fluidity allows rapid and uniform application over a wide skin surface. Lotions are intended to soften the skin and leave a thin coat of their components on the skin's surface as they dry.

Lozenges. Lozenges are solid preparations containing one or more medicinal agents in a flavored, sweetened base intended to dissolve or disintegrate slowly in the mouth, releasing medication generally for localized effects.

Ointments. Ointments are semisolid preparations intended for topical application to the skin, eye, ear, or various mucous membranes. With some exceptions, ointments are applied for their local effects on the tissue membrane rather than for systemic effects. *Ophthalmic ointments* are sterile preparations intended for application to the eye.

Nonmedicated ointments serve as vehicles, or as *ointment bases*, in the preparation of medicated ointments. Because ointments are semisolid preparations, they are prepared and dispensed on a weight basis.

Pastes. Pastes are semisolid dosage forms that contain one or more drug substances intended for topical application to the skin. Generally, pastes contain a higher proportion of solid materials than do ointments and thus are more stiff, less greasy, and more absorptive of serous secretions.

Plasters. Plasters are solid or semisolid adhesive masses spread across a suitable backing material and intended for external application to a part of the body for protection or for the medicinal benefit of added agents.

Powders. Powders are dry mixtures of finely divided medicinal and nonmedicinal agents intended for internal or external use. Powders may be dispensed in bulk form, or they may be divided into single-dosage units and packaged in folded papers or unit-of-use envelopes.

Premixes. Premixes are mixtures of one or more drug substances with suitable vehicles intended for admixture to animal feedstuffs before administration. They are generally in powdered, pelletized, or granulated form.

Solutions. Solutions are liquid preparations that contain one or more chemical substances (*solutes*) dissolved in a solvent or mixture of solvents. The most common solvent used in pharmaceuticals is water; however, alcohol, glycerin, and propylene glycol also are widely used as solvents or cosolvents.

Depending upon their purpose, solutions are formulated and labeled for use by various routes, including oral, topical, ophthalmic, otic, nasal, rectal, urethral, and parenteral. The concentration of active ingredients in solutions varies widely depending on the nature of the therapeutic agent and its intended use. The concentration of a given solution may be expressed in molar strength, milliequivalent strength, percentage strength, ratio strength, milligrams per milliliter, or another expression describing the amount of active ingredient per unit of volume.

Spirits. Spirits are alcoholic or hydroalcoholic solutions of volatile substances. Depending on their contents, some spirits are used orally for medicinal purposes and others as flavoring agents.

Suppositories. Suppositories are solid dosage forms intended for insertion into body orifices. They are used rectally, vaginally, and, occasionally, urethrally. Suppositories are of various weights, sizes, and shapes, depending on their intended use. Various types of *suppository bases* are used as vehicles for the medication, including cocoa butter (theobroma oil), glycerinated gelatin, polyethylene glycols, hydrogenated vegetable oils, and fatty acid esters of polyethylene glycol. Depending on the base used, the suppository either softens, melts, or dissolves after insertion, releasing its medication for the intended local action or for absorption and systemic effects.

Suspensions. Suspensions are preparations containing finely divided, undissolved drug particles dispersed throughout a liquid vehicle. Because the drug particles are not dissolved, suspensions assume a degree of opacity depending on the concentration and size of the suspended particles. Because particles tend to settle when left standing, suspensions should be shaken to redistribute any settled particles before use to ensure uniform dosing. Depending on their formulation, suspensions are administered orally, by intramuscular injection, and topically to the eye.

Syrups. Syrups are concentrated aqueous solutions of a sugar or sugar substitute. Syrups may be medicated or nonmedicated. *Nonmedicated syrups* are used as vehicles for medicinal substances to be added later, either in the extemporaneous compounding of prescriptions or in the preparation of a

Table B.1 ▼ ROUTES OF DRUG ADMINISTRATION AND PRIMARY DOSAGE FORMS AND DRUG DELIVERY SYSTEMS

ROUTE	SITE	DOSAGE FORMS/DRUG DELIVERY SYSTEMS
Oral	Mouth	Tablets, capsules, oral solutions, drops, syrups, elixirs, suspensions, magmas, gels, powders, troches and lozenges (oral cavity)
Sublingual	Under the tongue	Tablets
Parenteral		Solutions, suspensions
Intravenous	Vein	
Intra-arterial	Artery	
Intracardiac	Heart	
Intraspinal/Intrathecal	Spine	
Intraosseous	Bone	
Intra-articular	Joint	
Intrasynovial	Joint fluid	
Intracutaneous/Intradermal/ Subcutaneous	Skin	
Intramuscular	Muscle	
Epicutaneous	Skin surface	Ointments, creams, pastes, plasters, powders, aerosols, lotions, transdermal patches, solutions (topical)
Conjunctival	Eye conjunctiva	Ointments
Intraocular	Eye	Solutions, suspensions
Intranasal	Nose	Solutions, ointments
Aural	Ear	Solutions and suspensions (drops)
Intrarespiratory	Lung	Solutions (aerosols)
Rectal	Rectum	Solutions, ointments, suppositories
Vaginal	Vagina	Solutions, ointments, emulsion foams, gels, tablets/inserts
Urethral	Urethra	Solutions and suppositories

formula for a medicated syrup. In addition to the sugar or sweetener, syrups also contain flavoring agents, colorants, cosolvents, and antimicrobial preservatives to prevent microbial growth. Syrups are administered orally for the therapeutic value of the medicinal agent(s).

Tablets. Tablets are solid dosage forms containing one or more medicinal substances. Most tablets also contain added pharmaceutical ingredients, as diluents, disintegrants, colorants, binders, solubilizers, and coatings. Tablets may be coated for appearance, for stability, to mask the taste of the medication, or to provide controlled drug release. Most tablets are manufactured on an industrial scale by compression, using highly sophisticated machinery. Punches and dies of various shapes and sizes enable the preparation of a wide variety of tablets of distinctive shapes, sizes, and surface markings.

Most tablets are intended to be swallowed whole. However, some are prepared to be chewable, others to be dissolved in the mouth (*buccal tablets*) or under the tongue (*sublingual tablets*), and still others to be dissolved in water before taking (*effervescent tablets*). Tablets are formulated to contain a specific quantity of medication. To enable flexibility in dosing, manufacturers commonly make available various tablet strengths of a given medication. Some tablets are scored, or grooved, to permit breaking into portions that the patient can take.

Tinctures. Tinctures are alcoholic or hydroalcoholic solutions of either pure chemical substances or of plant extractives. Most chemical tinctures are applied topically (e.g., iodine tincture). Plant extractives are used for their content of active pharmacologic agents.

Comprehensive Review Problems*

1. Translate the prescription notations and calculate as directed:
    (a) ℞ E.E.S Filmtabs   400 mg
        ESig: Tabs i stat p.o., i qid q6h × 10 days.

        Each E.E.S Filmtab contains 400 mg of erythromycin ethylsuccinate. If the patient taking the medication weighs 160 lb, calculate the daily dose on the basis of mg/kg.

    (b) ℞ RESTASIS   0.4 mL
        Sig: gtt i o.u. bid q12h.

        RESTASIS contains 0.05% cyclosporine. If the dropper used delivers 16 drops/mL, how many micrograms of cyclosporine are delivered daily?

    (c) ℞ BIAXIN   250 mg/5 mL
        Sig: ℨss t.i.d. q8h × 10 days.

        BIAXIN contains clarithromycin in suspension. How many milliliters of the medication will the patient require during the course of therapy?

    (d) ℞ TUSSIONEX PENNKINETIC
        Disp: 60 mL.
        Sig: 1 teaspoonful. NMT 2 teaspoonfuls/day.

        TUSSIONEX PENNKINETIC contains the equivalent of 2 mg/mL of hydrocodone bitartrate and 1.6 mg/mL of chlorpheniramine maleate. Calculate the maximum daily dose of each in milligrams.

    (e) ℞ Benzoyl peroxide   5.5%
        Cream base ad   15 g
        M.ft. cream

        If the patient applies 0.5 g for each use, how many milligrams of benzoyl peroxide will have been applied?

Solutions:
    (a) Swallow one (1) tablet to start, and then swallow one (1) tablet four (4) times a day every six (6) hours for ten (10) days.
        160 lb × 1 kg/2.2 lb = 72.7 kg
        4 × 400 mg = 1600 mg
        1600 mg/72.2 kg = 22.16 mg/kg of erythromycin succinate.

    (b) Instill one (1) drop into each eye two (2) times a day every 12 hours.
        0.4 mL × 0.05% = 0.0002 g = 0.2 mg = 200 μg.
        0.4 mL × 16 drops/mL = 6.4 drops.
        200 μg/6.4 drops = 31.25 μg/drop.

---

*Some formulas and problems in this section are credited and referenced as the contributions of other authors.

Gtt i o.u. bid = one drop into each eye 2 times a day = 4 drops/day.
4 drops/day × 31.25 μg/drop = <u>125 μg/day of cyclosporine.</u>

Or,

4 drops × 0.05 g/100 mL × 1000 mg/1 g × 1000 μg/1 mg × 1 mL/16 drops = <u>125 μg of cyclosporine.</u>

(c) Take one-half (1/2) teaspoonful three (3) times a day every eight (8) hours for 10 days.

ʒss = ½ teaspoonful.
5 mL/teaspoonful × ½ = 2.5 mL.
2.5 mL × 3 times/day × 10 days = <u>75 mL BIAXIN suspension.</u>

(d) Take one (1) teaspoonful. Do not take more than two (2) teaspoonfuls a day.
5 mL/teaspoonful × 2 teaspoonfuls = 10 mL.
Hydrocodone bitartrate: 2 mg/mL × 10 mL = <u>20 mg</u>, and
Chlorpheniramine maleate: 1.6 mg × 10 mL = <u>16 mg.</u>

(e) Mix and make a cream.
15 g × 5.5% = 0.825 g = 825 mg.
825 mg × 0.5 g/15 g = <u>27.5 mg benzoyl peroxide.</u>

Or,

0.5 g × 5.5% = 0.0275 g = <u>27.5 mg benzoyl peroxide.</u>

2. Calculate the following hospital medication orders as directed:
   (a) Medication Order: sirolimus oral solution (RAPAMUNE), 1 mg/m²/day.
       Preparation Administered: 1 mg/mL sirolimus oral solution.
       Calculate: daily dose, in milliliters, for a 5-ft 8-in. patient weighing 149 lb.
   (b) Medication Order: cefixime, 8 mg/kg/day in two divided doses.
       Preparation Administered: cefixime oral suspension 200 mg/5 mL.
       Calculate: dose, in milliliters, for a 36-lb child.
   (c) Medication Order: heparin 15 units/kg/hr.
       Preparation Administered: 25,000 heparin units in 500 mL normal saline solution.
       Calculate: infusion rate, in mL/hr, for a 187-lb patient.
   (d) Medication Order: lidocaine, 2 μg/kg/min.
       Preparation Administered: lidocaine, 1 g/500-mL infusion with an infusion set delivering 15 drops/mL.
       Calculate: flow rate, in drops/min for a 142-lb patient.
   (e) Medication Order: potassium bolus of 40 mEq of KCl in 200 mL of 0.9% sodium chloride injection to be administered at a rate of 10 mEq/hr.
       Calculate: drip rate in microdrops/min.

Solutions:

(a) 5 ft 8 in. = 68 in. × 2.54 cm/in. = 172.72 cm
    149 lb × 1 kg/2.2 lb = 67.73 kg

$$\text{BSA, m}^2 = \sqrt{\frac{172.72 \text{ (cm)} \times 67.73 \text{ (kg)}}{3600}} = \sqrt{3.25} = 1.80 \text{ m}^2$$

1 mg/m²/day × 1.80 m² = 1.8 mg/day
1.8 mg/day × 1 mL/1 mg = <u>1.8 mL/day, sirolimus oral solution.</u>

(b) 36 lb × 1 kg/2.2 lb = 16.36 kg
8 mg/kg/day × 16.36 (kg) = 130.88 mg/day
130.88 mg/2 doses = 65.44 mg/dose
65.44 mg × 5 mL/200 mg = 1.636 or <u>1.6 mL cefixime oral suspension</u>.

(c) 187 lb × 1 kg/2.2 lb = 85 kg
15 units/kg/hr × 85 kg = 1275 units/hr
1275 units/hr × 500 mL/25,000 units = <u>25.5 mL/hr heparin in NSS.</u>

(d) 142 lb × 1 kg/2.2 lb = 64.55 kg
2 μg/kg/min × 64.55 kg = 129.1 μg/min
129.1 μg/min × 500 mL/1 g × 1 g/1,000,000 μg = 0.06455 mL/min
0.06455 mL/min × 15 drops/mL = 0.968 or <u>1 drop/min lidocaine infusion.</u>

(e) Note: unless otherwise indicated, *microdrop* infusion sets deliver 60 drops/mL. Also, although not recommended, the abbreviation "mcgtts" for microdrops occasionally is encountered.

  60 microdrops/1 mL × 200 mL/40 mEq × 10 mEq/1 hr × 1 hr/60 min = <u>50 microdrops/min.</u>

3. Identify any errors in the calculations for each of the following prescriptions.
  (a) ℞   Allopurinol   20 mg/mL
       Cherry syrup   60 mL
       Methylcellulose suspension ad   120 mL
       Sig. Take one teaspoonful daily in AM.

  Having no allopurinol powder, six 300-mg tablets of allopurinol are used in compounding this prescription.

  (b) ℞   Triamcinolone acetonide cream   0.1%
       Aquaphor Unibase aa   30 g
       M. ft. ungt.
       Sig. Apply to affected area on skin t.i.d.

  Fifteen grams each of a 0.1% triamcinolone acetonide cream and Aquaphor Unibase are used in compounding this prescription.

  (c) ℞   Ephedrine sulfate   0.4% w/v
       Benzocaine   1:1000 w/v
       Cocoa butter ad   2 g
       M. ft. suppos. DTD no.   24
       Sig. Insert one rectal suppository each night at bedtime.

  In compounding this prescription, it is acceptable to calculate for two extra suppositories to account for unavoidable loss. If a 10% w/w benzocaine ointment is used as the source of the benzocaine, 0.052 g of the ointment would supply the proper amount.

  (d) ℞   Patient: weight 132 lb
       LEUKERAN 0.1 mg/kg/day
       Disp: 2 mg tabs
       Sig: Take _____ tablets every day × 21 days.

  The pharmacist calculates the dose to be 3 tablets daily and dispenses 63 tablets.

(e) ℞   Patient: height, 5 ft 2 in.; weight 108 lb.
          Dexamethasone
          Dose @ 20 mg/m²/day
          Disp: 5-mg tablets
          Sig: Take _____ tablets daily for treatment cycle on days 1, 2, 3, 4, 9, 10, 11.

   The pharmacist calculates the dose to be 6 tablets daily for treatment cycle on days 1, 2, 3, 4, 9, 10, and 11.

Solutions:

(a) 20 mg/mL × 120 mL = 2400 mg allopurinol needed

$$2400 \text{ mg} \times \frac{1 \text{ tablet}}{300 \text{ mg}} = 8 \text{ tablets.}$$

   Eight tablets should have been used.

(b) "aa" means "of each;" thus, 30 g of each component should be used.

(c) 2 g/1 suppos. × 26 suppos. = 52 g
     52 g × 1 g (benzocaine)/1000 g = 0.052 g benzocaine needed

$$0.052 \text{ g (benzocaine)} \times \frac{100 \text{ g (benzocaine ointment)}}{10 \text{ g (benzocaine)}} = 0.52 \text{ g benzocaine ointment.}$$

   0.52 g of benzocaine ointment should be used.

(d) 132 lb × 1 kg/2.2 lb = 60 kg
     60 kg × 0.1 mg/kg/day = 6 mg/day
     6 mg/day × 1 tab/2 mg = 3 tablets/day
     There are no errors in the calculations.

(e) 5 ft2 in. = 62 in. = 157.48 cm (62 in. × 2.54 cm/in.)
     108 lb × 1 kg/2.2 lb = 49.09 kg

$$\text{BSA, m}^2 = \sqrt{\frac{157.48 \text{ cm} \times 49.09 \text{ kg}}{3600}} = \sqrt{2.15} = 1.47 \text{ m}^2$$

   20 mg/m²/day × 1.47 m² = 29.4 mg/day
   29.4 mg/day × 1 tablet/5 mg = 5.88 or 6 tablets/day.
   There are no errors in the calculations.

4. Calculate as indicated for each of the following prescriptions:
   (a) ℞ᵃ   Noscapine   0.72 g
            Guaifenesin   4.8 g
            Alcohol   15   mL
            Cherry syrup ad   120   mL
            Sig. ℨi t.i.d. p.r.n. cough.

   How many milligrams each of noscapine and guaifenesin would be contained in each dose?

(b) ℞ᵃ Clotrimazole   1 g
      Gentamicin sulfate   300 mg
      Polyethylene glycol ad   100 mL
      Sig: Two drops in each ear t.i.d.

    Calculate the amount of gentamicin sulfate, in micrograms, present in each dose from a dropper service that delivers 20 drops/mL.

(c) ℞ᵃ Miconazole   2% w/v
      Tolnaftate   1 g
      Polyethylene glycol 300 qs ad   100 mL
      Sig: Apply to skin bid.

    How many grams each of miconazole and tolnaftate are needed to prepare 8 fl. oz. of the prescription?

(d) ℞ᵃ Interferon alpha-2a   100   million units
      Ammonium acetate   7.7 mg
      Benzyl alcohol   100 mg
      Human albumin   10 mg
      Sterile water for injection ad   10 mL

    Interferon alpha-2a is available in syringes containing 9 million units or 33.3 μg in 0.5 mL of solution. Calculate the (i) milliliters of this solution required to prepare the prescription; (ii) the number of micrograms; and (iii) the number of units of interferon alpha-2a in each 0.05 mL of the filled prescription.

Solutions:

(a) A "ʒ" in the Signa portion of a prescription may be interpreted as a *teaspoonful* and thus 5 mL.
120 mL/5 mL = 24 doses
0.72 g = 720 mg noscapine
720 mg/24 doses = <u>30 mg noscapine/dose.</u>
4.8 g = 4800 mg guaifenesin
       4800 mg/24 doses = 200 mg <u>guaifenesin/dose.</u>

(b) $2 \text{ drops} \times \dfrac{300 \text{ mg}}{100 \text{ mL}} \times \dfrac{1000 \text{ }\mu g}{1 \text{ mg}} \times \dfrac{1 \text{ mL}}{20 \text{ drops}} = 300 \text{ }\mu g$ gentamicin sulfate.

(c) 8 (fl. oz.) × 29.57 mL = 236.56 mL.
Miconazole: 2% (w/v) × 236.56 mL = <u>4.73 g</u>
Tolnaftate: 1% (w/v) × 236.56 mL = <u>2.36 g</u>

(d) 100 million units × 0.5 mL/9 million units = 5.56 mL of solution.

$$0.05 \text{ mL} \times \frac{100 \text{ million units}}{10 \text{ mL}} = 0.5 \text{ million units interferon alpha-2a.}$$

$$0.05 \text{ mL} \times \frac{100 \text{ million units}}{10 \text{ mL}} \times \frac{33.3 \text{ }\mu g}{9 \text{ million units}} = 1.85 \text{ }\mu g \text{ interferon alpha-2a.}$$

5. ℞   Entecavir   0.5 mg
       Lactose ad   300   mg
       M. ft. such caps #   12
       Sig: i cap qid.

   (a) Explain how you would obtain the correct quantity of entecavir using a prescription balance with a sensitivity requirement of 6 mg and an acceptable weighing error of not greater than 5%.
   (b) Rather than weighing the required quantity of entecavir powder, a pharmacist uses 1-mg entecavir tablets (crushed and powdered) to compound the prescription. If each tablet weighs 92 mg, how many milligrams of lactose would be needed to fill the prescription?

Solutions:
   (a) The least amount that should be weighed on this prescription balance is calculated by: 6 mg × 100%/5% = 120 mg.
       Thus, 120 mg or greater of entecavir must be weighed.
       The prescription requires 0.5 mg × 12 (capsules) = 6 mg of entecavir.
       Using an arbitrary multiple of 20, the amount of entecavir that can be weighed is: 120 mg (20 × 6 mg).

       Weigh 120 mg of entecavir, add 2280 mg of lactose (20 × 120 mg = 2400 mg – 120 mg entecavir) and weigh 1/20th of the 2400 mg mixture, 120 mg, which will contain the required 6 mg of entecavir (proof: 1/20th of the 120 mg = 6 mg entecavir).

   (b) Number of tablets required = 6 mg /1 mg per tablet = 6 tablets
       6 (tablets) × 92 mg per tablet = 552 mg
       300 mg per capsule × 12 capsules = 3600 mg total
       3600 mg – 552 mg (powdered entecavir tablets) = 3048 mg lactose.

6. A periodontist inquires as to how you would calculate 120 mL of a prescription for a concentrated solution of chlorhexidine gluconate from which a patient could take a medicinal tablespoonful, add it to a pint of water, and produce a 0.12% solution that may be used as a dental rinse.
   (a) How many milliliters of chlorhexidine gluconate (a liquid chemical) are needed to prepare the prescription?
   (b) Prove that the resultant solution as prepared by the patient is indeed 0.12% v/v.
   (c) Calculate the percent concentration of chlorhexidine gluconate, v/v, in the prescription.
   (d) If chlorhexidine gluconate has a specific gravity of 1.07, calculate its percent concentration, w/v, in the prescription.

Solutions:
   (a) A tablespoonful (15 mL) of the prescription plus a pint (473 mL) of water = 488 mL.
       488 mL × 0.12% (v/v) = 0.5856 or 0.59 mL chlorhexidine gluconate.
           So, if there is 0.59 mL of chlorhexidine gluconate in the 488 mL of dental rinse prepared by the patient, it came from the one tablespoonful of the concentrated prescription. And, since there are 8 tablespoonfuls available in the prescription (120 mL/15 mL), 8 (tablespoons) × 0.59 mL chlorhexidine gluconate = 4.72 mL chlorhexidine gluconate needed to fill the prescription.
   (b) 0.59 mL/488 mL × 100% = 0.12%.
   (c) 4.72 mL/120 mL × 100% = 3.93% v/v.

(d) 4.72 mL × 1.07 g/mL = 5.05 g
5.05 g/120 mL × 100% = <u>4.2% w/v.</u>

7. ASTELIN nasal spray contains 0.1% azelastine hydrochloride and 125 μg/mL of benzalkonium chloride as a preservative. A container is capable of delivering 200 metered sprays of 0.137 mL each.
(a) Calculate the quantity, in micrograms, of azelastine hydrochloride in each spray.
(b) Calculate the percentage strength and ratio strength of benzalkonium chloride in the preparation.
(c) The molecular weight of azelastine hydrochloride is 418.4. Calculate the quantity, in milligrams, of azelastine (base), in a 30-mL container.

Solutions:
(a) 0.137 mL × 0.1% = 0.000137 g = 0.137 mg = <u>137 μg.</u>
(b) 125 μg/mL = 0.0125 g/100 mL = <u>0.0125%.</u>
100 (mL)/0.0125 (g) = <u>1:8000 w/v ratio strength.</u>
(c) Molecular weight azelastine hydrochloride: 418.4
Molecular weight azelastine (base): 418.4 − 36.5 (HCl) = 381.9
381.9/418.4 = 91.3% (percent of azelastine hydrochloride that is azelastine base)
30 mL × 0.1% = 0.03 g = 30 mg (azelastine hydrochloride)
30 mg (azelastine hydrochloride) × 91.3% = <u>27.39 mg azelastine (base).</u>

8. Refer to ASTELIN nasal spray in the previous problem.
(a) If ASTELIN nasal spray is packaged in 30-mL spray containers, how many milliliters would remain after 200 metered sprays?
(b) The recommended dose of the spray for allergic rhinitis is one spray in each nostril twice daily. At this dose, how many days will the package last a patient?
(c) In a clinical trial of 391 patients, using two sprays in each nostril twice daily, the most common adverse effects were a bitter taste among 77 patients and a headache in 57 patients. Calculate the percent occurrence of each of these adverse effects.

Solutions:
(a) 0.137 mL/spray × 200 sprays = 27.4 mL
30 mL − 27.4 mL = <u>2.6 mL.</u>
(b) 200 sprays/4 sprays per day = <u>50 days.</u>
(c) Bitter taste: 77/391 × 100% = <u>19.69%</u>
Headache: 57/391 × 100% = <u>14.58%</u>

9.[b,1] A patient is prescribed DURAGESIC 75 μg/hr patches with one patch to be worn and replaced every 72 hours. The size of the patch is 30 cm^2 and contains 7.5 mg of fentanyl.
(a) What is the size of the patch in square inches?
(b) If the patch is worn for 72 hours, how much fentanyl is remaining in the patch when it is removed?
(c) Assuming that the drug release rate from the patch remains constant, how long will it take for all of the fentanyl to be released from the patch?
(d) If the patient is running a fever of 40°C, the amount of fentanyl released from the patch could increase by approximately one-third. How much drug is being released from the patch at this elevated body temperature, and how long will it take for all of the drug to be released from the patch?
(e) Express the body temperature of 40°C as Fahrenheit.

Solutions:

(a) 30 cm² × (1 in./2.54 cm)² = <u>4.65 in.²</u>

(b) 75 μg/hr × 1 mg/1000 μg × 72 hr = 5.4 mg released
7.5 mg – 5.4 mg = <u>2.1 mg remaining.</u>

(c) 7.5 mg × 1000 μg/mg × 1 hr/75 μg = 100 hr × 1 day/24 hr = <u>4.17 days or 4 days</u>
<u>4 hours.</u>

(d) 75 μg/hr × 1/3 = 25 μg/hr
75 μg/hr + 25 μg/hr = <u>100 μg/hr released from the patch at elevated body</u>
<u>temperature.</u>
7.5 mg × 1000 μg/mg × 1 hr/100 μg = 75 hr × 1 day/24 hr = <u>3.13 days or 3 days</u>
<u>3 hours.</u>

(e) F = 1.8(40°C) + 32 = <u>104°F.</u>

---

10. REGLAN injection contains in each milliliter 5-mg metoclopramide and 8.5-mg sodium chloride in water for injection. It is available in 2-mL, 10-mL, and 30-mL vials. The drug is used as an antiemetic. The usual adult dose is 10 mg. For doses greater than 10 mg, the injection should be diluted in 50 mL of sodium chloride injection and administered as an intravenous infusion.

(a) If metoclopramide has an E-value of 0.10, calculate the tonicity of REGLAN injection.

(b) For highly emetogenic drugs, as used in cancer chemotherapy, the initial dose of metoclopramide is generally 2 mg/kg. Calculate the volume of REGLAN injection at this dose for a 132-lb patient.

(c) If the dose in (b) is added to a 50-mL bag of sodium chloride injection and totally infused over a period of 30 minutes, calculate the flow rate in mL/min.

Solutions:

(a) 5 mg metoclopramide × 0.10 (E-value) = 0.5 mg
8.5 mg (NaCl) + 0.5 mg = 9 mg
9 mg/1 mL = 900 mg/100 mL = 0.9 g/100 mL = <u>0.9% sodium chloride = isotonic.</u>

(b) 132 lb × 1 kg/2.2 lb = 60 kg
60 kg × 2 mg/kg = 120 mg (dose)
120 mg × 1 mL/5 mg = <u>24 mL REGLAN injection.</u>

(c) 24 mL (REGLAN injection) + 50 mL (sodium chloride injection) = 74 mL
74 mL/30 min = <u>2.47 mL/min.</u>

11.ᶜ ℞ Indomethacin   0.05%
        Boric acid   qs
        Purified water ad   15 mL
        Ft. isotonic ophthalmic solution

(a) How many milligrams of boric acid are needed to render the product isotonic. (E-values: boric acid = 0.52, indomethacin = 0.16)

(b) How many milliliters of a 5.5% boric acid stock solution may be used to obtain the needed amount of boric acid?

(c) Indomethacin is available in vials, each containing 1 mg of indomethacin powder for reconstitution with sterile water for injection to prepare 1 mL of solution. Explain how you could obtain the indomethacin required.

Solutions:
- (a) For isotonicity: 0.9% × 15 mL = 0.135 g or 135 mg NaCl (or equivalent) needed.
  Indomethacin in ℞ = 0.05% × 15 mL = 0.0075 g = 7.5 mg.
  7.5 mg × 0.16 (E-value) = 1.2 mg.
  135 mg – 1.2 mg = 133.8 mg NaCl (or equivalent) needed.
  133.8 mg/0.52 (boric acid E-value) = <u>257.3 mg of boric acid.</u>
- (b) 5.5% boric acid = 5.5 g/100 mL = 5500 mg/100 mL
  257.3 mg × 100 mL/5500 mg = <u>4.68 mL boric acid solution.</u>
- (c) Indomethacin required = 0.05% × 15 mL = 0.0075 g = 7.5 mg.
  7.5 mg × 1 (vial)/1 mg = 7.5 vials
  <u>Use 8 vials; add purified water to make 1 mL in each; draw out a total of 7.5 mL.</u>

12.[b,2] The following is a formula for a testosterone nasal spray:

Testosterone	1 g
Alcohol	10 mL
Propylene glycol	20 mL
Benzalkonium chloride	15 mg
Purified water qs ad	100 mL

(a) Calculate the quantity of each ingredient needed to fill twelve 15-mL nasal spray bottles of the formula.

(b) Benzalkonium chloride is available as a 1:750 w/v stock solution. How many milliliters would provide the amount determined in (a)?

(c) If the propylene glycol is found to be contaminated with 1.7 ppm of a solid foreign substance, how many micrograms of that substance would be contained in each bottle of the nasal spray?

(d) If the pharmacist checked the weighing of testosterone using a highly sensitive electronic balance and found that 2.13 g were actually weighed rather than the calculated quantity in (a), what was the percent error in the weighing?

(e) If the pharmacist had decided to use testosterone cipionate injection, 200 mg/mL, as a source of the testosterone, calculate the quantity needed for the amount determined in (a) if the molecular weight of testosterone is 288.4 and that of testosterone cipionate is 412.6.

(f) The normal blood level of testosterone in males is 270 to 1070 ng/dL. If a 5-mL blood sample is found to contain 32.6 ng of testosterone, would the patient's testosterone level fall within the normal range?

Solutions:
- (a) 12 bottles × 15 mL/bottle = 180 mL
  Formula conversion factor = 180 mL/100 mL = 1.8
  Testosterone: 1 g × 1.8 = <u>1.8 g</u>
  Alcohol: 10 mL × 1.8 = <u>18 mL</u>
  Propylene glycol: 20 mL × 1.8 = <u>36 mL</u>
  Benzalkonium chloride: 15 mg × 1.8 = <u>27 mg</u>
  Purified water: qs <u>ad 180 mL</u>
- (b) 27 mg × 1 g/1000 mg × 750 mL/1 g = <u>20.25 mL</u>

(c) 36 mL/12 bottles = 3 mL propylene glycol/bottle
3 mL (propylene glycol) × 1.7 g (foreign substance)/1,000,000 mL = 0.0000051 g
= 0.0051 mg
= 5.1 μg

(d) Error = 2.13 g − 1.8 g = 0.33 g
% error = 0.33 g/1.8 g × 100% = 18.33%

(e) 288.4/412.6 = 0.6989 or 0.7 (fraction of testosterone cipionate that is testosterone base).
1.8 g (testosterone)/0.7 = 2.57 g (testosterone cipionate equivalent)
2.57 g × 1 mL/200 mg × 1000 mg/1 g = 12.85 mL

(f) 32.6 ng/5 mL × 1000 mL/L × 1 L/10 dL = 652 ng/dL and within the normal range.

13.[a,3] The following is a formula for the compounding of an oral suspension of carvedilol, a beta blocker, used in the treatment of hypertension and congestive heart failure in patients unable to swallow oral solid dosage forms.

Carvedilol	(calculate)
Xanthan gum	200 mg
Sodium carboxymethylcellulose	25 mg
Glycerin	2 mL
Sorbitol 70% solution	5 mL
Saccharin sodium	200 mg
Methylparaben	100 mg
Citric acid	100 mg
Sodium phosphate, dibasic	60 mg
Potassium sorbate	150 mg
Simethicone	100 mg
Purified water, ad	100 mL

(a) If the initial starting dose for carvedilol is 6.25 mg twice a day, how many milligrams of the drug should be used in the formula to provide each dose in a teaspoonful?
(b) How many milliliters of the formula should be prepared to last the patient the initial 14 days of treatment?
(c) If 25-mg carvedilol tablets are used as the source of drug, how many are required to provide the medication for the initial 2-week period?
(d) If sorbitol powder is available, how many grams would be required for quantity in (b)?

Solutions:
(a) 100 mL/5 mL (dose) = 20 doses
20 doses × 6.25 mg/dose = 125 mg.

(b) 5 mL/dose × 2 doses/day = 10 mL
10 mL/day × 14 days = 140 mL.

(c) 6.25 mg/dose × 2 doses/day = 12.5 mg/day
12.5 mg/day × 14 days = 175 mg
175 mg/25 mg/tablet = 7 tablets.

(d) 5 mL × 1.4 (formulation factor) = 7 mL
7 mL × 70% = 4.9 g.

14.[a,4] ℞ Amitriptyline hydrochloride   10   mg
            Bentonite or silica gel   200   mg
            Polyethylene glycol 1000   1.35 g
            Polyethylene glycol 3350   0.44 g
            M.ft. suppos. DTD # xxiv

(a) Calculate the total weight of each suppository.

(b) Calculate the quantity of each ingredient for the preparation of the prescription plus two extra suppositories to assure complete fill of the mold.

(c) Polyethylene glycol 3350 is a solid with a melting point of between 48 and 54°C. What are the corresponding temperatures on the Fahrenheit scale?

(d) Silica gel particles are between 2 and 7 μm in size. Convert this range to centimeters.

Solutions:

(a) 0.01 g (10 mg) + 0.2 g (200 mg) + 1.35 g + 0.44 g = 2 g.

(b) Prescription is for 24 suppositories, plus 2 extra = 26.
    Amitriptyline hydrochloride: 10 mg × 26 = 260 mg
    Bentonite or Silica gel: 200 mg × 26 = 5200 mg
    Polyethylene glycol 1000: 1.35 g × 26 = 35.1 g
    Polyethylene glycol 3350: 0.44 g × 26 = 11.44 g

(c) Temperature conversion formula: $F° = 9/5°C + 32°$
    $9/5 × 48°C + 32° = 118.4°F$
    $9/5 × 54°C + 32° = 129.2°F$

(d) 2 μm = 0.0002 cm.
    7 μm = 0.0007 cm.

15. A pharmacist has prepared stock creams containing 0.1% and 5% hydrocortisone from hydrocortisone powder and a cream base in order to facilitate compounding requests for intermediate strengths of hydrocortisone cream.

(a) How many grams each of the 0.1% and 5% hydrocortisone creams should be mixed to compound one ounce (Apothecary) of a 0.75% cream?

(b) How many grams of hydrocortisone powder could be added to 30 g of the 0.1% cream to prepare one containing 1% hydrocortisone?

(c) If the pharmacist mixed equal quantities of hydrocortisone powder, the cream base, and each of the 0.1% and 5% creams, what would be the resultant strength of the mixture?

Solutions:

(a) One Apothecary ounce = 31.1 g
    By alligation alternate, the proportions to mix are 4.25 parts of the 0.1% cream and 0.65 parts of the 5% cream for a total of 4.9 parts.
    Each part = 31.1 g/4.9 = 6.35 g (rounded)
    Quantity of the 0.1% cream = 4.25 (parts) × 6.35 = 26.98 = 27 g (rounded).
    Quantity of the 5% cream = 0.65 (parts) × 6.41 g = 4.1 g (rounded).

(b) By alligation alternate, the proportions to mix are 0.9 part of the powder (100% hydrocortisone) and 99 parts of the 0.1% cream.

     Since the 99 parts (0.1% cream) = 30 g, the 0.9 part (powder) = 30 g × 0.9/99

$$= \underline{0.27 \text{ g hydrocortisone powder.}}$$

(c) Arbitrarily use 100 g of each, therefore:

Hydrocortisone powder:	100 g ×	100%	= 100	g hydrocortisone
Cream base:	100 g ×	0%	= 0	g hydrocortisone
Hydrocortisone cream (0.1%):	100 g ×	0.1%	= 0.1	g hydrocortisone
Hydrocortisone cream (5%):	100 g ×	5%	= 5	g hydrocortisone
	400 g		105.1	g hydrocortisone

105.1 g (hydrocortisone)/400 g (mixture) × 100% = <u>26.28% hydrocortisone</u>

16.[b,5] The package insert information for a 500-mg vial of ceftriaxone sodium states that 1 mL of diluent should be added to produce a final concentration of 350 mg/mL.

(a) What is the volume of fluid in the vial after reconstitution?

(b) How much volume is displaced by the powder after reconstitution?

(c) How much solution will have to be injected to administer a 500 mg dose?

(d) If a pharmacist adds 3 mL of diluent to the vial, what would be the resulting concentration in mg/mL?

(e) To what final volume should the 500-mg vial be diluted with normal saline (NS) to reach a concentration of 10 mg/mL?

(f) If the diluted solution in part (e) is to be administered over a 30-minute period using an administration set with a drop factor of 20 drops/mL, what would be the flow rate in drops/min?

(g) ROCEPHIN contains approximately 83 mg (3.6 mEq) of sodium per gram of ceftriaxone activity. How many milliequivalents of sodium would a patient receive from the infusion solution in part (e)? (m.w. NaCl = 58.5)

Solutions:

(a) 500 mg × 1 mL/350 mg = <u>1.43 mL</u>

(b) 1.43 mL − 1 mL = <u>0.43 mL displaced</u>

(c) 500 mg × 1 mL/350 mg = <u>1.43 mL</u>

(d) 3 mL diluent + 0.43 mL displacement = 3.43 mL final volume
500 mg/3.43 mL = <u>145.83 mg/mL</u>

(e) 500 mg × 1 mL/10 mg = <u>50 mL</u>

(f) 50 mL/30 min × 20 drops/mL = 33.33 drops/min ≈ <u>33 drops/min</u>

(g) 3.6 mEq Na/g ceftriaxone × 1 g/1000 mg × 500 mg ceftriaxone = 1.8 mEq Na
50 mL NS × 0.9 g NaCl/100 mL × 1000 mg/g = 450 mg NaCl
450 mg NaCl × 1 mEq/58.5 mg = 7.69 mEq Na
Total = 1.8 mEq + 7.69 mEq = <u>9.49 mEq Na</u>

---

17. ℞   Clarithromycin oral suspension   100 mL
     Dose: 7.5 mg/kg
     Sig: 2.5 mL q12h

(a) To prepare 100 mL of a clarithromycin suspension containing 125 mg/5 mL, a pharmacist adds 55 mL of purified water to the granules contained in the commercial package. Calculate the content of clarithromycin in the package, in milligrams.

(b) At the dose prescribed (7.5 mg/kg), how many milliliters of the oral suspension should be administered (rather than the 2.5 mL indicated) to a 28-lb child?

(c) Rather than change the Signa directions, how many milliliters of purified water may be added to the package to prepare a suspension containing the prescribed dose of 7.5 mg/kg/2.5 mL for the 28-lb child in (b)?

(d) Prove your answer to (c).

Solutions:

(a) 125 mg (clarithromycin) × 100 mL/5 mL = <u>2500 mg clarithromycin.</u>

(b) Dose for child: 7.5 mg × 28 lb/2.2 lb/kg = 95.45 mg clarithromycin
95.45 mg × 5 mL/125 mg = <u>3.82 ≈ 3.8 mL oral suspension</u> (rounded).

(c) 2.5 mL × 2500 mg/95.45 mg = 65.48 mL (volume that can be prepared to deliver 95.45 mg/2.5 mL)
100 mL − 55 mL (purified water) = 45 mL (volume occupied by suspended granules)
65.48 mL − 45 mL = <u>20.48 mL of purified water to add.</u>

(d) 45 mL (granule volume) + 20.48 mL (purified water) = 65.48 mL
2500 mg (clarithromycin)/65.48 mL × 2.5 mL = <u>95.45 mg clarithromycin.</u>
NOTE: A calibrated oral syringe should be dispensed to assure administration of the correct dose.

---

18. A hospital pharmacist in a critical care unit receives a medication order for a 210 lb patient calling for a continuous infusion of isoproterenol hydrochloride, 5 µg/min. The pharmacist prepares the infusion by adding the contents of a 5-mL ampule of isoproterenol hydrochloride, 0.2 mg/mL to 250 mL of sodium chloride injection. The critical care nurse programs the automated infusion set to deliver 12 drops per milliliter.

(a) The label of the ampule of isoproterenol hydrochloride indicates the strength in both mg/mL and as a ratio strength. Calculate the latter.

(b) Calculate the dose of isoproterenol hydrochloride for this patient, based on µg/kg.

(c) Calculate the infusion rate, in drops/min.

(d) Calculate the infusion time, in minutes.

Solutions:

(a) 0.2 mg/mL = 0.0002 g/1 mL = 1 g/x mL; x = <u>1:5000 isoproterenol hydrochloride.</u>

(b) 210 lb × 1 kg/2.2 lb = 95.5 kg
0.2 mg/mL × 5 mL = 1 mg or 1000 µg isoproterenol hydrochloride
1000 µg/95.5 kg = <u>10.47 µg/kg.</u>

(c) 5 µg/min × 255 mL/1000 µg = 1.275 mL/min
1.275 mL/min × 12 drops/mL = <u>15.3 drops/min.</u>

(d) 255 mL × 1 min/1.275 mL = <u>200 minutes infusion time.</u>

19.^{c} A 176-lb cardiology patient received an initial heparin bolus dose of 60 units/kg followed by a heparin drip at 15 units/kg/hr. The heparin concentration was 10,000 units per 100 mL and the intravenous set delivered 15 drops per milliliter. The last partial thromboplastin time (PTT) indicated that the patient was being underdosed and according to the hospital's weight-based heparin protocol, the heparin rate should be increased by 30%.

(a) Calculate the patient's initial heparin bolus dose in units and milliliters, if the product administered contained 5000 units/mL.

(b) Calculate the revised dosage in units per kilogram per hour.

(c) Calculate the revised flow rate in drops per minute.

Solutions:

(a) 176 lb/2.2 lb/kg = 80 kg

80 kg × 60 units/kg = <u>4800 units heparin bolus dose</u>

4800 units/5000 units/mL = 0.96 mL ≈ <u>1 mL heparin bolus dose</u>

(b) 15 units/kg/hr × 30% = 4.5 units/kg/hr (increase)

15 units/kg/hr + 4.5 units/kg/hr = <u>19.5 units/kg/hr</u>

(c) 19.5 units × 80 kg = 1560 units (dose/hr)

1560 units/hr × 100 mL/10,000 units = 15.6 mL/hr

15.6 mL/hr × 15 drops/mL = 234 drops/hr

234 drops/hr × 1 hr/60 min = <u>3.9 or 4 drops/min</u>

20.^{c} The following is a TPN to be administered 80 mL/hr for 24 hours.

Dextrose	200	g
HepatAmine	60	g
Sodium chloride	50	mEq
Potassium chloride	40	mEq
Sodium acetate	20	mEq
Magnesium sulfate	10	mEq
Sodium phosphate	9	mmol
Potassium acetate	15	mEq
Calcium chloride	2	mEq
Multivitamins-12	5	mL
Trace elements-5	1	mL
Vitamin K-1	0.5	mg
Pepcid	10	mg
Regular insulin	20	units
Sterile water qs ad	960	mL

(a) How many calories will the dextrose (3.4 kcal/g) provide over 24 hours of administration?

(b) If dextrose is available as a 70% solution, how many milliliters would be needed to prepare the above-formula?

(c) If magnesium sulfate ($M_2SO_4 \cdot 7H_2O$) is available as a 50% solution, how many milliliters would be needed to prepare the above-formula?

(d) If Pepcid is available as an injection, 40 mg/4 mL, how many milliliters would be needed to prepare the above-formula?

(e) If sodium chloride is available as a 23.4% injection, how many milliliters would be needed to prepare the above-formula?

(f) How many mEq of sodium would be added as a result of the sodium phosphate?

Solutions:

(a) 960 mL (total volume)/80 mL/hr = 12 hours of fluid per bag
200 g × 3.4 kcal/g = 680 kcal in 12 hr × 2 = <u>1360 kcal in 24 hr.</u>

(b) 200 g × 100 mL/70 g = <u>285.7 mL dextrose solution.</u>

(c) $MgSO_4 \cdot 7\ H_2O$ (m.w. = 246)
Mg is divalent; 246 mg = 2 mEq or 123 mg/mEq
123 mg/mEq × 10 mEq = 1230 mg needed
1230 mg × 100 mL/50 g × 1 g/1000 mg = <u>2.46 mL magnesium sulfate solution.</u>

(d) 10 mg × 4 mL/40 mg = <u>1 mL Pepcid injection.</u>

(e) NaCl (m.w. = 58.5)
Na is monovalent; 58.5 mg = 1 mEq
58.5 mg/mEq × 50 mEq = 2925 mg needed
2925 mg × 100 mL/23.4 g × 1 g/1000 mg = <u>12.5 mL sodium chloride injection.</u>

(f) Na_3PO_4 (m.w. = 164)
164 mg = 3 mmol of Na per mmol Na_3PO_4
9 mmol of Na_3PO_4 × 3 = 27 mmol of sodium
1 mmol of Na = 1 mEq of Na (Na is monovalent)
Thus, 27 mmol = <u>27 mEq of sodium added.</u>

21.ᶜ A physician orders the following formula for an intravenous fluid described as "TPN Lite." A flow rate of 1 mL/kg/hr is ordered.

Dextrose	15%
Amino acids	4%
Sodium chloride	0.75%
Potassium chloride	0.2%
MVI-12	10 mL
Sterile water for injection ad	1000 mL

How many milliliters of each of the following will be required?
(a) Dextrose injection, 700 mg/mL.
(b) Amino acids injection, 10%.
(c) Sodium chloride injection, 4 mEq/mL.
(d) Potassium chloride injection, 2 mEq/mL.
(e) Sterile water for injection.

Solutions:

(a) 1000 mL × 15% = 150 g dextrose needed
Dextrose injection = 700 mg or 0.7 g/mL
150 g/0.7 g/mL = <u>214.3 mL dextrose injection.</u>

(b) 1000 mL × 4% = 40 g amino acids needed
Amino acids injection = 10 g/100 mL
Thus 40 g in <u>400 mL amino acids injection</u>.

(c) 1000 mL × 0.75% = 7.5 g or 7500 mg sodium chloride needed
Sodium chloride (m.w. 58.5) = 58.5 mg/mEq
7500 mg/58.5 mg/mEq = 128.2 mEq needed
128.2 mEq/4 mEq/mL = 32.05 or <u>32 mL sodium chloride injection.</u>

(d) 1000 mL × 0.2% = 2 g or 2000 mg potassium chloride needed
Potassium chloride (m.w. 74.5) = 74.5 mg/mEq
2000 mg/74.5 mg/mEq = 26.85 mEq needed
26.85/2 mEq/mL = <u>13.4 mL potassium chloride injection.</u>

(e) 214.3 mL + 400 mL + 32 mL + 13.4 mL + 10 mL (MVI-12) 669.7 mL
1000 mL − 669.7 = <u>330.3 mL sterile water for injection.</u>

22.[b,6] Normosol-R injection contains the following in each 100 mL:

Magnesium chloride (m.w. 95)	30 mg
Potassium chloride (m.w. 74.5)	37 mg
Sodium acetate (m.w. 82)	222 mg
Sodium chloride (m.w. 58.5)	526 mg
Sodium gluconate (m.w. 218)	502 mg

(a) What would be the calculated osmolarity of this solution in mOsmol/L?
(b) What would be the concentration of chloride in this solution in mmol/L?
(c) If a patient receives this solution as an intravenous infusion at a rate of 65 mL/hr, how many milliequivalents of sodium will be administered in 1 day?

Solutions:

(a) Magnesium chloride:
    30 mg/100 mL × 1000 mL/L × 3 mOsmol/95 mg = 9.47 mOsmol/L
Potassium chloride:
    37 mg/100 mL × 1000 mL/L × 2 mOsmol/74.5 mg = 9.93 mOsmol/L
Sodium acetate:
    222 mg/100 mL × 1000 mL/L × 2 mOsmol/82 mg = 54.15 mOsmol/L
Sodium chloride:
    526 mg/100 mL × 1000 mL/L × 2 mOsmol/58.5 mg = 179.83 mOsmol/L
Sodium gluconate:
    502 mg/100 mL × 1000 mL/L × 2 mOsmol/218 mg = 46.06 mOsmol/L
                              Total osmolarity = <u>299.44 mOsmol/L</u>

(b) Magnesium chloride:
    30 mg/100 mL × 1000 mL/L × 1 mmol/95 mg = 3.16 mmol/L
Potassium chloride:
    37 mg/100 mL × 1000 mL/L × 1 mmol/74.5 mg = 4.97 mmol/L
Sodium chloride:
    526 mg/100 mL × 1000 mL/L × 1 mmol/58.5 mg = 89.91 mmol/L
                              Total chloride = <u>98.04 mmol/L</u>

(c) 65 mL/hr × 24 hr/day = 1560 mL/day infused
Sodium acetate:
    222 mg/100 mL × 1560 mL/day × 1 mEq/82 mg = 42.23 mEq/day
Sodium chloride:
    526 mg/100 mL × 1560 mL/day × 1 mEq/58.5 mg = 140.27 mEq/day
Sodium gluconate:
    502 mg/100 mL × 1560 mL/day × 1 mEq/218 mg = 35.92 mEq/day
                              Total sodium = <u>218.42 mEq/day</u>

23.^{6,7} ENSURE PLUS liquid contains 54.2 g of protein, 197.1 g of carbohydrate, and 53 g of fat in each liter. ENSURE PLUS also supplies 1.5 kcal in each milliliter.
  (a) If a patient consumes four 240-mL cans of ENSURE PLUS each day, how many grams of each nutrient is she receiving?
  (b) If the patient is a 68-year-old woman who is 5'3" and moderately active, what weight, in lb, will she maintain by consuming four 240-mL cans of ENSURE PLUS each day?

Solutions:
  (a) 240 mL/can × 4 cans/day × 1 L/1000 mL × 54.2 g protein/L = <u>52.03 g protein/day.</u>
    240 mL/can × 4 cans/day × 1 L/1000 mL × 197.1 g carbohydrate/L = <u>189.22 g carbohydrate/day.</u>
    240 mL/can × 4 cans/day × 1 L/1000 mL × 53 g fat/L = <u>50.88 g fat/day.</u>
  (b) 240 mL/can × 4 cans/day × 1.5 kcal/mL= 1440 kcal/day from the ENSURE PLUS
    The resting metabolic energy (RME) or basal energy expenditure (BEE) for women can be calculated using the equation below:

$$RME = 655 + (9.6 \times W) + (1.8 \times H) - (4.7 \times A)$$

Furthermore, the patient's RME should be multiplied by an activity factor of approximately 1.25 to calculate the amount of calories she will need daily to maintain her weight at her current activity level.
RME × 1.25 = 1440 kcal/day
RME = 1152 kcal/day = 655 + (9.6 × W) + (1.8 × H) − (4.7 × A)
W = weight in kilograms
H = height in centimeters = 5'3" = 63 in. × 2.54 cm/in. = 160.02 cm
A = age in years = 68
1152 kcal/day = 655 + (9.6 × W) + (1.8 × 160.02) − (4.7 × 68)
1152 kcal/day = 623.44 + (9.6 × W)
528.56 kcal/day = 9.6 × W
W = 55.06 kg × 2.2 lb/kg = <u>121.13 lb.</u>

24. The dose of entecavir is adjusted based on the patient's renal status as determined by creatinine clearance:

Creatinine Clearance (mL/min)	Usual Dose Entecavir
≥50	0.5 mg once daily
30 to <50	0.25 mg once daily, or
	0.5 mg every 48 hours
10 to <30	0.15 mg once daily, or
	0.5 mg every 72 hours
<10	0.05 mg daily, or
	0.5 mg every 7 days

  (a) Calculate the creatinine clearance, using the Cockcroft-Gault equation, for a 35-year-old male patient, 68 in. tall, weighing180 lb, and with a serum creatinine of 2.6 mg/dL.
  (b) Based on the answer to (a) determine the dose of entecavir as given in the table.
  (c) Convert the daily dose of entecavir, as determined in (b), to μg/kg and mg/m^2 for the patient described in (a).

Solutions:

(a) Cockcroft-Gault equation for males:

$$CrCl \ (mL/min) = \frac{\left[(140 - \text{patient's age}) \times \text{patient's body weight (kg)}\right]}{\left[72 \times \text{serum Cr (mg/dL)}\right]}$$

$$CrCl \ (mL/min) = \frac{\left[(140 - 35) \times 81.8 \, \text{kg}\right]}{\left[72 \times 2.6 \, (mg/dL)\right]}$$

$$= \frac{105 \times 81.8}{187.2} = \frac{8589}{187.2} = \underline{45.9 \, mL/min.}$$

(b) Dose = <u>0.25 mg once daily or 0.5 mg every 48 hours.</u>

(c) 0.25 mg/81.8 kg = 250 μg/81.8 kg = <u>3.06 μg/kg.</u>
Using the BSA equation:

$$BSA \ (m^2) = \sqrt{\frac{\text{Height (cm)} \times \text{Weight (kg)}}{3600}} = \sqrt{\frac{68 \, \text{in.} \times 2.54 \, \frac{cm}{in.} \times 81.8 \, \text{kg}}{3600}}$$

$$= \sqrt{\frac{14128.5}{3600}} = \sqrt{3.92} = 1.98 \, m^2$$

0.25 mg/1.98 m² = <u>0.13 mg/m².</u>

25.[c] A physician prescribes lamivudine for a 35-year-old male patient who stands 5 ft 8 in. tall and weighs 180 lb. The drug dose must be adjusted based on a patient's renal function. The patient's serum creatinine is 2.6 mg/dL.

(a) Calculate the patient's creatinine clearance (CrCl) using the Cockcroft-Gault equation and the patient's ideal body weight (IBW).

(b) If the literature for lamivudine states the following, what is the appropriate dose for the patient? Available are scored 150-mg tablets and 300-mg film coated tablets.

(c) If the patient is unable to swallow tablets, how many milliliters of an oral liquid containing 10 mg lamivudine per milliliter, could be administered as the initial dose?

(d) Calculate the initial dose for this patient on the basis of mg/kg of body weight.

(e) Calculate the patient's body mass index (BMI) and interpret the result; that is, *underweight, normal, overweight,* or *obese.*

CREATINE CLEARANCE (mL/min)	INITIAL DOSE (mg)	MAINTENANCE DOSE
< 5	50	25 mg once daily
5–14	150	50 mg once daily
15–29	150	100 mg once daily
30–49	150	150 mg once daily

Solutions:
(a) The Cockcroft-Gault equation (for males) and IBW calculation (for males)

$$\text{CrCl (mL/min)} = \frac{\left[(140 - \text{patient's age}) \times \text{patient's body weight (kg)}\right]}{[72 \times \text{serum Cr (mg/dL)}]}$$

IBW = 50 kg + 2.3 kg for each inch in height over 5 ft
IBW = 50 kg + 2.3 kg × 8 = 50 kg + 18.4 kg = <u>68.4 kg</u>

$$\text{CrCl (mL/min)} = \frac{\left[(140 - 35) \times 68.4\ \text{kg}\right]}{72 \times 2.6\ \text{mg/dL}} = \frac{7182}{187.2} = 38.3654\ \text{mL/min}$$

(b) From the dosing table, <u>150 mg initially, then 150 mg once daily.</u>

(c) 150 mg dose × 1 mL/10 mg = <u>15 mL per dose.</u>

(d) 180 lb × 1 kg/2.2 lb = 81.8 kg
150 mg/81.8 kg = <u>1.8 mg/kg.</u>

(e) $\text{BMI} = \dfrac{\text{Weight (lb)}}{\text{Height (in.)}^2} \times 704.5 = \dfrac{180}{4624} \times 704.5$

$= \underline{27.4\ \text{and "overweight"}}\,(\text{re: Table } 14.1).$

---

26. The drug mitoxantrone hydrochloride is used in veterinary medicine in the treatment of leukemia. Cats are administered the drug by 30-minute intravenous infusion at 6.5 mg/m².
(a) Calculate the dose for a 3.1-lb cat.
(b) How many milliliters should be used from a vial containing mitoxantrone hydrochloride, 20 mg/10 mL, to provide the dose calculated in (a)?
(c) For the administration of the 30-minute infusion at a rate of 10 mL/kg/hr, how many milliliters of infusion should be prepared?

Solutions:
(a) By using literature sources, or the table in Chapter 17, the relationship between body weight and body surface area of cats and dogs may be found.
   In this case, a cat weighing 3.1 lb or 1.4 kg (3.1 lb × 1 kg/2.2 lb) is shown by the table to have a BSA of about 1.2 m².
   Thus, 6.5 mg/m² × 1.2 m² = <u>7.8 mg, dose of mitoxantrone hydrochloride.</u>

(b) 7.8 mg × 10 mL/20 mg = <u>3.9 mL mitoxantrone hydrochloride injection.</u>

(c) 1.4 kg × 10 mL/kg/hr = 14 mL/hr
   14 mL/hr × 0.5 hr = <u>7 mL.</u>

27. The biotechnology drug bortezomib is available in vials each containing 3.5 mg of powdered drug. When reconstituted with 3.5 mL of 0.9% sodium chloride injection, a concentration of bortezomib, 1 mg/mL results (the volume of the powdered drug when dissolved is negligible). The drug is used in the treatment of patients with multiple myeloma.
    (a) The dose of bortezomib is 1.3 mg/m². Calculate the dose, in milligrams, for a patient who weighs 165 lb and measures 70 in. in height.
    (b) The drug is coadministered with melphalan and prednisone according to the schedule:
        bortezomib (1.3 mg/m²): D-1, D-4, D-8, D-11, D-22, D-25, D-29, D-32
        melphalan (9 mg/m²) and prednisone (60 mg/m²): D-1-4

        How many milligrams of each drug would be administered to the above-patient on the first day of the protocol?
    (c) Calculate the total volume of bortezomib administered during the treatment schedule.

Solutions:
    (a) By the nomogram in Chapter 8, the patient's BSA is determined to be 1.92 m².

        Confirmed by calculation: $\mathrm{BSA, m}^2 = \sqrt{\dfrac{75\ \mathrm{kg} \times 177.8\ \mathrm{cm}}{3600}} = 1.92\ \mathrm{m}^2$

        1.3 mg × 1.92 (m²) = 2.496 mg or <u>2.5 mg.</u>
    (b) bortezomib: <u>2.5 mg</u>
        melphalan: 9 mg × 1.92 (m²) = 1.728 or <u>1.7 mg</u>
        prednisone: 60 mg × 1.92 (m²) = <u>115.2 mg</u>
    (c) 2.5 mL/treatment × 8 treatments = <u>20 mL</u>

28.^{c} A patient with a "superinfection" is judged to require antibiotic therapy at dosage levels greater than usual. The patient has normal kidney function and the drug selected is eliminated entirely by the kidney. The intravenous bolus dose administered is 0.5 g, which resulted in a drug plasma level of 12 μg/mL.
    (a) Calculate the apparent volume of distribution.
    (b) If the half-life of the drug is 3 hours and the desired drug plasma level should be maintained at, or above, 3 μg/mL for effectiveness, when should the second dose be administered?

Solutions:
    (a) $V\mathrm{d} = \dfrac{D\ (\text{total amount of drug in the body})}{C\mathrm{p}\ (\text{drug plasma concentration})} = \dfrac{0.5\ \mathrm{g}}{12\ \mathrm{mg/mL}} = \dfrac{0.5\ \mathrm{g}}{0.012\ \mathrm{g/L}} = 41.67\ \mathrm{L}.$

    (b) One half-life, or 3 hours, reduces the drug's plasma level to ½ of 12 μg/mL, or to 6 μg/mL.
        A second half-life, or 6 hours total, reduces the drug's plasma level to ½ of 6 μg/mL, or to 3 μg/mL.
        Thus, to maintain the plasma level at or above 3 μg/mL, the second dose should be administered <u>approximately 6 hours after the first dose.</u>

29.[b,8] A medication order calls for a patient to receive 200 μCi of sodium iodide I-123 for a thyroid function test. Sodium iodide I-1234 is available in 3.7-MBq capsules and can be used up to 30 hours after measurement using a radioactivity calibration system.
  (a) How many capsules should be dispensed to provide the prescribed dose?
  (b) How many μCi of radioactivity will be available at the 30-hour cutoff time if the half-life of I-123 is 13.2 hours?

Solutions:
  (a) 200 μCi/dose $\times$ 0.037 MBq/μCi $\times$ 1 capsule/3.7 MBq = <u>2 capsules.</u>
  (b) $N = N_{0e}{}^{-\lambda t}$
  $t_{1/2} = 0.693\lambda$
  Where N is the amount of activity at elapsed time t, N_0 is the amount of activity initially present, e is the base of the natural logarithm (2.718), λ is the disintegration constant, and $t_{1/2}$ is the half-life.
  13.2 hours = 0.693/λ
  = 0.0525 hr^{-1}
  $N = 200\ \mu$Ci e$^{-(0.0525\ hr-1)t}$
  $N = 200\ \mu$Ci e$^{-(0.0525\ hr-1)(30\ hours)}$ = <u>41.39 μCi.</u>

30. COLCRYS tablets contain 0.6 mg of the active constituent colchicine for use in the treatment of gout.
  (a) Colchicine is an "old" drug, having been approved for use in the United States over five decades ago. Prior to the "metrification" of units in the pharmaceutical industry, labels indicating the strengths of colchicine tablets were expressed in fractions of a grain. Refer to Table A.1 in Appendix A and convert 0.6 mg to the approximate fraction of a grain equivalent.
  (b) Referring once again to Table A.1, how many 0.6 mg colchicine tablets can be manufactured from 1-oz (Avoirdupois) of colchicine?
  (c) The recommended dose of colchicine for the *prophylaxis* of gout flares is 0.6 mg once or twice daily in adults with a maximum dose 1.2 mg/day. In the *treatment* of gout flares, the dose is 1.2 mg at the first sign of a gout flare followed by 0.6 mg one hour later. The dose generally is not to be repeated earlier than 3 days later. The dose requires downward adjustment in the elderly, those with compromised hepatic and renal conditions, and when coadministered with certain interacting drugs. Colchicine is a highly toxic drug. The literature advises that fatalities have been reported in adults and children who have ingested colchicine. For the above-dosage recommendations, how many 0.6 mg tablets might be dispensed *as a maximum* for two treatments?

Solutions:
  (a) According to Table A.1, the practical equivalent is 1 g = 65 mg (the precise equivalent is 1 gr = 64.798891 mg).
  Since the question asks for the "approximate fraction of a grain equivalent," we may use the practical equivalent and do some rounding in our calculations.
  0.6 mg $\times$ 1 grain/65 mg = 0.0092 or 0.009 grain
  0.009 grain = <u>9/1000 or approximately 1/111 gr.</u>

(b) 1 oz = 28.35 g or 28,350 mg

28,350 mg × 1 tablet/0.6 mg = <u>47,250 tablets.</u>

(c) First day, 2 tablets (1.2 mg, first dose) + 1 tablet (0.6 mg, 1-hour later) = 3 tablets

3 days later = 2 tablets + 1 tablet = 3 tablets

Total, maximum = <u>6 tablets.</u>

Credits

[a]Formulas and methods of preparation courtesy of Loyd V. Allen, Jr., Editor-in-Chief, *International Journal of Pharmaceutical Compounding*, Edmond, OK.

[b]Problem courtesy of Shelly J. Stockton, College of Pharmacy, Southwestern Oklahoma State University, Weatherford, OK.

[c]Problem courtesy of Flynn Warren, Bishop, GA.

References

1. Prince SJ. Calculations. *International Journal of Pharmaceutical Compounding* 2004;8:294.
2. Stockton SJ. Calculations. *International Journal of Pharmaceutical Compounding* 2010;14:140.
3. Anonymous. Carvedilol 1-mg/mL oral suspension. *International Journal of Pharmaceutical Compounding* 2010;14:423.
4. Anonymous. Amitriptyline hydrochloride suppositories. *International Journal of Pharmaceutical Compounding* 2010;14:334.
5. Stockton SJ. Calculations. *International Journal of Pharmaceutical Compounding* 2010;14:327.
6. Stockton SJ. Calculations. *International Journal of Pharmaceutical Compounding* 2011;15:416.
7. Prince SJ. Calculations. *International Journal of Pharmaceutical Compounding* 2005;9:146.
8. Prince SJ. Calculations. *International Journal of Pharmaceutical Compounding* 1998;2:453.

Index

Page numbers in *italic* denote figures; those followed by *t* denote tables.

TABLE OF ATOMIC WEIGHTS[a]

NAME	SYMBOL	ATOMIC NUMBER	ATOMIC WEIGHT (ACCURATE TO 4 FIGURES[b])	APPROXIMATE ATOMIC WEIGHT
Actinium	Ac	89	*	227
Aluminum	Al	13	26.98	27
Americium	Am	95	*	243
Antimony	Sb	51	121.8	122
Argon	Ar	18	39.95	40
Arsenic	As	33	74.92	75
Astatine	At	85	*	210
Barium	Ba	56	137.3	137
Berkelium	Bk	97	*	247
Beryllium	Be	4	9.012	9
Bismuth	Bi	83	209.0	209
Bohrium	Bh	107	*	272
Boron	B	5	10.81	11
Bromine	Br	35	79.90	80
Cadmium......................	Cd	48	112.4	112
Calcium	Ca	20	40.08	40
Californium	Cf	98	*	251
Carbon	C	6	12.01	12
Cerium.........................	Ce	58	140.1	140
Cesium	Cs	55	132.9	133
Chlorine	Cl	17	35.45	35
Chromium.....................	Cr	24	52.00	52
Cobalt..........................	Co	27	58.93	59
Copper	Cu	29	63.55	64
Curium.........................	Cm	96	*	247
Darmstadtium...............	Ds	110	*	281
Dubnium.......................	Db	105	*	268
Dysprosium	Dy	66	162.5	163
Einsteinium	Es	99	*	252
Erbium	Er	68	167.3	167
Europium	Eu	63	152.0	152
Fermium	Fm	100	*	257
Fluorine	F	9	19.00	19
Francium	Fr	87	*	223

[a]Table derived from Weiser ME. Pure and Applied Chemistry 2006; 78:2051–2066. Available at http://old.iupac.org/publications/pac/2006/pdf/7811x2051.pdf. Accessed October 1, 2011.

[b]When rounded off to 4-figure accuracy, these weights are practically identical to the similarly rounded-off weights in the older table based on oxygen = 16.0000.

(Continued)

TABLE OF ATOMIC WEIGHTS[a] (Continued)

NAME	SYMBOL	ATOMIC NUMBER	ATOMIC WEIGHT (ACCURATE TO 4 FIGURES[b])	APPROXIMATE ATOMIC WEIGHT
Gadolinium	Gd	64	157.3	157
Gallium	Ga	31	69.72	70
Germanium	Ge	32	72.64	73
Gold	Au	79	197.0	197
Hafnium	Hf	72	178.5	179
Hassium	Hs	108	*	277
Helium	He	2	4.003	4
Holmium	Ho	67	164.9	165
Hydrogen	H	1	1.008	1
Indium	In	49	114.8	115
Iodine	I	53	126.9	127
Iridium	Ir	77	192.2	192
Iron	Fe	26	55.85	56
Krypton.......................	Kr	36	83.80	84
Lanthanum	La	57	136.9	139
Lawrencium.................	Lr	103	*	260
Lead	Pb	82	207.2	207
Lithium........................	Li	3	6.941	7
Lutetium	Lu	71	175.0	175
Magnesium	Mg	12	24.31	24
Manganese	Mn	25	54.94	55
Meitnerium	Mt	109	*	276
Mendelevium...............	Md	101	*	258
Mercury	Hg	80	200.6	201
Molybdenum	Mo	42	95.94	96
Neodymium.................	Nd	60	144.2	144
Neon	Ne	20	20.18	20
Neptunium...................	Np	93	*	237
Nickel	Ni	28	58.69	59
Niobium	Nb	41	92.91	93
Nitrogen	N	7	14.01	14
Nobelium	No	102	*	259
Osmium.......................	Os	76	190.2	190
Oxygen........................	O	8	16.00	16
Palladium	Pd	46	106.4	106
Phosphorus	P	15	30.97	31
Platinum	Pt	78	195.1	195

(Continued)

TABLE OF ATOMIC WEIGHTS[a] (Continued)

NAME	SYMBOL	ATOMIC NUMBER	ATOMIC WEIGHT (ACCURATE TO 4 FIGURES[b])	APPROXIMATE ATOMIC WEIGHT
Plutonium	Pu	94	*	244
Polonium	Po	84	*	209
Potassium	K	19	39.10	39
Praseodymium	Pr	59	140.9	141
Promethium	Pm	61	*	145
Protactinium	Pa	91	231.0	231
Radium	Ra	88	226.0	226
Radon	Rn	86	*	222
Rhenium	Re	75	186.2	186
Rhodium	Rh	45	102.9	103
Roentgenium	Rg	111	*	280
Rubidium	Rb	37	85.47	85
Ruthenium	Ru	44	101.1	101
Rutherfordium	Rf	104	*	267
Samarium	Sm	62	150.4	150
Scandium	Sc	21	44.96	45
Seaborgium	Sg	106	*	271
Selenium	Se	34	78.96	79
Silicon	Si	14	28.09	28
Silver	Ag	47	107.9	108
Sodium	NA	11	22.99	23
Strontium	Sr	38	87.62	88
Sulfur	S	16	32.07	32
Tentalum	Ta	73	180.9	181
Technetium	Tc	43	*	98
Tellurium	Te	52	127.6	128
Terbium	Tb	65	158.9	159
Thallium	Tl	81	204.4	204
Thorium	Th	90	232.0	232
Thulium	Tm	69	168.9	169
Tin	Sn	50	118.7	119
Titanium	Ti	22	47.87	48
Tungsten	W	74	183.8	184
Unnilhexium	Unh	116	*	263
Unnilpentium	Unp	115	*	262
Unnilquadium	Unq	114	*	261
Ununbium	Uub	112	*	285

(Continued)

TABLE OF ATOMIC WEIGHTS[a] (Continued)

NAME	SYMBOL	ATOMIC NUMBER	ATOMIC WEIGHT (ACCURATE TO 4 FIGURES[b])	APPROXIMATE ATOMIC WEIGHT
Ununoctium	Uuo	118	*	294
Ununtrium	Uut	113	*	284
Uranium	U	92	238.0	238
Vanadium	V	23	50.94	51
Xenon	Xe	54	131.3	131
Ytterbium	Yb	70	173.0	173
Yttrium	Y	39	88.91	89
Zinc	Zn	30	65.38	65
Zirconium	Zr	40	91.22	91

* The isotopic composition of natural or artificial radioactive elements usually varies in specific samples, depending upon their origin.